DIAGNOSIS AND TREATMENT OF DISEASES IN ĀYURVEDA

TODARĀNANDA—ĀYURVEDA SAUKHYAM SERIES

Ed. and tr. by *Vaidya Bhagwan Dash & Vaidya Lalitesh Kashyap*

No. 1 Materia Medica of Āyurveda

No. 2 Basic Principles of Āyurveda

No. 3 Diagnosis and Treatment of Diseases in Āyurveda
Part One

No. 4 Diagnosis and Treatment of Diseases in Āyurveda
Part Two

No. 5 Diagnosis and Treatment of Diseases in Āyurveda
Part Three

No. 6 Diagnosis and Treatment of Diseases in Āyurveda
Part Four

No. 7 Diagnosis and Treatment of Diseases in Āyurveda
Part Five (*In Press*)

No. 8 Five Specialised Therapies of Āyurveda
(*Pañca Karma*) (*In Progress*)

No. 9 Iatro-Chemistry of Āyurveda (*Rasa Śāstra*)
(*In Progress*)

By the same author

A Hand Book of Āyurveda, (Concept, 1986)

Studies in the Medicine of Ancient India : Osteology or the Bones of the Human Body, by **A.F. Rudolf Hoernle, C.I.E.** with An Introduction by **Vaidya Bhagwan Dash**. (Concept, 1986)

Todarānanda-Āyurveda Saukhyaṁ Series No. 6

DIAGNOSIS AND TREATMENT OF DISEASES IN ĀYURVEDA

BASED ON

ĀYURVEDA SAUKHYAṀ OF ṬOḌARĀNANDA
PART FOUR

by

VAIDYA BHAGWAN DASH
D.A.M.S., H.P.A., M.A., Ph.D.
Former Deputy Advisor (Ayurveda)
Ministry of Health & Family Welfare
Govt. of India
and
Consultant in Traditional Medicine, WHO.
&
VAIDYA LALITESH KASHYAP
B.I.M.S., Ph.D.
Medical Superintendent
Ayurvedic Hospital
Central Govt. Health Scheme
Directorate General of Health Services,
New Delhi

CONCEPT PUBLISHING COMPANY, NEW DELHI

ISBN 81-7022-024-6 (Set)
ISBN 81-7022-007-6 (Series No. 6)

First Published 1987
Reprinted 1996

Vaidya Bhagwan **Dash** (*b.* 1934)
Vaidya (Miss) Lalitesh Kashyap (*b.* 1939)

Published and Printed by
Ashok Kumar Mittal
CONCEPT PUBLISHING COMPANY
A/15-16, Commercial Block, Mohan Garden,
NEW DELHI-110059 (India).
Phones : 5554042, 5504042

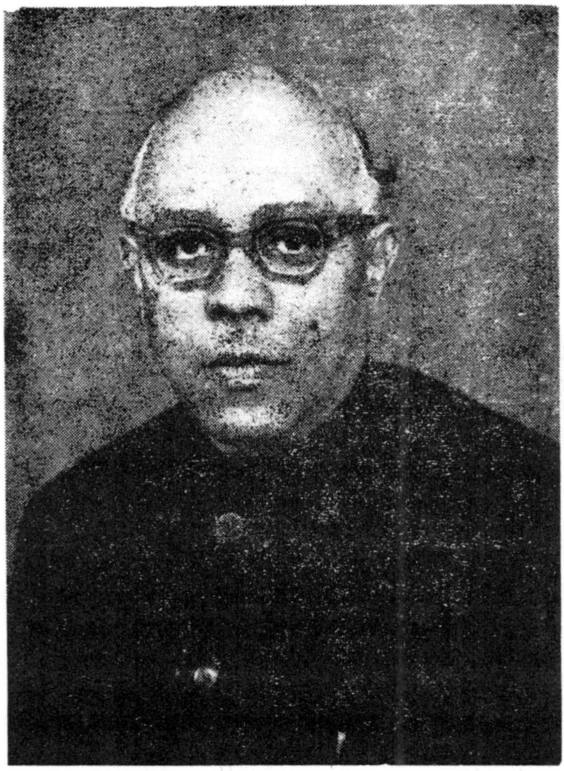

Dedicated
to

Late Prof. C. Dwarakanath
Ex-Prof. and Head of the Deptt of Kāyacikitsā
Post-Graduate Training Centre in Ayurveda
Jamnagar, India
Ex-Adviser in Ayurveda to Govt. of India

by his humble student

PREFACE

In the preface to 'Basic Principles of Āyurveda' (*Ṭoḍarānanda, Āyurveda Saukhyam* series, no. II) we have already described the availability and difference in the arrangement as well as numbering of the chapters in the six manuscripts which we have consulted for the preparation of this work. Out of these six mss, chapters included in the present volume, are available only in five manuscripts excluding the third one. As we have discussed there, the invocation (which, for the most part, is erroneous) is available only in the mss. no. 6 and the colophon is lacking there. The colophon, however, is available in the remaining four manuscripts. The arrangement of the chapters and the numbers thereof in the sixth ms. is entirely different from the remaining ones. Therefore, our readers will notice discrepancies in the numbers of chapters at the beginning (before the invocation) and also at the end (the colophon). The invocations are so full of errors that we preferred not to correct them and to leave them as such in the footnotes at the beginning of each chapter.

All our manuscripts have several grammatical and syntactical errors and these errors are found more and more, as we are going ahead, in subsequent volumes. We have of course, corrected some of these obvious errors in the text and the variant readings are given in the footnotes. This being a book of medical science, we are however, very careful not to temper with the text too much, lest it may give an erratic meaning to our readers and research workers. Therefore, our readers will find some errors left out in the text and draw their own judgement about the correct textual reading. In future, if we come across better manuscripts, then corrections would be carried out on the basis of those mss. in subsequent editions.

In this book, for the convenience of readers, we have given chapter numbers seriatim. This is an editorial device and has nothing to do with the chapter numbers given in various mss. of this work.

In this volume, we are mostly dealing with surgical ailments In ancient India, *Śalya tantra* or surgery was in practice and was treated as a specialised branch of ayurveda. There are many references to the practice of surgery in the VEDAS and PURĀṆAS. Many surgical performances like transplantation of the head of a horse to the trunk of a human being and its subsequent replacement by human head, providing artificial limbs, connecting the head of Yajña to his trunk etc., are described in the Vedas. Similarly, in puraṇas we come across the transplantation of an elephant's head with the trunk of Gaṇeśa. In *Rāmāyaṇa*, there is the description of war-surgery. When Lakṣmaṇa became unconscious being injured by a weapon, Suṣeṇa, the surgeon, revived his consciousness by surgery and administration of a plant called *sanjīvanī*.

During the life time of Lord Buddha, there was a famous physician by the name Jīvaka. Because of his proficiency in the art and science of surgery, he was thrice crowned as the king of physicians and surgeons. He was an expert pediatrician and even excelled in brain surgery. He successfully performed major abdominal operations. There are several anecdotes about this Jīvaka and his exploits in the Tibten literature.

Even in *Bhoja prabandha* (11th century A.D.), we have the description of the King Bhoja's suffering from a serious type of headache. He was anesthetized by *sammohana cūrṇa*, his cranial bone was opened, the foreign body was removed, the bone was replaced, stitched and he was made to regain his conciousness by the use of another powder called *sanjīvani cūrṇa*.

Whether these descriptions and anecdotes have to be believed or not is a different matter. But there is no doubt that several major surgical operations were in practice in ancient India and it reached the apogee of its development in the field of surgery during seventh century B.C.

The original texts of *Agniveśa saṃhitā*, *Suśruta saṃhitā* and several other texts on surgery and treatment of diseases of eye ear, nose and throat are not available now because of historical reasons. What is available now is *Caraka saṃhitā* and *Suśruta saṃhitā*, both in redacted and supplemented versions. Even in the extant *Caraka saṃhitā,* we have references to surgical performances, and for surgery, he has suggested patients to be referred to the practitioners of *Dhānvantara* school. The extant edition of *Suśruta saṃhitā* provides us an elaborate description of surgical equipments, methods and performances along with the description of ailments needing surgery. Description of rhinoplasty, Caesarean section provided in the text are the evidence of the high skill to which surgery developed in ancient India.

Unfortunately, Buddhism which was patronised by the rulers and subjects of India alike prohibited the practicc of surgery among several other professions. This gave a death blow to the medical practitioncrs. They have to give relief to suffering humanity. When the religion prohibited them to practise surgery they made efforts to develop medicines for correcting these surgical ailments. These drugs and recipes are in successful practice in India and its neighbouring countries even today. Therefore, one often comes across patients of cancer, stone in urinary tract, stone in gall bladder, peptic ulcer, heart diseases and the like who were directed for surgery but successfully treated by medicines by the ayurvedic physicians of this country.

Regarding the English translation given in this volume, we would like to mention that in the 6th manuscript there are brief notes in Hindi to some of the difficult terms described in the text. Some of these interpretations, given in the note, are unconventional. However, we have followed them in our translation.

We are extremely thankful to Ku. Kanchan Gupta, M.A., M. Ed., who was of great help in each and every stage of the preparation of this work. We express our gratitude to Shri Naurang Rai, the publisher who in spite of his pre occupation entertained the publication of this work for the welfare of the suffering humanity and encouraged us in each and every step of our endeavour. We will fail in our duty if we do not express our thanks to Shri Manjit Singh, the printer, for printing it expeditiously and for taking personal pains. Mr. Madhava Rao deserves our thanks for all the help he rendered in proof reading etc., of this book.

Both of us are extremely busy in our professional activities and we have very little free time to devote for this monumental work. The work is, therefore, done at midnight. If it proves beneficial to patients, physicians, teachers and research workers we will feel amply rewarded. At the end, we would like to quote the great poet Kālidāsa who, in his monomental play '*Abhijñāna Śākuntalam*', says :

"I will not consider my efforts to be meritorious until and unless the wise readers (audience) for whom this work is meant, are satisfied."

We share his sentiments.

BHAGWAN DASH
LALITESH KASHYAP

INDO-ROMANIC EQUIVALENTS OF DEVANĀGARI

अ	a	क	ka	ढ	ḍha	र	ra
आ	ā	ख	kha	ण	ṇa	ल	la
इ	i	ग	ga	त	ta	व	va
ई	ī	घ	gha	थ	tha	श	śa
उ	u	ङ	ṅa	द	da	ष	ṣa
ऊ	ū	च	ca	ध	dha	स	sa
ऋ	ṛ	छ	cha	न	na	ह	ha
ए	e	ज	ja	प	pa		
ऐ	ai	झ	jha	फ	pha		
ओ	o	ञ	ña	ब	ba		
औ	au	ट	ṭa	भ	bha		
अं	ṁ/ṃ	ठ	ṭha	म	ma		
अः	ḥ	ड	ḍa	य	ya		

CONTENTS

---

* Numbers given in the square brackets of "contents" indicate the verse/paragraph number of the concerned chapter.

Chapter : IV

Chapter XII

[157-158], *Jātyādya Ghṛta* [159-160], *Gaurādya Ghṛta* [161-164], *Gaurādya* and *Jātikādya Tailas* [165], *Karañjādya Ghṛta* [166-168], *Prapauṇḍarīkādya Ghṛta* [169], *Tiktādya Ghṛta* [170], *Viparīta Malla Taila* [171-172], *Aṅgāraka Taila* [173-174], *Prapauṇḍarīkādya Taila* [175], *Dūrvādya Taila* and *Dūrvādya Ghṛta* [176-177], *Mañjiṣṭhādya Ghṛta* [178], *Pāṭalā Taila* [179], *Candanādya Yamaka* [180-181], Recipes for correcting skin colour [182-186].

Fractures and Dislocations [187], Characteristic Features [188-192], Prognosis [193], Prohibitions [194-198], Management of Fracture [199-200], According to *Suśruta* [201-203], Splint [204], Recipes [205-206], Diet and Regimens [207-208], Wholesome Diet [209-210], Bandage [211], Line of Treatment [212-217], According to Kṛṣṇātreya [218], Open Fracture [219-220], Methods of curing Fracture [221-231], Crushing of Nail Joint [232-234], Finger bones broken or dislocated [235], Fracture in the Sole of the Feet [236], Fracture of the Bones of Leg or Thigh [237-238], Fracture in the Lumber Region [239], Fracture of the Rib Bones [240-241], Injury or Dislocation of Shoulder Joint [242], Dislocation of the Elbow Joint [243-244], Fracture in the Palm [245-246], Breakage in Clavicle [247], Fracture in the Arm [248], Fracture in the Neck [249-250], Fracture of the Jaw Bone [251-253], Fracture of the Nasal Bone [254], Breakage in Ear Cartilage and Skull [255-257], Injuries on Body [258-259], Fracture of Leg or Thigh Bones [260-264], Signs of Proper Healing [265], Ulcers above the bones or joints [266], Fracture in the Head and Neck [267], *Gandha Taila* [268-279], *Mahā Gandha Taila* [280-282], *Vajrā Guṭikā* [283], *Vajra Śekhara Rasa* [284-286], According to *Gorakṣa* [287-291], *Ābhā Guggulu* [292], Recipe [293], *Lākṣā Guggulu* [294], Recipe [295].

Rhinoplasty [296-300], Repairing Lip [301], Colophon [302].

CHAPTER I

॥ अथ शूलनिदानं चिकित्सा च ॥

Diagnosis and Treatment of Colic Pain

"[1]दोषैः पृथक् समस्तामद्वन्द्वैः शूलोऽष्टधा भवेत् ।
सर्वेष्वेतेषु शूलेषु प्रायेण पवनः प्रभुः ॥१॥

Classification

Depending upon the causative factors, *śūla* or colic pain is classified into eight categories, viz.

(1) *vātika*
(2) *paittika*
(3) *kaphaja*
(4) *vāta-pittaja*

---

1. This is the beginning of fortieth chapter of ***Āyurveda Saukhya*** in Ṭodarānanda and the invocation reads as follows :
वेणु प्रकुर्वंतमण सुखं यद्ब्रह्मानुभूतावखयानुग किम् ।
संवर्ण्य गोप्योनुरताभुक्त देसुखं सदद्यान्नृपटोडरेन्द्रम् ॥

(5) *vāta-kaphaja*

(6) *pitta-kaphaja*

(7) *sānnipātika* (caused by the simultaneous vitiation of all the three *doṣas*) and

(8) *āmaja* (caused by the *āma* which is the product of improper digestion and metabolism). *Vāyu*, however, predominates in the general pathogenesis of all these varieties of colic pain.

व्यायामयानादतिमैथुनाच्च प्रजागराच्छीतजलातिपानात्[1] ।
कलायमुद्गाढकिकोरदूषादत्यर्थरूक्षाध्यशनाभिघातात् ॥२॥
कषायतिक्तातिविरूढका[2]न्नविरुद्धवल्लूरकशुष्कशाकात् ।
विट्शुक्रमूत्रानिल[3]संनिरोधा[4]च्छोकोपवासादतिहास्यभाष्यात् ॥३॥

Etiology and Pathogenesis of Vātika Śūla

Vātika type of colic pain is caused by the aggravation of *vāyu* because of the following :

1. Exercise, riding over vehicles and sexual intercourse in excess;
2. Remaining awake at night and intake of cold water in excess;
3. Excessive intake of *kalāya*, *mudga*, *āḍhakī* and *koradūṣa* in excess;
4. Excessive intake of ununctuous food, habitual intake of food before the previous meal is digested and injury;
5. Excessive intake of astringent and bitter food, germinated corns and pulses, mutually contradictory ingredients of food, dried meat and dried vegetables;

---

1. ०जलाभिपानात् इति प्रथमपंचमपुस्तकयोः पाठः ।
2. ०विरूढजान्न० इति आकरे पाठः ।
3. ०मूत्रानिलवेगरोध० इति प्रथमपंचमषष्ठपुस्तकेषु आकरे च पाठः ।
4. ०च्शोको० इति प्रथमपंचमषष्ठपुस्तकेषु पाठः ।

6. Suppression of the manifested urges for defecation, ejaculation of semen, urination and passing of flatus; and
7. Grief, fasting, laughing and talking in excess.

वायुः प्रवृद्धो जनयेद्धि शूलं हृत्पार्श्वपृष्ठत्रिकबस्तिदेशे[1] ।
जीर्णप्रदोषे च घनागमे च शीते च कोपं समुपैति गाढम् ॥४॥
मुहुर्मुहुश्चोपशमप्रकोपौ[2] विण्मूत्रसंस्तम्भनतोदभेदैः[3] ।
संस्वेदनाभ्यञ्जनमर्दनाद्यैः स्निग्धोष्णभोज्यैश्च[4] शमं प्रयाति ॥५॥

Signs and Symptoms of Vātika Śūla

The aggravated *vāyu* causes pain in cardiac region, sides of chest, back, lumber region and the region of urinary bladder. This pain gets excessively aggravated after digestion of food, during evening, at the onset of rain and during the winter. The pain gets aggravated and alleviated very frequently. It causes retention of stool and urine. It is characterised by pricking and cracking pain. The pain gets alleviated by fomentation, massage, kneading etc., and by food which is unctuous and hot.

[5]क्षारातितीक्ष्णोष्णविदाहितैलनिष्पावपिण्याककुलित्थयूषैः[6] ।
कट्वम्लसौवीरसुराविकारैः क्रोधानलायासरविप्रतापैः ।

---

1. हृत्पार्श्वपृष्ठस्त्रिकबस्तिदेशे इति षष्ठपुस्तके पाठः ।
2. प्रकोपी विड्वातसंस्तम्भनतोदभेदैः इति आकरे पाठः ।
3. वनतोदभेदैः इति षष्ठपुस्तके पाठः ।
4. ०भोप्यैश्च इति प्रथमपंचमषष्ठपुस्तकेषु पाठः ।
5. क्षीरातितीक्ष्णोष्ण० इति द्वितीयपुस्तके पाठः ।
6. ०कुलत्थ इति प्रथमपंचमषष्ठपुस्तकेषु आकरे च पाठः ।

ग्राम्यातियोगादशनैर्विदग्धैः पित्तं प्रकुप्याशु करोति शूलम् ॥६॥

Etiology and Pathology of Paittika Śūla

Paittika type of colic pain is instantaneously caused by the aggravation of *pitta* because of the following :

1. Excessive intake of alkalies, *tīkṣṇa* (ingredients having sharp attribute), hot and *vidāhi* (ingredients causing burning sensation) food, oil, *niṣpāva* (legumes), oil cakes, soup of *kulattha*, pungent and sour food, *sauvīra* (a type of vinegar) and alcoholic preparations;
2. Excessive anger, exposure to the heat of fire, exhaustion and exposure to the hot sun-rays; and
3. Excessive indulgence in sex.

Because of the above mentioned factors, the food of the individual becomes *vidagdha* (undigested) which produces *paittika* type of colic pain.

तृण्मोहदाहार्त्तिकरं हि नाभ्यां संस्वेदमूर्च्छाभ्रमचोषयुक्तम् ।
मध्यंदिने कुप्यति चार्द्धरात्रे निदाघकाले जलदात्यये च ।
शीतेतिशीते[1] समुपेति शान्तिं सुस्वादुशीतैरपि भोजनैश्च ॥७॥

Signs and Symptoms of Paittika Śūla

Signs and symptoms of *paittika* type of colic pain are thirst, unconsciousness, burning sensation, sawing pain in the umbilical region, excessive perspiration, fainting, giddiness and *coṣa* (a sensation as if getting parched by strong heat). The pain gets aggravated during mid-day, mid-night, summer season and after the rainy season (i.e. during autumn). The pain gets alleviated during winter season, because of excessively cold regimens and by sweet as well as cooling food.

आनूप वारिजकिलाटपयोविकारै-
र्मांसेक्षुपिष्टकृशरातिलशष्कुलीभिः ।

---

1. शीते च शीतै इति आकरे पाठः ।

अन्यैर्बलासजनकैरपि हेतुभिश्च

श्लेष्माप्रकोपमुपगम्य करोति शूलम् ॥८॥

Etiology and Pathogenesis of Kaphaja Śūla

Kaphaja type of colic pain is caused by the aggravation of *kapha* because of the following :

1. Excessive intake of the meat of animals living in marshy land and water, cheese, milk-preparations, meat (of other animals), pastries prepared of sugar cane juice, *kṛśarā* (a type of gruel), preparations of sesame seed and *śaṣkulī* (a type of pastry); and
2. Such other food and regimens which aggravate *kapha*.

हृल्लासकाससदनारुचिसम्प्रसेकै-

रामाशयेस्तिमितकोष्ठशिरोगुरुत्वैः ।

भुक्ते सदैव हि रुजं कुरुतेऽतिमात्रं

सूर्योदये च[1] शिशिरे कुसुमागमे च ॥९॥

Signs and Symptoms of Kaphaja Śūla

Signs and symptoms of *kaphaja* type of colic pain are nausea cough, prostration, anorexia, salivation, constipation, heaviness and pain in the gastric region (upper abdomen). Whenever, the patient takes food, he gets pain. This pain gets aggravated at the time of sun rise, during *śiśira* (first half of winter) and during spring season.

[2]'द्विदोषलक्षणैरेतैर्विद्याच्छूलं द्विदोषजम् ॥१०॥'

---

1. सूर्योदयेऽथ इति आकरे पाठः ।
2. 'द्विदोष --द्विदोषजम्' पाठोऽयं आकरे नोपलभ्यते ।

Signs and Symptoms of Śūla caused by Two Doṣas

Colic pain caused by the simultaneous vitiation of two *doṣas* viz. *vāta-pitta*, *vāta-kapha* and *pitta-kapha* is characterised by the combination of the signs and symptoms of the concerned individual *doṣas*. For example, in *vāta-paittika śūla*, signs and symptoms of both *vātika śūla* and *paittika śūla* are manifested.

सर्वेषु दोषेषु[1] च सर्वलिंगं विद्याद्भिषक् सर्वभवं हि शूलम् ।
सुकष्टमेनं विषवज्रकल्पं विवर्जनीयं प्रवदन्ति तज्ज्ञाः ॥११॥"

[माधवनिदानः शूलादिनिदान २६:१-११]

Signs and Symptoms of Sānnipātika Śūla

In the colic pain caused by the simultaneous vitiation of all the three *doṣas*, signs and symptoms of *vātika śūla*, *paittika śūla* and *kaphaja śūla* are manifested. It is one of the extremely difficult conditions, like affliction by acute poisoning or thunderbolt, for treatment. Therefore, experts on this subject advise not to undertake treatment of such patients.

अतिमात्रं यदा भुक्तं पावके मूढतां गते ।
स्थिरीकृतं भवेत्कोष्ठे वायुरावृत्य तिष्ठति ॥
अविपाकगतं ह्यन्नं शूलं तर्हि करोति च ॥१२॥

Etiology and Pathogenesis of Āmaja Śūla

If a person takes food in excess when his power of digestion is sluggish, the food remains stagnant in the gastro-intestinal tract being surrounded by *vāyu*. Thus, this undigested food gives rise to colic pain.

---

1. पाठोऽयं द्वितीयपुस्तके नोपलभ्यते ।

मूर्च्छाध्मानं विदाहं च हृदि क्लेदो विलम्बिका[1]।
विषूच्यते छर्दयति कम्पते च प्रमुह्यति ।
अविपाकाद्भवेच्छूलमन्नदोषसमुद्भवम् ॥१३॥

Signs and Symptoms of Āmaja Śūla

Āmaja type of colic pain which is caused by faulty food and its indigestion is characterised by signs and symptoms like fainting, distension of the abdomen, burning sensation in the cardiac region (chest), feeling of stickiness, *vilambikā* (absence of peristaltic movement resulting in the stagnation of food), pricking pain, vomiting, trembling and unconsciousness.

"आटोपहृल्लासवमीगुरुत्वस्तैमित्यमा[2]नाहकफप्रसेकैः ।
कफस्य लिंगेन समानलिंगमामोद्भवं शूलमुदाहरन्ति[3] ॥१४॥"

[माधवनिदान : शूलादिनिदान २६ : १२]

Āmaja type of colic pain also shares the signs and symptoms of *kaphaja* colic pain resulting in the manifestation of *āṭopa* (gurgling noise in the abdomen), nausea, vomiting, heaviness, *staimitya*, (absence of peristaltic movement), abdominal distension and salivation.

निगृह्यमानः[4] स[5] श्लेष्मा कुक्षिपार्श्वे व्यवस्थितः ।
आध्मानाटोपसंरुद्धः सूचीभिरिव निस्तुदन् ॥१५॥

---

1. विलम्बिकाः इति प्रथमपुस्तके पाठः ।
2. ०स्तैमित्यकानाह० इति आकरे पाठः ।
3. "आटोप—शूलमुदाहरन्ति" पाठोऽयं द्वितीयपुस्तके नोपलभ्यते ।
4. निगृह्यमानं इति प्रथमपंचमपुस्तकयोः पाठः ।
5. सं इति प्रथमपंचमपुस्तकयोः पाठः ।

उच्छ्वसत्यथ[1] वक्त्रेण[2] न चान्नमभिनन्दति ।
न च निद्रामुपैत्येव पार्श्वशूलमिहोच्यते ॥१६॥

Pathogenesis, Signs and Symptoms of Pārśva Śūla (Pleurisy)

When the aggravated *kapha* located in the sides of the chest and abdomen gets vitiated, it causes *ādhmāna* (abdominal distension), *āṭopa* (gurgling noise in the abdomen), stiffness, pain as if being pricked by needles, taking out deep breath through mouth, lack of appetite and sleeplessness. This condition is called *pārśva śūla* (pain in the sides of the chest).

प्रकुप्यति यदा कुक्षौ वह्निमाक्रम्य[3] मारुतः ।
तदास्य भोजनं भुङ्क्त[4] दोषस्तब्धं न पच्यते ॥१७॥

मुहुः श्वसिति चात्यर्थं[5] शूलेनापीडितो[6] मुहुः ।
नैवासने शयने[7] च तिष्ठंश्चालभते सुखम् ।
कुक्षिशूल इति ख्यातो ग्रामवातसमुद्भवः ॥१८॥

Pathogenesis, Signs and Symptoms of Kukṣī Śūla (Pain in Pelvic region)

When the aggravated *vāyu* located in the pelvic region

---

1. क. उत्थसित्पथ इति पंचमपुस्तके पाठः ।
   ख. उच्छ्वसित्पथ इति प्रथमपुस्तके पाठः ।
2. वक्त्रेन तथान्नमयिनिन्दति इति षष्ठपुस्तके पाठः ।
3. वह्निमासाद्य० इति षष्ठपुस्तके पाठः ।
4. भुक्ते इति प्रथमपुस्तके पाठः ।
5. चात्यर्थ० इति द्वितीयपुस्तके पाठः ।
6. पीड्यते इति प्रथमपंचमपुस्तकयोः पाठः ।
7. स्वयं इति द्वितीयपुस्तके पाठः ।

afflicts the power of digestion, then the indigested food becomes stagnant and does not get digested. The person breaths hurriedly and frequently gets afflicted with pain. He never gets comfort either in sitting, sleeping or standing. This condition is called *kukṣi śūla* (colic pain in the pelvic region). This is caused by *āma* (product of indigestion) and aggravated *vāyu.*

कफपित्तावरुद्धस्तु मारुतः सममूर्छितः ।
हृदिस्थः कुरुते शूलमुच्छ्वासारोधनं परम् ॥
स हृच्छूल इति ख्यातो रसमारुतसंभवः ॥१६॥

Pathogenesis, Signs and Symptoms of Hṛt Śūla (Pain in Cardiac region)

When the aggravated *vāyu* located in the cardiac region gets obstructed by *kapha* and *pitta*, then the patient gets cardiac pain which is associated with extremely difficult or arrested breathing. This condition is called *hṛt śūla* or cardiac pain. This is caused by aggravated *vāyu* and vitiated *rasa* (plasma).

संरोधात्कुपितो वायुर्वह्निमावृत्य तिष्ठति ।
बस्तिवंक्षणनाभीषु ततः शूलोऽस्य[1] जायते ॥
विण्मूत्रवातसंरोधाद्बस्तिशूल स संज्ञितः[2] ॥२०॥

Pathogenesis, Signs and Symptoms of Basti Śūla (pain in the region of Urinary Bladder)

When the aggravated *vāyu* gets obstructed, it afflicts the power of digestion and causes colic pain in the region of urinary bladder and in pelvic as well as umbilical regions. It causes obstruction to the movement of stool, urine and flatus. This condition is called *basti śūla* (colic pain in the region of the urinary bladder).

1. शूलऽस्य इति पंचमपुस्तके पाठः ।
2. सन्वितः इति प्रथमपुस्तके पाठः ।

नाभ्यां वंक्षणमूलेषु कुक्षौ मेढ्रानुवर्तकः ।
मूत्रमावृत्य गृह्णाति मूत्रशूलं स मारुतः[1] ॥२१॥

Signs and Symptoms of Mūtra Śūla (pain in the Urinary Tract)

Aggravated *vāyu*, having arrested the flow of micturition, causes pain in the umbilical, lower hip and pelvic regions which radiates towards the pudendum. This condition is called *mūtra śūla* (colic pain in the urinary tract).

वायुः प्रकुपितो यस्य रूक्षाहारस्य[2] देहिनः ।
वातं रुणद्धि कोष्ठस्थं मंदीभूतं[3] च पावकम् ॥२२॥

शूलं संजनयेच्छीघ्रं स्रोतमावृत्य मारुतः ।
दक्षिणं[4] यदि वा वामं कुक्षिमादाय जायते ॥२३॥

सर्वत्र[5] वर्तते शीघ्रं भ्रामन्नथ[6] सदोषवत् ।
पिपासा वर्द्धते तीव्रा भ्रमो मूर्च्छा च जायते ॥२४॥

उच्चारितो मूत्रितश्च न शान्तिमधिगच्छति ।
विट्शूलमेतज्जानीयाद्भिषक् परमदारुणम् ॥२५॥

---

1. समारुतम् इति प्रथमपंचमपुस्तकयोः पाठः ।
2. क. रूक्षाद्वायस्य इति प्रथमपुस्तके पाठः ।
   ख. रूक्षायामच्च इति पंचमपुस्तके पाठः ।
3. मंदीकृत्यं इति पंचमपुस्तके पाठः ।
4. दक्षं वा इति षष्ठपुस्तके पाठः ।
5. चर्चा इति षष्ठपुस्तके पाठः ।
6. त्वामंऽथ स दोषवित् इति पंचमपुस्तके पाठः ।

Etiology, Pathogenesis, Signs and Symptoms of Viṭ Śūla (pain caused by intestinal obstruction)

Because of the excessive intake of ununctuous food, *vāyu* gets aggravated. If the digestive power of the individual is sluggish then this aggravated *vāyu* obstructs the passage of flatus in the intestine. This intestinal obstruction instantaneously gives rise to colic pain. The pain may originate from the right or the left side of the pelvic region. But immediately, it spreads to the entire abdomen and moves inside violently. There is excessive thirst, giddiness and fainting. The pain does not subside even after passing stool and urine. This serious type of colic pain is called *viṭ śūla* (colic pain caused by the obstruction of feces and flatus in the intestine).

"वातात्मकं बस्तिगतं वदन्ति पित्तात्मकं चापि वदन्ति नाभ्याम् ।
हृत्पार्श्वकुक्षौ तु[1] कफात्प्रदिष्टं सर्वेषु देशेषु च सन्निपातात् ॥२६॥"

[योगरत्नाकर : शूलचिकित्सा (उत्तरार्द्धम) : पृष्ठ ३]

Locations of Colic pain According to Doṣas

Colic pain caused by aggravated *vāyu* is generally located in the region of the urinary bladder, the pain caused by *pitta* is in umbilical region, the pain caused by *kapha* is located in the cardiac region, sides of the chest and sides of the abdomen and the colic pain caused by the simultaneous aggravation of all the three *doṣas* (*sannipāta*) is located all over the abdomen and chest.

"बस्तौ हृत्पार्श्वपृष्ठेषु[2] स शूलः कफवातिकः ।
कुक्षौ हृन्नाभिमध्येषु[3] स शूलः कफपैत्तिकः ॥

1. कफसन्निविष्टं इति आकरे पाठः ।
2. हृत्कण्ठपार्श्वेषु इति आदर्शपुस्तकेषु पाठः ।
3. पार्श्वेषु इति आदर्शपुस्तकेषु पाठः ।

दाहज्वरकरो[1] घोरो विज्ञेयो वातपित्ततः[2] ॥२७॥

Characteristic Features of Dvandvaja Śula

Colic pain caused by the simultaneous vitiation of *kapha* and *vāta* is located in the region of urinary bladder, cardiac region, sides of the chest and back. Colic pain caused by the simultaneous vitiation of *kapha* and *pitta* is located between the heart and umbilicus. Colic pain caused by the simultaneous vitiation of *vāyu* and *pitta* is associated with serious types of burning sensation and fever.

"एकदोषोत्थितः साध्यः कृच्छ्रसाध्यो द्विदोषजः ।

सर्वदोषोत्थितो घोरस्त्वसाध्यो भूर्युपद्रवः ॥२८॥"

[योगरत्नाकर : शूलचिकित्सा : पृष्ठ ३]

[माधवनिदान : शूलादिनिदान २६:१३-१५]

Prognosis

Colic pain caused by the aggravation of only one of the *doṣas* is curable. Colic pain caused by the simultaneous vitiation of two *doṣas* is difficult of cure. Colic pain which is associated with several complications and which is caused by the simultaneous vitiation of all the three *doṣas* is of serious nature and is incurable.

"वेदनातितृषा मूर्च्छा आनाहो गौरवारुचिः ॥"

[योगरत्नाकर : शूलचिकित्सा : पृष्ठ ३]

कासः श्वासश्च हिक्का च शूलस्योपद्रवाः स्मृताः ॥२९॥

1. महाज्वरकरो इति आदर्शपुस्तकेषु पाठः ।
2. वातपैत्तिकः इति आकरे पाठः ।

आनाहो गौरवं छर्दिर्ज्वरस्तृषा भ्रमोऽरुचिः ।
कृशत्वं बलहानिश्च वेदनातिप्रवर्तनम् ।
उपद्रवा दशैते च यस्य शूले च नास्ति सः ॥३०॥

॥ इति शूलनिदानम् ॥

Complications

Excruciating pain, excessive thirst, fainting, *ānāha* (obstruction to the passage of stool and urine), heaviness, anorexia, cough, dyspnoea and hic cup—these are the complications of *śūla roga* (colic pain).

If the patient of colic pain is afflicted with ten complications, viz. *ānāha* (obstruction to the passage of stool and urine), heaviness, vomiting, fever, morbid thirst, giddiness, anorexia, emaciation, weakness and excruciating pain, then he is surely to succumb to the disease.

Thus, ends the diagnosis of *Śūla* (Colic pain).

"वमनं लंघनं स्वेदः पाचनं फलवर्त्तयः ।
क्षार [1] चूर्णानि गुटिकाः शस्यन्ते शूलशान्तये ॥३१॥"

[भैषज्यरत्नावली : शूलरोगाधिकारः१]

Line of Treatment in General

Emetic therapy, fasting, fomentation, carminatives, suppository, alkalies, powders and tablets are useful for the treatment of a patient suffering from colic pain.

[2] ज्ञात्वा तु वातजं शूलं स्नेहस्वेदैरुपाचरेत् ।

---

1. क्षारचूर्णञ्च इति आकरे पाठः ।
2. "ज्ञात्वा—मार्गं" पाठोऽयं पंचमपुस्तके अधिकमुपलभ्यते ।

"पुंसः[1] शूलाभिपन्नस्य स्वेद एव सुखावहः ।"

[योगरत्नाकर : शूलचिकित्सा (उत्तरार्द्धम्) : पृष्ठ ४]

पायसैः कृशरापिण्डैः[2] स्निग्धैर्वा पिशितोत्करैः ॥३२॥"

[भैषज्यरत्नावली : शूलरोगाधिकार २]

Line of Treatment of Vātika Śūla

For a patient suffering from *vātika* type of colic pain, oleation and fomentation therapies are useful. For all types of colic pain fomentation therapy, which is useful, should be administered with the help of *pāyasa* (milk and rice preparation), bolus of *kṛśarā* (thick gruel) or meat of animals containing fat.

विश्वौषधेन रुचिकेन सदाडिमेन

स्यादम्लवेतसयुक्त कृतहिंगुभागं ।

तद् हिंगुपञ्चकमिदं हृदयामदघ्नं

भेदाभिधानमुनिना गदितं मुनीशं ॥३३॥

Hiṅgu Pañcaka

The recipe containing the powders of *śuṇṭhī*, *rucaka*, *dāḍima*, *amla vetasa* and *hiṅgu*—all taken in equal quantities is called *Hiṅgu pañcaka*. It cures heart diseases. It is propounded by Bheda muni.

"मृतिकां[3] सजलां पाकाद् घनीभूतां पटे क्षिपेत् ।

1. "पुंसः—सुखापहः" पाठोऽयं योगरत्नाकरे नोपयभ्यते ।
2. क. कृशरैः पिण्डैः इति प्रथमपुस्तके पाठः ।
   ख. कृशरैः पिष्टैः इति आकरे पाठः ।
3. "मृकिकां—निधापयेत्" पाठोऽयं पंचमपुस्तके अधिकमुपलभ्यते ।

कृत्वा तत्पोटलीं शूली तया[1] स्वेदं निधापयेत् ॥३४॥"

[भैषज्यरत्नावली : शूलरोगाधिकारः१६]

Mud Fomentation

Mud should be mixed with water and boiled till it becomes semi-solid. This may be kept in a piece of cloth and tied to a round bolus mass. With this, fomentation should be given to a patient suffering from colic pain.

"तुम्बुरूणि त्रिलवणं यवानी पुष्कराह्वयम् ।
यवक्षाराभयाहिंगुविडङ्गानि समानि च ॥३५॥
त्रिवृत्त्रिभागा विज्ञेया सूक्ष्मचूर्णानि कारयेत् ।
पिबेदुष्णेन तोयेन यवक्वाथेन वा पिबेत् ॥
जयेत्सर्वाणि शूलानि गुल्माध्मानोदराणि च ॥३६॥
॥ इति तुम्बुराद्यं चूर्णम् ॥"

[भारतभैषज्यरत्नाकर : द्वितीयभाग : पृष्ठ ३३७]

Tumburādya Cūrṇa

One part each of *tumburu*, rocksalt, sonchal salt, sea salt, *yavānī*, *puṣkara mūla*, *yava kṣāra*, *abhayā*, *hiṅgu* and *viḍaṅga*, and three parts of *trivṛt* should be made to a fine powder. This should be taken by the patient along with hot water or decoction of barley. This recipe cures all varieties of colic pain, *gulma* (phantom tumour), abdominal distension and *udara* (obstinate abdominal disorders including ascites).

"वातात्मकं हन्त्यचिरेण शूलं स्नेहेन युक्तस्तु कुलित्थयूषः ।

1. यथास्वेदं इति आकरे पाठः ।

ससैन्धवव्योषयुतः सलावः सहिंगुसौवर्चलदाडिमाढ्यः ॥३७॥

[कुलत्थयूषः][1]

Soup of Kulattha

The soup prepared of *kulattha* and meat of *lāva* by adding ghee, rock salt, *śuṇṭhī, pippalī, marica, hiṅgu,* sonchal salt and sufficient quantity of the juice of *dāḍima* instantaneously cures *vātika* type of colic pain.

बलापुनर्नवैरण्डबृहतीद्वयगोक्षुरैः ।

सहिंगुलवणं पीतं सद्यो वातरुजापहम् ॥३८॥

[बलादिक्वाथः][2]

Balādi Kvātha

The decoction of *balā, punarnavā, eraṇḍa, bṛhatī, kaṇṭakāri* and *gokṣura* should be taken by adding *hiṅgu* and rock salt. This potion instantaneously cures colic pain caused by the aggravated *vāyu.*

शूली निबद्धकोष्ठोऽद्भिरुष्णाभिश्चूर्णिताः पिबेत् ।

हिंगुप्रतिविषाव्योषवचासौवर्चलाभया ॥३९॥

[हिंग्वादिचूर्णम्]

Hiṅgvādi Cūrṇa

The patient suffering from colic pain associated with constipation should take the powder of *hiṅgu, prativiṣā, śuṇṭhī, pippalī, marica, vacā,* sonchal salt and *abhayā* along with hot water.

---

1. पाठोऽयं आदर्शपुस्तकेषु नोपलभ्यते ।
2. पाठोऽयं आदर्शपुस्तकेषु नोपलभ्यते ।

तुम्बुरूण्यभया हिंगु पौष्करं लवणत्रयम् ।
पिबेदुष्णाम्बुना[1] वातशूलगुल्मापतन्त्रकी ॥४०॥"

॥[2] इति तुम्बुराद्यं चूर्णम् ॥

[भैषज्यरत्नावली : शूलरोगाधिकार : ४-७]

Tumburādya Cūrṇa

The powder of *tumburu*, *abhayā*, *hiṅgu*, *puṣkara mūla*, rock salt, sonchal salt and sea salt should be taken along with hot water by the patient suffering from *vātika* type of colic pain, *gulma* (phantom tumour) and *apatantra* (tetanic convulsions).

"श्यामा विडं शिग्रुफलानि पथ्या विडंग कम्पिल्लकमश्वमूत्री ।
कल्कं समं मद्ययुतं च पीतं[3] शूलं निहन्यादनिलात्मकं च[4] ॥४१॥"

[श्यामादिचूर्णम्]

[भैषज्यरत्नावली : शूलरोगाधिकार : १२]

Recipes for Vātika Śūla

The paste of *śyāmā* (*vṛddhadāra*), *viḍa* type of salt, fruits of *śigru*, *pathyā*, *viḍaṅga*, *kampillaka* and *aśva mūtrī* (*śallakī*), taken with alcohol cures *vātika* type of colic pain.

---

1. पिबेत्सुराम्बुना इति प्रथमपुस्तके पाठः ।
2. तुम्बुर्वादि चूर्णम् इति आकरे पाठः ।
3. पीत्वा इति आकरे पाठः ।
4. निहन्यादनिलात्मकन्तु इति आकरे पाठः ।

[5] “यवानीहिंगुसिंधूत्थक्षारसौवर्चलाभयाः ।
सुरामण्डेन पातव्या वातशूलनिसूदनाः[1] ॥४२॥”

[भैषज्यरत्नावली : शूलरोगाधिकार : ८]

The powder of *yavānī*, *hiṅgu*, rock salt, *yava kṣāra*, sonchal salt and *abhayā* should be taken with *surā maṇḍa* (upper portion of the alcoholic preparation) which cures *vātika* type of colic pain.

“विश्वमेरण्डजं मूलं क्वाथयित्वा जलं पिबेत् ।
हिंगुसौवर्चलोपेतं सद्यः शूलनिवारणम् ॥४३॥

The decoction of *śuṇṭhī* and root of *eraṇḍa*, if taken by adding *hiṅgu* and sonchal salt, instantaneously cures colic pain.

हिंगुपुष्करमूलाभ्यां हिंगुसौवर्चलेन वा ।
विश्वैरण्डयवक्वाथः सद्यः[2] शूलनिवारणः ॥”

[भैषज्यरत्नावली : शूलरोगाधिकार : ९-१०]

तद्वद्रुबुयवक्वाथो हिंगुसौवर्चलान्वितः ॥४४॥

[भैषज्यरत्नावली : शूलरोगाधिकार : ९ (विशेषवचन)]

The decoction of *śuṇṭhī*, *eraṇḍa* and *yava* (barley) taken with either *hiṅgu* and sonchal salt or *hiṅgu* and *puṣkara mūla* instantaneously cures colic pain. Similarly, the decoction of *eraṇḍa* and *yava* (barley) taken along with *hiṅgu* and sonchal salt cures colic pain instantaneously.

---

1. वातशूलनिषूदनाः इति आकरे पाठः ।
2. पीत्वा इति आकरे पाठः ।

"हिंग्वम्लकृष्णामलकं यवानी क्षाराभयासैन्धवतुल्यभागम् ।
चूर्णं पिबेद्वारुणिमण्डं मिश्रं शूले प्रवृद्धेऽनिलजे शिवाय ॥४५॥"

[हिंग्वादिचूर्णम्]

[भैषज्यरत्नावली : शूलरोगाधिकार : ११]

The powder of *hingu*, *amla vetasa*, *pippalī*, *āmalakī*, *yavānī*, *yava kṣāra*, *abhayā* and rock-salt, all taken in equal quantities, should be given with the *vāruṇī maṇḍa* (upper layer of an alcoholic preparation). This cures acute form of colic pain caused by *vāyu*.

"सौवर्चलाम्लिकाजाजीमरिचैर्द्विगुणोत्तरः[1] ।
मातुलुंगरसैः[2] पिष्ट्वा गुटिकाऽनिलशूलनुत् ॥४६॥"

[भैषज्यरत्नावली : शूलरोगाधिकार : १३]

Sauvarcala (one part), *amlikā* (two parts), *ajājī* (four parts) and *marica* (eight parts) should be triturated with the juice of *mātuluṅga* and made to pills. Intake of these pills cures *vātika* type of colic pain.

'शुण्ठीसैन्धवटंकणखारः[3] हिंगुकरंजबीजः ।
समभागमुष्णाम्बुना पीतमुदरशूलं नाशयति ॥४७॥'

The powder of *śuṇṭhī*, rock-salt, fried borax, *hingu* and seed of *karañja*—all taken in equal quantities, should be given along with hot water which cures colic pain in the abdomen.

---

1. क. सवर्चलाम्लजाजाजी० इति द्वितीय पुस्तके पाठः ।
   ख. सवर्चलाम्रकाजाती० इति षष्ठपुस्तके पाठः ।
2. मातुलिङ्ग इति द्वितीय पुस्तके पाठः ।
3. "शुण्ठी......नाशयति" पाठोऽयं प्रथमपंचमपुस्तकयोः नोपलभ्यते ।

"हिंग्वम्लवेतसव्योषयवानीलवणत्रिकैः ।
बीजपूररसोपेतैर्गुटिका वातशूलनुत् ॥४८॥"

[हिंग्वादिगुटिका]

[भैषज्यरत्नावली : शूलरोगाधिकार : १४]

Hingu, amla vetasa, śuṇṭhī, pippalī, marica, yavānī, rock-salt, sonchal salt and sea-salt should be triturated with the juice of *bīja-pūra* and made to pills. Intake of these pills cures *vātika* type of colic pain.

"बीजपूरकमूलं च घृतेन सह पाययेत् ।
जयेद्वातभवं शूलं कर्षमेकं[1] प्रमाणतः ॥४९॥"

[भैषज्यरत्नावली : शूलरोगाधिकार : १५]

The root of *bīja pūraka* in one *karṣa* dose should be given along with ghee. It cures *vātika* type of colic pain.

"बिल्वमूलतिलैरण्डं पिष्ट्वा चाम्लतुषाम्भसा ।
गुटिकां[2] भ्रामयेदुष्णां वातशूलविनाशिनीम् ॥५०॥

The root of *bilva, tila, eraṇḍa* should be triturated with *tuṣāmbu* and made to pills. These pills, when warm, should be rolled over the abdomen which cures *vātika* type of colic pain.

---

1. माषमेकं इति आकरे पाठः ।
2. शुंठिकां इति द्वितीय पुस्तके पाठः ।

तिलैश्च गुटिकां कृत्वा भ्रामयेज्जठरोपरि ।
'गुडिका[1] शमयत्येषा शूलं चैवातिदुःसहम्[2] ॥५१॥'

A pill made of *tila* should be rolled over abdomen which cures serious type of colic pain caused by *vāyu.*

"नाभिलेपाज्जयेच्छूलं मदनं काञ्जिकान्वितम् ।
जीवन्तीमूलकल्को वा सतैलः पार्श्वशूलनुत् ॥५२॥"
[भैषज्यरत्नावली : शूलरोगाधिकार : १७-१९]

Madana should be made to a paste by triturating with *kāñjī* (a type of vinegar). This paste, when applied over the umbilical region, cures colic pain. Application of the paste of the root of *jīvantī* along with sesame oil cures *pārśva śūla* (pain in the sides of the chest).

"गुडः शालिर्यवाः क्षीरं सर्पिः पानं विरेचनम् ।
जांगलानि च मांसानि भेषजं पित्तशूलिनाम् ॥५३॥

Recipes for Paittika Śūla

Guḍa (jaggery), *śāli* (ordinary rice), *yava* (barley), milk, ghee, purgation therapy and meat of *jāṅgala* type of animals (inhabiting arid land)—these are the remedies for *paittika* type of colic pain.

पैत्ते तु शूले वमनं पयोऽम्बु रसैस्त्वथेक्षो सपटोलनिम्बैः ।
शीतावगाहाः पुलिनाः सवाताः कांस्यादिपात्राणि जलप्लुतानि ॥५४॥

---

1. गुटिका इति द्वितीय पुस्तके पाठः ।
2. क. चैवातिदुस्तरम् इति आकरे पाठः ।
   ख. "गुडिका.........चैवातिदुःसहम्" पाठोऽयं षष्ठ पुस्तके नोपलभ्यते ।

विरेचनं पित्तहरं च शस्तं रसाश्च शस्ताः शशलावकानाम् ।

संतर्पणं लाजमधूपपन्नं योगाः सुशीता मधुसम्प्रयुक्ताः ॥५५॥

In *paittika* type of colic pain, emetic therapy should be administered with the help of milk, water or sugar-cane juice boiled with *paṭola* and *nimba.* The patient should take cold bath. He should enjoy cold wind of ponds. Bronze vessel, etc. with cold water should be applied over the body. Purgative therapies which help in the elimination of *pitta* (bile) are useful. He should take soup of the meat of animals like *śaśa* (rabbit) and *lāvaka.* He should take *samtarpaṇa* (refreshing drinks) prepared of *lājā* (fried paddy) by adding honey. Cooling recipes added with honey are also useful in this condition.

छर्द्यां ज्वरे पित्तभवे च[1] शूले घोरे विदाहे त्वतितर्षिते च ।

यवस्य पेयां मधुना विमिश्रां पिबेत्सुशीतां मनुजः[2] सुखार्थी ॥५६॥

Use of Yava Peyā

The *peyā* (thin gruel), prepared of barley mixed with honey and made cool, is refreshing and useful for patients suffering from vomiting, fever, colic pain caused by *pitta*, serious type of burning sensation and acute form of thirst.

धात्र्या रसं विदार्या वा त्रायन्तीगोस्तनाम्बु वा ।

पिबेत्सशर्करं सद्यः पित्तशूलनिषूदनम् ॥५७॥

The juice of *āmalakī*, *vidārī*, *trāyantī* or *gostanī* (a variety of grape), added with sugar should be taken. It instantaneously relieves *paittika* type of colic pain.

---

1. पित्तभवेऽथ इति प्रथमपंचमपुस्तकयोः आकरे च पाठः ।
2. मधुनः इति द्वितीयपुस्तके पाठः ।

शतावरीरसं क्षौद्रयुतं प्रातः पिबेन्नरः।

दाहशूलोपशान्त्यर्थं सर्वपित्तामयापहम् ॥५८॥"

[भैषज्यरत्नावली : शूलरोगाधिकार : २३-२८]

The juice of *śatāvarī*, added with honey should be taken in the morning for the alleviation of the colic pain associated with burning sensation, and for the cure of all diseases caused by *pitta.*

"बृहत्यौ गोक्षुरैरण्डकुशकाशेक्षुवालिकाः ।

पीताः पित्तभवं शूलं सद्यो हन्युः सुदारुणम् ॥५९॥"

[भैषज्यरत्नावली : शूलरोगाधिकार : ३१]

Intake of (the decoction) of *bṛhatī*, *kṣudrā*, *gokṣura*, *eraṇḍa*, *kuśa*, *kāśa* and *ikṣu vālikā* instantaneously cures all serious types of colic pain caused by *pitta.*

"सशतावरी[1] यष्ट्याह्ववाट्यालकुशगोक्षुरैः ।

श्रृतशीतं पिबेत्तोयं सगुडक्षौद्रशर्करम् ॥

पित्तासृग्दाहशूलघ्नं सद्यो दाहज्वरापहम्[2] ॥६०॥"

[भैषज्यरत्नावली : शूलरोगाधिकार : २९]

The decoction of *śatāvarī*, *madhu yaṣṭi*, *vāṭyālaka*, *kuśa* and *gokṣura* should be cooled and taken along with jaggery, honey and sugar. It cures *rakta pitta* (an ailment characterised by bleeding from different parts of the body), burning sensation and colic pain. It also instantaneously cures fever associated with burning sensation.

---

1. शतावरीसयष्टयाह्व० इति आकरे पाठः ।
2. हन्युः सुदारुणं इति प्रथमपंचमपुस्तकयोः पाठः ।

"त्रिफलानिम्बयष्ट्याह्वकटुकारग्वधैः श्रृतम्[1] ।
पाययेन्मधुसंमिश्रं दाहशूलोपशान्तये ॥६१॥"

[भैषज्यरत्नावली : शूलरोगाधिकार : ३०]

The decoction of *triphalā*, *nimba*, *madhu yaṣṭi*, *kaṭukā* and *āragvadha* should be mixed with honey and given for the alleviation of colic pain associated with burning sensation.

"तैलमैरण्डजं वापि मधुकक्वाथसंयुतम् ।
शूलं पित्तोद्भवं हन्याद्[2]गुल्मं पैत्तिकमेव च ॥६२॥"

[भैषज्यरत्नावली : शूलरोगाधिकार : ३२]

Castor oil mixed with the decoction of *yaṣṭi madhu* cures colic pain as well as *gulma* (phantom tumour) caused by *pitta*.

"त्रिफलारग्वधक्वाथं सक्षौद्रं शर्करान्वितम् ।
पाययेद्रक्तपित्तघ्नं दाहशूलनिवारणम् ॥
प्रलिह्यात् पित्तशूलघ्नं[3] धात्रीचूर्णं समाक्षिकम् ॥६३॥

The decoction of *triphalā* and *āragvadha* should be mixed with honey and sugar and given. It cures *rakta pitta* (an ailment characterised by bleeding from different parts of the body, and colic pain associated with burning sensation. Similarly, the linctus prepared of the powder of *āmalakī* and honey should be given for the cure of *paittika* type of colic pain.

---

1. त्रिफलाग्निं चयष्ट्याह्व० इति द्वितीयपुस्तके पाठः ।
2. हन्ति गुल्मं इति आकरे पाठः ।
3. रक्तपित्तघ्नं इति द्वितीयपुस्तके पाठः ।

श्लेष्मात्मके छर्दनलंघनानि शिरोविरेकं मधुसीधुपानम् ।
मधूनि गोधूमयवान्नारिष्टान्सेवेत रूक्षान्कटुकांश्च सर्वान् ॥६४॥"

[भैषज्यरत्नावली : शूलरोगाधिकार : ३३-३४]

Treatment of Ślaiṣmika Śūla

Emetic therapy, fasting, *śiro virecana* (elimination of *doṣas* from the head with the help of inhalation therapy, etc.) intake of *madhu sidhu* (a type of alcoholic drink prepared of honey), different types of honey, wheat, barley, *ariṣṭas* (a variety of alcoholic drink) and all types of ununctuous as well as pungent food are useful in the treatment of *kaphaja* type of colic pain.

पिप्पलीपिप्पलीमूलं चव्यचित्रकनागरैः ।
यवागूर्दीपनी या स्याच्छूलघ्नी तोयसाधिता ॥६५॥

Yavāgū (thick gruel) prepared by boiling (rice) in water and adding *pippalī*, *pippalī mūla*, *cavya*, *citraka* and *nāgara* is stimulant of digestion. It cures [*kaphaja* type of] colic pain.

"लवणत्रयसंयुक्तं पञ्चकोलं सरामठम् ।
सुखोष्णेनाम्बुना पीतं कफशूलविनाशनम्[1] ॥६६॥

The powder of *pañca kola* (*pippalī*, *pippalī mūla*, *cavya*, *citraka* and *nāgara*) should be mixed with asafoetida, sea-salt, rock-salt and *viḍa* type of salt and taken with luke-warm water. It cures *kaphaja* type of colic pain.

बिल्वमूलमथैरण्डं चित्रकं विश्वभेषजम् ।
हिंगुसैन्धवसंयुक्तं सद्यःशूलनिवारणम् ॥६७॥

The powder of the root of *bilva*, *eraṇḍa*, *citraka* and *viśva*

---

1. कफशूलनिवारणम् इति आकरे पाठः ।

bheṣaja added with asafoetida and rock-salt instantaneously cures [*kaphaja* type of] colic pain.

मुस्तां[1] वचां तिक्तकरोहिणीं च तथाऽभयां निर्दहनां च तुल्याम् ।
पिबेच्च[2] गोमूत्रयुतां कफोत्थे शूले तथाऽमस्य च पाचनार्थम् ॥६८॥"

[भैषज्यरत्नावली : शूलरोगाधिकार : ३६-३८]

Mustā, vacā, tiktaka rohiṇī, abhayā and *nirdahanā*—all these drugs taken in equal quantities should be made to a powder. Intake of this powder along with cow's urine cures *kaphaja* type of colic pain. It also helps in the digestion of *āma* (byproduct of improper digestion and metabolism).

(बिल्व)वचाभयातिक्ताचूर्णं गोमूत्रसंयुतम् ।
सक्षारं वा पिबेत्क्वाथं बिल्वादेः कफशूलवान् ॥६९॥

The patient suffering from *kaphaja* type of colic pain should take either the powder of *bilva, vacā, abhayā* and *tiktā* along with cow's urine or the decoction of the above mentioned drugs along with *kṣāra* (alkali preparation).

"मातुलुंगरसो वापि शिग्रुक्वाथस्तथाऽपरः ।
सक्षारो मधुना पीतः पार्श्वहृद्बस्तिशूलनुत् ॥७०॥"

[भैषज्यरत्नावली : शूलरोगाधिकार : ४०]

Intake of either the juice of *mātuluṅga* or the decoction of *śigru* along with *kṣāra* (alkali preparation) and honey cures pain in the sides of the chest cardiac region and urinary bladder.

---

1. मुस्ताकवचां रोहिणी च इति द्वितीयपुस्तके पाठः ।
2. पिबेत्तु गोमूत्रयुतां इति आकरे पाठः ।

"आमशूले क्रिया कार्या कफशूलविनाशिनी ।
सेव्यमामहरं सर्वं यदग्निबलवर्द्धनम् ॥७१॥"

[योगरत्नाकर : शूलचिकित्सा (उत्तरार्द्धम्) : पृष्ठ ७]

Treatment of Āmaja Śūla

In the *āmaja* type of colic pain, all the recipes prescribed for the treatment of *kaphaja* type of colic pain should be used. The patient should take all such diet and drugs as are capable of removing *āma* (product of improper digestion and metabolism) from the body and which promote the power of digestion as well as metabolism.

सहिंगुतुम्बुरुव्योषयवानीचित्रकाभयाः ।
सक्षारलवणः चूर्णं पिबेत्प्रातः सुखाम्बुना ॥
विण्मूत्रानिलशूलघ्नं पाचनं वह्निदीपनम् ॥७२॥

Intake of the powder of *hiṅgu, tumburu, vyoṣa, yavānī, citraka, abhayā kṣāra* (alkali preparation) and rock-salt along with luke-warm water in the morning, cures colic pain caused by improper excretion of stool, urine and flatus. It is carminative and stimulant of digestion.

चित्रकं ग्रंथिकैरण्डशुण्ठीधान्यं[1] जले श्रृतम् ।
शूलानाह[2]विबन्धेषु सहिंगुविडसैन्धवम् ॥७३॥

Intake of the decoction of *citraka, granthika, eraṇḍa, śuṇṭhī* and *dhānya* along with asafoetida, *viḍa* (a type of salt) and

1. धान्य इति पंचमपुस्तके पाठः ।
2. शूलोनाह० इति द्वितीयपुस्तके पाठः ।

rock-salt is useful in colic pain, distension of abdomen and constipation.

"दीप्यकं[1] सैन्धवं पथ्या नागरं च चतुःसमम् ।
चूर्णं शूलं जयत्याशु मन्दस्याग्नेश्च दीपनम् ॥७४॥

[चतुसमः चूर्णम्]

The powder of *dīpyaka*, rock-salt, *pathyā* and *nāgara*—all taken in equal quantities—instantaneously cures colic pain. It also stimulates the suppressed power of digestion.

समाक्षिकं बृहत्यादिं पिबेत्पित्तानिलात्मके ।
द्व्यामिश्रं वा विधिं कुर्यात् शूलं पित्तानिलात्मके ॥७५॥

Treatment of Dvandvaja Śūla

Bṛhatyādi kvātha along with honey should be given for the colic pain caused by *pitta* and *vāyu* together. Alternatively, for the treatment of this type of colic pain, recipes meant for *paittika* and *kaphaja* types of colic pain should be mixed together and administered.

पित्तजे कफजे चापि या क्रिया कथिता पृथक् ।
एकीकृत्य प्रयुञ्जीत क्रियां कफजपित्तजे ॥७६॥

Recipes prescribed for *paittika* and *kaphaja* types of colic pain should be mixed together and administered for the treatment of colic pain caused by *pitta* and *kapha* together.

1. दीपनं इति षष्ठपुस्तके पाठः ।

पटोलत्रिफलारिष्टक्वाथं मधुयुतं पिबेत् ।
पित्तश्लेष्मज्वरच्छर्दिदाहशूलोपशान्तये ॥७७॥

[पटोलादिक्वाथ]

The decoction of *paṭola*, *triphalā* and *ariṣṭa* mixed with honey should be given for the alleviation of fever, vomiting, burning sensation and colic pain caused by both *kapha* and *pitta*.

रसोनं [1]चव्यसंमिश्रं पिबेत्प्रातः सकाजिकम् ।
वातश्लेष्मभवं शूलं निहन्ति वह्निदीपनम् ॥७८॥"

[भैषज्यरत्नावली : शूलरोगाधिकार : ४६-५०]

Rasona and *cavya* should be taken along with *kāñjī* (a type of vinegar) in the morning. This cures colic pain caused by *vāyu* and *kapha* together. It also stimulates the power of digestion.

"विश्वोरुबूकदशमूलयवांभसा तु
द्विक्षारहिंगुलवणत्रयपुष्करम् च ।
चूर्णं पिबेद्धृदयपा[2]र्श्वकटिग्रहाम-
पक्वाशया[3]र्तिभृशरुग्ज्वरगुल्मशूली ॥७९॥"

[योगरत्नाकर : शूलचिकित्सा (उत्तरार्द्धम्) : पृष्ठ ६]

क्वाथेन चूर्णपानं यत्तत्रक्वाथप्रधानता ।
प्रवर्तते च तेनात्र चूर्णापेक्षी चतुर्द्रवः ॥८०॥

॥ इति विश्वादि : ॥

---

1. मद्यसंमिश्रं इति प्रथमपंचमषष्ठपुस्तकेषु आकरे च पाठः ।
2. ०पृष्ठ० इति आकरे पाठः ।
3. पक्वाशयार्तिभृश० इति आकरे पाठः ।

Viśvādi Kvātha

With the decoction of *viśva, urubūka, daśa mūla* and *yava*, the powder of *svarji kṣāra, yava kṣāra,* sea-salt, rock-salt, *viḍa* (a type of salt) and *puṣkara mūla* should be taken. This cures pain in cardiac region, sides of the chest, lumber region, *āmāśaya* (small intestine including stomach) and *pakvāśaya* (large intestine). This recipe is specially useful when there is excessive pain, fever, *gulma* (phantom tumour) and colic pain.

When a recipe of powder is prescribed to be taken along with a decoction, it is the latter which predominates. Therefore, the decoction should be four times the quantity of the powder.

"चूर्णं समं रुचकहिंगुमहौषधानां
शुण्ठ्यम्बुना कफसमीरणसंभवासु ।
हृत्पार्श्वपृष्ठज्वरार्तिविषूचिकासु
पेयं तथा यवरसेन विड्विबन्धेषु ॥८१॥"

[भैषज्यरत्नावली : शूलरोगाधिकार : ५१]

"समं शुण्ठ्यम्बुनेत्येवं[1] योजना क्रियते बुधैः ।
तेनाल्पं मानमेवात्र हिंगुमुपरि[2] दीयते ॥८२॥
॥ इति रुचकादिः[3] ॥"

Rucakādi Cūrṇa

The powder of *rucaka, hiṅgu* and *mahauṣadha* should be taken along with the decoction of *śuṇṭhī* for [colic pain caused

1. समशुद्धाम्बुना पेयं इति षष्ठपुस्तके पाठः ।
2. हिंगुसंपरि इति प्रथमपुस्तके पाठः ।
3. "विश्वोरुबूक.........इति रुचकादिः ॥" पाठोऽयं षष्ठपुस्तके नोपलभ्यते ।

by] *kapha* and *vāyu* together. This powder taken along with the decoction of barley is useful in pain in cardiac region, sides of the chest and back, fever, *viṣūcikā* (choleric diarrhoea) and constipation.

This recipe is prescribed to be taken along with the decoction of *śuṇṭhī*. A small quantity of *hiṅgu* (in addition to what is prescribed in the recipe) should be added to the decoction while administering the recipe.

"तीक्ष्णायश्चूर्णसंयुक्तं[1] त्रिफलाचूर्णमुत्तमम् ।
प्रयोज्यं मधुसर्पिभ्यां सर्वशूलनिवारणम् ॥८३॥"

॥ त्रिफलालौहः ॥

[योगरत्नाकर : उत्तरार्ध : पृष्ठ ६]

Triphalā Lauha

The powder or *bhasma* of *tīkṣṇa* type of iron (steel) and the powder of *triphalā* should be taken along with honey and ghee. It cures all types of colic pain.

"घृताच्चतुर्गुणो देयो मातुलुंगरसो दधिः ।
शुष्कमूलककोलाम्लकषायो दाडिमाद्रसः ॥८४॥
विडंग-लवणक्षारपंचकोलयवादिभिः ।
पाठामूलककल्कैश्च सिद्धं शूलिघृतं मतम् ॥८५॥
हृत्पार्श्वशूलं वैस्वर्यकासहिक्कां तथैव च ।
ब्रध्नगुल्मप्रमेहार्शोवातव्याधींश्च नाशयेत् ॥८६॥

॥ इति शूलिघृतम् ॥"

[भारतभैषज्यरत्नाकर : पञ्चम भाग : पृष्ठ ५१]

---

1. "तीक्ष्णाय .... सर्वशूलनिवारणम्" पाठोऽयं पंचमपुस्तके अधिकमुपलभ्यते ।

Śūli Ghṛta

Ghee cooked with four times of the juice of *mātuluṅga*, curd, decoction of dry *mūlaka* and sour variety of *kola*, juice of *dāḍima* and [one fourth in quantity of] the paste of *viḍaṅga*, salt, *kṣāra*, (alkali preparation), *pippalī*, *pippalī mūla*, *cavya*, *citraka*, *nāgara*, *yava* (barley), *pāṭhā* and *mūlaka* is called *Śūli ghṛta*. It cures pain in cardiac region, sides of the chest, hoarseness of voice, cough, hic-cup, *bradhna* (inguinal lymphadenitis), *gulma* (phantom tumour), *prameha* (obstinate urinary disorders including diabetes), piles and *vāta vyādhis* (diseases of nervous system).

"हिंगु सौवर्चलं पथ्या विडं सैन्धव तुम्बुरु ।
पौष्करं च पिबेच्चूर्णं दशमूलयवाम्भसा ॥८७॥
पार्श्वहृत्कटिपृष्ठांसशूले तन्द्रापतानके ।
शोथे श्लेष्मप्रसेके च कर्णरोगे च शस्यते ॥८८॥"

[भैषज्यरत्नावली : शूलरोगाधिकार : ४२-४३]

The powder of *hiṅgu*, *sauvarcala*, *pathyā*, *viḍa*, rock-salt, *tumburu* and *puṣkara mūla* should be taken along with the decoction of *daśa mūla* and *yava* (barley). It is useful for the pain in the sides of the chest, cardiac region, lumber region and shoulder region, *tandrā* (drowsiness), *apatānaka*, oedema, excessive salivation and ear diseases.

"एरण्डबिल्वबृहतीद्वयमातुलुंग-
पाषाणभेदत्रिकटुमूलकृतः[1] कषायः ।
सक्षारहिंगुलवणो रुबुतैलमिश्रः

---

1. ०भित्त्रिकटु० इति आकरे पाठः ।

श्रोण्यंसमेढ्रहृदयस्तनरुक्षुपेयः[1] ॥८९॥

॥ एरण्डसप्तकम् ॥"

[भैषज्यरत्नावली : शूलरोगाधिकार : ४१]

Eraṇḍa Saptaka

The decoction of *eraṇḍa*, *bilva*, *bṛhatī*, *kaṇṭakārī*, *mātuluṅga*, *pāṣāṇa bheda*, *trikaṭu* and *puṣkara mūla* should be added with *kṣāra* (alkali preparation), asafoetida, rock-salt and castor oil. This should be taken by a patient suffering from pain in hip region, shoulder region, cardiac region, *meḍhra* (male genital organ) and breasts.

"हिंगु त्रिकटुकं कुष्ठं यवक्षारोऽथ सैन्धवम् ।

मातुलुंगरसोपेतं प्लीहशूलापहं[2] रजः ॥९०॥"

[भैषज्यरत्नावली : शूलरोगाधिकार : ४४]

The powder of *hiṅgu*, *trikaṭuka*, *kuṣṭha*, *yava kṣāra* and rock salt should be taken along with the juice of *mātuluṅga* which cures pain in the splenic region.

"दग्धमनिर्गतधूमं मृगश्रृंगं गोघृतेन सह पीतम्[3] ।

हृदयनितम्बजशूलं हरति शिखी दारुनिवहमिव ॥९१॥

[भैषज्यरत्नावली : शूलरोगाधिकार : ५७]

The ash of deer horn collected by burning in an airtight container should be mixed with cow's ghee. Intake of this cures pain in heart and hip regions as fire engulfs logs of wood.

---

1. ०रुक्षु इति आकरे पाठः ।
2. प्लीहशूलापहा शुटी इति आकरे पाठः
3. लीढम् इति आकरे पाठः ।

कृमिरिपु चूर्णं लीढं स्वरसेन वङ्गसेनस्य ।

क्षपयत्यचिरान्नियतं लोहाजीर्णोद्भवं शूलम् ॥६२॥

Intake of the powder of *kṛmi ripu* along with the juice of *vaṅga sena* instantaneously cures colic pain caused by the intake of unprocessed iron.

"विदारीदाडिमरसः सव्योष[1]लवणान्वितः ।

क्षौद्रयुक्तो जयत्याशु शूलं दोषत्रयोद्भवम् ॥६३॥

Treatment of Tridoṣaja Śūla

Intake of the juice of *vidāri* and *dāḍima* along with *trikaṭu*, rock-salt and honey instantaneously overcomes colic pain caused by the simultaneous vitiation of all the three *doṣas*.

एरण्डफलमूलानि बृहतीद्वयगोक्षुरम् ।

पर्णिन्यः सहदेवा[2] च सिंहपुच्छीक्षुवालिका ॥६४॥

तुल्यैरेभिः शृतं तोयं यवक्षारयुतं पिबेत् ।

पृथग्दोषोद्भवं[3] हन्याच्छूलं सर्वभवं तथा ॥६५॥

॥ इति एरण्डद्वादशः ॥"

[भैषज्यरत्नावली : शूलरोगाधिकार : ५४-५६]

Eraṇḍa Dvādaśa Kvātha

Fruits and roots of *eraṇḍa*, *bṛhatī*, *kaṇṭakārī*, *gokṣura*, *śāla parṇī*, *pṛśni parṇī*, *māṣa parṇī*, *mudga parṇī*, *sahadevi*, *siṁha pucchī* and *ikṣu vālikā*—all these drugs should be taken in equal

1. सव्योषो इति आकरे पाठः ।
2. सहदेवी इति द्वितीयपुस्तके पाठः ।
3. पृथग्दोषभवं इति आकरे पाठः ।

quantities and a decoction should be prepared. Intake of this decoction along with *kṣāra* (alkali preparation) cures colic pain caused by *doṣas* individually or together.

"गोमूत्रशुद्धं[1] मण्डूरं त्रिफलाचूर्णसंयुतम् ।
विलिहन् मधुसर्पिभ्यां शूलं हन्ति त्रिदोषजम् ॥६६॥"

[भैषज्यरत्नावली : शूलरोगाधिकार : ५३]

[योगरत्नाकर : शूलचिकित्सा (उत्तरार्द्धम्) पृष्ठ ६]

Maṇḍūra (rust iron) purified by boiling with cow's urine and the powder of *triphalā* should be made to a linctus by adding honey and ghee. Intake of this cures colic pain caused by the simultaneous vitiation of all the three *doṣas*.

शंखयोग :—

"शंखचूर्णं सलवणं सहिंगुव्योषसंयुतम् ।
उष्णोदकेन तत्पीतं शूलं हन्ति त्रिदोषजम् ॥६७॥"

[भैषज्यरत्नावली : शूलरोगाधिकार : ५२]

Śaṅkha Yoga

Intake of the powder or *bhasma* of conch shell mixed with rock salt, asafoetida and *trikaṭu* along with hot water cures colic pain caused by the simultaneous vitiation of all the three *doṣas*.

"मूत्रान्तःपाचितां 'शुष्कां[2] लोहचूर्णसमन्विताम् ।

---

1. क. गोमूत्रशुद्धं···त्रिदोषजम्" पाठोऽयं पंचमपुस्तके अधिकमुपलभ्यते
   ख. गोमूत्रसिद्धमण्डूरं इति आकरे पाठः ।
2. 'शुष्कां·········चित्रकम्' पाठोऽयं पंचमपुस्तके नोपलभ्यते ।

सगुडामभयां दद्यात्[1] सर्वशूलप्रशान्तये[2] ॥९८॥"

[योगरत्नाकर : शूलचिकित्सा : (उत्तरार्द्धम्) पृष्ठ ८]

Abhayā should be cooked in cow's urine and dried. Powder of this *abhayā* should be mixed with the powder or *bhasma* of *lauha* (iron). Intake of this powder along with jaggery cures all types of colic pain.

"पिप्पली नागरं बिल्वं कारवी चव्यचित्रकम्' ।
हिङ्गु दाडिमवृक्षाम्लं वचाक्षाराम्लवेतसम् ॥९९॥
वर्षाभूकृष्णलवणमजाजीबीजपूरकम् ।
दधित्रिगुणितं सर्पिस्तत्सिद्धं दाधिकं स्मृतम् ॥१००॥
गुल्मार्शःप्लीहहृत्पार्श्वशूलयोनिरुजापहम् ।
दोषप्रशमनं श्रेष्ठं दाधिकं परमं स्मृतम् ॥१०१॥

॥ इति दाधिकं घृतम् ॥ '

[भैषज्यरत्नावली : शूलरोगाधिकार : ९३-९५]

Dādhika Ghṛta

Ghee boiled with three times of *dadhi* (curd) and [one fourth in quantity of the paste of] *pippalī*, *nāgara*, *bilva*, *kāravī*, *cavya*, *citraka*, *hiṅgu*, *dāḍima*, *vṛkṣāmla*, *vacā*, *kṣāra* (alkali preparation), *amla vetasa*, *varṣābhū*, *kṛṣṇa lavaṇa* (a variety of salt, black in colour), *ajājī* and *bīja pūraka* is called *dādhika ghṛta*. It is an excellent recipe for the treatment of *gulma*

1. सगुडाममयामद्यात् इति ग्रादर्शपुस्तकेषु पाठः ।
2. सर्वशूलोपशान्तये इति आकरे पाठः ।

(phantom tumour), piles and pain in splenic region, cardiac region, sides of the chest and female genital tract. It is also useful for the alleviation of the vitiated *doṣas.*

"मृतसूतस्य भागैकं[1] षड्भागां शोधितां शिलां[2] ।
दिनं जंबीरजद्रावैर्मर्द्यो[3] रुध्वा धमेल्लघु[4] ॥
शिलावद्धो रसो नाम गुञ्जैकः पित्तशूलनुत्[5] ॥१०२॥
॥ इति शिलाबद्धोरसः[6] ॥"

[भारतभैषज्यरत्नाकर : पंचमभाग : पृष्ठ १२९]

Śilā baddha Rasa

One part of the *bhasma* of *pārada* and six parts of purified *manaḥ śilā* should be triturated with the juice of *jambīra.* The paste, thus prepared, should be kept in a sealed container and cooked in *laghu puṭa.* This is called *śilā baddha rasa.* Administration of this recipe in the dose of one *guñjā* (125 mg.) cures *paittika* type of colic pain.

एकं[7] हिंगु चतुः[8] पथ्या त्रि शुण्ठी द्वि सुवर्चलम्[9] ।

---

1. भागैकं इति आकरे पाठः ।
2. शोधिता शिला इति आदर्शपुस्तकेषु पाठः ।
3. जम्बीरजैर्द्रावैर्मर्द्यं इति आकरे पाठः ।
4. च मे लघु इति आदर्शपुस्तकेषु पाठः ।
5. पित्तशूलजित इति पंचमषष्ठपुस्तकयोः आकरे च पाठः ।
6. शिलाबद्धरस इति आकरे पाठः ।
7. एक इति आकरे पाठः ।
8. शतं इति आकरे पाठः ।
9. सुवर्चला इति आकरे पाठः ।

भागान्विचूर्ण्य[1] कर्षकमनुस्याच्छूलनाशनम्[2] ॥१०३॥

Hiṅgu (one part), *pathyā* (four parts), *śuṇṭhī* (three parts) and *sauvarcala* (two parts) should be made to a powder and administered in the dose of one *karṣa* after the administration of *śīla baddha rasa* which cures colic pain.

"सूतं गन्धं समं शुद्धं सूतांशं मृतताम्रकम्[3] ।
मर्दयेदातपे 'तीव्रे[4] रुध्वा लघुपुटत्रयम्[5] ॥१०४॥
दत्त्वादाय च तच्चूर्णं[6] सूतांशं त्रिकटुं क्षिपेत् ।
षण्मूखोऽयं रसो नाम्ना त्रिगुंजः[7] सर्वशूलनुत् ॥१०५॥

Ṣaṇmukha Rasa

Purified *pārada*, purified *gandhaka* and *bhasma* of *tāmra*, all taken in equal quantities, should be triturated by exposing to hot sun, kept in a *śarāva sampuṭa* and cooked in *laghu puṭa* three times. This powder should then be triturated by adding the powder of *trikaṭu* (taken in quantity equal to that of *pārada*). This is called *Ṣaṇmukha rasa.* It should be administered in the dose of three *guñjās* (375 mg) which cures all types of colic pain.

---

1. एतच्चूर्णञ्च इति आकरे पाठः ।
2. ०शान्तये इति आकरे पाठः ।
3. "सौवर्चलञ्च सूतांशं जम्बीरैर्दिनसप्तकम्" पाठोऽयं आकरे अधिकमुपलभ्यते ।
4. तीक्ष्णे इति आकरे पाठः ।
5. लघुपुटेत्त्रयम् इति आकरे पाठः ।
6. समं त्रिकटुकं पचेत् इति आकरे पाठः ।
7. त्रिगुञ्जेनामशूलनित् इति आकरे पाठः ।

एरण्डतैलषड्भागान्[1] लशुनस्य दशांशकम्[2] ।
एकं हिंगु त्रिसिन्धूत्थं सर्वमेकत्र मर्दयेत्[3] ॥
त्रिनिष्कं भक्षयेच्चानु आमशूलहरं[4] परम् ॥१०६॥
॥ इति षण्मुखरस:[5] ॥"

[भारतभैषज्यरत्नाकर : पञ्चमभाग : पृष्ठ १८८]

Eraṇḍa taila (six parts), *laśuna* (ten parts), *hiṅgu* (one part) and rock salt (three parts)—all these should be triturated together. Intake of three *niṣkas* of this recipe cures colic pain caused by *āma* (product of improper digestion).

ताम्रयोग:

मृतताम्रस्य भागैकं पिबेदुष्णजलेन वा ।
शुण्ठीक्वाथं पिबेच्चानु हिंगुसौवर्चलान्वितम् ॥१०७॥

Tāmra Yoga

[For getting relief from *āmaja* type of colic pain], the patient should take [one *guñja*=125 mg of] *tāmra bhasma* along with hot water. Thereafter, he should take the decoction of *śuṇṭhī* mixed with *hiṅgu* and *sauvarcala*.

[6]'क्षारं कपर्दाद्विषसैन्धवे च व्योषं च संमर्द्य भुजङ्गवल्या: ।

---

1. ०षड्भागं इति आकरे पाठ: ।
2. दशाष्टकम् इति आकरे पाठ: ।
3. कारयेत् इति आकरे पाठ: ।
4. आमशूलप्रशान्तये इति आकरे पाठ: ।
5. षण्मुखो रस: इति आकरे पाठ: ।
6. 'क्षारं..........शूलगजकेसरी' पाठोऽयं प्रथमपंचमपुस्तकयो: नोपलभ्यते ।

रसेन गुंजाप्रमितः प्रदिष्टः समीरशूलेभहरिः प्रचण्डः ॥१०८॥

॥ शूलगजकेसरी ॥'

Śūla Gaja Kesarī

Kṣāra (alkali preparation) [or *bhasma*] of cowri shells, *viṣa* (aconite), rock salt and *trikaṭu* should be triturated in the juice of betel leaf. It should be administered in a dose of one *guñjā* (125 mg) which effectively cures *vātika* type of colic pain.

"शुद्धसूतं द्विधा गन्धं यामैकं मर्दयेद्दृढम् ।
द्वयोस्तुल्यं ताम्रपत्रं[1] सम्पुटे तन्निरोधयेत् ॥१०९॥
ऊर्ध्वाधो लवणं दत्त्वा मृद्भाण्डे धारयेद्भिषक्[2] ।
रुध्वा गजपुटे[3] पच्यात्स्वांगशीतं[4] समुद्धरेत् ॥११०॥
सम्पुटं चूर्णयेत्सूक्ष्मं[5] पर्णखण्डे द्विगुञ्जकम्[6] ।
भक्षयेत्सर्वशूलार्त्तं हिंगुशुण्ठी च जीरकम्[7] ॥१११॥
वचा मरीचजं चूर्णं कर्षमुष्णाजलैः[8] पिबेत् ।

1. शुद्धताम्रसंपुटे इति आकरे पाठः ।
2. स्थापयेद् बुधः इति आकरे पाठः ।
3. गजपुटं इति आकरे पाठः ।
4. दत्वा स्वाङ्गशीतं इति आकरे पाठः ।
5. चूर्णयेच्छुलक्ष्णं इति आकरे पाठः ।
6. पर्णखण्डेऽर्धगुञ्जकम् इति आकरे पाठः ।
7. सजीरकम् इति आकरे पाठः ।
8. सममुष्णजलैः इति आकरे पाठः ।

आसाध्यं[1] नाशयेच्छूलं[2] रसोऽयं शूलकेसरी ॥११२॥"

॥ इति शूलगजकेसरी रसः ॥

[भैषज्यरत्नावली : शूलरोगाधिकार : २११-२१४]

Śūla Gaja Kesarī Rasa (*second variety*)

Purified *pārada* (one part) and purified *gandhaka* (two parts) should be triturated well for three hours. This should be added with thin leaves of *tāmra* (three parts) and kept inside a *śarāva samputa* (two earthen plates the joint of which is sealed by mud smeared cloth). This *śarāva samputa* containing the drugs should be kept in the middle of an earthen vessel with salt all around it. This earthen vessel should then be sealed and cooked in *gaja puṭa*. After cooking, the powder collected from *śarāva samputa* should be further triturated to make a fine powder. This should be administered in the dose of two *guñjās* (250 mg) which cures all types of colic pain. After taking this, the patient should take one *karṣa* (5 gms.) of the powder of *hiṅgu*, *śuṇṭhī*, *jīraka*, *vacā* and *marica* with hot water. This is called *śūla kesarī* and it cures even the incurable types of colic pain.

कंबलावृतगात्रस्य प्राणायामं प्रकुर्वतः ।
कटुतैलाक्तसक्तूनां धूम शूलहरः परः ॥११३॥

The patient's body should be covered with a blanket and he should then perform *prāṇāyāma* (breathing exercise). His body should then be fumigated by igniting *saktu* (corn flour) mixed with mustard oil. This is an excellent recipe for curing colic pain.

"व्यायामं मैथुनं मद्यं लवणं[3] कटुवैदलम् ।
वेगरोधं शुचं क्रोधं वर्जयेच्छूलवान्नरः ॥११४॥"

[भैषज्यरत्नावली : शूलरोगाधिकार:२०३]

1. साध्येच्छूलं इति आकरे पाठः।
2. श्री शूलजलकेसरी इति आकरे पाठः।
3. वैदलं लवणं तिलान् इति आकरे पाठः ।

Prohibitions

The patient suffering from colic pain should avoid exercise, sexual intercourse, alcoholic drinks, salt, pungent food, *vaidala* (pulses having two cotyledons), suppression of the manifested natural urges, worry and anger.

भवेच्छिम्बीधान्यातिशयभजानाच्छूलमनिलप्रधानम् ।
तान्यष्टौत्रिभिरथ समस्तैश्च युगलैः ॥११५॥
अजीर्णेऽन्ने ह्यस्मिन्भवति जठरे कुक्षियुगले-
यदि[1] प्रौढाटोपो रुगति न मलानां विसरणम् ॥११६॥

Eight types of colic pain caused by three *doṣas*, viz. *vāyu*, *pitta* and *kapha*, individually or two of them together or all the three *doṣas* together is generally dominated by *vāyu* [in the *sāmānya samprāpti*] and excessive intake of *simbī dhānya* (pulses and beans) is the causative factor of all of them. Excessive intake of these pulses and beans leads to indigestion, distension in the abdomen and pelvic regions, excessive pain and constipation [as a prelude to colic pain].

"भागौ रसस्य भागोऽथ[2] हेम्नः पिष्टीं विधाय च ।
तथा द्वादशभागानि ताम्रपत्राणि लेपयेत् ॥११७॥
ऊर्ध्वाधो गन्धकं दत्वा पलमात्रं समन्ततः ।
[3]'क्षारस्य मृगशृंगस्य चूर्णं योज्यं समं ततः ॥११८॥'
सिञ्चेन्मत्स्याक्षिनीरेण रुन्ध्याद्यामचतुष्टयम् ।

1. ह्यादि इति पंचमपुस्तके पाठः ।
2. भागाश्च इति आकरे पाठः ।
3. 'क्षारस्य ··········समं ततः' पाठोऽयं भारत भैषज्यरत्नाकरे नोपलभ्यते प्रथमपंचमपुस्तकयोः च ।

पचेच्छूलहरः सूतो[1] भवेत्त्रिपुरभैरवः ॥११९॥
माषो मध्वाज्यसंयुक्तो देयोऽस्य परिणामजे ।
अन्येष्वेरण्डतैलेन हिंगुत्रययुतो हितः ॥१२०॥"

॥ इति त्रिपुरभैरवी रसः ॥

[योगरत्नाकर : शूलचिकित्सा : (उत्तरार्द्धम्) पृष्ठ १७]

[भारतभैषज्यरत्नाकर : द्वितीय भाग : पृष्ठ ८५]

Tripura Bhairavi Rasa

Pārada (one part) and *svarṇa* (one part) should be triturated together to make an amalgam (*piṣṭi*). To this, thin leaves of *tāmra* (twelve parts) should be added and further triturated. This paste should be kept inside an earthen vessel and all around this paste, purified *gandhaka* (one *pala*—48 gms.), *kṣāra* or alkali preparation (one part) and the powder or *bhasma* of deer horn (one part) should be kept. Over this, the juice of *matsyākṣī* should be sprinkled. The earthen vessel should then be cooked for twelve hours [in *gaja puṭa*]. This is called *Tripura bhairava rasa.* This should be administered in the dose of one *māṣa* (6 gms.) along with castor oil and asafoetida which is useful in *pariṇāma śūla* and other types of colic pain.

"रसबलिगगनार्कं वेतसाम्लं विषंस्यात् ।
सावरमिति पृथक्तद्भावयेद्धस्तमेतैः ।
कनकभुजगवल्लीकंटकारीजयाद्भिः ।
कमलशशिकवासा[2]मुष्टिरुष्णाम्बुपूरैः[3] ॥१२१॥

1. शूलो इति द्वितीयपुस्तके पाठः ।
2. कमलसलिलवासाः इति आकरे पाठः ।
3. मुष्टिबज्राम्बुपूरैः इति आकरे पाठः ।

अरुणसदृशशाकैः[1] मातुलान्यथ योज्यः ।
पटुगण इह तुल्यो भावयेदार्द्रकाद्भिः ।
दहनवदनसंज्ञो[2] बल्लमात्रो निहन्ति ।
प्रबलपवनशूलं तद्विकारानशेषान्[3] ॥१२२॥

॥ इत्यग्निमुखो रसः ॥"

[भारतभैषज्यरत्नाकर : प्रथमभाग : पृष्ठ ७४]

Agni Mukha Rasa

Purified *pārada*, purified *gandhaka*, purified *abhra*, purified *tāmra*, *vetasāmla*, *viṣa* and *sāvara sṛṅga*—all these should be impregnated and triturated with the juice or decoction of *kanaka*, *bhujaga vallī*, *kaṇṭakārī*, *jayā*, *kamala*, *śaśika* (*kumuda*), *vāsā*, *muṣṭi*, *uṣṇāmbu* (latex of *snūhī*), *pura* (*guggulu*), red leaves of *mātulānī*, *trikaṭu* and *ārdraka*. This preparation is called *Dahana vadana* (*Agni mukha*). It should be administered in the dose of one *balla* which cures serious type of colic pain caused by *vāyu* along with all the attending complications.

शिवावचाहिंगुविषाकलिंगरुचकं समम् ।
कर्षमुष्णाम्बुना पेयमनुपानं हि शूलिभिः ॥१२३॥

Śivā, *vacā*, *hiṅgu*, *viṣā*, *kaliṅga* and *rucaka*—all these drugs taken in equal quantities should be made to a powder. This should be administered in the dose of one *karṣa* (6 gms.) along with the *anupāna* (post-prandial drink) of hot water. This cures colic pain.

---

1. अरुणसदृशपाकैः इति आकरे पाठः ।
2. दहनवदननाम्ना इति आकरे पाठः ।
3. तद्विकाराननेकान् इति द्वितीयपुस्तके पाठः ।

सूतगन्धविषव्योषवराभार्ग्यब्दवेल्लकैः ।
द्विपचातिविषावह्निः सर्वतुल्यगुडेन च ॥
गुटिका चणकोन्माना सर्वशूलनिकृन्तनी ॥१२४॥

॥ इति शूलनिकृन्तनी वटी[1] ॥

Śūla Nikṛntanī Vaṭī

Purified *pārada*, purified *gandhaka*, purified *viṣa*, *vyoṣa*, *varā*, *bhārgī*, *abda*, *bellaka*, *dvipa* (*gaja pippalī*), *ativiṣā* and *vahni* should be made to a powder. To this, jaggery in quantity equal to that of all these drugs should be added and pills should be made out of the size of peas. This cures all types of colic pain.

'युग(पत्तु)[2]संख्यानि दलानि भानोश्चत्वारि खण्डानि सुधाद्रुमस्य ।
रसेन्द्रवल्या[3] दश वै फलानि पञ्चैव पत्राणि कुमारिकायाः ॥१२५॥
व्याघ्री चतुःषष्टिपलानि दद्याच्चत्वारि वृन्ताकतरो[4] फलानि ।
पञ्चाङ्गमेकं हरिकन्दचूर्णं सिद्धार्थतैलं तु पलप्रमाणम् ॥१२६॥
यवानि सौवर्चलसैन्धवं च विडं यवक्षारसमुद्रजं च ।
सर्जो[5] ह्यपामार्गसकोरणं[6] च पलं पलं स्यात्क्रमशश्च चूर्णम् ॥१२७॥

---

1. "इति श्री महाराजाधिराजटोडरमल्लविरचिते टोडरानन्दे आयुर्वेदसौख्ये शूलनिदानचिकित्सा कथनं नाम सप्तत्रिंशत्तामो हर्षः ।" पाठोऽयं प्रथमपंचमपुस्तकयोः अधिकमुपलभ्यते ॥
2. क. 'युगपत्तु ....०पादेन निर्मितः' पाठोऽयं प्रथमपंचमपुस्तकयोः नोपलभ्यते ।
   ख. युगपत्तुं इति षष्ठपुस्तके पाठः ।
3. रसेन्द्रवल्याद्र इति षष्ठपुस्तके पाठः ।
4. वृन्तावितरोः इति द्वितीयपुस्तके पाठः ।
5. सज्जों इति षष्ठपुस्तके पाठः ।
6. त्वपामार्गं० इति षष्ठपुस्तके पाठः ।

भाण्डे पचेद्यामचतुष्टयेन तीव्राग्निना क्षारसमं च पचेत् ।
संभाव्य निम्बूरसबीजपूरैः संभक्षयेदर्धपलप्रमाणम् ॥१२८॥
पिबेत्कदुष्णोदकगोजलं च संनाशयेद्गुल्मं महातितीव्रम् ।
प्लीहोदरं विद्रधिशूलमुग्रं अजीर्णमूत्रग्रहनाशनं च ॥
आमप्रवृद्धं ग्रहणीमलं च दुष्टान्विकारान्हरतेऽतिशीघ्रम् ॥१२९॥

॥ इत्यर्कक्षारः ॥

Arka Kṣāra

Leaves of *arka* (12), pieces of *sudhā* (4), fruits of *rasendra vallī* (12), leaves of *kumārī* (5), *vyāghri* (64 *palas*), fruits of *vṛntāka* (4), entire plant of *hari kanda* (one), mustard oil (one *pala*), *yavānī* (one *pala*), *sauvarcala* (one *pala*), *saindhava* (one *pala*), *sāmudra lavaṇa* (one *pala*) *svarji kṣāra* (one *pala*), *apāmārga* (one *pala*) and *koraṇa* (?) (one *pala*)—all these drugs (the dried ones are to be made to powder) are to be cooked in a vessel for 12 hours on the line prescribed for *ksāra pāka* (alkali preparation) with the help of strong fire. The *kṣāra* (alkali preparation), thus obtained should be impregnated with lemon juice and the juice of *bīja pūra*. This recipe should be administered in the dose of half *pala* (24 gms.) along with luke-warm water or cow's urine which instantaneously cures serious type of *gulma* (phantom tumour), *plīhodara* (splenomegaly), serious types of abscess and colic pain, indigestion, anuria, *grahaṇī* (sprue syndrome) with excess of mucus and other obstinate diseases.

क्षारो मुष्कर्कांकिशुकार्जुनधवापामार्गरम्भातिलाः
जीवन्ती कनकाह्वयः(सह)च रजनी कूष्माण्डवल्ली तथा ॥१३०॥
वासासूरण[1] तीव्रमेव दहने प्रज्वाल्य भस्मीकृतम् ।

---

1. ०क्षुरण इति षष्ठपुस्तके पाठः ।

तोयेन प्रतिसेवितं शृतपयः पानं विधेयं सकृत्[1] ॥१३१॥

शूलानाहविबन्धगुल्मकफजान्रोगाञ्जयेत्कामलान् ।

अन्तर्वृद्धिमजीर्णकं ग्रहणिकांहृच्छूलपाण्डवर्शसाम्[2] ॥१३२॥

ग्रन्थ्यष्ठीलके शोफविद्रधिगदान्नानाविधान् पीनसान् ।

मन्दाग्निं जठरस्य पीडनगुरुप्लीहार्तिमेदादिकान् ॥१३३॥

॥ इत्यमृतक्षारः ॥

Amṛta Kṣāra

Kṣāra (alkali preparation) should be made out of *muṣkaka, kiṃśuka, arjuna, dhava, apāmārga, rambhā, tila, jivantī, kanaka, rajanī, kuṣmāṇḍa, vāsā* and *sūraṇa* by cooking over strong fire. This *kṣāra* (alkali preparation) should be taken with boiled water (only once ?) which cures colic pain, *ānāha* (abdominal distension), constipation, *gulma* (phantom tumour), diseases caused by *kapha, kāmalā* (jaundice), *antaḥ vṛddhi* (inguinal hernia), indigestion, *grahaṇī* (sprue syndrome), cardiac pain, anemia, piles, *granthi* (enlarged lymph glands), *aṣṭhīlā* (hard tumour), oedema, abscess, different types of *pīnasa* (chronic rhinitis), suppression of the power of digestion, pain and heaviness in abdomen, splenic disorders and adiposity.

सामुद्रं सैन्धवं काचं यवक्षारं सुवर्चलम् ।

टंकणं स्वर्जिकाक्षारं तुल्यं चूर्णं च कारयेत् ॥१३४॥

अर्कक्षीरैः स्नुहीक्षीरैरातपे भावयेत्त्र्यहम् ।

अर्कपत्रं लिपेत्तेन रुध्वा खाते पुटे पचेत् ॥१३५॥

ततः क्षारं चूर्णयेच्च त्र्यूषणं त्रिफलां तथा ।

---

1. सकृत् इति चतुर्थपुस्तके पाठः ।
2. हृच्छूलपाण्डवर्शसः इति षष्ठपुस्तके पाठः ।

जीरकं रजनी वह्नि नवकर्षसमं समम् ॥१३६॥
क्षारार्द्धमेतदर्द्धं च एकीकृत्य प्रयोजयेत् ।
वज्रक्षारमिदं ख्यातं स्वयं प्रोक्तं पिनाकिना ॥१३७॥
सर्वोदरेषु गुल्मेषु शूले शोफे च योजयेत् ।
अग्निमान्द्येष्वजीर्णेषु भक्षयेन्निष्ककद्वयम् ॥१३८॥

॥ इति वज्रक्षारः ॥

Vajra Kṣāra

Sāmudra lavaṇa, *saindhava lavaṇa*, *kāca lavaṇa*, *yava kṣāra*, *sauvarcala lavaṇa*, *ṭaṅkaṇa* and *svarjikā kṣāra*—all taken in equal quantities should be made to a powder. This should be impregnated and triturated by adding the milky latex of *arka* and *snūhī* while exposing to sun. Leaves of *arka* should be smeared with this paste, kept in a vessel, sealed and cooked by keeping in a pit. The *kṣāra* (alkali preparation), thus obtained, should be made to a powder. Separately, a powder should be made of *tryūṣaṇa*, *triphalā*, *jīraka*, *rajanī* and *vahni*—all taken in equal quantities. Then this powder and the alkali preparation made earlier should be mixed together in equal quantities. This is called *vajra kṣāra* and it was propounded by Lord Śiva himself. It is useful in all types of *udara rogas* (obstinate abdominal diseases including ascites), *gulma* (phantom tumour), colic pain, oedema, suppression of the power of digestion and indigestion. It should be administered in a dose of two *niṣkas*.

सुराह्वा प्राकृतक्षारो यवक्षारस्तथैव च ।
फटक्या नवसारेण क्षारं ज्येष्ठागरं पुनः ॥१३९॥
मर्दयेत्समभागानि कश्चिन्नीरं च दापयेत् ।
औषधाद्यधितो द्वारं नालं चैका विशेषयेत् ॥१४०॥

नालमुग्रस्य शंखस्य द्रवते तत्क्षणादपि ।
रसानां नाथकश्चैव शंखद्रावो महारसः ॥१४१॥
भक्षितेऽतिकृशे देहे पुष्टिर्नीरोगता भवेत् ।
आढ्यवाते हनुस्तम्भे मन्यास्तम्भे गलग्रहे ॥१४२॥
सर्वेषां वातरोगाणां निहन्ति गुल्मकस्य च ।
प्रमेहानि च सर्वाणि ग्रहणीदीपनं परम् ॥१४३॥

॥ इति शंखद्रावः ॥

Śaṅkha Drāva

Surā kṣāra (obtained from nature), *yava kṣāra*, *sphaṭikā kṣāra*, *navasāra* and *jyeṣṭhāgara*—all these taken in equal quantities should be triturated, and to this a small quantity of water should be added. To this, a piece of *śaṅkha* should be inserted which gets dissolved immediately. This is the best of recipes and is called *śaṅkha drāva*. If taken even by a person having an extremely emaciated body, he becomes nourished and free from diseases. It is useful in *āḍhya vāta*, *hanu stambha* (lock-jaw), *manyā stambha* (torticolis), obstruction in the throat, all types of *vāta rogas*, *gulma* (phantom tumour) and all types of *pramehas* (obstinate urinary disorders including diabetes). It stimulates the activities of *grahaṇī* (small intestine including duodenum).

स्फटिका च यवक्षारं सोरोऽथ[1] नवसादरः[2] ।

[भारतभैषज्यरत्नाकर : पंचमभाग : पृष्ठ ९९]

पर्पटी झर्झरोद्भूतं भूक्षारश्चाम्लवेतसः ॥१४४॥

---

1. शुरोऽथ इति आदर्शपुस्तिकासु पाठः।
2. नवसादरम् इति आकरे पाठः ।

एतानि समभागानि काचकुप्यान्तरे द्रवेत् ।
निश्चयं द्रवेत शंखं लोहं द्रवति तत्क्षणात् ॥१४५॥
पीतवर्णो महाजातो धातुद्रावी महारसः ।
कफकंठरोगशमनं दुर्नाम विनिवर्तनम् ॥१४६॥
कृमिरोगहरं चैव पञ्चगुल्मनिवारणम् ।
मन्दाग्निं नाशयेन्नूनं कंदर्पं वर्द्धते दृढम् ॥१४७॥
नातः परतरं लोके त्रिषुलोकेषु निश्चितम् ।
शंखद्रावेति विख्यातो रसस्त्रैलोक्यदुर्लभः ॥१४८॥

॥ इति शखद्रावः ॥

Śaṅkha Drāva (second recipe)

Sphaṭikā bhasma, yava kṣāra, sorā, nava sādara, bhū kṣāra (which is collected from the mountain crevices) and *amla vetasa*—all these drugs, taken in equal. quantities, should be kept in a glass bottle till it becomes a liquid. Conch shell and iron, if kept inside this liquid, will certainly get dissolved. It is yellow in colour, effective and is capable of dissolving metals. It alleviates diseases caused by *kapha*, diseases of the throat, piles, parasitic infestation, five varieties of *gulma* (phantom tumour) and suppression of the power of digestion. It promotes virility. No other drug can excel this recipe in therapeutic efficacy. This is called *śaṅkha drāva*. It is very rare in this universe.

अथान्यप्रकारः

त्रिक्षारं पटुपंचकं च गिरिजं लोणासुरोथा वरम् ।
फेनो ब्रह्मगरं समुद्रलवणं क्षारो ह्यपामार्गजम् ॥१४९॥

वज्रीक्षार तथैव मुष्ककपटुः पालाशमर्कोद्भवम् ।
सौराष्ट्री समभागमशितो गर्भाग्निना भावयेत् ॥१५०॥
तं कटुसर्षपांबुपृथुकैः संसिच्य रूक्ष क्षिपेत् ।
यन्त्रे तं नलिकाभिधे शुभदिने संस्वेदयेन्मद्यवत् ॥१५१॥
शंखद्रावरसायनं गदवतां वल्लैकमात्रं दहेत् ।
जिह्वाग्रे हविषा विलेप्य विबुधैः देयो न दन्तान्स्पृशेत् ॥१५२॥
शूलं तु घ्राणमात्रेण पञ्चगुल्मविनाशनम् ।
क्षणमात्रेण शंखं च लोहं द्रवति तत्क्षणात् ॥
कफकंठरोगशमनं दुष्टव्याधिविनाशनम् ॥१५३॥

॥ इति शंखद्राव रसः ॥

Śaṅkha Drāva (*third recipe*)

Three varieties of *kṣāras*, five varieties of *lavaṇas*, *girija lavaṇa*, *sorā*, *brahmagara phena*, *sāmudra lavaṇa*, *apāmārga kṣāra*, *vajrī kṣāra*, *muṣkaka kṣāra*, *palāśā kṣāra*, *arka kṣāra* and *saurāṣṭrī*—all these drugs taken in equal quantities, should be cooked by placing in a pit. The *kṣāra*, thus prepared should be sprinkled with pungent mustard oil and distilled [in a *vaka yantra*] like alcohol in an auspicious day. This elixir is called *śaṅkha drāva*, and should be administered to the patient in a dose of one *valla*. While administering, the tongue of the patient should be smeared with ghee and care should be taken so that the drug does not come in contact with teeth. Even the smell of this drug cures colic pain and it cures five varieties of *gulma* (phantom tumour). Conch shell and iron get dissolved in this liquid in a moment. It cures diseases caused by *kapha*, throat diseases and other obstinate types of ailments.

अन्यतमः

प्रत्येकं पञ्चलवणं वाणं तुत्थं च खर्परम् ।
कुडवार्द्धं स्फटिकं च स्यात्तदर्ध्वं नवसादरम् ॥१५४॥
कासीसं टंकणं सर्जो यवक्षारं पलार्द्धकम् ।
कुडवाः पञ्चभूसारं सर्वमेकत्र कारयेत् ॥१५५॥
भृष्ट्वा च खर्परे सम्यक् काचकुप्यां विनिःक्षिपेत् ।
तन्मुखे कूपिकां दत्वा स्थापयेच्चुलिलकोपरि ॥१५६॥
यमार्द्धं ज्वालयेदग्निं रसं द्रवति नान्यथा ।
शंखद्राव इति ख्यातः सर्वव्याधिविनाशनः ॥१५७॥
नाशाभिनायकश्चैव शंखद्रावाभिधो रसः ।
भक्षितः कुरुते देहे तुष्टि पुष्टिं निरोगताम् ॥१५८॥
सर्वेषां वातरोगाणां निहन्ता हि गुल्मस्य च ।
प्रमेहापि हरः सर्वे ग्रहणीहरणक्षमः ॥१५९॥
कालजं प्लीहजं जीर्णं सर्वधातुक्षयापहम् ।
अखिलान्वातरोगांश्च हन्ति चात्र न संशयः ॥
बुभुक्षाय सदा सेव्यो जठराग्निप्रदीपकः ॥१६०॥
अयःसहित पोषाय सेव्यः शंखद्रावो रसः ।
शंखं गालयते शीघ्रं लोहं द्रवति तत्क्षणात् ॥१६१॥
सूर्यं दहति मुंचेन्नो उदकं भवति निश्चितम् ।
कार्या सर्वात्तिकां लग्नं पिवेत्तालुकयोरपि ॥१६२॥

दन्ताः पतन्ति लग्नेन शेषरोगस्य का कथा ।
कांतिं ददाति संसेव्यः श्वासकासज्वरापहः ॥१६३॥
आमवातं च कुष्ठं च मूलरोगांश्च नाशयेत् ।
बलवान्कुरुते नित्यं बाजीकरणमेव च ॥१६४॥
स्त्रीणां च वल्लभो नित्यं याममेकेन द्रावयेत् ।
नराणामुपकाराय पूज्यपादेन निर्मितः ॥१६५॥'

Śaṅkha Drāva (*fourth recipe*)

One *kuḍava* (*vāṇa*) of each of five varieties of *lavaṇas*, half *kuḍava* of each of *tuttha* and *kharpara*, 1/4th *kuḍava* of *sphaṭika*, half *pala* of each of *nava sādara*, *kāsīsa*, *ṭaṅkaṇa*, *svarjī kṣāra* and *yava kṣāra* and one *kuḍava* of each of five varieties of *bhūsāra*—all these taken together should be roasted over an earthen pan and kept in a glass bottle [wrapped with mud smeared cloth]. To the mouth of this bottle a tube should be attached and the bottle should be placed over an oven. Fire should be employed for half an hour when the ingredients kept in the bottle turn to a liquid. Insufficient heat will not bring out this result. This is called *śaṅkha drāva* which cures all types of diseases. Intake of this recipe gives satisfaction, nourishment and freedom from diseases. It cures all *vāta rogas* (nervous ailments), *gulmas* (phantom tumour), *pramehas* (obstinate urinary disorders including diabetes), *grahaṇī* (sprue syndrome) and diminution of tissues of the body because of temporal factors, splenic disorders and aging. It undoubtedly cures all *vāta rogas*. Since it stimulates the power of digestion, it should invariably be given to a person for the promotion of appetite. For the purpose of nourishment, this *śaṅkha drāva* should be taken along with *lauha bhasma*. It immediately dissolves conch shell and iron. If it is exposed to strong sun rays, it certainly gets liquified. It should be taken with the help of a pipe by which only palates come in contact with this medicine. Teeth fall down if they come in contact with this drug, what to speak of the cure of other diseases. It promotes complexion and cures asthma, cough, fever, *āma vāta* (rheumatism), *kuṣṭha* (obstinate skin diseases including leprosy) and ***mūla rogas*** (anal diseases). It daily promotes strength. It is aphrodisiac. It makes the man lovable by ladies who get exhausted in three hours. For the welfare of human beings, this recipe is propounded by ***Pūjya pāda***.

इति श्रीमहाराजाधिराजटोडरमल्लविरचिते टोडरानन्दे आयुर्वेद-सौख्ये शूलनिदानचिकित्साकथनं नाम षष्ठत्रिंशत्तमो हर्षः ॥१६६॥

Thus, ends the 36th Chapter dealing with the diagnosis and treatment of colic pain of *Āyurveda saukhya* in *Ṭoḍarānanda* composed by the great king Ṭoḍara Malla.

CHAPTER II

अथपरिणाम-अन्नद्रवशूलनिदानं चिकित्सा च ।

(*Diagnosis and Treatment of Pariṇāma and Annadrava types of colic pain*)

"स्वैर्निदानैः[1] प्रकुपितो वायुः सन्निचितस्तदा[2] ।
कफपित्ते समावृत्य शूलकारी भवेद्बली ॥
भुक्ते जीर्यति यच्छूलं तदेव परिणामजम् ॥१॥"

[माधवनिदान : शूलनिदान २६ : १५-१६]

---

1. This is the beginning of 41st Chapter of *Āyurveda saukhya* in *Toḍarānanda* and the invocation reads as follows:

   कात्पयिना भक्ति कृशी कृतानां कृष्णाशयानां व्रजकन्यकानां ।
   जहारवासांसि हिमे सहन्याहृतावरीन् श्री नृपटोडरस्य ॥

2. संनिहितस्तदा इति आकरे पाठः ।

Pathogenesis

Vāyu, being extremely aggravated by the causative factors, gets localized and having afflicted the *kapha* and *pitta*, produces colic pain at the time of digestion of food which is called *pariṇāmaja śūla*.

'बलासः प्रच्युतः स्थानात्पित्तेन सह मूर्च्छितः ।
वायुमादाय कुपितः शूलं जीर्यति भोजने ॥२॥
बस्तौ नाभ्यां च जठरे पार्श्वपृष्ठस्तनान्तरे[1] ।
कट्यां[2] वा पृष्ठवंशे वा सर्वेष्वेतेषु वा पुनः ॥३॥
भुक्तमात्रे तथा चान्ने जीर्णे वाऽन्ने प्रशाम्यति ।
षष्टिकव्रीहिशालीनामोदनेन विवर्धते ।
पक्तिजं शूलमित्याहुः स विज्ञेयो महागदः ॥४॥'

[माधवनिदानः शूलनिदान : २६ : १६ मधुकोश टीका]

The displaced *kapha* gets afflicted by *pitta* and the aggravated *kapha* along with *vāyu* causes colic pain in the region of urinary bladder umbilicus, abdomen, sides of the chest, back, space between two breasts, lumber region or vertibral column or in all these places simultaneously at the time of the digestion of the food. This colic pain gets subsided by taking food or after the digestion of food. It gets aggravated by the intake of food ingredients like *ṣaṣṭika*, *brīhi* and *śālī*. This serious type of ailment is also known as *paktija śūla*.

---

1. पार्श्वपृष्ठतलान्तरे इति प्रथमपंचमपुस्तकयोः पाठः ।
2. कुक्षौ इति द्वितीयपुस्तके पाठः ।

"तस्य[1] लक्षणमप्येतत्समासेनभिधीयते ॥५॥

Signs and Symptoms

Signs and symptoms of different varieties of *paktija śūla* are described below in brief.

आटोपाध्मानविण्मूत्रविबन्धारतिवेपनैः ।
स्निग्धोपशमनं[2] प्रायं वातिकं तद्वदेद्भिषक् ॥६॥'

Vātika type

Vātika type of *pakti śūla* is characterised by *āṭopa* (gurgling sound in the abdomen), *ānāha* (abdominal distension), constipation, anuria, disliking for every thing and trembling. It generally gets alleviated by unctuous therapy.

तृष्णादाहारतिस्वेदं कट्वम्ललवणोत्तरम् ।
शूलं शीतशमं प्रायं पैत्तिकं लक्षयेद्बुधः ॥७॥

Paittika type

Paittika type of *pakti śūla* is characterised by thirst, burning sensation, disliking for every thing and sweating. It gets aggravated by pungent, sour and saline things, and alleviated by cold things.

छर्दिहृल्लासमम्मोहस्वल्परुक् दीर्घसन्ततिः ।
कटुतिक्तोपशान्तौ[3] च तच्च ज्ञेयं कफात्मकम् ॥८॥

---

1. 'तस्य............तद्वदेद्भिषक्' पाठोऽयं पंचमपुस्तके नोपलभ्यते ।
2. स्निग्धोष्णोपशमप्रायं इति आकरे पाठः ।
3. कटुतिक्तोपशान्तं इति आकरे पाठः ।

Kaphaja type

Kaphaja type of *pakti śūla* is characterised by vomiting, nausea, unconsciousness, mild pain and continuous pain for a long time. It gets alleviated by pungent and bitter things.

संसृष्टं लक्षणं ज्ञात्वा[1] द्विदोषं परिकल्पयेत्[2] ।
त्रिदोषजमसाध्यं तु[3] क्षीणमांसबलानलम् ॥९॥"

[माधवनिदान : शूलनिदान २६ : १७-२१]

एतद्द्विल्वणभेदेन[4] त्रयोदशविधस्तु[5] सः ॥१०॥

Dvandvaja and Sānnipātika types

In *dvandvaja* type of *pakti śūla*, signs and symptoms of the concerned two *doṣas* are simultaneously manifested. Similarly, in *sānnipātika* type, signs and symptoms of all the three *doṣas* are simultaneously manifested. *Sānnipātika* type is incurable if the patient is reduced of his muscle tissue, strength and power of digestion. This *sānnipātika* type of *pakti śūla* is again of 13 types depending upon the predominance of two *doṣas* (*dvilvaṇa*), etc.

"जीर्णे जीर्यत्यजीर्णे वा यच्छूलमुपजायते ।
पथ्यापथ्यप्रयोगेण भोजनाभोजनेन वा ॥

---

1. बुध्वा इति आकरे पाठः ।
2. परिलक्षयेत् इति षष्ठपुस्तके पाठः ।
3. स्यात् इति पंचमपुस्तके पाठः ।
4. एतदुल्वण० इति षष्ठपुस्तके पाठः ।
5. त्रयोदशविधं ततः इति षष्ठपुस्तके पाठः ।

"न[1] शमं याति नियमात्सोऽन्नद्रव उदाहृतः ॥११॥"

[माधवनिदान : शूलनिदान २६ : २१-२२]

Annadrava Śūla

The colic pain which is manifested irrespective of the digestive process i.e. after digestion, during digestion and before digestion, irrespective of the wholesome or unwholesome food and irrespective of taking or not taking any food and which does not get alleviated by any of these factors is called *anna drava śūla.*

स कष्टोऽन्नद्रवः केचिज्जरत्पित्ते च तद्विदुः ॥१२॥

Annadrava śūla is a serious ailment. According to some physicians, this condition is caused by excessive metabolic transformation (*jaraṇa*=cooking) of the *pitta.*

"वेदना च तृषा मूर्छा आनाहो[2] गौरवारुचिः ।
कासः श्वासो वमी हिक्का शूलस्योपद्रवाः[3] दश ॥१३॥"

[माधवनिदान : शूल २६ : १४ (मधुकोश टीका)]

Complications

Ten complications of colic pain are pain, thirst, fainting, abdominal distension, heaviness, anorexia, cough, asthma, vomiting and hiccup.

॥ इति परिणामशूल [अन्नद्रवशूल] निदानम् ॥१४॥

---

1. "न⋯⋯⋯उदाहृतः" पाठोऽयं पंचमपुस्तके नोपलभ्यते ।
2. ह्यानाहो इति आकरे पाठः ।
3. शूलस्योपद्र वाः स्मृताः इति आकरे पाठः ।

Thus, ends the description of the diagnosis of *pariṇāma* and *annadrava* types of colic pain.

"वमनं तिक्तमधुरैर्विरेकश्चात्र शस्यते ।
बस्तयश्च हिताः शूले परिणामसमुद्भवे ॥१५॥"

[भैषज्यरत्नावली : शूलरोगाधिकार : ५६]

Line of Treatment

Administration of emetic, purgation and enema therapies with the help of bitter and sweet drugs are useful in the treatment of *pariṇāma* type of colic pain.

"विडंगतंडुलं व्योषं त्रिवृद्दन्ती सचित्रकम् ।
सर्वाणि[1] तानि संहृत्य श्लक्ष्णचूर्णानि कारयेत् ।
[2]'गुडेन मोदकान् कृत्वा भक्षयेत्प्रातरुत्थितः ।
उष्णोदकानुपानश्च दद्यादग्निं विवर्द्धनं ॥'
जयेत्त्रिदोषजं शूलं परिणामसमुद्भवम् ॥१६॥"

॥ इति विडङ्गाद्यो मोदकः ॥

[योगरत्नाकर : शूलचिकित्सा : पृष्ठ १५]

[भैषज्यरत्नावली : शूलरोगाधिकार : १०२-१०३]

Viḍaṅgādya Modaka

Seeds of *viḍaṅga*, *trikaṭu*, *trivṛt*, *dantī*, *citraka*—all these drugs should be made to a powder and by cooking in jaggery syrup, *modakas* (large pills) should be prepared. In the morning,

---

1. सर्वाण्येतानि इति आकरे पाठः ।
2. "गुडेन·········विवर्द्धनं" पाठोऽयं द्वितीयपुस्तके नोपलभ्यते ।

after getting up from the bed one such *modaka* should be taken along with hot water. It promotes the power of digestion and cures *pariṇāma śūla* caused by the simultaneous vitiation of all the three *doṣas*.

"नागरतिलगुडकल्कं पयसा संसाध्य यः पुमानद्यात् ।
उग्रं परिणितिशूलं तस्योपैति[1] सप्तरात्रेण ॥१७॥

The patient who takes the paste of *nāgara*, *tila* and *guḍa* by boiling with milk, he becomes free from serious type of *pariṇāma śūla* within seven nights.

शंबूकजं भस्मपीतं जलेनोष्णेन तत्क्षणात् ।
पक्तिजं विनिहन्त्येव[2] शूलं विष्णुरिवासुरान् ॥१८॥"

[भैषज्यरत्नावली : शूलरोगाधिकार : ६०-६१]

Intake of the *bhasma* of *sambūka* along with hot water instantaneously cures *paktija* type of colic pain as demons were destroyed by Lord *Viṣṇu*.

अक्षधात्र्यभयाकृष्णाचूर्णं मधुयुतं लिहन् ।
[3]"दध्यन्नभुङ्तरो खादन्सतीनयवकोद्रवान् ॥
अचिरान्मुच्यते शूलान्नरोऽनुपरिणामजान् ॥१९॥

The powder of *akṣa*, *dhātrī*, *abhayā* and *kṛṣṇā* should be made to a linctus by adding honey. The patient should use this linctus, and as food, he should take rice mixed with curd,

---

1. सप्ताहाज्जयति चावश्यम् इति योगरत्नाकरे पाठः ।
2. विनिहन्त्येतत् शूलं इति आकरे प्रथमपंचमपुस्तकयोः च पाठः ।
3. क. दध्नालूनसरेणाद्यात् सतिलशक्तुकान् इति प्रथमपुस्तके पाठः ।
   ख. दध्नान्यूनसरेणाद्यात् सतीनयवशक्तुकान् इति आकरे पाठः ।

satīna, *yava* and *kodrava*. This makes him instantaneously free from *pariṇāmaja* type of colic pain.

तिलनागरपथ्यानां भागं शंबुकभस्मनः[1] ।
द्विभागगुडसंयुक्तां गुटीं[2] कृत्वाऽक्षभागिकाम् ॥२०॥
शीताम्बुपानं पूर्वाह्णे भक्ष येत्क्षीरभोजनम् ।
सायाह्ने[3] रसकं पीत्वा नरो मुच्येत दुर्जयात्[4] ॥
परिणामसमुत्थाच्च शूलाच्चिरभवादपि ॥२१॥

[तिलादिगुडिका]

Tilādi Guṭikā

Tila, *nāgara*, *pathyā* and *bhasma* of *śambūka* should be added with double the quantity of jaggery and pills of one *akṣa* each should be prepared. One such pill should be taken along with cold water. The patient should take milk and milk preparations as food in the morning, and meat soup in the afternoon. This makes him free from serious type of *pariṇāma śūla* even if it is of chronic onset.

शंबूकं त्र्यूषणं चैव पञ्चैव लवणानि च ।
समांशं गुटिकां कृत्वा कलंबुकरसेन वा ॥२२॥
प्रातर्भोजनकाले वा भक्षयेत्तु यथाबलम् ।
शूलाद्विमुच्यते जन्तुः सहसा परिणामजात् ॥२३॥"

[शम्बूकादि गुटिका]

[भैषज्यरत्नावली : शूलरोगाधिकार : ६२-६६]

1. शम्बूकभस्मनाम् इति आकरे पाठः ।
2. गुडीं शार्णकसम्मिताम् इति आकरे पाठः ।
3. सायाह्ने इति आकरे पाठः ।
4. दुर्जयात् इति आकरे पाठः ।

Śambūkādi Guṭikā

Bhasma of *śambūka, tryūṣaṇa,* five varieties of *lavaṇa*—all these should be taken in equal quantities and made to a powder. This should be impregnated by the juice of *kalambu* and triturated. From this paste, pills should be prepared. Depending upon the strength of the patient, this recipe should be used in appropriate dose by which he instantaneously becomes free from *pariṇāma* type of colic pain.

"यः पिबति सप्तरात्रं सक्तूनेतान्[1]कलाययूषेण ।
[2]जयति परिणामरुजं चिरजमपि किमुत नूतनजाम् ॥२४॥"

[भैषज्यरत्नावली : शूलरोगाधिकार : ७३]

The patient, who takes *saktū* (roasted corn flour) along with the soup of *kalāya*, for seven nights, becomes free from even chronic *pariṇāma śūla* what to speak of freshly occurring one.

वचालोहयोगः

"लोहचूर्णं [3]वचायुक्तं विलीढं मधुसर्पिषा ।
शमयेत्परिणामशूलं [4]तन्मलं वा प्रयोजितम् ॥२५॥"

[भैषज्यरत्नावली : शूलरोगाधिकार : ७४]

Vacā Loha Yoga

Powder or *bhasma* of *loha* and *vacā* should be mixed with honey and ghee. Intake of this alleviates *pariṇāma śūla.* In the place of *lauha* (iron), *maṇḍūra* (rust of iron) can also be used.

---

1. सक्तूनेकान्कलाय इति प्रथमपुस्तके पाठः ।
2. स जयति इति प्रथमपुस्तके पाठः ।
3. वरायुक्तं इति पंचमपुस्तके पाठः ।
4. तन्मयं इति द्वितीयपुस्तके पाठः ।

कृष्णाद्यलोहम्

"कृष्णाभयालोहचूर्णं गुडेन सह भक्षयेत् ।
पक्तिशूलं निहन्त्येतज्जाठरानग्निमान्द्यताम् ॥
आमवातविकारांश्च स्थौल्यं चैवापकर्षति ॥२६॥

Kṛṣṇādya Loha

Kṛṣṇā, *abhayā* and *lauha bhasma* should be taken along with jaggery. It cures *pakti śūla*, *jaṭhara* (obstinate abdominal diseases including ascites), suppression of the power of digestion, *āma vāta* (rheumatism) and obesity.

[1]पथ्यालोहरजः शुंठीचूर्णं माक्षिकसर्पिषा ।
परिणामरुजं हन्ति वातपित्तकफात्मकम्[2] ॥२७॥"

[भैषज्यरत्नावली : शूलरोगाधिकार : ७५-७६]

Intake of the powder of *pathyā*, *bhasma* of *lauha* and the powder of *śuṇṭhī* along with honey and ghee cures *pariṇāma śūla* caused by *vāyu*, *pitta* and *kapha*.

"सामुद्रं सैन्धवं क्षारो रुचकं रोमकं विडम् ।
दन्तीलोहरजः किट्टं त्रिवृच्छूरणकं समम् ॥२८॥
दधिगोमूत्रपयसा मन्दपावकपाचितम् ।
तद्यथाग्निबलं चूर्णं पिबेदुष्णेन वारिणा ॥२९॥
जीर्णेऽजीर्णे तु भुञ्जीत मांसादि घृतसाधितम् ।
नाभिशूलं प्लीहशूलं यकृद्गुल्मकृतं च यत् ॥३०॥

---

1. "पथ्यालोहरजः..............कफात्मकम्" पाठोऽयंषष्ठपुस्तके नोपलभ्यते ।
2. कफात्मिकम् इति प्रथमपुस्तके पाठः ।

विद्रध्यष्ठीलकं[1] हन्ति कफवातोद्भवं तथा ।
शूलानामपि सर्वेषामौषधं नास्ति तत्परम् ॥
परिणामसमुत्थस्य विशेषेणान्तकृन्मतम् ॥३१॥

॥ इति सामुद्राद्यं चूर्णम् ॥

Sāmudrādya Cūrṇa

Sāmudra lavaṇa, saindhava lavaṇa, kṣāra (alkali preparation), *rucaka, romaka, viḍa, dantī, lauha bhasma, maṇḍūra bhasma, trivṛt* and *sūraṇa*—all these drugs taken in equal quantities should be cooked over mild fire by adding curd, cow's urine and cow's milk. Depending upon the power of digestion, this powder should be taken in a suitable dose by the patient along with hot water. Whether there is proper or improper digestion, the patient should take meat, etc. cooked by adding ghee. This cures colic pain in umbilical region, splenic region and hepatic region, *gulma* (phantom tumour), abscess, hard tumour caused by *kapha* and *vāyu*, and all types of colic pain. There is no medicine better than this for the cure of colic pain. It is specially useful in curing *pariṇāma* type of colic pain.

नारिकेलं सतोयं च लवणेन प्रपूरितम् ।
'विपक्वमग्निना सम्यक् परिणामजशूलनुत्'[2] ॥
वातिकं पैत्तिकं चैव श्लैष्मिकं सान्निपातिकम् ॥३२॥

[नारिकेललवणम्]

---

1. विद्रध्यष्ठीलिकां इति आकरे पाठः ।
2. क. पिप्पल्या भक्षितं हन्ति शूलं विविधहेतुजम् । पाठोऽयं आकरे अधिकमुपलभ्यते ।
   ख. 'विपक्वाग्निन .... शूलनुत्' पाठोऽयं प्रथमपुस्तके नोपलभ्यते ।

Nārikela Lavaṇa

Coconut along with its water should be filled with rock salt and cooked on fire. After it is well cooked, a powder should be made out of the pulp. This cures *paniṇāmaja* type of colic pain and colic pain caused by *vāyu, pitta, kapha* and all the three *doṣas* vitiated simultaneously (*sānnipātika*).

मधुकं त्रिफलाचूर्णमयोरजः समं लिहन् ।
मधुसर्पिर्युतं सम्यक् गव्यं क्षीरं पिवेदनु ॥३३॥
छर्दिं सतिमिरं शूलमम्लपित्तं ज्वरं क्लमम् ।
अनाहं मूत्रकृच्छ्रं[1] च शोथं चैव निहन्ति सः[2] ॥३४॥"

[भैषज्यरत्नावली : शूलरोगाधिकार : ७७-८४]

Madhuka, triphalā and *bhasma* of *lauha*—all these drugs taken in equal quantities should be made to a powder. It should be taken along with ghee and honey, and thereafter, the patient should take cow's milk. It cures vomiting, *timira* (cataract), colic pain, *amla pitta*, fever, *klama* (mental fatigue), abdominal distension, dysuria and oedema.

पलानि त्रीणि शम्बूकाल्लोहचूर्णं पलद्वयम् ।
रसाञ्जनात्पलं चैकं लोहसिंघाणकात्पलम् ॥३५॥
सर्वैः समा शर्करा व मधुना च परिप्लुतम् ।
सर्वमेतत्समाहृत्य मोदकान् कारयेद्भिषक् ॥३६॥
भक्षयेच्च प्रयत्नेन शूले गुल्मे गुदामये ।
विशेषतः पक्तिशूले शोथपाण्डूदरे भ्रमे ॥३७॥

1. मूत्रसङ्गं इति आकरे प्रथमपुस्तके च पाठः ।
2. तत् इति आकरे पाठः ।

दुर्नाम्नि कासे कृच्छ्रे च प्रमेहाश्मरि वृद्धिषु ।
अग्निमान्द्ये स्मृतिभ्रंशे पीनसेऽर्द्धावभेदके ॥३८॥

॥ इति शम्बूकाद्याः मोदकाः ॥

Śambūkādya Modaka

Bhasma of *śambuka* (three *palas*), *lauha bhasma* (two *palas*), *rasāñjana* (one *pala*), *maṇḍūra bhasma* (one *pala*) and sugar (seven *palas*) should be mixed together and added with honey in adequate quantity. From out of this, *modakas* (large size pills) should be prepared. Appropriate intake of this cures colic pain, *gulma* (phantom tumour) and piles. It is specially useful in *paktija* type of colic pain, oedema, anemia, *udara* (obstinate abdominal diseases including ascites), giddiness, piles, cough, dysuria, *prameha* (obstinate urinary disorders including diabetes), stone in the urinary tract, *vṛddhi* (enlarged scrotum including hernia), suppression of the power of digestion, loss of memory, *pīnasa* (chronic rhinitis) and hemicrania.

"सपिप्पलीगुडं सर्पिः पचेत्[1]क्षीरं चतुर्गुणम् ।
विनिहन्त्यम्लपित्तं च शूलं च परिणामजम् ॥३९॥"

॥ इति गुडपिप्पलीघृतम् ॥

[भैषज्यरत्नावली : शूलरोगाधिकार : ८५]

Guḍa Pippalī Ghṛta

Ghee should be boiled by adding *pippalī*, jaggery and four times of milk. This medicated ghee cures *amla pitta* (excessive acidity in the stomach) and *pariṇāmaja* type of colic pain.

---

1. पिबेत् क्षीरं चतुर्गुण इति प्रथमपुस्तके पाठः ।

"क्वाथेन कल्केन च पिप्पलीनां सिद्धं घृतं माक्षिकसम्प्रयुक्तम् ।
क्षीरानुपानस्य निहन्त्यवश्यं शूलं प्रवृद्धं परिणामसंज्ञम् ॥४०॥"

॥ इति पिप्पलीघृतम् ॥

[भैषज्यरत्नावली : शूलरोगाधिकार : ८६]

Pippalī Ghṛta

Ghee cooked with the decoction as well as paste of *pippalī* and taken by adding honey followed by milk certainly cures acute form of *pariṇāmaja śūla.*

कोलग्रंथिकशृंगवेरचपलाक्षारैः समं चूर्णितम् ।
मण्डूरं सुरभीजलेऽष्टगुणिते पक्त्वा[1] च सान्द्रीकृतम् ॥४१॥
[2]तत्खादेदशनादिमध्यविरतौ प्रायेण दुग्धान्नभुक् ।
जेतुं वातकफामया[3] परिणतौ शूलं च शूलानि च ॥४२॥

॥ इति कोलादिमाण्डूरम् ॥

[भैषज्यरत्नावली : शूलरोगाधिकार : १०६]

Kolādi Maṇḍūra

The powder of *maṇḍūra* should be boiled by adding eight times of cow's urine and the powder of *kola, granthika, śṛṅga-vera, capalā* and *kṣāra* (each taken equal to that of *maṇḍūra*) till it becomes semi solid. This should be taken before, during and after food and the patient should take only milk and rice as food. It cures diseases caused by *vāyu* and *kapha, pariṇāma* and all other types of colic pain.

---

1. पक्त्वाथ इति आकरे पाठः ।
2. तं खादेद० इति प्रथमपुस्तके पाठः ।
3. क. वातकफामयान् इति आकरे प्रथमपुस्तके च पाठः ।
   ख. वातकफामया परिणतं इति षष्ठपुस्तके पाठः ।

"कोलग्रंथिकसहितैर्विश्वौषधमागधीयवक्षारैः ।
प्रस्थमयोमलरजसः[1] पलिकांशैश्चूर्णितैर्मिश्रैः ॥४३॥
अष्टगुणमूत्रयुक्ते[2] क्रमपाकात्पिण्डतां नयेत् ।
सर्वं[3] कोलप्रमाणवटिकास्तिस्रो भोज्यादिमध्यविरतौ च ॥४४॥
रससर्पिर्यूषपयोमांसैरश्नन्नरो निवारयति ।
अन्नविवर्त्तनशूलं गुल्मप्लीहाग्निमान्द्यानि[4] ॥४५॥"

॥ इति भीममण्डूरम्[5] ॥

[भैषज्यरत्नावली : शूलरोगाधिकार : १२१-१२३]

Bhīma Maṇḍūra

One *prastha* of *maṇḍūra* should be boiled in eight times of cow's urine by adding one *pala* of each of the powder of *kola*, *granthika*, *viśvauṣadha*, *māgadhī* and *yava kṣāra*. The boiling should be first of all over mild fire, then over moderate fire and at the end over strong fire till the ingredients become semi solid. From out of this, pills of the size of *ber* fruit should be prepared. One such pill should be taken in the beginning, one in the middle and one at the end of the food. The patient should eat meat soup, ghee and vegetable soup. This recipe cures *anna vivartana* (*annadrava*) type of colic pain, *gulma* (phantom tumour), splenic disorders and suppressed power of digestion.

---

1. प्रस्थमयोरजसां इति आकरे पाठः ।
2. अष्टगुणमूत्रयुक्तं इति आकरे प्रथमपुस्तके च पाठः ।
3. माषप्रमाणवटिकास्तिस्रो इति आकरे पाठः ।
4. ०सादांश्च इति आकरे पाठः ।
5. भीमवटक मण्डूरम् इति आकरे पाठः ।

"लोहकिट्टपलान्यष्टौ गोमूत्रार्द्धाढके पचेत् ।
क्षीरप्रस्थेन तत् सिद्धं पक्तिशूलहर नृणां ॥४६॥
॥ क्षीरमण्डूरम् ॥"

[भैषज्यरत्नावली : शूलरोगाधिकार : १०७]

Kṣīra Maṇḍūra

Eight *palas* of *maṇḍūra* should be boiled with half *āḍhaka* of cow's urine and one *prastha* of milk. This cures *pakti śūla*

"लोहकिट्टपलान्यष्टौ गोमूत्रेऽष्टगुणे पचेत् ।
चविकानागरक्षारपिप्पलीमूलपिप्पली ॥४७॥
संचूर्ण्य निःक्षिपेत्तस्मिन् पलांशान्[1] सान्द्रतां गते ।
गुटिका कल्पयेत्तेन पक्तिशूलनिवारणी ॥४८॥
॥ चविका[2]मण्डूरम् ॥"

[भैषज्यरत्नावली : शूलरोगाधिकार : १२४-१२५]

Cavikā Maṇḍūra

Eight *palas* of *maṇḍūra* should be boiled with eight times of cow's urine. One *pala* of each of the powder of *cavikā*, *nāgara*, *kṣāra*, *pippalī mūla* and *pippalī* should be added to it. When it becomes semi solid, pills should be made out which, when administered cures *pakti śūla*.

"गुडामलक[3]शुण्ठीनां चूर्णं प्रत्येकशः पलम् ।
त्रिपलं लोहकिट्टस्य तत्सर्वं मधुसर्पिषा ॥४६॥

---

1. पलांशाः इति आकरे पाठः ।
2. मण्डूरवटिका इति आकर पाठः ।
3. गुडामलकपथ्यानां इति प्रथमपुस्तके आकरे च पाठः ।

समालोड्य ततः[1] खादेदक्षमात्रं प्रमाणतः ।
आदिमध्यावसानेषु भोजनस्य निहन्ति ताम् ॥५०॥
अन्नद्रवं[2] जरत्पित्तमम्लपित्तं सुदारुणम् ।
परिणामसमुत्थं च शूलं संवत्सरोत्थितम् ॥५१॥"

॥ इति गुडाद्यं[3] मण्डूरम् ॥

[भैषज्यरत्नावली : शूलरोगाधिकार : १३४-१३६]

Guḍādya Maṇḍūra

One *pala* of each of the powder of *guḍa*, *āmalaka* and *śuṇṭhī* and three *palas* of *maṇḍūra* should be mixed together by adding honey and ghee. It should be administered in a dose of one *akṣa* in the beginning, during and after food. It cures *anna-drava* type of *śūla*, *jarat pitta* (*pariṇāma śūla*) and *amla pitta*. It even cures *pariṇāma śūla* which is one year old.

मण्डूरं साधितं धात्रीं[4] लोहजां वा गुडेन तु ।
भक्षयन्मुच्यते शूलात्परिणामसमुद्भवात् ॥५२॥

Maṇḍūra cooked with *dhāṭrī* or with jaggery, when taken, cures *pariṇāma* type of colic pain.

"संशोध्य चूर्णितं कृत्वा मण्डूरस्य पलाष्टकम् ।
शतावरीरसस्याष्टौ दध्नस्तु[5] पयसस्तथा ॥५३॥

---

1. समश्नीयाच्चतुर्गुञ्जाप्रमाणतः इति आकरे पाठः ।
2. अन्नद्रवजरत्पित्तमस्त्रपित्तं इति आकरे पाठः ।
3. गुडमण्डूरम् इति आकरे पाठः ।
4. यत्ना इति षष्ठपुस्तके पाठः ।
5. दध्नश्च इति आकरे पाठः ।

पलान्यादाय चत्वारि तथा गव्यस्य सर्पिषः ।

विपचेत्सर्वमेकस्थं[1] यावत्पिण्डत्वमागतम् ॥५४॥

सिद्धं तु भक्षयेन्मध्ये भोजनस्याग्रतोऽपि वा ।

वातात्मकं पित्तभवं शूलं च परिणामजम् ॥

निहन्त्येव हि योगोऽयं मण्डूरस्य न संशयः[2] ॥५५॥"

॥ इति शतावरी मण्डूरम् ॥

[भैषज्यरत्नावली : शूलरोगाधिकार : ११४-११६]

Śatāvarī Maṇḍūra

Eight *palas* of purified *maṇḍūra* powder should be added with juice of *śatāvarī* (eight *palas*), curd (four *palas*), milk (four *palas*) and cow's ghee (four *palas*) and cooked till the ingredients become semi-solid. This should be taken before or during food. It undoubtedly cures *vātika* and *paittika* types of colic pain and *pariṇāmaja* type of colic pain.

"विडङ्गं चित्रकं चव्यं त्रिफलात्र्यूषणानि च ।

नवभागानि चैतानि लोहकिट्टसमानि च ॥५६॥

गोमूत्रं द्विगुणं दत्त्वा मूत्रार्द्धकगुडान्वितम् ।

शनैर्मृद्वग्निना पक्त्वा सुसिद्धं पिण्डतां गतम् ॥५७॥

स्निग्धे भाण्डे विनिःक्षिप्य भक्षयेत्कोलमात्रया[3] ।

प्राङ्[4]मध्यान्ते क्रमेणैव भोजनस्य प्रयोजितः ॥५८॥

---

1. सर्वमेकत्र इति आकरे पाठः ।
2. "रसोगंडः शुभपाके वर्त्ति स्यादति मर्द्दनात्" पाठोऽयं षष्ठपुस्तके अधिकमुपलभ्यते ।
3. माषकोन्मितमात्रया इति आकरे पाठः ।
4. मध्यान्तक्रमेणैव इति आकरे पाठः ।

योगोऽयं शमयत्याशु पक्तिशूलं सुदारणम्[1] ।
कामलां पाण्डुरोगं च शोथं मन्दाग्नितामपि ॥५९॥
अर्शांसि ग्रहणीरोगं कृमिगुल्मोदराणि च ।
नाशयेदम्लपित्तं च स्थौल्यं[2] चैवापकर्षति ॥६०॥
वर्जयेच्छुष्कशाकानि गुरू[3]ष्णानि कटूनि च ।
पक्तिशूलान्तको ह्येष गुडो मण्डूरसंज्ञितः ॥
शूलार्तानां क्रिया[4]हेतोस्तारया परिकीर्तितः ॥६१॥

॥ तारामण्डूरगुडः ॥"

[भैषज्यरत्नावली : शूलरोगाधिकार : १०८-११३]

Tārā Maṇḍūra Guḍa

One part of each of *viḍaṅga*, *citraka*, *cavya*, *triphalā* and *tryūṣaṇa*, nine parts of *maṇḍūra*, 18 parts of cow's urine and nine parts of jaggery—all these should be boiled together till the ingredients become semi-solid. This should be kept in a vessel smeared with ghee. It should be administered in the dose of one *kola* before, during and after food. This cures serious type of *pakti śūla*, *kāmalā* (jaundice), anemia, oedema, suppressed power of digestion, piles, *grahaṇī* (sprue syndrome), parasitic infestation, *gulma* (phantom tumour), *udara* (obstinate abdominal diseases including ascites), *amla pitta* (hyperacidity) and obesity. The patient should avoid dried vegetables, heavy, hot and pungent things. This is specifically an effective

---

1. सुदारुणम् इति आकरे पाठः ।
2. स्थौल्यञ्चापि नियच्छति इति आकरे पाठः ।
3. विदह्यम्लकटूनि च इति आकरे पाठः ।
4. कृपाहेतो० इति आकरे पाठः ।

cure for *pakti śūla*. For the benefit of patients suffering from colic pain, the goddess Tārā has propounded this recipe.

वसिरं श्वेतवाट्यालं मधुपर्णी मयूरकम् ।
तण्डुलीयं च वर्षाह्वं दत्त्वाधश्चोर्ध्वमेव च ॥६२॥
पाच्यं सुजीर्णमण्डूरं गोमूत्रेण दिनद्वयम् ।
अन्तर्बाष्पमदग्धं च तथा स्थाप्यं दिनत्रयम् ॥६३॥
विचूर्ण्य द्विगुणेनैव गुडेन च सुमर्दितम् ।
भोजनस्यादिमध्यान्ते भक्ष्यं कर्षत्रिभागतः ॥६४॥
तक्रानुपानं योज्यं च वर्ज्यमम्लकमत्र तु ।
अम्लपित्ते च शूले च हितमेतद्यथाऽमृतम् ॥६५॥

॥ राममण्डूरम् ॥

Rāma Maṇḍūra

Very old *maṇḍūra* should be kept in the centre of a pot. The space above and below it should be filled with *vasira*, *śveta vāṭyālaka*, *madhu parṇī*, *mayūraka*, *taṇḍulīyaka* and *varṣāhva*. To this, cow's urine should be added and the pot should be sealed to avoid contact with air. This should then be cooked for two days. If the ingredients are not properly cooked, then the process should be continued for one day more. Thereafter, ingredients should be triturated to reduce to a powder form. This should be administered in the dose of one *karṣa* before, during and after food with butter-milk. Other sour ingredients of food should be avoided. It works like ambrosia in the treatment of *amla pitta* (hyper-acidity of stomach) and colic pain.

"कुडवं पथ्याचूर्णं द्विपलं गन्धाश्मलोहकिट्टं च ।
शुद्धरसस्यार्द्धपलं रसं[1] केशराजस्य ॥६६॥
प्रस्थोन्मितं च दत्त्वा पात्रे लौहे च दण्डं संघृष्टम् ।
शुष्कं घृतमधुसंयुक्तं मृदितं स्थाप्यं च भाजने स्निग्धे ॥६७॥
उपयुक्तमेतदचिरान्निहन्ति कफपित्तजान्रोगान् ।
शूलं तथाम्लपित्तं ग्रहणीं सकामलामुग्राम्[2] ॥६८॥
॥ इति रसमण्डूरम् ॥"

[भैषज्यरत्नावली : शूलरोगाधिकार : १३९-१४१]

Rasa Maṇḍūra

Powder of *pathyā* (one *kuḍava*), *gandhaka* (two *palas*), *maṇḍūra* (two *palas*) and purified *pārada* (half *pala*) should be kept in an iron vessel to which one *prastha* of the juice of *keśarāja* should be added and triturated with the help of a rod till the ingredients become dry. Thereafter, honey and ghee should be mixed and the preparation should be stored in a ghee smeared container. Intake of this cures diseases caused by *kapha* and *pitta*, colic pain, *amla pitta* (hyper-acidity), *grahaṇī* (sprue syndrome) and serious type of jaundice.

अक्षामलकशिवानां स्वरसैः पक्वं सुलोहरजः ।
सगुडं यद्युपभुङ्क्ते मुञ्चति शूली त्रिदोषजं शूलम् ॥६९॥
॥ इति त्रिफलागुडमण्डूरम् ॥

Triphalā Guḍa Maṇḍūra

Lauha or *maṇḍūra bhasma* should be boiled with the decoc-

---

1. भृङ्गस्यरसं इति आकरे पाठः ।
2. च कामलामुग्राम् इति आकरे पाठः ।

tion of *haritakī*, *bibhitakī* and *āmalakī*. This should be taken along with jaggery which cures colic pain caused by the simultaneous vitiation of all the three *doṣas* (*sānnipātika*).

"लोहस्य रजसो भागस्त्रिफलायास्तथा त्रयः ।
गुडस्याष्टौ तथा भागा गुडान्मूत्रं चतुर्गुणम् ॥७०॥
एतत्सर्वं च विपचेद्गुडपाकविधानवत् ।
लिहेच्चैव तथा शक्तिक्षये शूले च पाकजे ॥७१॥
॥ इति लोहगुटिका ॥"

[भैषज्यरत्नावली : शूलरोगाधिकार : १०४-१०५]

Loha Guṭikā

Lauha bhasma (one part), *triphalā* (three parts), *guḍa* (eight parts and cow's urine (twenty four parts)—all these should be cooked on the line prescribed for *guḍa pāka*. This medicine (linctus) should be taken if there is diminution of strength and for the cure of *paktija śūla*.

"धात्री चूर्णस्याष्टौ पलानि चत्वारि लोहचूर्णस्य ।
यष्टीमधुकरजो[1] द्विपलं दद्यात्पटे घृष्टम् ॥७२॥
अमृताक्वाथेनैतच्चूर्णं भाव्यं च सप्ताहम् ।
चण्डातपेषु शुष्कं भूयः पिष्ट्वा नवे घटे स्थाप्यम् ॥७३॥
घृतमधुना संयुक्तं भक्तादौ मध्यतोऽन्ते[2] च ।
त्रीनपि वारान् खादेत्पथ्यं दोषानुबन्धेन ॥७४॥

1. ०मधुकरजश्च इति आकरे पाठः ।
2. मध्यस्तथान्ते इति आकरे पाठः ।

भुक्तस्यादौ[1] शमयति व्याधीन् पित्तानिलोद्भूतान् ।
मध्येऽन्ने विष्टम्भं जयति च नृणां विदह्यते नान्नम् ॥७५॥
पानान्नकृतान्दोषान्भक्तान्ते शीलितो[2] जयति ।
एवं जीर्यति चान्ने[3] शूलं नृणां सुकष्टमपि[4] ॥७६॥
हरति च सहसा युक्तो योगश्चायं जरत्तिम् ।
चक्षुष्यः पलितघ्नः कफपित्तसमुद्भवान् जयेद्रोगान् ॥
प्रसादयत्यपि[5] रक्तं पाण्डुत्वं कामलां जयति ॥७७॥"

॥ धात्रीलोह : ॥

[भैषज्यरत्नावली : शूलरोगाधिकार : १४२-१४७]

Dhātrī Lauha

Powder of *dhātrī* (eight *palas*), *lauha bhasma* (four *palas*) and *yaṣṭi madhu* powder (two *palas*)—all these should be strained through a cloth and impregnated with the decoction of *amṛtā* for seven days. This should be dried in hot sun, triturated again and kept in a new jar. By adding ghee and honey, it should be taken before, during and after meals. The patient should take diet which is wholesome for the aggravated *doṣas*. If taken before meals, the medicine relieves diseases caused by *pitta* and *vāyu*. If taken in the middle of the meal, then it corrects *viṣṭambha* (arrested or reduced peristalsis of intestines) and the

1. भक्तस्यादौ इति आदर्शपुस्तकेषु पाठः ।
2. क. शीलितं इति आकरे पाठः ।
   ख. शीलातो इति षष्ठपुस्तके पाठः ।
3. चान्नं इति आकरे पाठः ।
4. सुकष्टमति इति आदर्शपुस्तकेषु पाठः ।
5. रक्तं प्रसादमत्यपि इति आदर्शपुस्तकेषु पाठः ।

food does not get putrified to cause burning sensation. If taken after meals, then it corrects the faults of food and drinks ingested. This recipe, thus cures serious type of *pariṇāma śūla* and *jarat pitta* (over metabolic transformation of *pitta*; it is also used as a synonym of *pariṇāma śūla*). This promotes eye sight, corrects graying of hair and cures diseases caused by *kapha* as well as *pitta*. It promotes pure blood formation and cures anemia as well as jaundice.

[1]"तनूनि लोहपत्राणि तिलोत्सेधसमानि च ।
कशिकामूलकल्केन संलिप्य सर्षपेण वा ॥७८॥
विशोष्य सूर्यकिरणैः पुनरेवावलेपयेत् ।
त्रिफलाया जले ध्मातं वापयेच्च पुनः पुनः ॥७९॥
ततः सञ्चूर्णितं कृत्वा कर्पटेन तु छानयेत् ।
भक्षयेन्मधुसर्पिभ्यां यथाग्नियस्ततप्रयोजयेत् ॥८०॥
गुञ्जार्द्धं गुञ्जकं वाथ द्विगुञ्जकमथापि वा ।
छागस्य पयसः कुर्यादनुपानमभावतः ॥८१॥
गवां घृतेन दुग्धेन चतुःषष्टिगुणेन च ।
पक्तिशूलं निहन्त्येतन्मासेनैकेन निश्चितम् ॥८२॥
लोहामृतमिदं श्रेष्ठं ब्रह्मणा निर्मितं पुरा ।
ककारपूर्वकं यच्च यच्चाम्लं परिकीर्त्तितम् ॥
सेव्यं तन्न भवेदत्र मांसं चानूपसम्भवम् ॥८३॥

॥ लोहामृतम् ॥"

1. पाठोऽयं षष्ठपुस्तके आकर च अधिकमुपलभ्यते ।

Lohāmṛta

Iron should be made to thin leaves of the thickness of sesame seed. These iron sheets should be smeared with the paste of either the root of *kaśikā* or mustard seed and dried in the sun. This process should be repeated. With the help of a blower these sheets should be made red hot and immersed in the decoction of *triphalā* repeatedly. Thereafter, a fine powder should be made out of these sheets by grinding and straining through a cloth. Depending upon the power of digestion, half *guñjā*, one *guñjā* or two *guñjās* of this powder should be administered with honey and ghee. Goat milk should be taken thereafter. In case of its non-availability, the patient should be given sixty four times of cow's ghee or cow's milk. It undoubtedly cures *pakti śūla* by taking for one month. This excellent recipe called *Lohāmṛta* was propounded in the days of yore by lord Brahmā. Ingredients of diet starting their names with the Sanskrit alphabet '*ka*', sour things and meat of aquatic animals should be avoided.

"स्विन्नं पीडितकूष्माण्डं तुलार्द्धं भृष्टमाज्यतः ।
प्रस्थार्द्धं तुल्यखण्डं च पचेदामलकी रसात् ॥८४॥
प्रस्थे तु[1] स्विन्नकूष्माण्डरसप्रस्थे विघट्टयेत्[2] ।
दर्व्या पाकं गते तस्मिञ्चूर्णीकृत्य विनिःक्षिपेत् ॥८५॥
द्वे द्वे पले कणाजा[3]जीशुण्ठीनां मरिचस्य च ।
पलंतालीसधान्याकचातुर्जातकमुस्तकम् ॥८६॥
कर्षप्रमाणं प्रत्येकं प्रस्थार्द्धं माक्षिकस्य च ।
पक्तिशूलं निहन्त्येतद्दोषत्रयकृतं च यत् ॥८७॥

1. सुस्विन्न० इति आकरे पाठः ।
2. विघट्टयन् इति आकरे पाठः ।
3. कणाजातीशुण्ठीनां इति आदर्शपुस्तकेषु पाठः ।

छर्द्यम्लपित्तमूर्छाश्च श्वासकासविरोचकम्[1] ।
हृच्छूलं रक्तपित्तं च पृष्ठशूलं च नाशयेत् ॥
रसायनमिदं श्रेष्ठं खंडामलकसंज्ञितम् ॥८८॥
॥ इति खण्डामलकम् ॥"

[भैषज्यरत्नावली : शूलरोगाधिकार : १६३-१६७]

Khaṇḍāmalaka

Half *tulā* of steam boiled and squeezed pulp of *kuṣmāṇḍa* should be fried with ghee. Half *prastha* of sugar should be cooked with one *prastha* of each of the juice of *āmalakī* and *kuṣmāṇḍa*. To this, the fried pulp of *kuṣmāṇḍa*, made earlier, should be added and cooked. When it reaches the stage of *darvī pāka* (*i.e.* when the preparation sticks to the stirrer), then the powder of two *palas* of each of *kaṇā*, *ajājī*, *śuṇṭhī* and *marica*, one *karṣa* of each of *tālīsa*, *dhānyāka*, *cāturjātaka* and *mustaka*, and half *prastha* of honey should be added. This cures *pakti śūla* caused by the simultaneous vitiation of all the three *doṣas*. It also cures vomiting, *amla pitta* (hyper-acidity), fainting, asthma, cough, anorexia, cardiac pain, *rakta pitta* (a disease characterised by bleeding from the different parts of the body) and pain in the back. This excellent rejuvenating recipe is called *Khaṇḍāmalaka*.

"कुडवमितमिह स्यान्नारिकेरं सुपिष्टम् ।
पलपरिमितसर्पिः पाचितं खण्डतुल्यम् ॥८९॥
निजपयसि तदेतत्प्रस्थमात्रे विपक्वम् ।
गुडवदथ सुशीते शाणभागान् क्षिपेच्च ॥९०॥

1. श्वासं कासमरोचकम् इति आकरे पाठः ।

धान्यकपिप्पलिपयोदतुगा-[1]द्विजीरान् ।
शाणं त्रिजातमिभकेसरवह्निचूर्ण्य ॥६१॥
हन्त्यम्लपित्तमरुचिं [2]क्षयमस्रपित्त ।
शूलं वमिं [3]सबलपौरुषकारि हारी ॥६२॥
॥इति नालिकेरखण्डः ॥"

[भैषज्यरत्नावली : शूलरोगाधिकार : १६८-१६६]

Nālikera Khaṇḍa

One *kuḍava* of coconut pulp should be made to a paste and fried with one *pala* of ghee. To this, one *kuḍava* of sugar as well as one *prastha* of the milk (juice) of coconut should be added and cooked till the state of *guḍa pāka* is attained. When cooled, one *śāṇa* of the powder of each of *dhānyaka*, *pippalī*, *payoda*, *tugā*, *śveta jīraka*, *kṛṣṇa jīraka*, *trijātaka* and *nāga kesara* should be added. It cures *amla pitta* (hyper-acidity), anorexia, consumption, *rakta pitta* (an ailment characterised by bleeding from different parts of the body), colic pain, and vomiting. It promotes strength and virility.

कलायवटी—कलायचूर्णभागौ द्वौ लोहचूर्णस्य चापरः ।
कारवेल्लपलाशानां रसेनैव विमर्दितः ॥६३॥
कर्षमात्रं ततश्चैकां भक्षयेद्गुटिकां नरः ।
मण्डानुपानाज्जयति जरत्पित्तसुदारणम् ॥६४॥

---

1. ०तुगाद्विजीरकम् इति ग्राकरे पाठः ।
2. क्षतमम्लपित्तं इति ग्रादर्शपुस्तकेषु पाठः ।
3. सकल० इति ग्राकरे पाठः ।

Kalāya Vaṭi

Two parts of the powder of *kalāya* and one part of *lauha bhasma* should be impregnated and triturated with the juice of *kāravella* and *palāśa*. From out of this paste, pills of one *kārṣa* each should be prepared. It should be administered in a dose of one pill each time along with the *maṇḍa* (scum which comes out while boiling rice) which cures serious type of *jarat pitta* (*pariṇāma śūla*).

लिह्याद्धात्रीफलं चूर्णमयश्चूर्णसमाश्रितम् ।
यष्टीचूर्णेन वा युक्तं लिह्यात्क्षौद्रेण तद्गदे ॥६५॥

Āmalakī powder or *yaṣṭi madhu* powder mixed with *lauha bhasma* should be taken by adding honey which cures colic pain.

"टंकणं[1] हारिणं श्रृंगं कर्षतुल्यं समं रसम् ।
आर्द्रकस्य रसैश्चाह्नो मर्द्यं रुध्वा पुटैः पचेत् ॥६६॥
त्रिनेत्राख्यं रसं नाम माषैकं मधुसर्पिषा ।
सैन्धवं सर्पिजीरकं मध्वाज्याभ्यां लिहेदनु ॥
पक्तिशूलहरं ख्यातं मासमात्रान्न संशयः ॥६७॥
॥ इति त्रिनेत्रो रसः ॥"

Trinetra Rasa

One *karṣa* of each of *ṭaṅkaṇa bhasma*, *mṛga śṛṅga bhasma* and purified *pārada* should be added with ginger juice and triturated for one day. This should be kept in a sealed pot and cooked by *puṭa pāka*. This is called *trinetra rasa*. It should be administered in the dose of one *māṣa* along with honey and

1. द्रष्टव्यम्—भारतभैषज्यरत्नाकरः द्वितीयभाग : पृष्ठ ४८२ ।

ghee. Thereafter, rock-salt, ghee and *jīraka* should be taken along with honey and ghee (?). It undoubtedly cures *pakti śūla* within one month.

"शुद्धं सूतं विषं गन्धं पलांशं मर्दयेद्दृढम् ।
मरिचं पिप्पली शुण्ठी हिंगु[1] चैव द्वयं द्वयम् ॥९८॥
पलाष्टकं पटूनां च चिंचाक्षारं पलाष्टकम् ।
सप्तवारं शंखभस्म जंबीराम्लेन[2] सेवयेत् ॥९९॥
पलाष्टकं च संयोज्यं तत्सर्वं निम्बुकोद्भवैः[3] ।
दिनं मर्द्यं कोलमात्रं भक्षयेत्सर्वशूलनुत् ॥१००॥
अजीर्णोदरमन्दाग्निमसाध्यमपि साधयेत् ।
शूलदावानलाख्योऽयं रसोऽजीर्णादिरोगहा ॥१०१॥"

॥ इति शूलदावानलः ॥

[योगरत्नाकर : शूलचिकित्सा (उत्तरार्द्ध) : पृष्ठ १७]

Śūla Dāvānala Rasa

Purified *pārada*, *viṣa*, *gandhaka* and *palāśa kṣāra* should be taken, one part each. To this, two parts of each of *marica*, *pippalī* and *hiṅgu*, eight parts of each of five varieties of *lavaṇas* and *ciñcā kṣāra* and seven parts of *śaṅkha bhasma* and eight parts of *jambīrāmla* should be added. All these should be impregnated and triturated for one day by adding lemon juice. It should be administered in the dose of one *kola*. It cures all types of colic pain, indigestion, *udara* (obstinate abdominal

---

1. हिंगु सौवर्चलं द्वयम् इति आकरे पाठः ।
2. जम्बीराम्ले निषेचयेत् इति आकरे पाठः ।
3. निम्बुकद्रवैः इति आकरे पाठः ।

diseases including ascites) and suppression of the power of digestion even if these ailments are considered to be incurable otherwise. This is called *śūla dāvānala rasa* which cures indigestion, etc.

शुल्वतुल्येन सूतेन बलिना तत्समेन च ।
तदर्द्धांशेन तालेन शीलया च तदर्द्धया ॥१०२॥
विधाय कज्जलीं श्लक्ष्णां भिन्नकज्जलसन्निभाम् ।
यन्त्राध्यायविनिर्दिष्टां गर्भयन्त्रोदरान्तरे ॥१०३॥
कज्जलीं ताम्रपत्राणि पर्यायेण विनिर्दिशेत् ।
प्रपचेद्यामपर्यन्तं स्वांगशीतं च चूर्णयेत् ॥१०४॥
तत्तद्रोगहरानुपानसहितं सार्द्धं हि वल्लोन्मितम् ।
सप्लीहं परिणामशूलमुदरं शूलं च पाण्डुज्वरम् ॥१०५॥
गुल्मप्लीहहरं क्षयादिशमनं मेहं च शूलामयम् ।
दुष्टां च ग्रहणीं हरेद् ध्रुवमिदं तत्सोमनाथाभिधम् ॥१०६॥

॥ इति सोमनाथताम्रेश्वरो रसः ॥

Somanātha Tāmreśvara Rasa

Purified *pārada* (one part). purified *gandhaka* (one part), purified *haratāla* (1/2 part) and purified *manaḥ śilā* (1/2 part)—all these taken together should be triturated till a fine powder like *kajjalī* (collyrium) is formed. This *kajjalī* including thin leaves of *tāmra* (one part) should be kept in layers in a *garbha yantra* and cooked for three hours. When cooled, these ingredients should be removed from *garbha yantra* and made to a powder. It is administered in a dose of one *valla*, along with vehicles appropriate to each of the diseases to be treated. It cures *pariṇāma* type of colic pain, *udara* (obstinate abdominal diseases including ascites), other types of colic pain, anemia, fever, *gulma* (phantom tumour), splenic disorders, consumption, *meha* (obstinate urinary disorders including diabetes) and *grahaṇī doṣa* (sprue syndrome). It is called *somanātha rasa.*

टंकणं मूर्छितं[1] सूतं यवक्षारं समं समम् ।
चूर्णितं भक्षयेन्माषं मधुना पक्तिशूलनुत् ॥
जम्बूमाषकृतं यूषमनुपानं सदा पिबेत् ॥१०७॥

Ṭaṅkaṇa bhasma, pārada bhasma and *yava kṣāra* taken in equal quantities should be triturated. It should be administered in the dose of one *māṣa* along with honey which cures *pakti śūla.* The soup of *jambū* and *māṣa* should invariably be taken as *anupāna* or post-prandial drink along with this recipe.

"[2]दग्धं शंखं वराटं वा मृतं ताम्रं समं समम् ।
निष्कार्द्धं नवनीतेन भक्षयेत्पक्तिशूलनुत् ।
पूर्वोक्तं च पिबेत्क्षीरमनु स्याच्छंखभास्करात् ॥१०८॥"

॥ इति शंखभास्करः ॥

Śaṅkha Bhāskara

Śaṅkha bhasma or *varāṭikā bhasma* should be mixed with equal quantity of *tāmra bhasma.* Half *niṣka* of this powder should be taken along with butter which cures *pakti śūla.* After the medicine, the patient should take milk as described before (?). This is called *śaṅkha bhāskara.*

---

1. चूर्णितं इति षष्ठपुस्तके पाठः ।
2. द्रष्टव्यम्—भारतभैषज्यरत्नाकर : पञ्चमो भाग : पृष्ठ १०३ ।

पित्तान्तं वमनं कृत्वा कफान्तं च विरेचनम् ।

अन्नद्रवे तु तत्कार्यां जरत्पित्ते यदीरितम् ॥

आमपक्वाशये शुद्धे गच्छेदन्नद्रवः समम् ॥१०९॥

Line of Treatment of Annadrava Śūla

The patient suffering from *annadrava śūla* should be first of all be given emetic therapy till *pitta* appears in the vomited substance and purgation therapy till *kapha* appears in the stool. Thereafter, therapies already described for *jarat pitta* (*pariṇāma*) type of *śūla* should be administered. *Annadrava śūla* is alleviated by the cleansing of *āmāśaya* (stomach including the upper part of small intestine) and *pakvāśaya* (large intestine).

"माषेण्डरी सतुषिका स्विन्ना सर्पिर्युता हिता ।

गोधूममण्डकं तत्र सर्पिषा गुडसंयुतम् ।

ससितं शीतदुग्धेन मृदितं वा हितं मतम् ॥११०॥

शालितण्डुलमण्डं वा कवोष्णं सिक्थवर्जितम् ।

वाट्यं क्षीरेण संसिद्धं घृतं यूषं सशर्करम् ॥१११॥

शर्करां भक्षयित्वा वा क्षीरमुत्क्वथितं पिबेत् ।

पटोलपत्रयूषेण खादेत् चणकशक्तुकान् ॥११२॥

Wholesome Diet

To patients suffering from colic pain, steam boiled *eṇḍari* type of cake prepared of *māṣa* along with its husk and ghee, should be given as food. Wheat flour mixed with ghee and jaggery is useful. It can be given along with sugar and cold milk. Luke warm *maṇḍa* (water which is strained out after boiling rice) of *śāli* rice free from *siktha* (sticky portion) is also useful. *Vāṭya* (barley) cooked in milk and added with ghee, vegetable soup and sugar may also be given. The patient can take boiled milk after taking sugar. He can also take *saktu* (roasted flour) of *caṇaka* along with the soup of leaves of *paṭola*.

अन्नद्रवे जरत्पित्ते वह्निर्मन्दो भवेद्यतः ।
तस्मादत्रानुपानानि मात्राहीनानि कल्पयेत् ॥११३॥"

[भैषज्यरत्नावली : शूलरोगाधिकार : २६५-२६८]

Annadrava and *jarat pitta* (*pariṇāma*) types of colic pain are invariably associated with *agni māndya* (suppression of the power of digestion). Therefore, the *anupāna* (post-prandial drink) prescribed in respect of each recipe should be given only in small quantity.

इति श्रीमहाराजाधिराजटोडरमल्लविरचिते टोडरानन्दे आयुर्वेद-सौख्ये परिणामशूलनिदानचिकित्साकथनं नाम अष्टत्रिंशत्तमो हर्षः ॥११४॥

Thus, ends the 38th Chapter dealing with the diagnosis and treatment of *pariṇāma* (and *annadrava*) *śūla* in the *Āyurveda saukhya* of *Ṭoḍarānanda* composed by the great king Ṭoḍara Malla.

CHAPTER III

अथ उदावर्त्त-आनाहनिदानं चिकित्सा च ।

Diagnosis and Treatment of Udāvarta (upward movement of vāyu) and Anāha (abdominal distension)

“[1]वातविण्मूत्रजृम्भा[2]श्रुक्षवोद्गारवमिन्द्रियैः ।
क्षुत्तृष्णोच्छ्वासनिद्राणां धृत्वो[3]दावर्त्तसम्भवः ॥१॥

Etiology

Udāvarta is caused by the suppression of the manifested natural urges for *vāta* (passing flatus), stool, urine, yawning,

---

1. This is the beginning of 42nd Chapter of *Āyurveda saukhya* in *Ṭoḍarānanda* and the invocation reads as follows :—
गोपालिकानां सुविबुध्य भावं दद्यान्नतानां प्रददौवरं यः ।
कामं तथा टोडरमल्लभूपे भूदेव संघेलन धर्म्मं रूपे ॥
2. ०जृंभास्त्रु० इति पंचमपुस्तके आकरे च पाठः ।
3. धृत्यो० इति आकरे पाठः ।

tear, sneezing, eructation, vomiting, seminal ejaculation, hunger, thirst, breathing and sleep.

वातमूत्रपुरीषाणां संगाध्मानं क्लमो रुजा ।
जठरे वातजाश्चान्ये रोगास्युर्वातनिग्रहात् ॥२॥

Udāvarta caused by Suppression of Vāta

Obstruction to the passage of flatus, urine and stool, wind formation in the stomach, fatigue, pain in abdomen and manifestation of other *vātika* diseases—these are caused by the suppression of the urge for passing flatus.

आटोपशूलौ परिकर्त्रका[1] च संगः पुरीषस्य तथोर्ध्ववातः ।
पुरीषमास्यादथवा निरेति पुरीषवेगेऽभिहते नरस्य ॥३॥

Udāvarta caused by Suppression of Stool

Āṭopa (gurgling sound in the abdomen), colic pain, *parikartikā* (sawing pain), obstruction to the passage of stool, *ūrdhva vāta* (upward movement of gas in the abdomen) and coming ou of fecal material through the mouth—these are caused by the suppression of the urge for defecation.

बस्तिमेहनयोः शूलं मूत्रकृच्छ्रं शिरोरुजा ।
विबंधो[2] वंक्षणानाहः स्याल्लिंगं मूत्रनिग्रहे ॥४॥

Udāvarta caused by Suppression of Urine

Colic pain in the region of urinary bladder and genital organ, dysuria, headache, constipation and distension in the pelvic region—these are caused by the suppression of the urge for urination.

1. परिकर्तिका इति आकरे पाठः ।
2. विनामो इति आकरे पाठः ।

मन्यागलस्तम्भशिरोविकारा जृम्भोपघातात् पवनात्मकाः स्युः ।
तथाक्षिनासावदनामयाश्च भवन्ति तीव्रा[1] सह कर्णरोगैः ॥५॥

Udāvarta caused by the Suppression of Yawning

Stiffness of sternomastoid region and neck, head-diseases caused by *vāyu* and serious diseases of eyes, nose, face as well as ears—these are caused by the suppression of the urge for yawning.

आनन्दजं बाष्पमथ शोकजं वा नेत्रोदकं प्राप्तममुंचतो हि ।
शिरोगुरुत्वं नयनामयाश्च भवन्ति तीव्राः सह पीनसेन ॥६॥

Udāvarta caused by the Suppression of Tears

Tears may appear in the eyes because of either pleasure or sorrow. Suppression of this urge may cause heaviness of head, serious type of eye diseases, and *pīnasa* (chronic rhinitis).

मन्यास्तम्भः शिरःशूलमर्दितार्द्धावभेदकौ ।
इंद्रियाणां च दौर्बल्यं क्षवथोः स्याद्विधारणात् ॥७॥

Udāvarta caused by Suppression of Sneezing

Torticolis, headache, facial paralysis, hemicrania and weakness of sense organs—all these are caused by the suppression of the urge for sneezing.

कंठास्यपूर्णत्वमतीव तोदः कूजश्च वायोरथवाऽप्रवृत्तिः ।
उद्गारवेगेऽभिहते भवन्ति घोरा विकाराः पवनप्रसूताः ॥८॥

---

1. तीव्राः इति आकरे पाठः ।

Udāvarta caused by Suppression of Eructation

Sense of fullness in throat and mouth, excessive pain, cooing sound, obstruction to the passage of the wind and other serious *vātika* diseases are caused by the suppression of the urge for eructation.

कंडूकोठारुचिव्यंगशोफपांड्वामयज्वराः ।

कुष्ठहृल्लासविसर्पाश्छर्दिनिग्रहजा गदाः ॥९॥

Udāvarta caused by Suppression of Vomiting

Itching , urticaria, anorexia, pigmented patches, oedema, anemia, fever, *kuṣṭha* (obstinate skin diseases including leprosy), nausea and erysipelas—these are caused by the suppression of the urge for vomiting.

मूत्राशये वै गुदमुष्कयोश्च शोफो रुजा मूत्रविनिग्रहश्च ।

शुक्राश्मरी तत्स्रवणं भवेच्च[1] रेतोविकारोऽभिहते तु शुक्रे ॥१०॥

Udāvarta caused by Suppression of Semen

Oedema and pain in urinary bladder, anus and testicles, anuria, stone in seminal channel, frequent seminal discharge and similar other seminal morbidities are caused by the suppression of the urge for seminal ejaculation.

तन्द्रांगमर्दावरुचिः श्रमश्च क्षुधाभिघातात् कृशता च दृष्टेः ।

कंठास्यशोषः श्रवणावरोधः तृष्णाभिघातात् हृदयव्यथा[2] च ॥११॥

---

1. भवेच्च ते ते विकारा विहते च शुक्रे इति आकरे पाठः ।
2. हृदये व्यथा इति आकरे पाठः ।

Udāvarta caused by Suppression of Hunger and Thirst

Drowsiness, malaise, anorexia, fatigue and impairment of vision—these are caused by the suppression of hunger. Dryness of throat and mouth, impairment of hearing and cardiac pain are caused by the suppression of thirst.

श्रांतस्य निश्वासविनिग्रहेण[1] हृद्रोगमोहावथवापि गुल्मः ।
जृम्भागंमर्दोऽक्षिसिरातिजाड्यं निद्राभिघातादथवाऽपि तंद्रा ॥१२॥

Udāvarta caused by Suppression of Breathing and Sleep

If a person, after exercise, suppresses the urge for (deep) breathing, he suffers from heart disease, unconsciousness and *gulma* (phantom tumour). Suppression of the urge for sleep causes yawning, malaise, stiffness of the vessels of eyes and drowsiness.

वायुः कोष्ठानुगो रूक्षैः[2] कषायकटुतिक्तकैः ।
भोजनैः कुपितः सद्य उदावर्त्तं करोति च[3] ॥१३॥

Other Causes

Udāvarta is also caused immediately after the intake of unctuous, astringent, pungent and bitter food in excess. These food ingredients aggravate the *vāyu* located in the colon which causes *udāvarta*.

वातमूत्रपुरीषासृक्कफमेदोवहानि[4] वै ।
स्रोतांस्युदावर्त्तयति पुरीषं चातिवर्त्तयेत् ॥१४॥

1. निःश्वास० इति आकरे पाठः ।
2. रूक्षः इति आकरे पाठः ।
3. हि इति आकरे पाठः ।
4. ०पुरीषास्तुफमेदोवहानि वै इति आदर्शपुस्तकेषु पाठः ।

ततो हृद्बस्तिशूलार्त्तो हृल्लासारतिपीडितः ।
वातमूत्रपुरीषाणि कृच्छ्रेण लभते नरः ॥१५॥
कासश्वासप्रतिश्यायदाहमोहतृषाज्वरान् ।
वमीहिक्काशिरोरोगमनःश्रवणविभ्रमान् ॥
बहूनन्यांश्च लभते विकारान् वातकोपजान् ॥१६॥

Signs and Symptoms

The aggravated *vāyu* obstructs (or causes movement in reverse order) the channels of circulation for flatus, urine, stool blood, *kapha* as well as adipose tissue, and causes excessive obstruction to the movement of stool. Thereafter, the patient suffers from pain in the heart and urinary bladder, nausea and dislike for any work. With considerable difficulty, he passes flatus, urine and stool. He also suffers from cough, dyspnoea, acute form of cold, burning sensation, unconsciousness, morbid thirst, fever, vomiting, hiccup, diseases of the head, impairment of the functioning of mind as well as ears and several other diseases caused by the aggravation of *vāyu.*

आमं शकृद्वा निचितं क्रमेण भूयो विबद्धं विगुणानिलेन ।
प्रवर्त्तमानं न यथास्वमेनं विकारमानाहमुदाहरंति ॥१७॥

Pathogenesis of Ānāha

Āma (product of improper digestion) and stool, gradually accumulated in the colon get further obstructed by aggravated *vāyu* as a result of which, their evacuation automatically becomes difficult. This ailment is called *ānāha.*

तस्मिन् भवन्त्यामसमुद्भवे तु तृष्णाप्रतिश्यायशिरोविदाहाः ।
आमाशये शूलमथो गुरुत्वं हृल्लासमुद्गारविघातनं[1] च ॥१८॥

1. हृत्स्तम्भ उद्गारविघातनं इति आकरे पाठः ।

स्तम्भः कटीपृष्ठपुरीषमूत्रे शूलोऽथ मूर्छा शकृतश्च छर्दिः ।
श्वासश्च पक्वाशयजे भवन्ति तथाऽलसोक्तानि[1] च लक्षणानि ॥१६॥

Signs and Symptoms of Ānāha

Signs and symptoms of *ānāha* are colic pain in epigastric region, heaviness, nausea, obstruction to eructation, stiffness of lumber region and back, obstruction to the passage of stool and urine, colic pain, fainting, vomiting of fecal matter, dyspnoea and affliction of the colon as it happens in *alasaka*.

तृष्णार्दितं परिक्लिष्टं क्षीणं शूलैरुपद्रुतम्[2] ।
शकृद्वमन्तं मतिमानुदावर्त्तिनमुत्सृजेत् ॥२०॥"

[माधवनिदान : उदावर्त्तनिदान : १-२०]

॥ इति उदावर्त्तानाहनिदानम् ॥

Prognosis of Udāvarta

Excessive morbid thirst, complete exhaustion, emaciation, excessive colic pain and vomiting of fecal matter—these symptoms in a patient of *udāvarta* are indicative of bad prognosis and such a patient should not be treated.

Thus, ends the diagnosis of *udāvarta* and *ānāha*.

"त्रिवृत्-सुधापत्रतिलादिशाकं ग्राम्यौदकानूपरसैर्यवान्नम् ।
अन्यैश्च सृष्टानिलमूत्रवड्भिरद्यात् प्रसन्नागुडसीधुपायी ॥२१॥

आस्थापनं मारुतजे स्निग्धस्विन्नस्य शस्यते ।
पुरीषजे तु कर्त्तव्यो विधिरानाहिकस्तु यः ॥२२॥"

[भैषज्यरत्नावली : उदावर्त्तानाहाधिकार : १-२]

क्षारवैतरणौ बस्तिं युंज्यात्तत्र चिकित्सकः ॥२३॥

1. तथाऽलसोक्तानि इति आकरे पाठः ।
2. शूलैरभिद्रुतम् इति आकरे पाठ :

Line of Treatment

Yava (barley) boiled with *trivṛt*, leaves of *sudhā* and *tila* or with the soup of the meat of animals which are domesticated, aquatic animals and animals inhabiting marshy land or with such other ingredients which help in the elimination of flatus as well as urine is useful. The patient should drink *prasannā*, *guḍa* and *sīdhu* types of alcoholic preparations. If there is aggravation of *vāyu*, such patients should be given *āsthāpana* type of medicated enema after oleation, and fomentation therapies. For the patient suffering from *purīṣaja* type of *udāvarta*, the line of treatment suggested for *ānāha* should be adopted. The patient should be given medicated enema containing alkali preparation [the meaning of the term '*kṣāravaitaraṇau*' is not clear].

श्यामादन्तीद्रवन्तीत्वक् महाश्यामास्नुहीत्रिवृत् ।
सप्तला शंखिनी श्वेता राजवृक्षः सतिल्वकः ।
कम्पिल्लकः करञ्जश्च हेमक्षीरी पयं गणः ॥२४॥
सर्पिस्तैलरजः क्वाथकल्कैरन्यतमेन तु ।
उदावर्त्तोदरानाहविषगुल्मादिनाशनः ॥२५॥

Śyāmā, *dantī*, *dravantī*, *tvak*, *mahāśyāmā*, *snuhī*, *trivṛt*, *saptalā śaṅkhinī*, *śvetā*, *rāja vṛkṣa*, *tilvaka*, *kampillaka*, *karañja*, *hema kṣīrī* and other drugs belonging to *kṣīrī vṛkṣa* group should be used for the preparation of medicated ghee, medicated oil, powder, decoction, paste and such other preparations. These are useful in the treatment of *udāvarta*, *udara* (obstinate abdominal diseases including ascites), *ānāha*, poisoning, *gulma* (phantom tumour), etc.

"त्रिवृत्कृष्णाहरीतक्यो द्विचतु:पञ्चभागिकाः ।
गुडिका गुडतुल्यास्ताः विड्विबन्धगदापहाः ॥२६॥"

॥ त्रिवृतादिगुडिका ॥

[भैषज्यरत्नावली : उदावर्त्तानाहाधिकार : ३१]

Trivṛtādi Guḍikā

Trivṛt (two parts), *kṛṣṇā* (four parts) and *harītakī* (five parts) should be mixed with jaggery (eleven parts) and pills should be made out of these ingredients. These pills cure diseases caused by the obstruction to the passage of stool.

"हरीतकीयवक्षारपीलुनि[1] त्रिवृता तथा ।
घृतश्चूर्णमिदं पेयमुदावर्त्तविनाशनम् ॥२७॥"

[भैषज्यरत्नावली : उदावर्त्तानाहाधिकार : ४]

The powder of *harītaki*, *yava kṣāra*, *pīlu* and *trivṛt* should be taken along with ghee for the cure of *udāvarta*.

'[2]हिंगुकुष्ठवचास्वर्जिविडञ्चेति द्विरुत्तमम् ।
पीतं मद्येन तत् चूर्णमुदावर्त्तविनाशनम् ॥२८॥'

The powder of *hiṅgu* (one part), *kuṣṭha* (two parts), *vacā* (four parts), *svarji kṣāra* (eight parts) and *viḍa* (16 parts) should be taken along with alcoholic drinks which cures *udāvarta*.

"खण्डात् पलं त्रिवृतासममुपकुल्याकर्षचूर्णितं श्लक्ष्णम् ।
प्राग्भोजने च समधुना विडालपदकं लिहेत्प्राज्ञः ॥२९॥
एतत् गाढपुरीषे वाते[3] पित्ते कफे च विनियोज्यम् ।
स्वादुर्न पयोग्योऽयं चूर्णो नाराचको नाम्ना ॥३०॥
॥ नाराचचूर्णम् ॥"

[भैषज्यरत्नावली : उदावर्त्तानाहाधिकार : २८-२९]

---

1. ०पीलूनि इति आकरे पाठः ।
2. द्रष्टव्यम्—भैषज्यरत्नावली : उदावर्त्तानाहाधिकार : २१ ।
3. वाते पाठोऽयं आकरे नोपलभ्यते ।

Nārāca Cūrṇa

One *pala* of sugar, one *pala* of *trivṛt* and one *karṣa* of *upakulyā* should be made to a fine powder. This should be administered in the dose of one *viḍāla padaka* along with honey before food. It should be given for the treatment of constipation caused by *vāyu*, *pitta* and *kapha*. This powder is sweet in taste and can be taken even by kings. This is called *Nārācaka*.

"रसोनं मद्यसंमिश्रं पिबेत् प्रातः प्रकांक्षितः ।
गुल्मोदावर्त्तशूलघ्न दीपन बलवर्द्धनम् ॥३१॥"

[भैषज्यरत्नावली : उदावर्त्तानाहाधिकार : ४]

Rasona mixed with alcoholic drinks should be taken by the patient as much as he likes. This cures *gulma* (phantom tumour), *udāvarta* and colic pain. This stimulates the power of digestion and promotes strength.

"हिंगुमाक्षिकसिंधूत्थैः पक्त्वा वर्ति सुवर्त्तिताम्[1] ।
घृताभ्यक्तां गुदे दद्यादुदावर्त्तविनाशिनीम्[2] ॥३२॥

॥ हिङ्ग्वादिवर्तिः ॥

Hiṅgvādi Varti

Asafoetida, honey and rock-salt should be cooked together and from this paste, *vartis* (elongated pills) should be prepared. This *varti* should be smeared with ghee and administered in the anus as suppository which cures *udāvarta*.

मदनं पिप्पली कुष्ठं वचा गौराश्च सर्षपाः ।
गुडक्षारसमायुक्ताः फलवर्त्तिः प्रशस्यते[3] ॥३३॥"

॥ फलवर्त्तिः ॥

[भैषज्यरत्नावली : उदावर्त्तानाहाधिकार : ३०-३१]

1. विनिर्मिताम् इति आकरे पाठः ।
2. न्यस्येदुदावर्त्त० इति आकरे पाठः ।
3. फलवर्त्तिरिहोच्यते इति आकरे पाठः ।

Phala Varti

Madana, *pippalī*, *kuṣṭha*, *vacā*, white variety of *sarṣapa*, *guḍa* and *kṣāra* (alkali preparation) should be triturated together and suppositories should be prepared. This is called *phala varti* and it is useful in the treatment of *udāvarta*.

"आगारधूमसिन्धूत्थस्तैलयुक्ताम्लमूलकम् ।
क्षुन्नं[1] निर्गुण्डिपत्रं वा स्विन्ने पायौ क्षिपेद् बुधः ॥३४॥"

[भैषज्यरत्नावली : उदावर्त्तानाहाधिकार : ६]

The paste of house shoot, rock-salt, oil and *amla mūlaka* or the paste of the leaves of *nirguṇḍi* should be applied over the anus after its fomentation [for the cure of *udāvarta*].

"सौवर्चलाढ्यां मदिरां मूत्रे त्वभिहते पिबेत् ।
एलां वा[ऽ]प्यथ मद्येन क्षारं[2] वारि पिबेच्च वा ॥३५॥
दुःस्पर्शास्वरसं वा[ऽ]पि कषायं ककुभस्य वा ।
एर्वारुबीजं तोयेन पिबेद्वा लवणीकृतम् ॥
पञ्चमूलीभृतं क्षीरं द्राक्षारसमथापि वा ॥३६॥"

[भैषज्यरत्नावली : उदावर्त्तानाहाधिकार : ७-९]

[3]सर्वथैवोपयुञ्जीतमूत्रकृच्छ्राश्मरीविधिम् ॥३७॥

Treatment of Mūtraja Udāvarta

If *udāvarta* is caused by the suppression of the urge for

---

1. क्षुण्ण इति आकरे पाठः ।
2. क्षीरवारि पिबेन्नरः इति आकरे पाठः ।
3, स्र्यर्थै० इति पंचमपुस्तके पाठः ।

urination, then the patient should be treated with the following recipes.

1. *Madirā* type of wine with profuse quantity of sonchal salt;
2. Alcoholic drinks mixed with cardamom;
3. Water mixed *kṣāra* (alkali preparation);
4. Juice of *duḥsparśā*;
5. Decoction of *kakubha*;
6. Seeds of *ervāruka* mixed with water and salt;
7. Milk boiled with the decoction of *pañca mūla* (*bilva*, *śyonāka*, *gambhārī*, *pāṭalī* and *gaṇi kārikā*); and
8. Grape juice.

In all such cases, procedures and recipes described for the treatment of *mūtra kṛcchra* (dysuria) and *aśmarī* (stone in urinary tract) should be followed.

"स्नेहस्वेदैरुदावर्त्तं जृम्भजं[1] समुपाचरेत् ।
अश्रुमोक्षोऽश्रुजे कार्यः स्वप्नो मद्यं प्रियाः[2] कथाः ॥३८॥

Treatment of Jṛmbhāja Udāvarta, etc.

If *udāvarta* is caused by the suppression of the urge for yawning, then the patient should be treated with oleation and fomentation therapies. If *udāvarta* is caused by the suppression of tears, then therapies should be administered for lacrimation and the patient should be asked to sleep and take alcoholic drinks. He should be consoled with pleasing talks.

क्षवजे क्षवपत्रेण घ्राणस्थेनानयेत्क्षवम् ।
तथोर्ध्वंजत्रुको[3]ऽभ्यङ्गः स्वेदो धूमः सनावनः ॥३९॥

---

1. जृम्भाजं इति आकरे पाठः ।
2. प्रियाकथा इति आदर्श पुस्तकेषु पाठः ।
3. तथोर्ध्वंजत्रुगोऽभ्यङ्गः इति आकरे पाठः ।

Treatment of Kṣavaja Udāvarta

If *udāvarta* is caused by the suppression of the urge for sneezing, then the patient should be made to sneeze by inhaling *kṣava patra* (*chikkiṇī*), and thereafter, oil should be applied and massaged over his head and neck. He should also take fomentation, smoking and inhalation therapies.

हितं वातघ्नमद्यश्च[1] घृतं चोत्तरभक्तकं ।
उद्गारजे क्रमोपेतं स्नैहिकं धूममाचरेत् ॥४०॥

Treatment of Udgāraja Udāvarta

If *udāvarta* is caused by the suppression of the urge for eructation, then he should be given such food as would alleviate *vāyu*, and ghee to take after food. He should be administered unctuous type of smoking therapy in appropriate time.

छर्द्याघाते यथादोषं नस्यस्नेहादिभिर्जयेत् ।
भुक्त्वा प्रच्छर्दनं धूमो लंघनं रक्तमोक्षणम् ।
रूक्षान्नपानं व्यायामो विरेकश्चात्र शस्यते ॥४१॥

Treatment of Chardija Udāvarta

If *udāvarta* is caused by the suppression of the urge for vomiting, then depending upon the *doṣas* involved, the patient should be given different types of inhalation and oleation therapies. He should be given emetic therapy after the intake of food. He should also be given smoking, fasting and blood-letting therapies. Ununctuous food and drinks, exercise and purgation therapies are useful for such patients.

बस्तिशुद्धिकरावापं चतुर्गुणजलं पयः ।
आवारिनाशात्क्वथितं पीतवन्तं प्रकामतः ॥४२॥

---

1. वातघ्नमाज्यं च घृतं इति आदर्शपुस्तकेषु पाठः ।

रमयेयुः प्रिया नार्यः शुक्रोदावर्त्तिनं नरम् ।
अत्राभ्यङ्गावगाहाश्च मदिराश्चरणायुधाः ॥
शीलः पयो निरूहाश्च शस्तं[1] मैथुनमेव च ॥४३॥

Treatment of Śukraja Udāvarta

Milk should be boiled with four times of water and reduced to one fourth. This milk should be given in sufficient quantity to drink to a patient suffering from *udāvarta* caused by the suppression of the urge for ejaculation of semen. Thereafter, fomentation therapy should be employed for cleansing the urinary bladder. He should indulge in sex acts with lovable ladies. Massage, *avagāha* type of fomentation therapy, alcohol, chicken meat, *śāli* rice, milk, *nirūha* type of enema and sexual intercourse are useful for such patients.

क्षुद्विघाते हितं स्निग्धमुष्णमल्पं च भोजनम् ।
तृष्णाघाते पिबेन्मन्थं यवागूं वाऽपि शीतलम्[2] ॥४४॥
रसेनाद्यात्सुविश्रान्तः श्रमश्वासातुरो नरः ।
निद्राघाते पिबेत्क्षीरं स्वप्नः संवाहनानि च ॥४५॥"

[भैषज्यरत्नावली : उदावर्त्तानाहाधिकार : १०-१८]

"उदावर्त्तक्रियानाहे सामे लंघनपाचनम् ॥४६॥

Treatment of Udāvarta caused by Kṣutvighāta, etc.

If *udāvarta* is caused by the suppression of hunger, then the patient should be given unctuous and hot food in small quantities. If *udāvarta* is caused by the suppression of thirst, then the patient should take *mantha* (thin gruel) or *yavāgū* (thick gruel)

1. हितं इति आकरे पाठः ।
2. शीतलाम् इति आकरे पाठः ।

repeatedly. The patient suffering from *udāvarta* because of the suppression of deep breathing after exercise, should be advised to take rest after which he should be given meat soup. If *udāvarta* is caused by the suppression of the urge for sleep, then the patient should be given milk, he should be allowed to sleep and his body should be gently massaged (*saṃvāhana*).

द्विरुत्तरा हिंगु वचा सकुष्ठा सुर्वाचका चेति विडंगचूर्णम् ।

सुखाम्बुनानाहविसूचिकाऽर्त्तिहृद्रोगगुल्मोर्ध्वसमीरणघ्नम् ॥४७॥

Treatment of Ānāha

Therapies prescribed for *udāvarta* should be administered appropriately to a patient suffering from *ānāha*. In the *āma* stage (first stage) of this ailment, fasting and carminative therapies are useful.

The powder of *hiṅgu* (one part), *vacā* (two parts), *kuṣṭha* (four parts), *suvarcikā* (eight parts) and *viḍaṅga* (sixteen parts), if taken with luke-warm water, cures *ānāha*, *visūcikā* (choleric diarrhoea), heart diseases, *gulma* (phantom tumour) and *udāvarta* (*ūrdhva samīraṇa*).

वचाऽभयाचित्रकयावशूकान् सपिप्पलीकातिविषान् सकुष्ठान् ।

उष्णाम्बुनानाहविमूढवातान् पीत्वा जयेदाशु हितौदनाशी ॥४८॥"

[भैषज्यरत्नावली : उदावर्त्तानाहाधिकार : २०-२२]

The powder of *vacā*, *abhayā*, *citraka*, *yava kṣāra*, *pippalī*, *ativiṣā* and *kuṣṭha* should be given with hot water which immediately cures *ānāha* and *vimūḍha vāta*. The patient should take wholesome diet along with this recipe.

"त्रिवृत् हरीतकीश्यामाः स्नुहीक्षीरेण भावयेत् ।

वटिका मूत्रपीतास्ताः श्रेष्ठाश्चानाहभेदिकाः ॥४९॥"

[भैषज्यरत्नावली : उदावर्तानाहाधिकार : ४२]

Trivṛt, *harītakī* and *śyāmā* should be impregnated and triturated by adding the milky latex of *snuhī* and pills should be made out of this paste. Intake of this pill with cow's urine is excellent for curing *ānāha* by purgation.

"फलं च मूलं च विरेचनोक्तं हिंग्वर्कमूलं दशमूलमग्र्यम् ।
स्नुक्चित्रकौ चैव पुनर्नवा च तुल्यानि सर्वैर्लवणानि पञ्च ॥५०॥
स्नेहैः समूत्रैः सह जर्जराणि
शरावसन्धौ विपचेत्सुलिप्ते ।
पक्वं सुपिष्टं लवणं तदन्नैः
पानैस्तथा[1][ऽ]नाहरुजाघ्नमग्र्यम्[2] ॥५१॥

Fruits and roots of drugs belonging to *virecaka gaṇa* (group of purgatives), *hiṅgu*, *arka* (root), *daśa mūla*, *snuhī*, *citraka* and *punarnavā* should be made to a coarse powder. To this, five salts in equal quantity should be added. This should then be mixed with ghee and cow's urine and kept in *śarāva sampuṭa* (two earthen plates), the joint of which should be sealed by smearing seven layers of mud-smeared cloth. This should then be cooked in *puṭa* appropriately. Thereafter, the powder of ingredients should be removed and further triturated to make a fine powder. Intake of this powder along with food and drinks effectively cures *ānāha*.

राठधूमविडव्योषगुडमूत्रैर्विपाचिता[3] ।
गुदेऽङ्गुष्ठसमा वर्तिर्निधेयानाहशूलनुत्[4] ॥५२॥"
[भैषज्यरत्नावली : उदावर्त्तानाहाधिकार : २३-२५]

1. पानैस्तदानाह० इति पंचमपुस्तके पाठः ।
2. ०रुजाघ्नमग्यम् इति आकरे पाठः ।
3. ०पाचित इति आदर्शपुस्तकेषु पाठः ।
4. वर्तिर्विधेयाऽऽनाहशूलनुत् इति आकरे पाठः ।

Rāṭha, house shoot, *viḍa*, *vyoṣa* and *guḍa* should be cooked with cow's urine, and suppositories of the shape and size of thumb should be prepared. Insertion of this suppository into the anus cures pain caused by *ānāha*.

"वर्तिस्त्रिकटुकसैन्धवसर्षपगृहधूमकुष्ठमदनफलैः ।
मधुनि गुडे वा[1]ऽङ्गुष्ठपरिमाणा ॥५३॥
वर्त्तिरियम् दृष्टफला शनैः शनैः प्रणिहिता घृताभ्यक्ता ।
आनाहोदावर्त्तप्रशमना[2] जठरगुल्मनिवारिणी[3] ॥५४॥"

[भैषज्यरत्नावली : उदावर्त्तानाहाधिकार : ४३-४४]

Trikaṭu, *saindhava*, *sarṣapa*, *gṛha dhūma*, *kuṣṭha* and *madana phala* should be cooked in honey or jaggery. From out of this, suppositories of the size and shape of thumb should be prepared. This suppository, smeared with ghee should be gradually inserted into the anus which cures *ānāha*, *udāvarta*, *jaṭhara* (obstinate abdominal diseases including ascites) and *gulma* (phantom tumour). Effect of this therapy is experienced in practice.

शुष्कमूलाद्यं घृतम्—

"मूलकं शुष्कमार्द्रञ्च वर्षाभूमूलपञ्चकम् ।
आरेवतफलञ्चापि पिष्ट्वा तेन पचेद् घृतम् ॥
तत्पीयमानं[4] शमयेदुदावर्त्तमशेषतः[5] ॥५५॥"

॥ शुष्कमूलाद्यं घृतम् ॥

[भैषज्यरत्नावली : उदावर्त्तानाहाधिकार : ४६]

1. वा पक्त्वा पार्थ्वीरिताङ्गुष्ठपरिमाणा इति आकरे पाठः ।
2. ०प्रशमनी इति आकरे पाठः ।
3. च पाठोऽयं आकरे अधिकमुपलभ्यते ।
4. तत्पतिमात्र इति आकरे पाठः ।
5. शमयेदुदावर्त्तमसंशयम् इति आकरे पाठः ।

Śuṣka Mūlādya Ghṛta

Ghee boiled with the paste of dry as well as fresh *mūlaka*, *varṣābhū*, *pañca mūla* and fruit of *ārevata* should be taken which cures all types of *udāvarta*.

स्थिराद्यं घृतम्

"स्थिरादिवर्गस्य पुनर्नवायाः
शम्पाक[1]पूतीककरञ्जयोश्च ।
सिद्धं[2] कषायो द्विपलांशिकानां प्रस्थं[3]
घृतं स्यात् प्रतिबद्धवाते ॥५६॥"

॥ स्थिराद्यं घृतम् ॥

[भैषज्यरत्नावली : उदावर्त्तानाहाधिकार : ४५]

Sthirādya Ghṛta

One *prastha* of ghee boiled with the decoction of two *palas* of each of the drugs belonging to *sthirādi varga*, *punarnavā*, *śampāka* and *pūtika karañja* is useful in *pratibaddha vāta* (*udāvarta* and *ānāha*).

इति श्रीमहाराजाधिराजटोडरमल्लविरचिते टोडरानन्दे आयुर्वेद-सौख्ये उदावर्त्तनिदानचिकित्साकथनं नाम नवत्रिंशत्तमो हर्षः ॥५७॥

Thus, ends the 39th Chapter dealing with the diagnosis and treatment of *udāvarta* and *ānāha* of *Āyurveda saukhya* in *Ṭoḍarānanda* composed by the great king Ṭoḍara Malla.

---

1. सम्पाक० इति आकरे पाठः ।
2. सिद्धः इति आकरे पाठः ।
3. प्रस्थो घृतास्यात्प्रतिरुद्धवाते इति आकरे पाठः ।

CHAPTER IV

अथ गुल्मनिदानं चिकित्सा च ।

Diagnosis and Treatment of Gulma (Phantom Tumour)

"दुष्टा[1] वातादयो[ऽ]त्यर्थं मिथ्याहारविहारतः ।

कुर्वन्ति पञ्चधा गुल्मं कोष्ठान्तर्ग्रन्थिरूपिणम्[2] ॥

तस्य पञ्चविधं स्थानं पार्श्वे[3] हृन्नाभिबस्तयः ॥१॥

---

1. This is the beginning of 43rd Chapter of *Āyurveda saukhya* in *Ṭoḍarānanda* and the invocation reads as follows :—

   यो यज्ञभुक् विप्रमखं विहाय तदंगनानां कृपयां चकार ।
   कुर्यात् कृपां टोडरमल्लभूपे दयान्विते स्वाश्रृत(श्रित) जीवरूपे ॥

2. रूपिणाम् इति आदर्शपुस्तकेषु पाठः ।
3. पार्श्वहृन्नाभि० इति आकरे पाठः ।

Etiology

Vāyu, etc., extremely vitiated by unwholesome diet and regimens give rise to five types of *gulma* which appear like tumours in the gastro-intestinal tract (*koṣṭha*) and located in five places, viz. two sides of the chest, cardiac region, umbilicus and urinary bladder.

'हृन्नाभ्योरन्तरे ग्रन्थिः संचारी यदि वा[ऽ]चलः ।
वृत्तश्चैवोपचयवान् स गुल्म इति कीर्तितः ॥२॥'

[सुश्रुत : उत्तरतन्त्र ४२ : ४]

Definition

Mobile or stationary tumour, round in shape with periodical increase or decrease in size and located between the heart and umbilicus is called *gulma*.

'स व्यस्तैर्जायते[1] दोषैः समस्तैरपि चोच्छ्रितैः ।
पुरुषाणां, तथा स्त्रीणां ज्ञेयो रक्तेन चापरः ॥३॥'

[सुश्रुत : उत्तरतन्त्र ४२ : ७-८]

Pathogenesis

It is caused by *vāyu*, *pitta* and *kapha*, vitiated individually or all the three vitiated simultaneously. The fifth variety which occurs only in females is caused by the vitiation of *rakta* (blood).

उद्गारबाहुल्यपुरीषबन्धतृप्त्यक्षमत्वान्त्रविकूजनानि ।
आटोपमाध्मान[2]मपक्तिशक्तिरासन्नगुल्मस्य वदन्ति चिह्नम् ॥४॥

---

1. यायते इति आदर्शपुस्तकेषु पाठः ।
2. आटोप आध्मानमपक्ति० इति आकरे पाठः ।

Premonitory Signs and Symptoms

Excessive eructation, constipation, sense of satisfaction, weakness, gurgling sound in the intestine, abdominal distension, *ādhmāna* (in percussion, producing a sound as if a drum is beaten) and absence of the power of digestion—these are the premonitory signs and symptoms of *gulma.*

अरुचिः कृच्छ्रविण्मूत्रवातताऽन्त्रविकूजनम्[1] ।
आनाहश्चोर्ध्ववातत्वं सर्वगुल्मेषु लक्षयेत् ॥५॥

General Symptoms

Anorexia, difficulty in passing urine, stool and flatus, gurgling sound in the intestines, abdominal distension and upward movement of abdominal wind—these are the general features of all types of *gulma.*

'रूक्षान्नपानं विषमातिमात्रं विचेष्टनं वेगविनिग्रहश्च ।
शोको[2] विघातो[ऽ]तिमलक्षयश्च निरन्नता चानिलगुल्महेतुः ॥६॥

Cause of Vātika Gulma

Intake of ununctuous food and drinks, irregular and excessive intake of food, wrong posture, suppression of *vegas* (natural urges), grief, injury, excessive excretion of waste products (*malas*) and fasting produce *vātika* type of *gulma.*

यः स्थानसंस्थानरुजा[3]विकल्पं विड्वातसङ्गं गलवक्त्रशोषम् ।
श्यावारुणत्वं शिशिरज्वरं च हृत्कुक्षिपार्श्वां[4]सशिरोरुजाश्च[5] ॥७॥

---

1. क. कृष्णविन् मूत्रं प्रततान्त्रविकूजनम् इति आदर्शपुस्तकेषु पाठः ।
   ख. कृष्णविन् मूत्रे प्रततान्त्रविकूजनम् इति चतुर्थपुस्तके पाठः ।
2. शोकोऽभिघातो० इति आकरे पाठः ।
3. ०रुजां इति आकरे पाठः ।
4. पार्श्वं इति आदर्शपुस्तकेषु पाठः ।
5. ०रुजं च इति आकरे पाठः ।

करोति जीर्णेऽभ्यधिकप्रकोपं[1] भुक्ते मृदुत्वं समुपैति यश्च ।

वातात्स गुल्मो न च तत्र रूक्षं कषायतिक्तं कटु चोपसेवेत्[2] ॥८॥

Signs and Symptoms of Vātika Gulma

Variability in location, shape and pain, obstruction to the passage of stool and flatus, dryness in the throat and mouth, grayish or pinkish colouration, fever with cold, pain in heart, pelvis, sides of the chest and head, more pain after the food is digested and reduction of pain after the intake of food—these are the characteristic features of *vātika gulma.* In such a condition, the patient should avoid ununctuous, astringent, bitter and pungent food and drinks.

कट्वम्लतीक्ष्णोष्णविदाहिरूक्षक्रोधातिमद्यार्क[3]हुताशसेवा ।

आमाभिघातो रुधिरं च दुष्टं पैत्तस्य गुल्मस्य निमित्तमुक्तम् ॥९॥

Causes of Paittika Gulma

Intake of pungent, sour, sharp, hot, *vidāhi* (which causes burning sensation) and ununctuous food as well as drinks, anger, intake of alcohol, exposure to sun and fire, affliction by *āma* (product of improper digestion and metabolism) and vitiation of blood are the causative factors of *paittika* type of *gulma.*

ज्वरः पिपासा वदनाङ्गरागः शूलं महज्जीर्यति भोजने च ।

स्वेदो विदाहो व्रणवच्च[4] गुल्मः स्पर्शासहः पैत्तिकगुल्मरूपम् ॥१०॥

Signs and Symptoms of Paittika Gulma

Fever, thirst, colouration of the face and body, excruciating colic pain during the digestion of food, sweating, burning

---

1. जीर्णे त्वधिकं इति आकरे पाठः ।
2. चोपशेते इति आकरे पाठः ।
3. मद्यार्कवहुताससेवा इति प्रथमपंचमषष्ठपुस्तकेषु पाठः ।
4. व्रणश्च इति आदर्शपुस्तकेषु पाठः ।

sensation, ulcer like growth and tenderness—these are the signs and symptoms of *paittika gulma.*

शीतं गुरु स्निग्धमचेष्टनं च सम्पूरणं[1] प्रस्वपनं दिवा च ।
गुल्मस्य हेतुः कफसंभवस्य सर्वस्तु दुष्टो निचयात्मकस्य ॥११॥

Causes of Kaphaja and Sānnipātika Gulma

Intake of cold, heavy and unctuous food, lack of exercise, over nourishment and sleep during the day time are the causative factors of *kaphaja gulma. Sānnipātika gulma* is caused by the simultaneous vitiation of all the three *doṣas* as a result of diet and regimens described in respect of each of them.

स्तैमित्यशीतज्वरगात्रसादहृल्लासकासारुचिगौरवाणि ।
शैत्यं रुगल्पा कठिनोन्नतत्वं गुल्मस्य रूपाणि कफात्मकस्य ॥१२॥

Signs and Symptoms of Kaphaja Gulma

Timidity, fever with cold, prostration, nausea, cough, anorexia, heaviness, feeling of cold, less of pain, hardness and increase in size are the signs and symptoms of *kaphaja gulma.*

निमित्तलिंगान्युपलभ्य[2] गुल्मे द्विदोषजे दोषबलाबलं च ।
व्यामिश्रलिङ्गानपरांस्तु[3] गुल्मान्[4] त्रीनादिशेदौषधकल्पनार्थम् ॥१३॥

Dvandvaja Gulma

Depending upon the causative factors and signs as well as symptoms, the physician should determine three varieties of *dvandvaja* i.e. *vāta-pittaja, vāta-kaphaja* and *kapha-vātaja gulma* which is relevant from the point of view of determining suitable medicaments.

---

1. संपूर्णं इति आदर्शपुस्तकेषु पाठः ।
2. ०रूपाण्युपलभ्य इति आकरे पाठः ।
3. ०लिङ्गानपरांश्च इति आकरे पाठः ।
4. गुल्मांस्त्रीनादिशेंदौषध० इति आकरे पाठः ।

महारुजं दाहपरीतमश्मवद्घनोन्नतं शीघ्रविदाहीदारुणम् ।
मनःशरीराग्निबलापहारिणं त्रिदोषजं गुल्ममसाध्यमादिशेत् ॥१४॥'

[चरक : चिकित्सा : ३ : ६-१७]

Sānnipātika Gulma

Excruciating pain, burning sensation, stone-like compact growth, quick suppuration, seriousness, reduction in the mental as well as physical strength, suppression of the power of digestion—these are the signs and symptoms of *gulma* caused by the simultaneous vitiation of all the three *doṣas*. This type of *gulma* is incurable.

'नवप्रसूता[ऽ]हितभोजना या या चामगर्भं[1] विसृजेदृतौ वा ।
वायुर्हि तस्याः परिगृह्य रक्तं करोति गुल्मं सरुजं सदाहम् ॥
पैत्तस्य लिङ्गेन समानलिङ्गं विशेषणं चाप्यपरं निबोध ॥१५॥'

[सुश्रुत : उत्तरतन्त्र : ४२ : १३-१४]

Raktaja Gulma in Females

If a lady takes unwholesome food immediately after delivery or after abortion or miscarriage and during the period of menstruation, *vāyu* in her body afflicts *rakta* (blood) and causes *gulma* with pain and burning sensation. Signs and symptoms of *paittika gulma* are manifested in this condition along with some others.

'यः सपन्दते पिण्डित एव
नाङ्गैश्चिरात्सशूलः समगर्भलिङ्गः ।
स रौधिरः स्त्रीभव एव गुल्मो मासे
व्यतीते दशमे चिकित्स्यः ॥१६॥'

[चरक : चिकित्सा : ३ : १६]

---

1. चामगर्भे इति प्रथमपुस्तके पाठः ।

Differential Diagnosis

In a lady suffering from *rakta gulma*, all the signs and symptoms of pregnancy are manifested. There will be *spandana* (palpitation or movement) but unlike pregnancy, the growth will have no limbs but it will appear like a round mass only. This is called *rakta gulma* which should be treated after the expiry of ten months.

'संचितः क्रमशो गुल्मो महावास्तुपरिग्रहः[1] ।
कृतमूलः[2] सिरानद्धो यदा कूर्म इवोन्नतः[3] ॥१७॥
दौर्बल्यारुचिहृल्लासकासवम्[4]यरतिज्वरैः ।
तृष्णातन्द्राप्रतिश्यायै[5]र्युज्यते स न सिध्यति ॥१८॥

Prognosis

If the growth in *gulma* gets gradually more and more accumulated and increased in size leading to the extension of the area of its location, if it is deeply seated, if it is surrounded by vessels, if it is elevated like the back of a tortoise and if the patient, in addition, suffers from weakness, anorexia, nausea, cough, vomiting, disliking for every thing, fever, thirst, drowsiness and acute form of cold, then the ailment is incurable.

गृहीत्वा सज्वरं श्वासच्छर्द्य[6]तीसारपीडितम् ।
हृन्नाभिहस्तपादेषु शोथः कर्षति गुल्मिनम् ॥१९॥'

[चरक : चिकित्सा : ५:१६६-१७१]

---

1. परिग्रहाः इति आदर्शपुस्तकेषु पाठः ।
2. क. कृतमूलं प्रथमपुस्तके पाठः ।
   ख. कृतशूलः पंचमपुस्तके पाठः ।
3. इवोत्थितः इति आकरे पाठः ।
4. ०कासच्छर्द्यरति० इति आकरे पाठः ।
5. ०प्रतिस्यायैर्यु० इति प्रथमपुस्तके पाठः ।
6. क. स्वासछर्द्यतोसार० इति प्रथमपुस्तके पाठः ।
   ख. सज्वरश्वासं वम्यतीसारपीडितम् इति आकरे पाठः ।

Fever, dyspnoea, vomiting, diarrhoea and oedema in the cardiac region, umbilical region, hands as well as legs lead to the death of the patient suffering from *gulma.*

श्वासशूलपिपासा[ऽ]न्नविद्वेषो ग्रन्थिमूढता ।
जायते दुर्बलत्वं च गुल्मिनो मरणाय वै ॥२०॥"

[माधवनिदान : गुल्मनिदान २८ : १-२०]

॥ इति गुल्मनिदानम् ॥२१॥

Dyspnoea, colic pain, thirst, disliking for food, immobility of the growth and weakness lead to the death of the patient suffering from *gulma.*

Thus, ends the diagnosis of *gulma.*

[गुल्मे क्रियाक्रम]—

"लङ्घनं दीपनं स्निग्धमुष्णं वातानुलोमनम् ।
बृंहणं यद्भवेत्सर्वं तद्धितं[1] सर्वगुल्मिनाम् ॥२२॥"

[भैषज्यरत्नावली : गुल्मरोगाधिकार : १]

Line of Treatment

Fasting, stimulation of the power of digestion and intake of unctuous, hot, *vātānulomana* (which helps in the downward movement of wind) as well as nourishing food and drinks—all these are wholesome for all types of *gulma.*

[गुल्मे स्वेदनम्]—

"स्निग्धस्य भिषजा स्वेदः कर्त्तव्यो गुल्मशान्तये ।
[2]स्रोतसां मार्दवं कृत्वा जित्वा मारुतमुल्वणम् ।
भित्वा विबन्धं स्निग्धस्य स्वेदो गुल्मान्[3] व्यपोहति ॥२३॥

1. वद्धितं इति आकरे पाठः ।
2. श्रोतसां इति आदर्शपुस्तकेषु पाठः ।
3. गुल्मं मपोहति इति आदर्शपुस्तकेषु पाठः ।

Fomentation Therapy

After oleation therapy, the patient suffering from *gulma* should be given fomentation therapy for getting relieved of the ailment. Fomentation, administered after oleation therapy softens the channels of circulation, alleviates the aggravated *vāyu* and relieves constipation as a result of which *gulma* is cured.

कुम्भीपिण्डेष्टकास्वेदान् कारयेत् कुशलो भिषक् ।
उपनाहाश्च कर्त्तव्याः सुखोष्णाः शाल्वणादयः ॥२४॥
स्थानावसेको[1] रक्तस्य बाहुमध्ये शिराव्यधः[2] ।
स्वेदो[ऽ]नुलोमनञ्चैव प्रशस्तं[3] सर्वगुल्मिनाम् ॥२५॥

The expert physician should administer *kumbhī*, *piṇḍa* and *iṣṭaka* types of fomentation in addition to *upanāha* (application of hot ointment) and luke-warm *śālvaṇa* type of fomentation. Blood-letting should be performed from the place where *gulma* is located and venesection should be done in the middle of the arm. Fomentation and *anulomana* (which helps in the downward movement of *vāyu*) therapies are useful for all types of *gulma*.

पेया वातहरैः सिद्धा कौलत्था जांगला[4] रसाः ।
खडाः सपञ्चमूलाश्च गुल्मिनां भोजने हिताः ॥२६॥

Diet

Peyā (thin gruel) prepared by boiling with drugs belonging to *vāta hara* (alleviator of *vāyu*) group, soup of *kulattha* and meat

---

1. गुल्मस्थाने रक्तमोक्षो इति आकरे पाठः ।
2. सिराव्यधः इति आकरे पाठः ।
3. प्रशस्तः इति प्रथमपंचमपुस्तकयोः पाठः ।
4. धान्वजा इति आकरे पाठः ।

of animals inhabiting arid land, and *khaḍa* (a sour preparation) made by boiling with *daśa mūla* are useful as diet of a patient suffering from *gulma*.

मातुलुङ्गरसो हिंगु दाडिमं विडसैन्धवम् ।
सुरामण्डेन पातव्यं वातगुल्मरुजापहम् ॥२७॥

The juice of *mātuluṅga* mixed with *hiṅgu*, *dāḍima*, *viḍa* and *saindhava* should be administered along with *surā maṇḍa* (alcoholic preparation) which cures the pain caused by *vātika* type of *gulma*.

नागरार्धपलं पिष्टं द्वे पले लुञ्चितस्य च ।
तिलस्यैकं गुडपलं क्षीरेणोष्णेन पाययेत् ॥
वातगुल्ममुदावर्त्तं योनिशूलञ्च नाशयेत् ॥२८॥

The paste of *nāgara* (half *pala*), dehusked sesamum seed (two *palas*) and jaggery (one *pala*) should be administered with hot milk which cures *vāta-gulma*, *udāvarta* and pain in the female genital tract.

पिबेदेरण्डतैलं वा वारुणीमण्डमिश्रितम् ।
तदेव तैलं पयसा वातगुल्मी पिबेन्नरः ॥२९॥

Castor oil should be administered either with *vāruṇī maṇḍa* (a type of alcoholic preparation) or water to a patient suffering from *vāta gulma*.

साधयेच्छुद्धशुष्कस्य रसोनस्य[1] चतुःपलम्[2] ।
क्षीरोदके त्रिगुणिते[3] क्षीरशेषञ्च पाययेत् ॥३०॥

---

1. लशुनस्य इति आकरे पाठः ।
2. चतुष्पलम् इति चतुर्थपुस्तके पाठः ।
3. क्षीरोदकेऽष्टगुणिते इति आकरे पाठः ।

वातगुल्ममुदावर्त्तं गृध्रसीं विषमज्वरम् ।
हृद्रोगं विद्रधिं शोषं साधयत्याशु[1] तत्पयः ।
एवं संसाधिते[2] क्षीरे स्तोकमप्यत्र[3] दीयते ॥३१॥

Four *palas* of dehusked and dried garlic should be boiled with three times (?) of each of milk and water, and reduced to the quantity of milk. This milk should be given for the immediate cure of *vāta gulma*, *udāvarta*, *gṛdhrasī* (sciatica), *viṣama jvara* (irregular fever), heart disease, abscess and consumption. This milk should be given in small quantities.

सर्जिका कुष्ठसहितः क्षारः केतकिजो[ऽ]पि[4] वा ।
तैलेन पीतः शमयेद् गुल्मं पवनसम्भवम् ॥३२॥

Intake of *svarji kṣāra*, *kuṣṭha* and alkali preparation of *ketakī* along with oil cures *vātika gulma*.

वातगुल्मे कफे वृद्धे वान्तिश्चूर्णादि शस्यते[5] ।
पित्ते विरेचनं स्निग्धं रक्ते रक्तस्य मोक्षणम् ॥३३॥"

[भैषज्यरत्नावली : गुल्मरोगाधिकार : ४-१५]

If *kapha* gets aggravated in a patient suffering from *vāta-gulma*, then emetic therapy should be administered. If *pitta* gets aggravated in a patient of *vāta gulma*, then unctuous purgative should be administered, and if *rakta* (blood) gets vitiated then blood letting therapy should be given.

1. नाशयत्याशु इति आकरे पाठः ।
2. एवन्तु साधिते इति आकरे पाठः ।
3. स्तोकमेवात्र इति आकरे पाठः ।
4. केतिकिजोपि इति प्रथमपुस्तके पाठः ।
5. चेष्यते इति आकरे पाठः ।

"स्निग्धोष्णेनोदिते गुल्मे पैत्तिके स्रंसनं हितम् ।
रूक्षोष्णेन तु सम्भूते सर्पिः प्रशमनं परम् ॥३४॥

Treatment of Pitta Gulma

If *pitta gulma* is caused by unctuous and hot things, then *sraṃsana* (mild laxative) is useful. If it is caused by ununctuous and hot things, then ghee is excellent for its alleviation.

काकोल्यादिमहातिक्तवासाद्यैः पित्तगुल्मिनम् ।
स्नेहितं स्रंसयेत्पश्चात् योजयेद्बस्तिकर्मणा[1] ॥३५॥

The patient of *pitta gulma* should be given oleation, mild purgation and medicated enema therapies and for all these, drugs belonging to *kākolyādi*, *mahātikta* and *vāsādi* groups should be used.

स्निग्धोष्णजे पित्तगुल्मे कम्पिल्लं मधुना लिहेत् ।
रे[2]चनार्थं[3] रसं वापि द्राक्षायाः सगुडं पिबेत् ॥३६॥

Pitta gulma caused by unctuous and hot things should be treated by the administration of *kampillaka* with honey. For purgation, the patient may be given the juice of *drākṣā* along with jaggery.

दाहशूलार्तिसंक्षोभस्वप्ननाशारु[4]चिज्वरैः ।

---

1. कर्मणि इति पञ्चमपुस्तके पाठः ।
2. 'द्राक्षारसोऽभया गुल्मे पैत्तिके सगुडां पिबेत् ।
मधुकं चन्दनं द्राक्षापयस्या मधुकं मधु ।
पिबेत्तंदुलतोयेन पित्तगुल्मप्रशान्तये' । पाठोऽयं पंचमपुस्तके अधिकमुपलभ्यते ।
3. रेचनार्थी इति आकरे पाठः ।
4. ०नाशारतिज्वरैः इति आकरे पाठः ।

विदह्यमानं[1] जानीयाद् गुल्मं तमुपनाहयेत् ॥३७॥"

[भैषज्यरत्नावली : गुल्मरोगाधिकार : २१-२४]

Burning sensation, colic pain, miserable feeling, sleeplessness, anorexia and fever—these signs and symptoms indicate the suppuration of *gulma*. Such patients should be treated with *upanāha* (hot ointment).

पक्वस्तु[2] पीडितोन्नामी[3] बहुतुंगोऽल्पवेदनः ।
श्यावो बस्तिनिभस्तत्रप्यधः शोधनरोपणे[4] ॥३८॥
"स्वयमूर्ध्वमधो वापि स चेद्दोषः[5] प्रपद्यते[6] ।
द्वादशाहमुपेक्षेत रक्षन्नन्यानुपद्रवान्[7] ॥३९॥"

[भैषज्यरत्नावली : गुल्मरोगाधिकार : २५]

If the growth in *gulma* is fully suppurated, then it takes a bolus form and gets elevated with several peaks. There will be reduction in pain. The area becomes grayish black and it feels as if a bladder is being palpated. In such a condition purgation and healing (*ropaṇa*) therapies should be administered. If the faulty material comes out of its own by upward or downward tracts, then the physician should wait for twelve days and during this period only complications, if any, should be treated.

---

1. विदाह्यमानं इति आकरे पाठः ।
2. पक्वसु इति पंचमपुस्तके पाठः ।
3. पीडितोन्नामी इति चतुर्थपुस्तके पाठः ।
4. रोपणा इति प्रथमद्वितीयपुस्तकयोः पाठः ।
5. क. चेदोषप्रपद्यते इति प्रथमपुस्तके पाठः ।
   ख. चेदोषः प्रपद्यते इति चतुर्थपुस्तके पाठः ।
6. प्रवर्त्तते इति आकरे पाठः ।
7. ०द्रवात् इति प्रथमपुस्तके पाठः ।

परन्तु शोधनं सर्पिः शुद्धं समधुतिक्तकम् ॥४०॥

The best healing therapy is pure ghee mixed with honey and bitter drugs. [The meaning of this line is not clear. Something appears to be missing here].

"रोहिणीकटुकानिम्बमधूकत्रिफलात्वचः ।
कर्षांशास्त्रायमाणा[1] च पलं च त्रिवृता पलम् ॥४१॥
द्विपलञ्च[2] मसूराणां साध्यमष्टगुणेऽम्भसि ।
शृताच्छेषं घृतसमं सर्पिषश्च चतुः पलम् ॥४२॥
पिबेत्संमूर्छितं तेन गुल्मः शाम्यति पैत्तिकः ।
ज्वरस्तृष्णा च शूलं च भ्रमो मूर्च्छाऽरुचिस्तमः[3] ॥४३॥"

[चरक : चिकित्सा : ५ : ११५-११७]

दीप्ताग्नयो महाकाया स्नेहसात्म्याश्च ये नराः ।
गुल्मिनः सर्पदष्टाश्च विषे[4]नोपहताश्च ये ।
जेष्ठां[5] मात्रां[6] पिबेयुस्ते पलान्यष्टौ विशेषतः ॥४४॥

[इति रोहिण्याद्यं[7] घृतम्]

1. शास्त्रायमाणा च पटोलत्रिवृतोः पले इति आकरे पाठः ।
2. द्वे पले च इति आकरे पाठः ।
3. ०ऽरुचिस्तथा इति आकरे पाठः ।
4. सर्प्पोपहताश्चये इति चतुर्थपुस्तके पाठः ।
5. जेष्ठं इति चतुर्थपुस्तके पाठः ।
6. मात्रंऽपि इति पंचमपुस्तके पाठः ।
7. पाठोऽयं आदर्शपुस्तकेषु नोपलभ्यते ।

Rohiṇyādya Ghṛta

One *karṣa* of each of *rohiṇī*, *kaṭukā*, *nimba*, *madhūka*, *triphalā* and *tvak*, one *pala* of each of *trāyamāṇā* and *trivṛt*, and two *palas* of *masūra* should be boiled with eight times of water and reduced to one fourth. To this decoction, equal quantity of ghee should be added and cooked. Intake of this medicated ghee in the dose of four *palas* cures *paittika gulma*, fever, thirst, colic pain, giddiness, fainting, anorexia and *tama* (a feeling as if entering into darkness). Persons having strong digestive power and robust physique and those who are habituated to taking ghee should take this recipe in a higher dose of eight *palas* if they suffer from *gulma*, snake bite and other forms of poisoning.

"लङ्घनोल्लेखने स्वेदे कृतेऽग्नौ संप्रधूक्षते[1] ।"

[चरक : चिकित्सा : ५ : ५२]

"घृतं सं[2]स्कारकटुकं पातव्यं कफगुल्मिनाम् ॥४५॥"

[भैषज्यरत्नावली : गुल्माधिकार : २७]

Treatment of Kaphaja Gulma

For the treatment of *kaphaja gulma*, ghee cooked with *kaṭuka* should be administered when the digestive power is stimulated after the administration of fasting, emetic and fomentation therapies.

"मन्दोऽग्निर्वेदना मन्दा गुरुस्तिमितकोष्ठता ।

सोत्क्लेशश्चारुचिर्यस्य स गुल्मी वमनोपगः ॥४६॥"

[चरक : चिकित्सा : ५ : ४९-५०]

[भैषज्यरत्नावली : गुल्माधिकार : २८]

---

1. संप्रधक्षिते इति श्राकरे पाठः ।
2. च क्षारकटुकं इति श्राकरे पाठः ।

Patients suitable for Emetic Therapy

The patient suffering from *gulma*, who has less of digestive power, less of pain, heaviness, sluggish digestive tract, nausea and anorexia, is suitable for the administration of emetic therapy.

"मन्देऽग्नावनिले मूढे ज्ञात्वा सस्नेहमाशयम् ।
गुटिकाचूर्णनिर्यूहाः प्रयोज्याः कफगुल्मिनाम् ॥४७॥"

[चरक : चिकित्सा : ५ : ५४-५५]

[भैषज्यरत्नावली : गुल्माधिकार : २६]

The patient suffering from *kaphaja gulma* has generally sluggish digestive power and sluggish movement of wind. To such patients, oleation therapy should be administered, and thereafter, other medicines in the form of pill, powder or decoction should be given.

क्षारारिष्टगणो वापि दाहः शेषेऽभिधीयते ॥४८॥

Cauterization (*dāha*) therapy, wherever necessary, should be employed. Thereafter, *kṣārāriṣṭa* (an alcoholic preparation containing alkalies) should be employed.

पञ्चमूलीशृतं तोयं पुराणं वारुणीरसम् ।
"कफगुल्मी पिबेत् काले जीर्णं[1] माध्वीकमेव वा ॥४९॥"

[चरक : चिकित्सा : ५ : ५३]

The patient suffering from *kaphaja gulma*, should be administered the decoction of *pañca mūla*, old *vāruṇi* (a type of alcoholic preparation) and old *mādhvīka* type of wine in appropriate time.

---

1. सक्षारकटुकं घृतम् इति आकरे पाठः ।

"तिलैरण्डातसीबीजसर्षपैः[1] परिपाल्य च ।
श्लेष्मगुल्ममयःपात्रैः[2] सुखोष्णैः स्वेदयेद्भिषक् ॥५०॥

In an iron pan, *tila, eraṇḍa, atasī* and *sarṣapa* seeds should be kept and ignited. With this (slightly worm pot), the patient suffering from *kaphaja gulma* should be fomented.

[3]यमानीचूर्णितं तक्रं विडेन लवणीकृतम् ।

---

1. अपामार्गपलशतं तथैव क्षुरकस्य च ।
स्नुह्यर्कयोर्मातुलंगकुष्ठस्य अग्निकस्य च ।
तिलसर्षपनालग्नि [नालानि] दग्धभस्मानि कारयेत् ।
गोजविडम् [विण्मूत्र] च सहितं सर्पिस्तैलसमन्वितम् ।
त्र्यूषणं पिप्पलीमूलं चित्रकं शुष्कमूलकम् ।
मूर्वामतिविषां पाठां कुष्ठभल्लातकानि च ।
चव्यं पूतिकरञ्जं च तिल्वकं कटुरोहिणी ।
द्वौ क्षारौ पंचलवणं समभागानि कारयेत् ।
सनीयचूर्णंलवणं शनैर्मृद्वग्निना पचेत् ।
तदग्निचूर्णनिर्धूमं कृत्वा चूर्णं सुशीतलम् ॥
अंगुलिग्रहमालोढ्य सुरामण्डेन पाययेत् ।
मस्त्वारनालयूषैस्तु युक्तस्याद्वातगुल्मनुत् ॥
शूलवातोदरे प्लीहपाण्ड्वामयकिलास [म]कम् ।
हन्यादारोग्यलवणं प्रशस्तं कफवातनुत् ॥—॥आरोग्यलवणम् ॥
पाठोऽयं चतुर्थपंचमपुस्तकयोः अधिकमुपलभ्यते ।
2. पत्रैः इति आकरे पाठः ।
3. "चित्रकत्रिवृतादन्तीत्रिफलारुष्करैः समैः ।
यावदेतानि चूर्णानि तावन्मात्रं सुसैन्धवम् ॥
भावितं तत् स्नुहीक्षीरमृद्भाण्डे च क्षिपेत्ततः ।
मृत्येकानुलिप्तं च तत्प्रक्षिपेज्जातवेदसि ॥
सुदग्धं तु ततः कृत्वाऽधरे तुरानैर्भिषक् ।
यकृत्प्लीहोदरानाहगुल्मपाण्ड्वामयादिहेत्॥
सेवितोग्निबलं मत्वा अर्शोभ्यः प्रतिमोचयेत् ।
लवणाग्निमुखोनाम वह्निदीप्तिकरः परः ॥—॥ अग्निमुखं लवणम ॥"
पाठोऽयं चतुर्थपचंमपुस्तकयोः अधिकमुपलभ्यते ।

पिबेत्सन्दीपनं वातमूत्रवर्चोऽनुलोमनम् ॥५१॥

Butter-milk added with *yamānī* powder and *viḍa* type of salt should be given. It stimulates the power of digestion and helps in the downward movement of flatus, urine and stool.

वि[1]मिश्रदोषे व्यामिश्र ए[2]ष एव क्रियाक्रमः ।
सन्निपातोद्भवे गुल्मे त्रिदोषघ्नो विधिर्हितः ॥५२॥"

[भैषज्यरत्नावली : गुल्माधिकार : ३३-३५]

If *gulma* is caused by the simultaneous vitiation of two *doṣas*, then treatment in respect of these two *doṣas* should be administered. If, however, all the three *doṣas* are simultaneously vitiated to cause *gulma*, then treatment in respect of all the three *doṣas* combined should be administered.

"वचाविडाभयाशुण्ठीहिंगुकुष्ठाग्निदी[3]पकाः ।
द्वित्रिषट्चतुरेकाष्टसप्तपंचांशिकाः क्रमात् ॥५३॥
चूर्णं मद्यादिभिः पीतं गुल्मानाहोदरापहम् ।
शूलार्शःश्वासकासघ्नं ग्रहणीदीपनं परम् ॥५४॥"

॥वचाद्यं[4] चूर्णम् ॥

Vacādya Cūrṇa

Vacā (two parts), *viḍa* (three parts), *abhayā* (six parts), *śuṇṭhī* (four parts), *hiṅgu* (eight parts), *kuṣṭha* (seven parts) and

1. व्यामिश्रदोषे इति आकरे पाठः ।
2. सर्वं इति आकरे पाठः ।
3. ०दीप्यकाः इति आकरे पाठः ।
4. पाठोऽयं आदर्शपुस्तकेषु नोपलभ्यते ।

agnidīpaka (five parts) should be made to a powder and administered along with alcoholic drinks, etc. It cures *gulma*, *ānāha* (abdominal distension), *udara* (obstinate abdominal diseases including ascites), colic pain, piles, asthma and cough. It is an excellent stimulant of the functioning of *grahaṇī* (small intestine including duodenum.)

"यमानीहिंगुसिन्धूत्थक्षारसौवर्चलाभयाः ।
सुरामण्डेन पातव्याः शूलगुल्मनिषूदनाः ॥५५॥"

[यमान्यादिचूर्णम्[1]]

[भैषज्यरत्नावली : गुल्माधिकार : ३९-४१]

Yamānyādi Cūrṇa

The powder of *yamānī*, *hiṅgu*, rock-salt, *kṣāra* (alkali preparation), *sauvarcala* and *abhayā* should be given along with *surā maṇḍa* (a type of alcoholic preparation) which cures *gulma* and colic pain.

"हिंगु[2] त्रिकटुकं पाठां हबुषा[3]मभयाशटीम् ।
अजमोदाजगन्धा[4] च तिन्तिडीकाम्लवेतसौ ॥५६॥

---

1. पाठोऽयं आदर्शपुस्तकेषु नोपलभ्यते ।
2. "शुक्ति क्षारनिशखिशालकदलो स्यात्शूरणं कोकिला ।
पामासंदहनार्जुनं सलवणापा मार्गकुष्मांडकम् ॥
दग्ध्वा क्षारविपाचितं परिशृतं हिंगुत्रिकद्वान्वितम् ।
गुल्मानाहविबन्धशूलहरणं सर्वोदराणां हितम् ॥
॥ क्षारामृतम् ॥"
पाठोऽयं चतुर्थपंचमपुस्तकयोः अधिकमुपलभ्यते ।
3. हपुषा० इति चरके पाठः ।
4. अजमोदाजगन्धे इति आकरे पाठः ।

दाडिमं पौष्करं धान्यमजाजीचित्रकं वचाम् ।
द्वौ क्षारौ लवणे द्वे च चव्यं चैकत्र चूर्णयेत् ॥५७॥
चूर्णमेतत् प्रयोक्तव्यमन्नपाने निरत्ययम् ।
प्रगभक्तमथवा पेयं मद्येनोष्णोदकेन वा ॥५८॥
पार्श्वहृद्वस्तिशूलेषु गुल्मे वातकफात्मके ।
आनाहे मूत्रकृच्छ्रे वा गुदयोनिरुजासु च ॥५९॥
ग्रहण्यर्शोविकारेषु प्लीह्नि पाण्ड्वामयेऽरुचौ ।
उरोविबन्धे हिक्कायां कासे[1] श्वासे गलग्रहे ॥६०॥
भावितं मातुलुङ्गस्य चूर्णमेतद्रसेन वा ।
बहुशो गुडिकाः[2] कार्याः कार्मुकाः स्युस्ततोऽधिकम्[3] ॥६१॥"

॥ इति हिंग्वादिचूर्णम्[4] ॥

[चरक : चिकित्सा : ५ : ७९-८४]

[भैषज्यरत्नावली : गुल्माधिकार : ४२-४७]

Hiṅgvādi Cūrṇa

Hiṅgu, trikaṭu, pāṭhā, habuṣā, abhayā, śaṭī, ajamodā, ajagandhā, tintiḍīka, amla vetasa, dāḍima, puṣkara mūla, dhānya, ajājī, citraka, vacā, svarjī kṣāra, yava kṣāra, saindhava, sāmudra

---

1. क. कासश्वासे इति प्रथमपुस्तके पाठः ।
   ख. काशे श्वासे इति चतुर्थपुस्तके पाठः ।
2. गुटिकाः इति चरके पाठः ।
3. ०धिकाः इति प्रथमपुस्तके पाठः ।
4. 'इति हिंग्वादि चूर्णं गुटिका च' इति आकरे पाठः ।

lavaṇa and *cavya*—all these drugs should be made to a powder. This powder should be given along with food and drinks or before food along with *madya* (alcoholic drink) or hot water for the alleviation of pain in the sides of the chest, heart as well as urinary bladder, *vātika gulma*, *kaphaja gulma*, *ānāha* (abdominal distension), dysuria, pain in anus as well as female genital tract, *grahaṇī* (sprue syndrome), piles, splenic disorder, anemia, anorexia, stiffness of the chest, hic-cup, cough, dyspnoea and obstruction in the throat.

This powder may be impregnated with the juice of *mātuluṅga* and pills should be prepared. These pills work better than the powder in the treatment of the above mentioned ailments.

[1]पूतीकपत्रगजचिर्भटचव्यवह्निव्योषश्च
संस्तरचितं लवणोपधानम् ।
दग्धं विचूर्ण्य दधिमस्तुयुतं प्रयोज्यं
गुल्मोदरश्वयथुपाण्डुगुदोद्भवेषु ॥६२॥

---

1. क. क्षारद्वयानलव्योषनीली लवण यवकम् ।
चूर्णितं सर्पिषा पेयं सर्वगुल्मोदरापहम् ।।
पाठोऽयं चतुर्थपुस्तके अधिकमुपलभ्यते ।

ख. "हिंगुग्रथिकधान्यजीरकवचाचव्याग्निपाठासटी ।
वृक्षाम्लं लवण त्रयं त्रिकटुकं क्षारद्वयं दाडिमम् ।।
पथ्यापौष्करवेतसाम्लहपुषाजाज्यस्तेदभि: कृत ।
चूर्णं भावितमतदाद्रकरसैः स्याद्बीजपूरद्रवै: ।
आध्मानं ग्रहणीविकारगुदजान्गुल्मानुदावर्तकाम् ।
प्रत्याध्मानगरोदरास्मीरयुतां स्तनो (स्तूणी) द्वयं रोचकान् ।
उरुस्तम्भमतिभ्रमं च मात्रसो वाधिर्यमष्ठिलिकान् ।
प्रत्यष्ठीलाकफामथापहरते: माकपोत (प्राक्यात) मुष्णाम्बुना ।
हृत्कुक्षिवंक्षणकटीजठरांतरेषुबस्तिहृन्नशफलकेषु च ।
पार्श्वयोश्च शूलानि नाशयति वातवतासजानि:
हिंग्वादिः मांद्यमिदं माश्विनं संहितायाम् ।
।। हिंग्वादि चूर्णम् ।।"
पाठोऽयं चतुर्थपंचमपुस्तकयोः अधिकमुपलभ्यते ।

Leaves of *pūtīka*, *gaja cirbhaṭa*, *cavya*, *vahni* and *vyoṣa* should be spread in layers intercepted by the layers of rock-salt in a jar and should be cooked. Thereafter, ingredients should be made to a powder. Administration of this with butter-milk is useful in *gulma*, *udara* (obstinate abdominal diseases including ascites), oedema, anemia and piles.

"हिंगुपुष्करमूलानि तुम्बुरूणि हरीतकी ।
श्यामा विडं सैन्धवञ्च यवक्षारं महौषधम् ॥६३॥
यवक्वाथोदकेनैतद् घृतभृष्टन्तु पाययेत् ।
तेनास्य भिद्यते गुल्मः सशूलः सपरिग्रहः ॥६४॥

[॥ अपरं हिङ्ग्वादिचूर्णम्[1] ॥]

Hiṅgvādi Cūrṇa (Second Recipe)

Hiṅgu, *puṣkara mūla*, *tumburu*, *harītakī*, *śyāmā*, *viḍa*, *saindhava*, *yava kṣāra* and *mahauṣadha* should be fried by adding ghee. This powder, administered along with the decoction of barley, cures *gulma*, deeply located and associated with colic pain.

वचा हरीतकी हिङ्गु सैन्धवं साम्लवेतसम् ।
यवक्षारं यमानीञ्च पिबेदुष्णेन वारिणा ॥६५॥
एतद्धि गुल्मनिचयं सशूलं सपरिग्रहम् ।
भिनत्ति सप्तरात्रेण वह्नेर्वृद्धिं करोति च ॥६६॥"

[॥ वचादिचूर्णम्[2] ॥]

[भैषज्यरत्नावली : गुल्माधिकार : ४८-५१]

---

1. पाठोऽयं आदर्शपुस्तकेषु नोपलभ्यते ।
2. क. पाठोऽयं आदर्शपुस्तकेषु नोपलभ्यते ।
 ख. वचाद्यं इति चतुर्थपुस्तके पाठः ।

Vacādi Cūrṇa

The powder of *vacā*, *harītakī*, *hiṅgu*, *saindhava*, *amla vetasa*, *yava kṣāra* and *yamānī* should be taken along with hot water. Within seven days, this cures *gulma* which is associated with colic pain and which is deeply located. It also promotes the power of digestion.

"पिप्पलीपिप्पलीमूलचित्रकाजाजिसैन्धवैः ।
युक्ता पीता सुरा हन्ति गुल्ममाशु सुदुस्तरम् ॥६७॥"

[भैषज्यरत्नावली : गुल्माधिकार : ३२]

Alcohol taken along with the powder of *pippalī*, *pippalī mūla*, *citraka*, *ajāji* and *saindhava* instantaneously cures even serious types of *gulma*.

"जवानी[1] जीरकं धान्यमरिचं[2] गिरिकर्णिका ।
अजमोदोपकुंची च चतुः शाणं[3] पृथक् पृथक् ॥६८॥
हिंगु षट्शाणिकं कार्यं क्षारौ लवणपंचकम् ।
त्रिवृदष्टमितैः[4] शाणैः प्रत्येकं कल्पयेत् सुधीः ॥६९॥
दंती शठी पौष्करं च विडङ्गं दाडिमं शिवा ।
चित्राम्लवेतसः शुंठी शाणैः षोडशभिः पृथक् ॥७०॥

---

1. क. "जवानी .... काङ्कायनवटी" पाठोऽयं प्रथमपुस्तके नोपलभ्यते ।
   ख. यवानी इति आकरे पाठः ।
2. धान्यं मरिचं इति आकरे पाठः ।
3. चतुः शाणा इति आकरे पाठः ।
4. त्रिवृच्चाष्टमितैः इति आकरे पाठः ।

बीजपूररसेनैषां गुटिकाः[1] कारयेत्[2] सुधी ।
घृतेन पयसा मद्यैरम्लैरुष्णोदकेन वा ॥७१॥
पिबेत् कांकायनप्रोक्तां गुटिकां गुल्मनाशिनीम्[3] ।
मद्येन वातिकं गुल्मं गोक्षीरेण च पैत्तिकम् ॥७२॥
मूत्रेण कफगुल्मं च दशमूलैस्त्रिदोषजम् ।
उष्ट्रीदुग्धेन[4] नारीणां रक्तगुल्मं निवारयेत् ॥
हृद्रोगं ग्रहणीशूलं[5] कृमीनर्शांसि नाशयेत् ॥७३॥
॥ काङ्कायन वटी[6] ॥"

[भारतभैषज्यरत्नाकर : प्रथमभाग : पृष्ठ १८७]

Kāṅkāyana Vaṭi (First Recipe)

Four *śāṇas* of each of *javānī*, *jīraka*, *dhānya*, *marica*, *giri karṇikā*, *ajamodā* and *upakuñcikā*, six *śāṇas* of *hiṅgu*, eight *śāṇas* of each of *svarji kṣāra*, *yava kṣāra*, *lavaṇa pañcaka* and *trivṛt* and sixteen *śāṇas* of each of *dantī*, *śaṭhī*, *puṣkara mūla*, *viḍaṅga*, *dāḍima*, *śivā*, *citra*, *amla vetasa* and *śuṇṭhī* should be impregnated and triturated with the juice of *bīja-pūra*. From out of this paste, pills should be prepared and administered along with ghee, milk, alcoholic drinks, sour juice or hot water. This pill is propounded by the sage *Kāṅkāyana* which cures

---

1. गुटिका इति ग्रादर्शपुस्तकेषु पाठः ।
2. कारयेद्बुध: इति ग्राकरे पाठः ।
3. गुल्मनाशिनम् इति पंचमपुस्तके पाठः ।
4. उष्ट्रदुग्धेन इति ग्राकरे पंचमपुस्तके च पाठः ।
5. ग्रहणीं शूलं इति ग्राकरे पाठः ।
6. काकायन गुटिका इति ग्राकरे पाठः ।

gulma. Along with alcoholic drinks, it cures *vātika gulma*, taken with cow's milk, it cures *paittika gulma*, along with cow's urine, it cures *kaphaja gulma*, along with the decoction of *daśa mūla*, it cures *tridoṣaja gulma* and along with camel milk, it cures *rakta gulma* of females. This pill also cures heart diseases, *grahaṇī* (sprue syndrome), colic pain, parasitic infestation and piles.

वासामुष्ककपाटलासलवणा दग्ध्वा जले पाचितम् ।
हिङ्ग्वादिप्रतिवापमेतदुदितं गुल्मोदराष्टीलिषु ॥७४॥

Vāsā, muṣkaka, pāṭalā and rock-salt should be burnt to ash and boiled with water. To this, small quantity of *hiṅgu* should be added. This is useful in the treatment of *gulma, udara* (obstinate abdominal diseases including ascites) and *aṣṭhilā* (hard tumour).

"हिङ्गूग्रगन्धाविडशुण्ठ्यजाजीहरीतकीपुष्करमूलकुष्ठम् ।
भागोत्तरं चूर्णितमेतदिष्टं गुल्मोदराजीर्णविसूचिकासु ॥७५॥"

॥ हिङ्ग्वादिचूर्णम्[1] ॥

[भैषज्यरत्नावली : गुल्माधिकार : ५२]

Hiṅgvādi Cūrṇa

Hiṅgu (one part), *ugragandhā* (two parts), *viḍa* (three parts), *śuṇṭhī* (four parts), *ajājī* (five parts), *harītakī* (six parts), *puṣkara mūla* (seven parts), and *kuṣṭha* (eight parts) should be made to a powder. It is useful in the treatment of *gulma, udara* (obstinate abdominal diseases including ascites), indigestion and *visūcikā* (choleric diarrhoea).

[2]'नादेयीकुटजार्कशिग्रुबृहतीस्नुक्बिल्वभल्लातकम् ।
व्याघ्रीकिंशुकपारिभद्रकजटापामार्गदीप्याग्निकम् ॥७६॥'

1. हिंग्वादिः इति आदर्शपुस्तकेषु पाठः ।
2. 'नादेयी० .... ०दीप्याग्निकम्' पाठोऽयं प्रथमपुस्तके नोपलभ्यते ।

The powder of *nādeyī*, *kuṭaja*, *arka*, *śigru*, *bṛhatī*, *snuk*, *bilva*, *bhallātaka*, *vyāghrī*, *kiṃśuka*, *pāribhadra* (root), *apāmārga*, *dīpyaka* and *agnika* [should be made to a powder and administered for the treatment of *gulma*. The recipe is incomplete.]

त्रिफलाकाञ्चनक्षीरी-सप्तलानीलिनी-वचा- ।
त्रायन्तीहबुषातिक्तात्रिवृत् सैन्धवपिप्पलीः ॥७७॥
पिबेद्विचूर्ण्यं मूत्रोष्णवारिमांसरसादिभिः ।
सर्वगुल्मोदरप्लीहकुष्ठार्शःशोथखेदितः ॥७८॥

॥ त्रिफलाद्यम् ॥[1][2]

Triphalādya Cūrṇa

Triphalā, *kāñcana kṣīrī*, *saptalā*, *nīlinī*, *vacā*, *trāyanti*, *habuṣā*,

---

1. पाठोऽयं प्रथमपुस्तके नोपलभ्यते ।
2. 'क्षीरं वज्रतरूद्भवं दशपलं तावत्पयोप्यर्कजम् ।
प्रत्येकं पलं पंचलवणं क्षारं च पंचात्मकम् ।
विशत्यार्कदलैर्युतं भवितेरोभिश्चैश्चतुर्भिः ।
पलैर्मृद्धांडेगुरुपागतो गजपुटेवह्नौ विपक्वीकृतम् ।
संचूर्ण्यथिकटुत्रयं त्रिफलमय्येकं रामठम् ।
सर्ववस्त्रपुनीतमेतदमले पात्रे सुखं स्थापयेत् ।
वज्रक्षारं मिदं निहंति सकलाल्गुल्मानुदग्रान्नृणाम् ।
पीतं तक्रयुतं प्रभातसमये कर्षप्रमाणं क्रमात् ।
मन्दाग्निसविषुचिकामरुचितामापांडुताम् क्षीणताम् ।
श्वासकासमजीर्णशैत्यपवनप्याधीन् बलासोद्भवान् ।
वज्रक्षारमिदं भिवार्यभिषजाम् कीर्तिं चदर्त्तशम् ।
मांसं दीप्यति स्फुटं घटिकयोर्द्धं द्वे किमन्नं पुनः ।
वाते कोष्णजलं पेयं घृतं पित्ताधिके पिबेत् ।
कफे गोमूत्रसंयुक्तं मारनालं त्रिदोषजे ।
वज्रक्षारानुपानम् ।
॥इति वज्रक्षारम्॥' पाठोऽयं चतुर्थपुस्तके अधिकमुपलभ्यते ।

tiktā, *trivṛt*, *saindhava* and *pippali* should be made to a powder and administered along with cow's urine, hot water, meat soup, etc. It cures all types of *gulma*, *udara* (obstinate abdominal diseases including ascites), splenic disorders, *kuṣṭha* (obstinate skin diseases including leprosy), piles and oedema.

"शटी पुष्करमूलञ्च दन्ती चित्रकमाढकीम् ।
शृंगवेरं वचाञ्चैव पलिकानि समाहरेत् ॥७९॥
त्रिवृतायाः पलञ्चैव[1] कुर्यात् त्रीणि च हिंगुनः ।
यव क्षारपले द्वे च द्वे पले चाम्लवेतसात् ॥८०॥
यमान्यजाजीमरिचं धान्यकञ्चेति कार्षिकम् ।
उपकुञ्च्यजमोदाभ्यां[2] तथा चाष्टमिकामपि ॥८१॥
मातुलुङ्गरसे चैताः गुडिकाः कारयेद्भिषक् ।
[3]आसाञ्चैकां पिबेद् द्वे वा तिस्रो वाथ सुखाम्बुना ॥८२॥
अम्लैश्च[4] मद्यैर्यूषैश्च घृतेन पयसाथवा ।
एषा कांकायनोक्ता च गुटिका[5] गुल्मनाशिनी ॥८३॥
अर्शोहृद्रोगशमनी कृमीणाञ्च विनाशिनी ।
गोमूत्रयुक्ता शमयेत् कफगुल्मं चिरोत्थितम्[6] ॥८४॥

---

1. पलञ्चैकं इति आकरे पाठः ।
2. ०जमोदाभ्यां इति प्रथमपुस्तके पाठः ।
3. तासामेकां इति प्रथमपुस्तके पाठः ।
4. अम्लैर्मद्यैश्च यूषैश्च इति आकरे पाठः ।
5. गुडिका इति आदर्शपुस्तकेषु पाठः ।
6. चिरोच्छ्रितम् इति पंचमपुस्तके पाठः ।

क्षीरेण पित्तगुल्मञ्च मद्यैरम्लैश्च वातिकम् ।
त्रिफलारसमूत्रैश्च नियच्छेत् सान्निपातिकम् ॥
रक्तगुल्मे च नारीणामुष्ट्रीक्षीरेण पाययेत् ॥८५॥
॥ काङ्कायनगुटिका[1] ॥"
[भैषज्यरत्नावली : गुल्माधिकार : ५६-६२]

Kāṅkāyana Guṭikā (Second Recipe)

One *pala* of each of *śaṭi*, *puṣkara mūla*, *dantī*, *citraka*, *āḍhakī*, *śṛṅgavera*, *vacā* and *trivṛt*, three *palas* of *hiṅgu*, two *palas* of each of *yava kṣāra* and *amla vetasa*, one *karṣa* of each of *yamānī*, *ajājī*, *marica* and *dhānyaka* and one *aṣṭamikā* of each of *upakuñcī* and *ajamodā* should be triturated along with the juice of *mātuluṅga* and pills should be made out. One or two or three of these pills should be administered along with luke-warm water, sour juice, alcoholic drinks, vegetable soup, ghee or milk. This recipe is propounded by the sage *Kāṅkāyana*. It cures *gulma*, piles, heart diseases and parasitic infestations. Along with cow's urine, it cures chronic *kaphaja gulma*. Along with milk, it is capable of curing *paittika gulma*. Along with alcoholic drinks and sour juice, it cures *vātika gulma*. Along with *triphalā* decoction or cow's urine, it cures *sānnipātika gulma*. For the *rakta gulma* in females, it should be administered along with camel-milk. [This recipe is a variant reading of the one given earlier in verses 68-73].

"हबुषा-व्योष-पृथ्वीका-चव्य-चित्रक-सैन्धवैः ।
[2]अजाजीपिप्पलीमूलदीप्यकैर्विपचेत् घृतम् ॥८६॥

1. ०गुडिका इति आकरे पाठः ।
2. सजाजीपिप्पलीमूलदीप्यकैः पाचयेद् घृतम् । इति आकरे पाठः ।

सकोलमूलकरसं सक्षीरदधिदाडिमम् ।
अत्यन्तवातगुल्मघ्नं[1] शूलानाहविबन्धनुत् ॥८७॥
योन्यर्शोग्रहणीदोषश्वासकासारुचिज्वरान् ।
पार्श्वहृद्वस्तिशूलञ्च घृतमेतद् व्यपोहति ॥८८॥

॥ हबुषाद्यं घृतम् ॥

Habuṣādya Ghṛta

Ghee cooked with the paste of *habuṣā*, *vyoṣa*, *pṛthvīkā*, *cavya*, *citraka*, *saindhava*, *ajājī*, *pippalī mūla* and *dīpyaka*, juice of *kola*, *mūlaka*, as well as *dāḍima* and milk as well as curd is very effective in curing *vāta gulma*, colic pain, *ānāha* (abdominal distension), constipation, diseases of the female genital tract, piles, *grahaṇī* (sprue syndrome), dyspnoea, cough, anorexia, fever and pain in the sides of the chest, heart as well as urinary bladder.

पिप्पल्याः पिचुरध्यर्द्धो दाडिमाद् द्विपलं पलम् ।
धान्यात् पञ्च घृताच्छुण्ठ्या कर्षं क्षीरचतुर्गुणम् ॥८९॥
सिद्धमेतद्घृतं सद्यो वातगुल्मं नियच्छति[2] ।
योनिशूलं शिरःशूलमर्शांसि विषमज्वरम् ॥९०॥

॥ पञ्चपलं घृतम् ॥"

[भैषज्यरत्नावली : गुल्माधिकार : ७५-७९]

Pañca Pala Ghṛta

Five *palas* of ghee should be cooked with one and half *palas* of *pippalī*, two *palas* of *dāḍima*, one *pala* of *dhānya*, one *karṣa* of *śuṇṭhī* and four times in quantity of milk. This cures *vātika gulma*, pain in female genital tract, headache, piles and *viṣama jvara* (irregular fever).

---

1. तत्परं इति आकरे पाठः ।
2. चिकित्सति इति आकरे पाठः ।

"त्र्यूषणत्रिफलाधान्यविडङ्गचव्यचित्रकैः ।
कल्कैरेतैर्घृ[1]तं सिद्धं सक्षीरं वातगुल्मनुत् ॥६१॥
॥ त्र्यूषणाद्यं घृतम् ॥"
[भैषज्यरत्नावली : गुल्माधिकार : ८८]

Tryūṣaṇādya Ghṛta

Ghee boiled with the paste of *tryūṣaṇa, triphalā, dhānya, viḍaṅga, cavya* as well as *citraka* and milk cures *vātika gulma.*

"जले दशगुणे साध्यं त्रायमाना चतुःपलम् ।
पञ्चभागस्थितं पूतं कल्कैः संयोज्य कार्षिकैः ॥६२॥
रोहिणी कटुका मुस्त त्रायमाणा दुरालभा ।
कल्कस्तथामलकीनां च क्षीरस्य च घृतस्य च ।
पला[2]नि पृथगष्टाष्टौ दत्वा सम्यग्विपाचयेत् ॥६३॥
[चरक : चिकित्सा : ५ : ११८-१२०]
पित्तगुल्मं रक्तपित्तं[3] वीसर्पं पैत्तिकज्वरम्[4] ।
हृद्रोगं कामलां कुष्ठं हन्यादेतद् घृतोत्तमम् ॥६४॥
पलोल्लेखागते माने न द्वैगुण्यमिहेष्यते ।
चत्वारिंशत् पलं तेन तोयं दशगुणं भवेत् ॥६५॥
॥ त्रायमाणाघृतम् ॥"
[भैषज्यरत्नावली : गुल्माधिकार : ८०-८४]

1. कल्कीकृतैर्घृतं इति आकरे पाठः ।
2. पलेकानि इति प्रथमपुस्तके पाठः ।
3. रक्तगुल्मं इति आकरे पाठः ।
4. पैत्तिकं ज्वरम् इति आकरे पाठः ।

Trāyamāṇā Ghṛta

Four *palas* of *trāyamāṇā* should be boiled with ten times of water till half remains. To this, the paste of one *karṣa* of each of *rohiṇī*, *kaṭukā*, *mustā*, *trāyamāṇā* and *durālabhā* should be added. In addition, eight *palas* of each of the paste of *āmalakī*, milk and ghee should be added and cooked. This cures *pitta gulma*, *rakta pitta* (an ailment characterised by bleeding from different parts of the body), erysipelas, *paittika* type of fever, heart diseases, jaundice and *kuṣṭha* (obstinate skin diseases including leprosy). According to general rule or *paribhāṣā*, if the quantity of any liquid is mentioned in *pala* as the unit of measurement, then while actually adding to the recipe, the quantity should be doubled. The present recipe is, however, an exception to this general rule and forty *palas* (ten times of *trāyamāṇā*) of water should be taken for the purpose of preparing the decoction.

"द्राक्षामधुकखर्जूरं विदारीं सशतावरीम् ।
परूषकाणि[1] त्रिफलां साधयेत्पलसम्मितम्[2] ॥९६॥
जलाढके पादशेषे रसमामलकस्य च ।
घृतमिक्षुरसं क्षीरमभयाकल्कपादिकम् ॥९७॥
साधयेत्तद्घृतं सिद्धं शर्कराक्षौद्रपादिकम् ।
प्रयोगात् पित्तगुल्मघ्नं सर्वपित्तविकारनुत् ॥९८॥

[चरक : चिकित्सा : ५ : १२३-१२५]

साहचर्यादिह पृथक्[3] घृतादेः क्वाथतुल्यता ॥९९॥"

॥ द्राक्षाद्यं घृतम् ॥

[भैषज्यरत्नावली : गुल्माधिकार : ९८-१००]

1. परुषकादि इति प्रथमपुस्तके पाठः ।
2. ०सम्मिताम् इति प्रथमपुस्तके पाठः ।
3. पृथग् इति आकरे पाठः ।

Drākṣādya Ghṛta

One *pala* of each of *drākṣā*, *madhuka*, *kharjūra*, *vidārī*, *śatāvarī*, *parūṣaka* and *triphalā* should be boiled in one *āḍhaka* of water and reduced to one fourth. To this, *āmalaka* juice, ghee, sugar-cane juice and milk, in quantities equal to that of the decoction should be added. Further, one fourth in quantity of the paste of *harītakī* should be added and cooked. Thereafter, one fourth in quantity of each of sugar and honey should be added. Administration of this recipe cures *pitta gulma* and all other diseases caused by *pitta*. Three liquids are mentioned to be used in this recipe. According to the general rule (*paribhāṣā*) of pharmaceutics, each one of these should have been taken four times in quantity of ghee. Since all these liquids are mentioned together (*sāhacaryāt*), the present recipe is an exception to this rule and each one of these liquids should be equal to the decoction in quantity.

"पिप्पलीपिप्पलीमूलचव्यचित्रकनागरैः ।
पलिकैः सयवक्षारैः सर्पिः[1] प्रस्थं विपाचयेत् ॥१००॥
क्षीरप्रस्थेन[2] तत्सर्पिः हन्ति गुल्मं कफात्मकम् ।
ग्रहणीपाण्डुरोगघ्नं प्लीहकासज्वरापहम् ॥१०१॥

॥ क्षीरषट्पलकं घृतम् ॥"

[चरक : चिकित्सा : ५ : १४७-१४८]

[भैषज्यरत्नावली : गुल्माधिकार : ८५-८६]

Kṣīr Ṣaaptalaka Ghṛta

One *prastha* of ghee should be cooked by adding one *pala* of each of *pippalī*, *pippalī mūla*, *cavya*, *citraka*, *nāgara* and *yava kṣāra* and one *prastha* of milk. This medicated ghee cures *grahaṇī* (sprue syndrome), anemia, splenic disorders, cough and fever.

---

1. सयवक्षारैर्घृतप्रस्थं इति आकरे पाठः ।
2. क्षीरप्रस्थं च तत् सर्पिर्हन्ति इति आकरे पाठः ।

"षड्भिः पलैर्मगधजाफलमूलचव्य-

विश्वौषधज्वलनयावकफलपक्वम् ।

प्रस्थं घृतस्य दशमूल्यु[1]रुबूकभार्ङ्गी-

क्वाथेऽप्यथो[2]पयसि दध्नि च षट्पलाख्यम् ॥१०२॥

गुल्मोदरारुचिभगन्दरवह्नि[3]साद-

कासज्वरक्षयशिरोग्रहणीविकारान्[4] ।

सद्यः शमं नयति ये च कफानिलोत्थाः

भार्ङ्ग्याख्यषट्पलमिदं प्रवदन्ति तज्ज्ञाः[5] ॥१०३॥

॥ भार्ङ्गी[6]षट्पलकं घृतम् ॥"

[भैषज्यरत्नावली : गुल्माधिकार : ८९-९०]

Bhārṅgī Ṣaṭpalaka Ghṛta

One *prastha* of each of ghee, decoction of *daśa mūli*, *urubūka* and *bhārṅgī*, milk and curd should be added with the paste of six *palas* of *pippalī*, *pippalī mūla*, *cavya*, *viśvauṣadha*, *jvalana* and *yava kṣāra* and cooked. This recipe of medicated ghee is called *bhārṅgī ṣaṭpalaka ghṛta* which cures *gulma*, *udara* (obstinate abdominal diseases including ascites), anorexia, fistula-in-ano, suppression of the power of digestion, cough, fever, consumption, diseases of the head, *grahaṇī* (sprue syndrome) and other diseases caused by the aggravated *kapha* and *vāyu*.

---

1. दशमूल्यरुबूक० इति प्रथमपुस्तके पाठः ।
2. ०प्यथा इति प्रथमपुस्तके पाठः ।
3. ०भगन्दरभग्निसाद० इति आकरे पाठः ।
4. विकारात् इति प्रथमपुस्तके पाठः ।
5. वैद्याः इति आकरे पाठः ।
6. भार्गीषटपलकं इति आदर्शपुस्तकेषु पाठः ।

"श्यामात्रिवृद्वह्निपलत्रयं च[2] हरीतकीनां तु शतार्द्धमन्यत् ।[1]
तोयार्मणोऽर्धेन विपाचितेन प्रस्थं पचेद्गव्यघृतस्य वैद्यः ॥१०४॥
कम्पिल्लकस्यापि पलप्रमाणं[3] सनीलिनीबीजपलद्वयं च ।
चतुःपलं स्नुक्पयसश्च दत्वा गुल्मापहं बिन्दुघृतं विरेकात् ॥१०५॥"

॥ बिन्दुघृतम् ॥

[भारतभैषज्यरत्नाकर : चतुर्थभाग : पृष्ठ ६४३]

Bindu Ghṛta

Three *palas* of *śyāmā, trivṛt* and *vahni*, and fifty fruits of *harītakī* should be boiled with half *armaṇa* of water. To this decoction, one *prastha* of cow's ghee, one *pala* of *kampillaka*, two *palas* of the seeds of *nīlinī* and four *palas* of the milky latex of *snuhī* should be added and cooked. This is called *bindu ghṛta*. It causes purgation, and thereby, cures *gulma*.

"भल्लातकानां द्विपलं पञ्चमूलं पलोन्मितम् ।
साध्यं विदारीगन्धाद्यमापोथ्य[4] सलिलाढके ॥१०६॥
पादावशेषे[5] पूते च पिप्पलीं नागरं वचाम् ।
विडङ्गं सैन्धवं हिंगु यावशूकं विडं शटीम् ॥१०७॥
चित्रकं मधुकं रास्नां[6] पिष्ट्वा कर्षसमान्[7] भिषक्[8] ।

1. 'श्यामा .... बिन्दुघृतम्', पाठोऽयं प्रथमपुस्तके नोपलभ्यते ।
2. हि इति आकरे पाठः ।
3. कम्पिल्लकस्यात्प्रसृति प्रमाणं इति आकरे पाठः ।
4. विदारीगन्धाज्यमापोथ्य इति आदर्शपुस्तकेषु पाठः ।
5. पादशेषे रसे तस्मिन् पिप्पली इति चरके पाठः ।
6. राष्णां इति आदर्शपुस्तकेषु पाठः ।
7. कर्षसमं इति चरके पाठः ।
8. पृथक् इति चतुर्थपुस्तके पाठः ।

प्रस्थञ्च पयसो दत्वा घृतप्रस्थं विपाचयेत ॥१०८॥

एतद्भल्लातकं नाम कफगुल्महरं परम् ।

प्लीहापाण्ड्वामयश्वासग्रहणीकासगुल्मनुत् ॥१०९॥

॥ भल्लातकघृतम्[1] ॥"

[भैषज्यरत्नावली : गुल्माधिकार : ९४-९७]

[चरक : चिकित्सा : ५ : १४३-१४६]

hallātaka Ghṛta

Two *palas* of *bhallātaka*, one *pala* of *pañca mūla* and drugs belonging to the *Vidārī gandhādi* group should be boiled in one *āḍhaka* of water till one fourth remains. This decoction should be added with the paste of one *karṣa* of each of *pippalī*, *nāgara*, *vacā*, *viḍaṅga*, *saindhava*, *hiṅgu*, *yava kṣāra*, *viḍa*, *śaṭī*, *citraka*, *madhuka* and *rāsnā*, one *prastha* of milk and one *prastha* of ghee and cooked. This is called *bhallātaka ghṛta*. It is an excellent recipe for curing *kapha gulma*, splenic disorder, anemia, dyspnoea, *grahaṇī* (sprue syndrome), cough and other types of *gulma*.

"त्रिवृतां त्रिफलां दन्ती दशमूलं पलोन्मितम् ।

जले चतुर्गुणे पक्त्वा चतुर्भागस्थितं[2] रसम् ॥११०॥

सर्पिरेरण्डजं तैलं क्षीरं चैकत्र साधयेत् ।

सःसिद्धो[3] मिश्रकः स्नेहः सक्षौद्रः[4] कफगुल्मनुत् ॥१११॥

---

1. क. भल्लातकं इति आकरे पाठः ।
   ख. भल्लातकाद्यं इति चरके पाठः ।
2. चतुर्भागोस्येते इति प्रथमपुस्तके पाठः ।
3. स सिद्धो मिश्रकस्नेहः इति आकरे पाठः ।
4. सक्षौद्रकफगुल्मनुत् इति प्रथमपुस्तके पाठः ।

कफवातविकारेषु[1] कुष्ठप्लीहोदरेषु च ।
प्रयोज्य मिश्रकस्नेहो[2] योनिशूलेषु चाधिकम् ॥११२॥
॥ मिश्रकः स्नेहः ॥"

[चरक : चिकित्सा : ५ : १४६-१५१]

Miśraka Sneha

One *pala* of each of *trivṛt*, *triphalā*, *dantī* and *daśa mūla* should be boiled in four parts of water till one fourth remains. To this decoction, ghee, castor oil and milk should be added and cooked together. This is called *miśraka sneha*. Taken along with honey, it cures *kapha gulma*. It is also useful in the treatment of diseases caused by *kapha* and *vāyu*, *kuṣṭha* (obstinate skin diseases including leprosy), splenic disorder, *udara* (obstinate abdominal diseases including ascites) and pain in the female genital tract.

"रसोनस्वरसे सर्पिः पञ्चमूलरसान्वितम् ।
सुरारनालदध्यम्लमूलकस्वरसैः सह ॥११३॥
व्योषदाडिमवृक्षाम्लयमानीचव्यसैन्धवैः ।
हिङ्ग्वम्लवेतसाजाजीदीप्यकैश्च पलांशिकैः[3] ॥११४॥
सिद्धं गुल्मग्रहण्यर्शःश्वासोन्मादक्षयज्वरान् ।
कासापस्मारमन्दाग्निप्लीहशूलानि[4] नाशयेत् ॥११५॥"
॥ रसोनाद्यं घृतम् ॥

[भैषज्यरत्नावली : गुल्माधिकार : ६१-६३]

---

1. कफवातविबन्धेषु इति आकरे पाठः ।
2. मिश्रकः स्नेहो इति आकरे पाठः ।
3. पलांशकैः इति आकरे पाठः ।
4. ०शूलानिलान् जयेत् इति आकरे पाठः ।

Rasonādya Ghṛta

One *pala* of the paste of each of *vyoṣa, dāḍima, vṛkṣāmla, yamānī, cavya, saindhava, hiṅgu, amla vetasa, ajājī* and *dīpyaka* should be added with juice of *rasona*, ghee, decoction of *pañca mūla, surā* (alcoholic preparation), *āranāla* (a type of vinegar), curd, sour juice and juice of *mūlaka*, and cooked. It cures *gulma, grahaṇī* (sprue syndrome), piles, asthma, insanity consumption, fever, cough, epilepsy, suppression of the power of digestion, splenic disorder and colic pain.

"जलद्रोणे विपक्तव्या विंशतिः पञ्च चाभयाः ।
दन्त्याः पलानि तावन्ति चित्रकस्य तथैव च ॥११६॥
तेनाष्टभागशेषेण पचेद्दन्तीसमं गुडम् ।
तच्चाभयास्त्रिवृत्चूर्णात्[1] तैलस्वापि चतुःपलम् ॥११७॥
पलमेकं कणाशुण्ठ्योः सिद्धे लेहे च शीतले ।
क्षौद्रतैलसमं[2] दद्याच्चतुर्जातपलं[3] तथा ॥११८॥
ततो लेहपलं[4] लीढ्वा जग्ध्वा चैकां हरीतकीम् ।
सुखं विरिच्यते स्निग्धो दोषप्रस्थमनामयः[5] ॥११९॥
प्लीहश्वयथुगुल्मार्शोहृत्पाण्डुग्रहणीगदाः ।
शाम्यन्त्युत्क्लेशविषमज्वरकुष्ठान्यरोचकाः ॥१२०॥"

॥ दन्तीहरीतकी ॥

[भैषज्यरत्नावली : गुल्माधिकार : १०१-१०५]

1. ताश्चाभयास्तृवृत् चूर्णा इति आदर्शपुस्तकेषु पाठः ।
2. क्षौद्रं तैलसमं इति आकरे पाठः ।
3. ०चातुर्जातपलं इति आदर्शपुस्तकेषु पाठः ।
4. द्विकोलकमितं लेहं जग्धवा इति आकरे पाठः ।
5. दोषः प्रस्थमनामयः इति आदर्शपुस्तकेषु पाठः ।

Dantī Harītakī

In one *droṇa* of water, twenty five fruits of *abhayā*, twenty five *palas* of each of *dantī* and *citraka* should be boiled till one eighth remains. To this decoction, twenty five *palas* of *guḍa*, twenty five fruits of *abhayā* boiled earlier, twenty five *palas* of the powder of *trivṛt*, four *palas* of *taila* and one *pala* of *kaṇā* and *śuṇṭhī* should be added and cooked. The linctus, thus prepared, should be allowed to cool down. Thereafter, four *palas* of honey and one *pala* of *caturjāta* should be added to the linctus and mixed well. The patient should take one *pala* of the *leha* along with one fruit of *harītakī* (added earlier to the linctus) by which there will be easy purgation. Before this recipe, the patient should have taken oleation therapy. By this recipe the patient voids one *prastha* of waste products. It cures splenic disorder, oedema, *gulma*, piles, heart disease, anemia, *grahaṇī* (sprue syndrome), nausea, *viṣama jvara* (irregular fever), *kuṣṭha* (obstinate skin diseases including leprosy) and anorexia.

"[1]चित्रकं त्रिफला दन्ती त्रिवृता कण्टकारिका ।
स्नुहीक्षीरं विडङ्गानि घृतं दशममुच्यते ॥१२१॥
एकैकस्य [2]तु कर्षेण घृतस्य कुडवं पचेत् ।
[3]'चतुर्गुणेन तोयेन सम्यगेतत्तुषाग्निना ॥१२२॥'
[4]अस्य काले पिबेन्मात्रा पलार्द्धसम्मितां नराः ।
उष्णोदकञ्चानुपिबेद्विल्व[5]त्वादस्य सर्पिषा ॥१२३॥

1. "चित्रकं ....नाराचघृतम् ॥" पाठोऽयं द्वितीयपुस्तके नोपलभ्यते ।
2. च इति आकरे पाठः ।
3. 'चतुर्गुणें.........ग्निना' पाठोऽयं आकरे नोपलभ्यते ।
4. अस्यमात्रां पिबेत्काले शाणार्द्धेन च सम्मिताम् इति आकरे पाठः ।
5, ०पिबेद्विरेकार्थं सदा नरः इति आकरे पाठः ।

पिबेद् यवागूं सर्पिषा[1] पेयां वा क्षीरसाधितम्[2] ।
[3]'वा रक्ते च यवागूस्यात्सर्पिषा परिमर्जिता ॥१२४॥'
रसेन जाङ्गलानां वा भोजयेन्मतिमान् भिषक् ।
वातगुल्ममुदावर्तप्लीहार्शो ब्रध्नकुण्डलम् ॥१२५॥
ग्रहणीं दीपयेन्मन्दां कुष्ठदोषांश्च नाशयेत् ।
[[4]नाराचकमिदं सर्पिः ख्यातं नाराचसन्निभम् ॥१२६॥]

॥ नाराचघृतम् ॥"

[भैषज्यरत्नावली : गुल्माधिकार : ७०-७४]

Nārāca Ghṛta

One *kuḍava* of ghee should be cooked with one *karṣa* of each of *citraka*, *triphalā*, *dantī*, *trivṛt*, *kaṇṭakāri*, latex of *snuhī* and *viḍaṅga* by adding four *kuḍavas* of water. Paddy husk should be used as fuel for this cooking. This recipe should be administered to the patient in appropriate time in a dose of half *pala* along with hot water [the meaning of the term '*vilvatvādasya sarpiṣā*' is not clear] or *yavāgu* (thick gruel) mixed with ghee or *peyā* (thin gruel) prepared with milk or with the meat soup or with the soup of the meat of animals inhabiting arid region. For the preparation of *yavāgu*, described above, rice should be fried with ghee and this is useful for *rakta gulma* (?). This recipe cures *vāta gulma*, *udāvarta*, splenic disorder, piles, inguinal lymphadenitis and *kuṇḍala* (movement of wind in the abdomen). It stimulates the suppressed activities

1. हविषा इति आकरे पाठः ।
2. क्षीसाधिताम् इति आकरे पाठः ।
3. 'वा·········परिमर्जिता' पाठोऽयं आकरे नोपलभ्यते ।
4. 'नाराच·········०सन्निभम्' पाठोऽयं आदर्शपुस्तकेषु नोपलभ्यते ।

of *grahaṇī* (small intestine including duodenum) and cures *kuṣṭha* (obstinate skin diseases including leprosy). This is called *nārāca ghṛta* and it attacks the disease like a *nārāca* (spear).

"वृश्चीवमुरुबूकं च वर्षाह्व[1] बृहतीद्वयम् ।
चित्रकं च जलद्रोणे पचेत्पादावशेषितम् ॥१२७॥
मागधीचित्रकक्षौद्रलिप्ते कुम्भे निधापयेत् ।
मधुनः प्रस्थमावाप्य पथ्याचूर्णार्द्धसंयुतम् ॥१२८॥
नि[2]शोषितं दशाहं तु जीर्णभक्तः पिबेन्नरः ।
अरिष्टोऽयं जयेद् गुल्मं विपक्वं च सुदुस्तरम् ॥१२९॥
॥ वृश्चीवा[3]द्यरिष्टः ॥"

[भारतभैषज्यरत्नाकर : चतुर्थभाग : पृष्ठ ६८४]

Vṛścīvādyariṣṭa

Vṛścīva, urubūka, varṣāhvā, bṛhatī, kaṇṭakārī and *citraka* should be boiled in one *droṇa* of water till one fourth remains. This decoction should be placed in a jar smeared with *pippalī*, *citraka* and honey. To this decoction, one *prastha* of honey and half *prastha* of the powder of *pathyā* should be added and kept for fermentation for 10 days. This should be taken after the digestion of food which cures suppurated and obstinate type of *gulma*.

---

1. वर्षाभूबृहती० इति आकरे पाठः ।
2. संस्थापितं इति आकरे पाठः ।
3. वृश्चीवाद्योऽरिष्टः इति आकरे पाठः ।

"रौधिरस्य तु गुल्मस्य गर्भकालव्यतिक्रमे ।
स्निग्धस्विन्नशरीरायै दद्यात् स्निग्धं[1] विरेचनम् ॥१३०॥

[चरक : चिकित्सा ५ : १७२]

Treatment of Rakta Gulma

The lady suffering from *rakta gulma*, after 10th month, should be given oleation and fomentation therapies, and thereafter, unctuous type of purgation therapy should be administered.

'शताह्वचिरबिल्वत्वग्दारुभार्ङ्गीकणोद्भवः ।
कल्कः पीतो हरेद्[2] गुल्मं तिलक्वाथेन रक्तजम् ॥१३१॥

The paste prepared of *śatāhvā*, *cirabilva*, *tvak*, *dāru*, *bhārṅgī* and *kaṇā* should be given with the decoction of *tila* which cures *rakta gulma.*

तिलक्वाथो गुडव्योषहिंगुभार्गीयुतो[3] भवेत् ।
पानं रक्तभवे गुल्मे नष्टे पुष्पे च योषितः ॥१३२॥'

[योगरत्नाकर : गुल्मचिकित्सा : पृष्ठ ३३]

Intake of the decoction of *tila*, mixed with *guḍa*, *vyoṣa*, *hiṅgu* and *bhārgī* cures *rakta gulma* and amenorrhea in ladies.

---

1. स्नेहविरेचनम् इति चरके पाठः ।
2. जयेद् इति योगरत्नाकरे पाठः ।
3. क. गुडघृतव्योषभार्ङ्गीरजोन्वितः इति योगरत्नाकरे पाठः ।
   ख. गुडव्योषहिंगुंपर्णीयुतो इति श्राकरे पाठः ।

सक्षारत्र्यूषणं मद्यं प्रपिबेदस्रगुल्मिनी ।
पलाशक्षारतोयेन सिद्धं सर्पि पिबेच्च सा ॥१३३॥"

[भैषज्यरत्नावली : गुल्माधिकार : १४५-१४८]

The lady suffering from *rakta gulma* should take *madya* (alcoholic drink) along with *kṣāra* (alkali preparation) and *tryūṣaṇa.* Such a patient can also take ghee cooked with the solution of *kṣāra* (alkali preparation) of *palāśa.*

"उष्णैर्वा भेदयेद्भिन्ने विधिरासृग्दर हितः ।
'न प्रभिद्येत यद्येवं दद्याद्योनिविशोधनम् ॥१३४॥
क्षारेण युक्तं पललं सुधाक्षीरेण वा पुनः ।'

[चरक : चिकित्सा : ५ : १७४]

'रुधिरेऽतिप्रवृत्ते तु रक्तपित्तहरी क्रिया ॥१३५॥'

[चरक : चिकित्सा : ५ : १८०]

The patient should be given purgation therapy which is hot in potency as a result of which the mass of *rakta gulma* may get burst, and thereafter, therapies prescribed for *asṛgdara* should be given to her. If, however, it does not get burst, then *yoni viśodhana* (vaginal douching) should be done with the help of *palala* mixed with *kṣāra* (alkali preparation) or the latex of *snuhī.* If, as a result of the bursting of *rakta gulma,* there is excess of bleeding, then therapies meant for curing *rakta pitta* (an ailment characterised by bleeding from different parts of the body) should be adopted.

भल्लातकात्कल्ककषायपक्वं सर्पिः पिबेत्[1] शर्करया विमिश्रम् ।

1. पिबेच्छर्करया इति आकरे पाठः ।

तद्रक्तगुल्मं विनिहन्ति पीतं बलासगुल्मं मधुना समेतम् ॥१३६॥"

॥ भल्लातकघृतम् ॥

[भैषज्यरत्नावली : गुल्माधिकार : १५०-१५२]

Bhallātaka Ghṛta

Ghee cooked with the paste and decoction of *bhallātaka* should be taken along with sugar which cures *rakta gulma.* If this medicated ghee is taken along with honey, then it cures *kaphaja gulma.*

गुल्मेऽपथ्यानि[1]

"वल्लूरं मूलकं मत्स्यान् शुष्कशाकानि वैदलम् ।
न खादेच्चालुकं गुल्मी मधुराणि फलानि च ॥१३७॥"

[भैषज्यरत्नावली : गुल्माधिकार : १६७]

Unwholesome Diet

Vallūra (dried meat), radish, fish, dried vegetables, pulses, *āluka* and sweet fruits should not be taken by a patient suffering from *gulma.*

"सूतं टङ्कणतुल्यांशं मरिचं सूततुल्यकम् ।
गंधकं पिप्पली शुण्ठी द्वौ द्वौ भागौ विचूर्णयेत् ॥१३८॥
सर्वतुल्यं क्षिपेद् दन्तीबीजं निस्तुषितं[2] भिषक् ।
द्विगुञ्जं[3] रेचनं सिद्धं नाराचो[ऽ]यं महारसः[4] ॥

1. पाठोऽयं चतुर्थपुस्तके नोपलभ्यते ।
2. निस्तुषमेव च इति ग्राकरे पाठः ।
3. द्विगुञ्जो रेचने सिद्धो इति ग्राकरे पाठः ।
4. महारथः इति प्रथमपुस्तके पाठः ।

गुल्मप्लीहोदरं हन्ति पिबेत्तण्डुलवारिणा[1] ॥१३६॥"

॥ नाराचरसः[2] ॥

[भारतभैषज्यरत्नाकर : तृतीयभाग : पृष्ठ २४०]

Nārāca Rasa

Purified *pārada* (one part), purified *ṭaṅkaṇa* (one part), *marica* (one part), purified *gandhaka* (two parts), *pippalī* (two parts) and *śuṇṭhī* (two parts) should be mixed together and made to a powder. To this, the powder of dehusked seeds of *dantī* (nine parts), should be added. This powder should be administered in a dose of two *guñjas* (250 mg) which causes purgation. It is called *Nārāca rasa*. It cures *gulma*, splenic disorder, and *udara* (obstinate abdominal diseases including ascites). The recipe should be given along with *taṇḍula vāri* (rice wash).

"सूतं गन्धं च मरिचं[3] टङ्कणं नागराभये[4] ।
जयपालबीजसंयुक्तं[5] इच्छाभेदीरसः[6] स्मृतः ॥१४०॥"

[भारतभैषज्यरत्नाकर : प्रथमभाग : पृष्ठ १३१]

---

1. पिवेत्त चोष्णवारिणा इति आदर्शपुस्तकेषु पाठः ।
2. पाठोऽयं प्रथमपुस्तके नोपलभ्यते ।
3. तथा व्योखं इति प्रथमपुस्तके पाठः ।
4. नागराभया इति आदर्शपुस्तकेषु पाठः ।
5. क. जयपालं बीजसंयुक्त इति प्रथमपुस्तके पाठः ।
   ख. जयपालेनसंयुक्त इति चतुर्थपुस्तके पाठः ।
6. क्रमोत्तरगुणं भवेत् । सर्वगुल्मोदरे देय इच्छाभेदी त्वयं रसः ।
   इति आकरे पाठः ।

क्रमात्तं द्विगुणं कुर्यान्मर्द्दयेत्तत्समं गुडम् ।
चतुर्गुंजावटीं कुर्याच्छीततोयेन पाययेत् ।
रेचने ज्वरगुल्मं च शोफशूलं विनश्यति ॥१४१॥

॥ इच्छाभेदीरसः ॥[1]

Icchā Bhedī Rasa

Purified *pārada* (one part), purified, *gandhaka* (two parts), *marica* (four parts), purified *ṭaṅkaṇa* (eight parts), *nāgara* (sixteen parts), *abhayā* (thirty two parts), and seeds of *jaya pāla* (sixty four parts) should be triturated by adding 127 parts of jaggery. Out of this paste, pills of the size of 4 *guñjās* (500 mg) should be prepared. It should be administered along with cold water. It causes purgation and cures fever, *gulma*, oedema and colic pain.

"[2]सूताभ्रगंधताप्यार्कं यवक्षारं च मर्द्दयेत् ।
अग्न्यम्बुना[ऽ]हिपत्रेण सेव्यो वल्लोनिलोद्भवे ॥१४२॥

Purified *pārada*, *bhasma* of *abhraka*, purified *gandhaka*, purified *tāpya*, purified *arka* (*tāmra*) and *yava kṣāra* should be triturated with the decoction of *agni* (*citraka*). This recipe should be administered in the dose of one *valla* along with the leaf of *nāga vallī* which is useful in *vātika gulma.*

हिंगुसौवर्चलं सिंधुदाडिमं वेल्लमंवुभिः ।
पिष्टं लुंगोद्भवैर्देयः कर्षोस्य सुरया सह ॥१४३॥

॥ वडवानलो रसः ॥"

---

1. पाठोऽयं प्रथमपुस्तके नोपलभ्यते ।
2. दृष्टव्यम्—भारतभैषज्यरत्नाकर : चतुर्थभाग : पृष्ठ ७२७ ।

Vaḍavānala Rasa

Hiṅgu, *sauvarcala*, *saindhava* and *dāḍima* should be triturated by adding the juice of *vella* and juice of *mātuluṅga*. This should be administered in the dose of one *karṣa* along with *surā* (alcoholic drink).

[1] 'सूतमर्कं शाकवृक्षस्य नीरैः सर्पाक्ष्यद्भिः पेष्येद्वस्त्रमेकम् [?]।
भूमेः कुक्षौ पंचधैव पुटित्वा युंज्यास्तुल्याः चारुनकुम्भबीजात् ॥१४४॥
उड्डामराख्यः स्याद्रसः सर्पिषोयं गुंजायुग्मः पित्तगुल्मं निहन्ति ।
द्राक्षापथ्याक्वाथमनुपानं वर्ज्यं सर्वं पित्तलं दाहकारि ॥१४५॥
॥ उड्डामरो रसः[2] ॥'

Uḍḍāmara Rasa

Purified *pārada* and *tāmra bhasma* should be triturated by adding the decoction of *śāka vṛkṣa* and *sarpākṣī*. Then it should be cooked in *bhūdhara puṭa* for five times. To this, equal quantity of the seeds of *nikumbha* should be added and further triturated. This is called *uḍḍāmara rasa*. It should be administered in the dose of two *guñjas* (250 mg) along with ghee which cures *paittika gulma*. The decoction of *drākṣā* or *pathyā* should be used as *anupāna* (post-prandial drink). While taking this recipe, the patient should avoid all such things as are aggravators of *pitta* and which cause burning sensation.

[3] 'सूतो गंधस्तालकस्ताम्रताप्यं
तुल्यं सर्वं मृच्छिला[4] चेति पिष्ट्वा ।

1. द्रष्टव्यम्—भारतभैषज्यरत्नाकर : प्रथमभाग : पृष्ठ १४१ ।
2. पाठोऽयं प्रथमपुस्तके नोपलभ्यते ।
3. द्रष्टव्यम्—भारतभैषज्यरत्नाकर : चतुर्थभाग : पृष्ठ ७६९ ।
4. हृच्छिलाचेति इति चतुर्थपुस्तके पाठः ।

कृष्णाक्वाथैः स्नुग्[1]भवक्षीरपूरैः

घस्त्रं [?] सतोनाम विद्याधरः स्यात् ॥१४६॥

निष्कार्द्धोयं श्लेष्मगुल्मं निहन्यात्

प्लीहानं च क्षौद्रयुक्तानुपानात् ।

आदौ गुल्मे रक्तमोक्षं विधाय प्रौढः

कार्योयं विधिः सर्वजेपि ॥१४७॥

तिलक्वाथे पिबेदाज्यं भार्गीव्योषगुडान्वितम् ।

पुष्परोधे रक्तगुल्मे स्त्रीभिर्विद्याधरादनु ॥१४८॥

॥ विद्याधरो[2] रसः ॥

Vidyādhara Rasa

Purified *pārada*, purified *gandhaka*, purified *tālaka*, *tāmra bhasma*, *tāpya bhusma* and purified *mṛt śilā* (?)—all these taken in equal quantities should be triturated by adding the decoction of *pippalī* and the latex of *snuhī*. This is called *Vidyādhara rasa*. This should be administered in a dose of half *niṣka* along with honey which cures *kaphaja gulma* and splenic disorder. This recipe can also be administered to a patient suffering from *sānnipātika gulma*. But before administering this, blood-letting therapy should be employed in such cases. For the treatment of amenorrhea and *rakta gulma* in ladies, this recipe should be taken along with the decoction of *tila* mixed with ghee, *bhārgī*, *vyoṣa* and jaggery.

---

1. पाठोऽयं प्रथमपुस्तके नोपलभ्यते ।
2. विद्याधररसः इति चतुर्थपुस्तके पाठः ।

सूतगंधकणापथ्यातुत्थारग्वधकान् द्दढम् ।
मर्दयेद्वज्रिदुग्धेन तन्माषं खादयेद्दिनम्[1] ॥१४९॥
स्त्रीणां जलोदरं हन्ति पथ्यं शाल्योदनं दधि ।
चिंचाफलरसं चानुपानमस्मिन्प्रयोजयेत् ॥१५०॥
॥उदरारिः[2] ॥

Udarāri Rasa (First Recipe)

Purified *pārada*, purified *gandhaka*, *kaṇā*, *pathyā*, *tuttha bhasma* and *āragvadha* should be triturated by adding the milky latex of *snuhī*. One *māṣa* of this recipe should be administered every day which cures *jalodara* (ascites) in ladies. *Śāli* type of rice and curd should be used as diet while taking this recipe. *Anupāna* (post-prandial drink) of the juice of the fruit of *ciñcā* should be taken along with this recipe.

"पारदं शिखितुत्थञ्च[3] जैपालं पिप्पलीसमम् ।
आरग्वधफलान्मज्जां[4] वज्रदुग्धेन मर्दयेत् ॥१५१॥
माषमात्रां[5] वटीं खादेद्धरेत्स्त्रीणां जलोदरम् ।
चिञ्चाफलरसञ्चानु पथ्यं दध्योदनं हितम् ॥

1. खादयेद्दिनाम् इति चतुर्थपुस्तके पाठः ।
2. पाठोऽयं प्रथमपुस्तके नोपलभ्यते ।
3. शुक्तितुत्थञ्च इति आकरे पाठः ।
4. क. आरग्वधभत्वान्मज्जां इति प्रथमपुस्तके पाठः ।
   ख. आरग्वधमवां मज्जां इति चतुर्थपुस्तके पाठः ।
5. माखमात्रां इति प्रथमपुस्तके पाठः ।

दकोदरं[1] हरेत् चैव कठिनं रेचनेन[2] तु ॥१५२॥

॥उदरारि[3] [रसः]॥"

[भारतभैषज्यरत्नाकर : प्रथमभाग : पृष्ठ १४५]

Udarāri Rasa (*Second Recipe*)

Purified mercury, *bhasma* of *mayūra grīva tuttha*, purified *jayapāla*, *pippalī* and pulp of the fruit of *āragvadha*—all these taken in equal quantities should be triturated by adding the milky latex of *snuhi*. Out of this paste, pills of one *māṣa* should be prepared. This is administered in the dose of one such pill which cures *jalodara* (ascites) in ladies. The juice of the fruit of *ciñcā* should be given as *anupāna* (post-prandial drink). Curd mixed rice is useful in this condition as wholesome diet. This cures ascites because of its strong purgative action. [This is a variant reading of the recipe described in verse nos. 149-150]

[4]'सुरेशयांग प्रीणहि पयोद्रेः स्वरूप धृक् सर्वभुजेतदीनाम् ।
गोवर्द्धनो हंसनृपं प्रयायादुन्त्कासदा टोडरमल्लकेशम् ॥१५३॥'

[This verse is full of mistakes. It seems to be a subsequent interpolation. Hence, not translated]

---

1. दकोदरहरञ्चैव तीव्रेण रेचनेन च इति ग्राकरे पाठः ।
2. रेचनं ननु इति प्रथमपुस्तके पाठः ।
3. पाठोऽयं प्रथमपुस्तके नोपलभ्यते ।
4. 'सुरेश०———टोडरमल्लकेशम्' पाठोऽयं चतुर्थपुस्तके नोपलभ्यते ।
5. 'श्री ———विरचिते' पाठोऽयं चतुर्थपुस्तके नोपलभ्यते ।

इति 'श्रीमहाराजाधिराजटोडरमल्लविरचिते'[5] टोडरानंदे आयुर्वेदसौख्ये गुल्मनिदानचिकित्सा'कथनं'[1] नाम '[2]एकोनचत्वारिंशत्तमो हर्षः ॥१५४॥

Thus, ends the 39th Chapter dealing with the diagnosis and treatment of *gulma* in the *Āyurveda saukhya* of *Ṭoḍarānanda* composed by the great king Ṭoḍara Malla.

---

1. कथनं पाठोऽयं चतुर्थपुस्तके नोपलभ्यत ।
2. 'एकोन———हर्षः' पाठोऽयं चतुर्थपुस्तके नोपलभ्यते ।

CHAPTER V

अथ हृद्रोगनिदानं चिकित्सा च ।

Diagnosis and Treatment of Heart Diseases

[1] कफपित्तावरुद्धस्तु[2] मारुतो रसमूर्छितः ।
हृदिस्थः[3] कुरुते शूलं मूर्च्छा संरोधनः परः ।
स हृच्छूल इति ख्यातो रसमारुतसंभवः ॥१॥

Pathogenesis

The *vāyu,* located in the heart being obstructed by *kapha*

---

1. This is the beginning of 44th Chapter of *Āyurveda Saukhya* in *Ṭoḍarānanda* and the invocation reads as follows:—
सुरेशयागं प्रणिहत्ययोद्रेः स्वरूप धृक् सर्वं भुजेतदानीं ।
गोवर्द्धनोहंसनृपं प्रयायादुक्ता सदा टोडरमल्लकेशं ॥
2. ०विरुद्धरक्तमारुतो इति प्रथमद्वितीयपुस्तकयोः पाठः ।
3. क. हृदिस्तु इति पंचमपुस्तके पाठः ।
ख. हृदये इति चतुर्थपुस्तके पाठः ।

and *pitta* interacts with *rasa*, thereby causing colic pain, fainting and (cardiac) obstruction. This condition is called cardiac pain (*hṛt śūla*) which is the result of vitiated *vāyu* and *rasa*.

ऊष्मा पित्तादृते नास्ति ज्वरो नास्त्यूष्मणा विना ।
तस्मात्पित्तविरुद्धानि त्यजेत्पित्ताधिकेऽधिकम् ॥२॥

There is no fever without rise in temperature (increase in bodily heat) and there is no bodily heat without *pitta*. Therefore, in an ailment caused by the aggravated *pitta*, the patient should specially avoid things which are aggravators of *pitta*. [The verse appears to be out of context here; may be an interpolation].

"अत्युष्णगुर्वम्लकषाय[1]तिक्तश्रमाभिघाताध्यशनप्रसङ्गैः ।
[2]संचिन्तनैर्वेगविधारणैश्च हृदामयः पञ्चविधः प्रदिष्टः ॥३॥

Causative Factors

Five types of heart diseases are caused by the intake of excessively hot, heavy, sour, astringent and bitter things, by physical exhaustion, injury, habitually taking food before the previous meal is digested, worry and suppression of natural urges.

दूषयित्वा रसं दोषा विगुणा हृदयं गताः ।
हृदि बाधां प्रकुर्वन्ति हृद्रोगं तं प्रचक्षते ॥४॥

Definition

When vitiated *doṣas* located in the heart afflict *rasa dhātu* to

1. ०गुर्वन्नकषाय० इति आकरे पाठः ।
2. क. सिञ्चितन्नैर्च्वेगविघारणैश्च इति प्रथमपुस्तके पाठः ।
ख. सिञ्चितस्तैर्वेगविधारणैश्च इति पंचमपुस्तके पाठः ।

cause pain in cardiac region, the condition is called *hṛd roga* (heart disease).

आयम्यते मारुतजे हृदयं[1] तुद्यते तथा ।
निर्मथ्यते दीर्यते[2] च स्फोट्यते पाटयतेऽपि च[3] ॥५॥

Vātika Hṛd Roga

Vātika type of *hṛd roga* is characterised by stretching, pinching, grinding, cracking and tearing types of pain in the heart.

तृष्णोष्मादाहचोषाः स्युः पैत्तिके हृदयक्लमः ।
धूमायनं च मूर्च्छा च स्वेदः शोषो मुखस्य च ॥६॥

Paittika Hṛd Roga

Paittika type of *hṛd roga* is characterised by morbid thirst, heating sensation, burning sensation, sucking sensation, cardiac fatigue, a feeling as if inside a smoky place, fainting, sweating and dryness of the mouth.

गौरवं कफसंस्रावो[ऽ]रुचिः स्तम्भो[ऽ]ग्निमार्दवम् ।
माधुर्यमपि चास्यस्य बलासावतते[4] हृदि ॥७॥

[सुश्रुत : उत्तरतन्त्र ४३ : ६-८]

Kaphaja Hṛd Roga

Kaphaja type of *hṛd roga* is characterised by heaviness, excessive salivation, anorexia, stiffness, suppression of the power of digestion and sweet taste in the mouth.

---

1. हृद्रोगं इति आकरे पाठः ।
2. दीप्यते इति आदर्शपुस्तकेषु पाठः ।
3. वा इति आदर्शपुस्तकेषु पाठः ।
4. बलासामते इति आदर्शपुस्तकेषु पाठः ।

विद्यात्त्रिदोषजं चापि सर्वलिंगं हृदामयम् ॥८॥

Sānnipātika Hṛd Roga

Sānnipātika type of *hṛd roga* is characterised by the manifestation of symptoms of all the three varieties of *hṛd roga* described above.

'त्रिदोषजे तु हृद्रोगे यो दुरात्मा निषेवते ।
तिलक्षीरगुडादीनि ग्रन्थिस्तस्योपजायते ॥९॥
मर्म्मैकदेशे संक्लेदं रसश्चाप्युपगच्छति[1] ।
संक्लेदात् कृमयश्चास्य भवन्त्युपहतात्मनः ॥१०॥

[चरक : सूत्रस्थान १७ : ३७-३८]

तीव्रार्तितोदं कृमिजं तं दोषत्रयसंकटम् ।
'उत्क्लेदष्ठीवनं[2] तोदः शूलं हृल्लासकस्तमः ॥
अरुचिः श्यावनेत्रत्वं शोषश्च कृमिजे भवेत् ॥११॥

Kṛmija Hṛd Roga

If the unwise patient suffering from *sānnipatika* type of *hṛd roga* indulges in *tila*, milk, jaggery, etc. then nodules (*granthis*) appear in a part of this vital organ (heart), and *rasa* located there becomes sticky. Because of this stickiness, germs appear there. It is as if the patient wants to kill himself.

This *kṛmija hṛd roga* is characterised by excruciating pain and discomfort as a result of the vitiation of all the three *doṣas* simultaneously, spitting of sticky material, stabbing pain, colic pain, horripilation, a sensation as if entering into darkness, anorexia, grayish colouration of eyes and dryness.

1. रसश्चास्योपगच्छति इति आकरे पाठः ।
2. उत्क्लेदःष्ठीवनं इति आकरे पाठः ।

क्लमः[1] सादो भ्रमः शोषो ज्ञेयास्तेषामुपद्रवाः ।

कृमिजे कृमिजातीनां श्लैष्मिकाणां च ये मताः ॥१२॥"

[सुश्रुत : उत्तरतन्त्र ४३ : ६-१०]

[माधवनिदान : हृद्रोगनिदान : १-७]

॥ हृद्रोगनिदानम् ॥१३॥

Complications

Mental fatigue, prostration, giddiness and feeling of dryness are the complications of different types of heart disease. In *kṛmija hṛd roga*, signs and symptoms of *kāphaja kṛmi* are manifested.

Thus, ends the diagnosis of *hṛd rogas*.

"वातोपसृष्टे हृदये वामयेत्स्निग्धमातुरम् ।

द्विपञ्चमूलीक्वाथेन सस्नेहलवणेन च[2] ॥१४॥

Treatment of Vātika Hṛd Roga

The patient of *vātika hṛd roga* should first of all be given oleation therapy followed by emetic therapy with the help of the decoction of *daśa mūla*, oil and rock-salt.

पिप्पल्यैलावचाहिंगुयवक्षारोऽथ[3] सैन्धवम् ।

सौवर्चलमथो शुण्ठी अजमोदा च चूर्णितम् ॥१५॥

---

1. क. क्लोम्नः इति आदर्शपुस्तकेषु योगरत्नाकरे च पाठः ।
   ख. भ्रमक्लमौ सादशोषौ इति आकरे पाठः ।
2. तु इति आकरे पाठः ।
3. पिप्पल्येलावचाहिङ्गुयवमस्मानि इति आकरे पाठः ।

फलधान्याम्लकौलत्थदधिमद्यासवादिभिः ।

पाययेच्छुद्धदेहञ्च स्नेहेनान्यतमेन वा ॥१६॥"

[सुश्रुत : उत्तरतन्त्र ४३ : ११-१३]

॥ पिप्पल्यादिचूर्णम्[1] ॥

Pippalyādi Cūrṇa

The powder of *pippalī*, *elā*, *vacā*, *hiṅgu*, *yava kṣāra*, *saindhava*, *sauvarcala*, *śuṇṭhī* and *ajmodā* should be given along with the decoction of *phala* (*triphalā*), *dhānyāmla* (a sour drink), decoction of *kulattha*, curd, *madya* (alcoholic drink), *āsava* (a type of fermented drink), etc. After the body is cleansed of impurities, the patient should be given the potion prepared of either of the unctuous substances to drink.

"नागरं वा पिबेदुष्णं कषायञ्चाग्निवर्द्धनम् ।

कासश्वासानिलहरं शूलहृद्रोगनाशनम् ॥१७॥"

[भैषज्यरत्नावली : हृद्रोगाधिकार : ४]

Alternatively, the patient should be given the hot decoction of *nāgara* to drink which stimulates the power of digestion and cures cough, dyspnoea, aggravated *vāyu*, colic pain and heart diseases.

"श्रीपर्णीमधुकक्षौद्रं सितागुडजलैर्वमेत् ।

पित्तोपसृष्टे हृदये सेवेत् मधुरकैः श्रृतम् ॥१८॥

Treatment of Paittika Hṛd Roga

The patient suffering from *paittika hṛd roga* should be given emetic therapy with *śrīparṇī madhuka*, honey, sugar and jaggery

---

1. इति पंचमपुस्तके अधिकः पाठः ।

mixed with water or with water boiled by adding drugs belonging to *madhura* (sweet) group.

घृतं कषायांश्चोद्दिष्टान् पित्तज्वरविनाशनान् ॥१९॥

The patient suffering from *paittika hṛd roga* should be given medicated ghees and decoctions prescribed for the treatment of *paittika* type of fever.

शीताः प्रदेहाः परिषेचनानि तथा विरेको हृदि पित्तदुष्टे ।

द्राक्षासिताक्षौद्रपरूषकैः स्यात् शुद्धे च पित्तापहमन्नपानम् ।

पिष्ट्वा पिबेद्वापि सिताजलेन यष्ट्याह्वयं तिक्तकरोहिणीञ्च ॥२०॥

Cooling ointments, sprinkling of cooling decoctions and purgation therapy prepared of cooling drugs are useful for the patient suffering from *paittika hṛd roga.* After the body is cleansed, the patient should be given food and drinks which alleviate *pitta*, viz. grape, sugar, honey and *parūṣaka.* The paste of *madhu yaṣṭi* and *tiktaka rohiṇī* along with sugar solution may also be given to him.

अर्जुनस्य त्वचा सिद्धं क्षीरं योज्यं हृदामये ।

सितया पञ्चमूल्या वा बलया मधुकेन वा ॥२१॥

Milk boiled with the decoction of the bark of *arjuna* along with sugar or decoction of *pañca mūla*, *balā* or *madhuka* should be given to the patient suffering from *hṛd roga* (heart diseases).

घृतेन दुग्धेन गुडाम्भसा वा पिबन्ति चूर्णं[1] ककुभत्वचो वा ।

हृद्रोगजीर्णज्वररक्तपित्तं हत्वा भवेयुश्चिरजीविनस्ते ॥२२॥

---

1. ये इति आकरे पाठः ।

Intake of the powder of the bark of *arjuna* along with ghee, milk or jaggery-water promotes the longevity of the patient by curing heart disease, chronic fever and *rakta pitta* (an ailment characterised by bleeding from different parts of the body).

वचानिम्बकषायाभ्यां वान्तं हृदि कफोत्थिते ।

वातहृद्रोगनुच्चूर्णं[1] पिप्पल्यादिञ्च योजयेत्[2] ॥२३॥"

[भैषज्यरत्नावली : हृद्रोगाधिकार : ८-१३]

Treatment of Kaphaja Hṛd Roga

The patient suffering from *kaphaja hṛd roga* should be given emetic therapy with the help of the decoction of *vacā* and *nimba*. *Pippalyādi cūrṇa* described for the treatment of *vātika hṛd roga* should also be administered to these patients.

"त्रिदोषजे लघंनमादितः स्यादन्नञ्च सर्वेषु हितं विधेयम् ।

हीनातिमध्यत्वमवेक्ष्य चैव कार्यं त्रयाणामपि कर्म शस्तम् ॥२४॥

Treatment of Sānnipātika Hṛd Roga

In *sānnipātika hṛd roga*, first of all, the patient should be given fasting therapy. Thereafter, he should take such diet which is wholesome for all the three *doṣas*. After ascertaining less aggravated, more aggravated and moderately aggravated *doṣas*, he should be given such therapies as would alleviate all these *doṣas*.

चूर्णं पुष्करजं लिह्यान्माक्षिकेण समायुतम् ।

हृच्छूलश्वासकासघ्नं क्षयहिक्कानिवारणम् ॥२५॥

The powder of *puṣkara mūla* should be taken along with

1. वातहृद्रोगहृच्चूर्णं इति आदर्शपुस्तकेषु पाठः ।
2. पाययेत् इति आकरे पाठः ।

honey which cures cardiac pain, dyspnoea, cough, consumption and hic-cup.

तैलाज्यगुडविपक्वं चूर्णं गोधूमपार्थजं वापि ।
पिबति च पयोऽन्न[1] च स भवेज्जितसकलहृदामयः पुरुषः[2] ॥२६॥"

[भैषज्यरत्नावली : हृद्रोगाधिकार : १६-१८]

Intake of wheat flour and *arjuna* bark powder boiled with oil, ghee and jaggery and diet of milk as well as rice makes the person free from all heart diseases.

"गोधूमककुभचूर्णं छागपयो गव्यसर्पिषा पक्वम् ।
मधुशर्करासमेतं शमयति हृद्रोगमुद्धतं पुंसाम् ॥२७॥"

[भैषज्यरत्नावली : हृद्रोगाधिकार : २१]

Wheat flour and *arjuna* bark powder cooked with goat-milk and cow's ghee should be taken along with honey and sugar which cures even serious types of heart disease.

"मूलं नागबलायास्तु चूर्णं दुग्धेन पाययेत् ।
हृद्रोगश्वासकासघ्नं ककुभस्य च वल्कलम् ॥२८॥
रसायनं परं बल्यं वातजिन्मासयोजितम् ।
संवत्सरप्रयोगेन जीवेद्वर्षशतं ध्रुवम् ॥२९॥"

[भैषज्यरत्नावली : हृद्रोगाधिकार : १९-२०]

1. पिबति पयोऽनु च इति आकरे पाठः ।
2. "उशीरमागधीमूलचूर्णं पीतं घृतान्वितम् ।
गुडेन बीजपूरस्य रसो हृदयशूलनुत् ॥" पाठोऽयं चतुर्थपुस्तके अधिकमुपलभ्यते ।

The powder of the root of *nāga balā* or the bark of *arjuna* should be given along with milk which cures heart disease, dyspnoea and cough. These recipes help in rejuvenation of the body, promotion of strength and alleviation of *vāyu* if used for one month. If this recipe is taken for one year, then the patient certainly lives for one hundred years.

"हिंगूग्रगन्धा विडविश्वकृष्णाकुष्ठाभयाचित्रकयावशूकम् ।
पिबेत्तसौवर्चलपुष्कराढ्यं यवाम्भसा शूलहृदामयघ्नम् ॥३०॥

Intake of the powder of *hiṅgu, ugra gandhā, viḍa, viśva, kṛṣṇā, kuṣṭha, citraka* and *yava kṣāra* mixed with sufficient quantity of *sauvarcala* and *puṣkara mūla* along with barley water cures colic pain and heart disease.

दशमूलकषायस्तु[1] लवणक्षारयोजितः ।
कासं श्वासञ्च हृद्रोगगुल्मशूलञ्च नाशयेत् ॥३१॥

Decoction of *daśa mūla* mixed with salt and *kṣāra* (alkali preparati) cures cough, asthma, heart disease, *gulma* (phantom tum) and colic pain.

पाठां वचां यवक्षारमभयां साम्लवेतसम्[2] ।
दुरालभां चित्रकञ्च त्र्यूषणं च फलत्रयम् ॥३२॥
शटीं पुष्करमूलञ्च तिन्तिडीकं सुदाडिमम् ।
मातुलुङ्गस्य मूलानि श्लक्ष्णचूर्णानि कारयेत् ॥३३॥

---

1. दशमूकषायन्तु इति आदर्शपुस्तकेषु पाठः ।
2. चाम्लवेतसम इति आकरे पाठः ।

सुखोदकेन ह्यम्लैर्वा[1] प्लुतान्येतानि पाययेत् ।
अर्शः शूलञ्च हृद्रोगं गुल्मञ्चाशु व्यपोहति[2] ॥३४॥

The powder of *pāṭhā*, *vacā*, *yava kṣāra*, *abhayā*, *amla vetasa*, *durālabhā*, *citraka*, *tryūṣaṇa*, *triphalā*, *śaṭī*, *puṣkara mūla*, *tintiḍī*, *dāḍima* and root of *mātuluṅga* should be made to a fine powder. This should be given with luke-warm water or sour juice which cures piles, colic pain, heart disease and *gulma* (phantom tumour) instantaneously.

पुटदग्धमश्मपिष्टं हरिणविषाणचूर्णं सर्पिषा पिबतः ।
हृत्पृष्ठशूलमुपशमपुपयात्यचिरेण[3] कष्टमपि ॥३५॥

Deer horn should be burnt in *puṭa* and made to a powder by grinding over stone. Intake of this powder with ghee cures cardiac pain and back pain even if these are of serious nature.

कृमिहृद्रोगिणं स्निग्धं भोजयेत्पिशितौदनम् ।
दध्ना च पललोपेतं त्र्यहं पश्चात् विरेचयेत् ॥३६॥

Treatment of Kṛmija Hṛd Roga

The patient suffering from *kṛmija hṛd roga* should take rice cooked with meat and ghee along with curd and *palala*. After three days, the patient should be given purgation therapy.

सुगन्धिभिः सलवणैर्योगैः साजाजिशर्करैः ।
विडङ्गगाढैर्धान्याम्लं पापयेद्धितमुत्तमम् ॥३७॥

1. मद्यैर्वा इति आकरे पाठः ।
2. नियच्छति इति आकरे पाठः ।
3. ०शूलमुपशमनमुपजात्यचिरेण इति आदर्शपुस्तकेषु पाठः ।

Dhānyāmla (a type of sour drink) mixed with fragrant drugs, salt, *ajāji*, sugar and *vidaṅga* should be taken by the patient suffering from *kṛmija hṛd roga.*

क्रिमिजे च पिबेन्मूत्रं विडङ्गामयसंयुतम् ।
हृदि स्थिताः पतन्त्येवमधस्थात्[1] क्रमयो नृणाम् ॥
यवान्नं वितरेच्चास्मै सविडङ्गमतः परम् ॥३८॥"

[भैषज्यरत्नावली : हृद्रोगाधिकार : २३-३०]

The patient suffering from *kṛmija hṛd roga* should drink cow's urine mixed with *viḍaṅga* and *kuṣṭha.* By this, the germs of the heart get excreted through downward tracts. Thereafter, the patient should be given barley along with *viḍaṅga.*

"मुख्यं शतार्द्धञ्च हरीतकीनां सौवर्चलस्यापि पलद्वयञ्च ।
पक्वं घृतं वल्लभकेति नाम्ना हृत्[2]श्वासशूलोदरमारुतघ्नम् ॥३९॥

॥ वल्लभ[3]घृतम् ॥

Vallabha Ghṛta

Ghee should be cooked with fifty matured fruits of *harītakī* and two *palas* of *sauvarcala* which is called *Vallabha ghṛta.* It cures heart diseases, *asthma*, colic pain, *udara* (obstinate abdominal diseases including ascites) and diseases caused by *vāyu.*

श्वदंष्ट्रो[4]शीरमञ्जिष्ठाबलाकाश्मर्यकत्तृणम् ।
दर्भमूलं पृथक्पर्णी पलाशर्षभकौ स्थिरा ॥४०॥

---

1. ०स्तात् इति आकरे पाठः ।
2. हृल्लासशूलोदर इति आकरे पाठः ।
3. वल्लभकं घृतम् इति आकरे पाठः ।
4. ०सीरम० इति आदर्शपुस्तकेषु पाठः ।

पलिकान् साधयेत्तेषां रसे क्षीरचतुर्गुणे[1] ।
कल्कैः स्वगुप्तर्षभकमेदाजीवन्तिजीवकैः[2] ॥४१॥
शतावर्यृद्धिमृद्वीका—शर्कराश्रावणीविषैः[3] ।
प्रस्थः सिद्धो घृताद्वातपित्तहृद्रोगशूलनुत्[4] ॥४२॥
मूत्रकृच्छ्रप्रमेहार्शःश्वासकासक्षयापहः ।
धनुस्त्रीमद्यभाराध्वक्षीणानां[5] बलमांसदः ॥४३॥

॥ श्वदंष्ट्राद्यं घृतम् ॥

Śvadaṃṣṭrādya Ghṛta

One *prastha* of ghee should be cooked with the decoction of *śvadaṃṣṭrā*, *uśīra*, *mañjiṣṭhā*, *balā*, *kāśmarya*, *kattṛṇa*, root of *darbha*, *pṛthak parṇī*, *palāśa*, *ṛṣabhaka* and *sthirā*, taken in the quantities of one *pala* each, four *prasthas* of milk and the paste of *svaguptā*, *ṛṣabhaka*, *medā*, *jīvanti*, *jīvaka*, *śatāvarī*, *ṛddhi*, *mṛdvīkā*, *śarkarā*, *śrāvaṇī* and *viṣa*. This medicated ghee cures *vātika hṛd roga*, *paittikā hṛd roga*, colic pain, dysuria, *prameha* (obstinate urinary disorders, including diabetes), piles, asthma, cough and consumption. It promotes strength and muscles of persons who are emaciated because of excessive use of bow and arrow and indulgence in women, alcohol, heavy weight-lifting and walking long distance.

1. क्षीरे चतुर्गुणे इति आकरे पाठः।
2. सुगुप्तर्षभमेदाजीवन्तिजीरकैः इति आदर्शपुस्तकेषु पाठः।
3. ०बिसैः इति आकरे पाठः।
4. ०हृद्भवशूलनुत् इति आकरे पाठः।
5. ०राध्वखिन्नानां इति आकरे चतुर्थपुस्तके च पाठः।

घृतं बलानागबलार्जुनाम्बुसिद्धं सयष्टीमधुकल्कपादम् ।
हृद्रोगशूलक्षतरक्तपित्तकासानिलासृक् शमयत्युदीर्णम् ॥४४॥

॥ बलाद्यं घृतम् ॥

Balādya Ghṛta

Ghee cooked with the decoction of *balā*, *nāga balā* and *arjuna*, and one fourth in quantity of the paste of *yaṣṭi maahu* cures serious types of heart disease, colic pain, phthisis, *rakta pitta* (an ailment characterised by bleeding from different parts of the body), cough and *vāta rakta* (gout).

पार्थस्य कल्कस्वरसेन सिद्धं शस्तं घृतं सर्वहृदामयेषु ॥४५॥

॥ अर्जुनघृतम् ॥"

[भैषज्यरत्नावली : हृद्रोगाधिकार : ३३-३९]

Arjuna Ghṛta

Ghee cooked with the paste and juice (or decoction) of *arjuna* is useful in all types of heart disease.

व्यायामं पिच्छिलं शोकं कुमद्यं परिषेचनम् ।
वीभत्सं गुडपिण्याकं त्याज्यं हृद्रोगिभिः सदा ॥४६॥

Diet and Regimens

The patient suffering from heart disease should always avoid physical exercise, slimy food, worry, *kumadya* (alcoholic preparations not prepared properly), sprinkling of water over the body, fearful sights, jaggery and oil cake.

इति श्रीमहाराजाधिराजटोडरमल्लविरचिते टोडरानन्दे आयुर्वेदसौख्ये हृद्रोगनिदानचिकित्साकथनं नाम चत्वारिंशत्तमो हर्षः ॥४७॥

Thus, ends the 40th Chapter dealing with the diagnosis and treatment of heart disease in *Āyurveda saukhya* of *Ṭoḍarānanda* composed by the great king Ṭoḍara Malla.

CHAPTER VI

अथ उरोग्रहमूत्रकृच्छ्रनिदानं चिकित्सा च ।

Diagnosis and Treatment of Urograha (*Stiffness in the sides of chest as well as abdomen*) *and Mūtra Kṛcchra* (*Dysuria*)

[1]"अत्यभिष्यंदिगुर्वन्नशुष्कपूत्यामिषाशनात् ।
स्निग्धं मांसं यकृत्प्लीह्नौ सद्यो वृद्धिं यदा गतं ॥
उरोग्रहं तदा कुक्षौ कुरुतः कफमारुतौ ॥१॥

---

1. क. This is the beginning of 45th Chapter of *Āyurveda saukhya* in *Ṭoḍarānanda* and the invocation reads as follows—
वृत्ती(त्त)घ्नकुप्तेहिघनार्दितं व्रजं योगं समुद्धृत्यररक्षदुःखितम् ।
रक्षत्व सौटोडरमल्ल भूमिपंस्वमूरगघ्नो भु (भू) विपारिजातकाम् ॥
ख. गुर्व्वभिष्यंदि० इति पंचमपुस्तके पाठः ।
ग. गम्यभिष्यंदि० इति षष्ठपुस्तके पाठः ।

Etiology and Pathogenesis

By the intake of excessively *abhiṣyandi* (which obstructs channels of circulation) and heavy food, and dry as well as putrified meat, the fat and muscle tissue of liver and spleen get increased suddenly which causes *urograha* (stiffness in the sides of the chest and abdomen) because of the affliction of the lumber regions by the aggravated *kapha* and *vāyu.*

[1]सस्तम्भं सरुजं घोरं रूक्षं स्पर्शासहं गुरुम् ।

[2]आध्मानं कुक्षिहृच्छोषः[3] वातविण्मूत्ररोधता ।

तन्द्रारोचकशूलानि तस्य लिंगानि निर्दिशेत् ॥२॥"

[योगरत्नाकर : उरोग्रहनिदान : (उत्तरार्द्ध) पृष्ठ ४६]

॥ उरोग्रहनिदानं ॥३॥

Signs and Symptoms

Stiffness, acute pain. ununctuousness, tenderness, heaviness, *ādhmāna* (abdominal distension), dryness of lumber and cardiac regions, obstruction to the passage of flatus, stool and urine, drowsiness, anorexia and colic pain—these are signs and symptoms of *urograha.*

Thus, ends the diagnosis of *urograha.*

"व्यायामतीक्ष्णौषधरूक्षमद्यप्रसङ्गनित्यद्रुतपृष्ठयानात् ।

---

1. क. संस्तम्भसं रुजं इति पंचमपुस्तके पाठः ।
   ख. सस्तम्भं सज्वरं इति आकरे पाठः ।
2. करोति इति षष्ठपुस्तके पाठः ।
3. क. कुक्षिहृत्सोषः इति पंचमपुस्तके पाठः ।
   ख. कुक्षिहृच्छोषो इति चतुर्थषष्ठपुस्तकयोः पाठः ।

आनूपमत्स्याध्यशनादजीर्णात्स्युर्मूत्रकृच्छ्राणि नृणामिहाष्टौ ॥४॥[1] [2]

Etiology of Mūtra Kṛcchra

Eight types of *mūtra kṛcchra* are caused by exercise, intake of medicines having *tīkṣṇa* (sharp) quality and ununctuous food, habitual intake of alcohol, daily travelling by riding a fast moving vehicle (animal back), intake of the meat of animals inhabiting marshy land and fish, intake of food before the previous meal is digested and indigestion.

पृथक्मलाः[3] स्वैः कुपिता निदानैः सर्वेऽथवा कोपमुपेत्य बस्तौ ।
मूत्रस्य मार्गं परिपीडयन्ति यदा तदा मूत्रयतीह कृच्छ्रात् ॥५॥

Pathogenesis

Doṣas, located in the urinary bladder, individually or together get aggravated by the respective causative factors and obstruct the urinary passage which cause difficulty in micturation.

तीव्रा[4] रुजो वंक्षणबस्तिमेढ्रे स्वल्पं मुहुर्मूत्रयतीह वातात् ।
पीतं[5] सरक्तं सरुजं[6] सदाहं कृच्छ्रान्मुहुर्मूत्रयतीह पित्तात् ॥६॥
बस्तेः सलिङ्गस्य गुरुत्वशोफौ[7]
मूत्रं सपिच्छं कफमूत्रकृच्छ्रे ।

---

1. आनूपमांसा० इति आकरे पाठः ।
2. नृणां तथाऽष्टौ इति आकरे पाठः ।
3. पृथङ्मला इति आकरे पाठः ।
4. क. तीक्ष्णरुजो इति षष्ठपुस्तके पाठः ।
   ख. तीव्रार्तिरुग्वंक्षण० इति आकरे पाठः ।
5. पित्तं इति पंचमपुस्तके पाठः ।
6. सहजं इति षष्ठपुस्तके पाठः ।
7. क. गुरुत्वशोथौ इति आकरे पाठः ।
   ख. गुरु च शोफौ इति षष्ठपुस्तके पाठः ।

सर्वाणि रूपाणि च सन्निपाताद्

भवन्ति तत्कृच्छ्रतमं तु कृच्छ्रम् ॥७॥"

[चरक : चिकित्सा २६:३२-३५]

Signs and Symptoms

Vātika mūtra kṛcchra is characterised by acute pain in the pelvic region, urinary bladder and *meḍhra* (pudendum) and the patient passes small quantities of urine very frequently. *Paittika mūtra kṛcchra* is characterised by yellow colour of the urine, blood in urine, pain and burning sensation. The patient passes urine very frequently with considerable difficulty. *Kaphaja mūtra kṛcchra* is characterised by heaviness and oedema of the bladder. The patient passes urine which is slimy in consistency. In *sānnipātika* type of *mūtra kṛcchra* signs and symptoms of all the above mentioned three types of *mūtra kṛcchra* are manifested and it is a serious condition.

'मूत्रवाहिषु शल्येन क्षतेष्वभिहतेषु वा ।'

[सुश्रुत : उत्तरतन्त्र ५९:८]

मूत्रकृच्छ्रं तदाघाताज्जायते भृशदारुणम् ।

वातकृच्छ्रेण तुल्यानि तस्य लिंगानि निर्दिशेत् ॥८॥

Kṣataja Mūtra Kṛcchra

If the urinary tract gets injured by weapons, then *kṣataja* type of dysuria is caused which is a very serious ailment. Signs and symptoms of *vātika* type of *mūtra kṛcchra* are manifested in this variety of dysuria.

'शकृतस्तु प्रतीघाताद्वायुर्विगुणतां गतः ।

आध्मानवातशूलौ[1] च मूत्रकृच्छ्रं करोति च ॥९॥'

[सुश्रुत : उत्तरतन्त्र ५९ : ९-१०]

Viḍ Vighātaja Mūtra Kṛcchra

Because of the obstruction to the passage of stool, the *vāyu* gets vitiated. This produces *ādhmāna* (abdominal distension) and *vātika* type of colic pain in this type of dysuria.

अश्मरीहेतु[2] तत्पूर्वं मूत्रकृच्छ्रमुदाहरेत् ॥१०॥

Aśmarīja Mūtra Kṛcchra

Dysuria may also be caused by *aśmarī* (stone) in the urinary tract.

शुक्रे दोषैरुपहते मूत्रमार्गे विधारिते[3] ।

सशुक्रं मूत्रयेत्कृच्छ्राद्बस्तिमेहनशूलवान् ॥११॥

Śukraja Mūtra Kṛcchra

When the semen, being afflicted by *doṣas*, gets lodged in the urinary tract, then the patient passes urine with difficulty along with semen and there is pain in the urinary bladder region and *mehana* (pudendum).

'अश्मरी शर्करा चैव तुल्ये सम्भवलक्षणैः ॥

शर्कराया विशेषं तु श्रृणु कीर्त्तयतो मम ॥१२॥'

[सुश्रुत : उत्तरतन्त्र ५९:११]

---

1. आध्मानं वातशूलं च मूत्रसङ्गं करोति हि इति आकरे पाठः ।
2. द्रष्टव्यम्---सुश्रुतः उत्तरतन्त्र ५९:१० ।
3. विधाविते इति आकरे पाठः ।

पच्यमानाऽश्मरी पित्ताच्छोष्यमाणा च वायुना ।
विमुक्तकफसंघाता क्षरन्ती शर्करा मता ॥१३॥
'हृत्पीडा वेपथुः शूलं कुक्षावग्निश्च दुर्बलः ।
तया[1] भवति मूर्च्छा च कृच्छ्रमूत्रं[2] च दारुणम् ॥१४॥'

[सुश्रुत : उत्तरतन्त्र ५६:१३]

[माधवनिदान : मूत्रकृच्छ्रनिदान : १-११]

॥ मूत्रकृच्छ्रनिदानं ॥१५॥"

Stone and Gravel in the Urinary Tract

The etiology and signs as well as symptoms of *aśmarī* (stone) and *śarkarā* (gravel) are similar. Specific features of *śarkarā* are as follows :—When *aśmarī* (stone) under goes metabolic changes being dried up by the vitiated *pitta* and *vāyu*, it loses its compactness caused by *kapha* as a result of which it gets broken and small gravels come out through the urinary flow. This causes pain in cardiac region, trembling, colic pain in the lumber region, weakness of the power of digestion, fainting and serious type of dysuria.

Thus, ends the diagnosis of dysuria.

"अभ्यञ्जनस्नेहनिरूहबस्तिस्वेदोपनाहोत्तरबस्तिसेकान् ।
स्थिरादिभिर्वातहरैश्च सिद्धान् दद्याद्रसांश्चानिलमूत्रकृच्छ्रे ॥१६॥"

[भैषज्यरत्नावली : मूत्रकृच्छ्राधिकार : १]

1. ताभिर्भवति इति आकरे पाठः ।
2. क. मूत्राघातश्च इति आकरे पाठः ।
ख. मूत्रकृच्छ्रं इति माधवनिदाने पाठः ।

Treatment of Vātika Mūtra Kṛcchra

Massage, oleation, *nirūha* type of medicated enema, fomentation, *upanāha* (application of hot ointment), medicated douching and *seka* (sprinkling of water)—all these therapies should be administered with the help of drugs which alleviate *vāyu,* viz. drugs belonging to *sthirādi* group, to the patient suffering from *vātika mūtra kṛcchra.*

"अमृता नागरं धात्री वाजिगन्धा त्रिकण्टकम् ।
प्रपिबेद् वातरोगार्त्तः सशूलो[1] मूत्रकृच्छ्रवान् ॥१७॥"

[भैषज्यरत्नावली : मूत्रकृच्छ्राधिकार : १५]

The patient suffering from *vātika mūtra kṛcchra* and having colic pain should take the decoction of *amṛtā*, *nāgara*, *dhātrī*, *vāji gandhā* and *tri kaṇṭaka.* The decoction is also useful in the treatment of other diseases caused by *vāyu.*

"सेकावगाहाः शिशिराः प्रदेहा ग्रैष्मोविधिर्वस्तिपयोविरेकाः[2] ।
द्राक्षाविदारीक्षुरसैर्घृतैश्च कृच्छ्रेषु पित्तप्रभवेषु कार्याः ॥१८॥"

[भैषज्यरत्नावली : मूत्रकृच्छ्राधिकार : २]

Treatment of Paittika Mūtra Kṛcchra

For the patient suffering from *paittika* type of *mūtra kṛcchra*, cooling *seka* (sprinkling of water), bath and ointment should be prescribed. The patient should resort to all diet and regimens prescribed for summer season. He should be given medicated enema and purgation therapy containing milk by adding *drākṣā*, *vidārī*, sugar cane juice and ghee.

---

1. सशूली इति पंचमपुस्तके पाठः ।
2. विकारः इति आकरे पाठः ।

"कुशः काशः शरो दर्भ इक्षुश्चेति तृणोद्भवम्[1] ।
पित्तकृच्छ्रहरं पञ्चमूलं बस्तिविशोधनम् ।
एतत् सिद्धं पयः पीतं मेढ्रगं हन्ति शोणितम् ॥१९॥"

[भैषज्यरत्नावली : मूत्रकृच्छ्राधिकार : १०-११]

॥ तृणपंचकम्[2] ॥

The decoction of *tṛṇa pañca mūla*, viz. *kuśa, kāśa, śara, darbha* and *ikṣu* is useful in the treatment of *paittika* type of dysuria. This decoction helps in the cleansing of the urinary bladder. If milk boiled with the roots of these plants is taken, then it cures bleeding from the *meḍhra* (pudendum).

[शतावर्य्यादिः]

"शतावरीकुशकाश[3]श्वदंष्ट्रा-
विदारिशालीक्षुकशेरुकाणाम् ।
क्वाथं सुशीतं मधुशर्करात्तं पिबन्
जयेत् पैत्तिकमूत्रकृच्छ्रम् ॥२०॥"

[भैषज्यरत्नावली : मूत्रकृच्छ्राधिकार : १६]

Śatāvaryādi Kvātha

Intake of the cooled decoction of *śatāvarī, kuśa, kāśa, svadaṃṣṭrā, vidāri, śāli, ikṣu* and *kaśeruka* added with honey and sugar cures *paittika* type of dysuria.

---

1. गणोद्भवम् इति षष्ठपुस्तके पाठः ।
2. क. तृणपंचकम् पाठोऽयं चतुर्थपुस्तके अधिकमुपलभ्यते ।
   ख. तृणपंचमूलम् इति आकरे पाठः ।
3. ०काशैः श्वदंष्ट्रा० इति आकरे पाठः ।

[हरीतक्यादिः]

"हरीतकीगोक्षुरराजवृक्षपाषाणभिद्धन्वयवासकानाम्[1] ।
क्वाथं पिबेन्माक्षिकसम्प्रयुक्तं कृच्छ्रे सदाहे सरुजे विबन्धे ॥२१॥"

[भैषज्यरत्नावली : मूत्रकृच्छ्राधिकार : १९]

Harītakyādi Kvātha

Intake of the decoction of *harītakī*, *gokṣura*, *rāja vṛkṣa*, *pāṣāṇa bheda* and *dhanva yavāsaka* along with honey cures dysuria associated with burning sensation and painful constipation.

"गुडेनामलकं[2] हृद्यं श्रमघ्नं तर्पणं प्रियम् ।
पित्तासृग्दाहशूलघ्नं मूत्रकृच्छ्रविनाशनम् ॥२२॥

Intake of *āmalakī* along with jaggery is cardiac tonic, alleviator of physical fatigue, refreshing and pleasing. It cures *rakta pitta* (an ailment characterised by bleeding from different parts of the body), burning sensation, colic pain and dysuria.

एर्वारुबीजं मधुकं सदार्वि पैत्ते पिबेत्तण्डुलधावनेन ।
दार्वीं तथैवामलकीरसेन समाक्षिकां पैत्तिकमूत्रकृच्छ्रे ॥२३॥"

[भैषज्यरत्नावली : मूत्रकृच्छ्राधिकार : १७-१८]

For the cure of *paittika* type of dysuria, seeds of *ervāruka*, *madhuka*, and *dārvī* should be taken along with rice-wash. Similarly, *dārvī* and the juice of *āmalakī* should be taken along with honey for the cure of *paittika* type of dysuria.

---

1. ०पाषाणभिद्बिल्वयवासकानाम् इति आदर्शपुस्तकेषु पाठः ।
2. गुडेनामलकीक्वाथं श्रमघ्नं तर्पणं परम् इति आकरे पाठः ।

"क्षारोष्णतीक्ष्णौषधमन्नपानं स्वेदो यवान्नं वमनं निरूहाः ।
तक्रं सतिक्तौषधसिद्धतैलमभ्यङ्गपानं कफमूत्रकृच्छ्रे[1] ॥२४॥"

[भैषज्यरत्नावली : मूत्रकृच्छ्राधिकार : ३]

Treatment of Kaphaja Mūtra Kṛcchra

For the treatment of *kaphaja* type of dysuria, the patient should be given drugs, diet and drinks which are alkaline, hot and *tīkṣṇa* (sharp). He should be given fomentation therapy, barley as food, emetic therapy, *nirūha* type of enema and butter-milk. Oil boiled with bitter drugs should be given for massage and drinking.

"मूत्रेण सुरया वापि कदलीस्वरसेन[2] वा ।
कफकृच्छ्रविनाशाय श्लक्ष्णं[3] पिष्ट्वा त्रुटिं पिबेत् ॥२५॥"

[योगरत्नाकर : मूत्रकृच्छ्रचिकित्सा : (उत्तरार्द्ध) पृष्ठ ५३]

[भैषज्यरत्नावली : मूत्रकृच्छ्राधिकार : २०]

Fine paste of *truṭi* should be given with either cow's urine, alcoholic drink or the juice of *kadalī* for the treatment of *kaphaja mūtra kṛcchra*.

---

1. "त्रिकंटकारग्वधदर्भकासदुरालभप्रस्तरभेदपथ्या: ।
निघ्नन्ति पीडां मधुनाश्मरीञ्च सम्प्राप्तमृत्योरपि मूत्रकृच्छ्रम् ॥
यवक्षार समायुक्तं पिबेत्ताक्रं प्रकामतः ।
मूत्रकृच्छ्रविनाशाय तथैवाश्मरिनाशनम् । पाठोऽयं चतुर्थपुस्तके अधिकमुपलभ्यते ।
2. कदलीसुरसेन इति आदर्शपुस्तकेषु पाठः ।
3. क. श्लक्ष्णां इति आकरे पाठ: ।
ख. सूक्ष्मां इति षष्ठपुस्तके योगरत्नाकरे च पाठः ।

"तक्रेण युक्तं सितिसारकस्य[1] बीजं पिबेत्कृच्छ्रविघातहेतोः ।
पिबेत् तथा तण्डुलधावनेन प्रवालचूर्णं कफमूत्रकृच्छ्रे ॥२६॥"

[योगरत्नाकर : मूत्रकृच्छ्रचिकित्सा : (उत्तरार्द्ध) पृष्ठ ५४]

Seeds of *sitisāraka* (*ervāruka*) should be given along with butter-milk for the cure of dysuria. Powder of coral taken along with rice-wash cures *kaphaja* type of dysuria.

श्वदंष्ट्राविश्वतोयं वा कफकृच्छ्रविनाशनम् ॥२७॥

Intake of the decoction of *śvadaṃṣṭrā* and *viśva* cures *kaphaja* dysuria.

"सर्वं त्रिदोषप्रभवे तु[2] वायोः[3]
स्थानानुपूर्व्या[4] प्रसमीक्ष्य कार्यम् ।
त्रिभ्योधिके प्राग्वमनं कफे स्यात्
पित्ते विरेकः पवने तु बस्तिः ॥२८॥"

[भैषज्यरत्नावली : मूत्रकृच्छ्राधिकार : ४]

Treatment of Sānnipātika Mūtra Kṛcchra

In *sānnipātika* type of dysuria treatment should first of all be given for the alleviation of *vāyu* followed by other *doṣas*. If, however, *kapha* is dominated, then emetic therapy should be given; if *pitta* is dominant, then purgation therapy should be administered; and if *vāyu* is dominant, then the patient should be given medicated enema.

---

1. सितावारुकस्य इति आकरे पाठः ।
2. त्त् इति पंचमपुस्तके पाठः ।
3. कृच्छ्रे यथाबलं कर्मसमीक्ष्य कार्यम् इति आकरे पाठः ।
4. क. पूर्व्वां इति पंचमपुस्तके पाठः ।
   ख. पूर्व्यं इति षष्ठपुस्तके पाठः ।

"बृहतीधावनीपाठायष्ठीमधुकलिङ्गकाः ।
पाचनीयो[1] बृहत्यादिः कृच्छ्रदोषत्रयापहः ॥२९॥
॥ बृहत्यादिक्वाथः ॥[2]"

[योगरत्नाकर : मूत्रकृच्छ्रचिकित्सा : (उत्तरार्द्ध) पृष्ठ ५४]

Bṛhatyādi Kvātha

The decoction of *bṛhati*, *dhāvanī*, *pāṭhā*, *yaṣṭi madhu* and *kaliṅgakā* promotes the process of digestion and it cures *sānnipātika* type of dysuria.

"तथाभिघातजे कुर्यात्सद्योव्रणचिकित्सितम् ।"

[भैषज्यरत्नावली : मूत्रकृच्छ्राधिकार : ५]

मूत्रकृच्छ्रे सदा चास्य कार्या वातहरक्रिया ॥३०॥

Treatment of Kṣataja Mūtra Kṛcchra

If dysuria is caused by injury to the urinary passage, then the therapies prescribed for the treatment of fresh wound should be adopted. In such cases also, therapies for the alleviation of *vāyu* should be administered.

"स्वेदचूर्णक्रियाभ्यङ्गाः वस्तयः स्युः पुरीषजे ॥३१॥"

[भैषज्यरत्नावली : मूत्रकृच्छ्राधिकार : ५]

Treatment of Viḍ Vighātaja Mūtra Kṛcchra

For the treatment of *viḍ vighātaja* type of dysuria, fomentation therapy, powdered drugs, massage and medicated enema should be administered.

---

1. पक्त्वा क्वाथं पिबेन्मर्त्यः कृच्छ्रे दोषत्रयोद्भवे इति ग्राकरे पाठः ।
2. पाठोऽयं प्रथमपंचमपुस्तकयोः नोपलभ्यते ।

"क्वाथं गोक्षुरबीजस्य यवक्षारयुतं पिबेत् ।
मूत्रकृच्छ्[1] शकृत्जं च पीतः शीघ्रं निवारयेत् ॥३२॥"

[भैषज्यरत्नावली : मूत्रकृच्छ्राधिकार : १२]

The decoction of the seeds of *gokṣura* should be taken by adding *yava kṣāra* which instantaneously cures dysuria caused by the obstruction of the urinary passage by lumps of stool (pressure from the colon).

"क्रिया हिता त्वश्मरीशर्करायां
या मूत्रकृच्छ्रे[2] कफमारुतोत्थे ॥३३॥

Treatment of Aśmarīja Mūtra Kṛcchra

For the treatment of dysuria, caused by *aśmarī* (stone) and *śarkarā* (gravels), therapies prescribed for the *kaphaja* and *vātika* types of dysuria should be adopted.

लेह्यं शुक्रविबन्धोत्थे शिलाजतु समाक्षिकम् ।
वृष्यैर्बृंहितधातोश्च[3] विधेयाः प्रमदोत्तमाः ॥३४॥"

[भैषज्यरत्नावली : मूत्रकृच्छ्राधिकार : ६-७]

Treatment of Sukraja Mūtra Kṛcchra

For the treatment of *śukraja* type of dysuria, the patient should be given the linctus prepared of *śilā jatu* and honey. After getting strength by aphrodisiac drugs, he may indulge in sex with ladies.

---

1. तथा रक्तं इति आकरे पाठः ।
2. त्वथमारुतोत्थे इति आदर्शपुस्तकेषु पाठः ।
3. ०धातूत्थे इति आकरे पाठः ।

एलाहिंगुयुतं क्षीरं सर्पिमिश्रं पिबेन्नरः ।
मूत्रदोषविशुद्ध्यर्थं शुक्रदोषहरञ्च तत्[1] ॥३५॥

For correcting the vitiated semen and for cleansing the vitiated urine, the patient should take milk added with *elā*, *hingu* and ghee.

यन्मूत्रकृच्छ्रे विहितं हि पैत्ते
तत्कारयेच्छोणितमूत्रकृच्छ्रे ।
"त्रिकण्टकारग्वधदर्भकास-
दुरालभाप्रस्तर[2]भेदपथ्याः ॥
निघ्नन्ति पीता मधुनाऽश्मरीञ्च[3]
सम्प्राप्तमृत्योरपि मूत्रकृच्छ्रम् ॥३६॥"

[योगरत्नाकर : मूत्रकृच्छ्रचिकित्सा : (उत्तरार्द्ध) पृष्ठ ५५]

[भैषज्यरत्नावली : मूत्रकृच्छ्राधिकार :११]

For dysuria associated with bleeding, therapies prescribed for *paittika* type of dysuria should be administered.

Intake of the decoction of *tri kaṇṭaka*, *āragvadha*, *darbha*, *kāsa*, *durālabhā*, *pāṣāṇa bheda* and *pathyā* mixed with honey cures *aśmarī* and serious type of dysuria.

कषायोऽतिबलामूलसाधितो शोषकृच्छ्रजित् ॥३७॥

The decoction of the root of *ati balā* cures consumption and dysuria.

1. यत् इति षष्ठपुस्तके पाठः ।
2. ०पर्वतभेद० इति आदर्शपुस्तकेषु पाठः ।
3. अश्मरीका इति योगरत्नाकरे पाठः ।

[एलादिचूर्णम्]

"एलाश्मभेदकशिलाजतुपिप्पलीनां
चूर्णानि तण्डुलजलैर्लु[1]लितानि पीत्वा ।
यद्वा गुडेन सहितान्यवलिह्य सम्यक्
[2]आसन्नमृत्युरपि जीवति मूत्रकृच्छ्री ॥३८॥"

[भैषज्यरत्नावली : मूत्रकृच्छ्राधिकार : २५]

Intake of the powder of *elā, aśma bheda, śilā jatu* and *pippalī* mixed with rice-wash or jaggery cures dysuria even if the patient is moribund.

अयोरजः श्लक्ष्णपिष्टं मधुना सहयोजितम् ।
मूत्रकृच्छ्रं निहन्त्याशु त्रिभिर्लेहैर्न्नसंशयः ॥३९॥

Intake of the fine powder or *bhasma* of *lauha* along with honey undoubtedly cures dysuria in three doses.

"सितातुल्यो यवक्षारः सर्वकृच्छ्रनिवारणः ।
निदिग्धिकारसो वापि सक्षौद्रः कृच्छ्रनाशनः ॥४०॥"

[योगरत्नाकर : मुत्रकृच्छ्रचिकित्सा : (उत्तरार्द्ध) पृष्ठ ५६]

[भैषज्यरत्नावली : मूत्रकृच्छ्राधिकार : २७]

Sugar and *yava kṣāra* taken in equal quantities cures all types of dysuria. Similarly, the juice of *nidigdhikā* mixed with honey cures dysuria.

---

1. ०जलैप्लुतानि इति पंचमपुस्तके पाठः ।
2. चैतानासन्नमृत्युरपि इति आकरे पाठः ।

"शतावरीकाश[1]कुशश्वदंष्ट्राविदारीकेक्ष्वामलकैः सुसिद्धम् ।
सर्पिः पयो वा सितया विमिश्रं कृच्छ्रेषु पित्तप्रभवेषु योज्यम् ॥४१॥
॥ इति शतावरीघृतं[2] क्षीरञ्च ॥"

[भैषज्यरत्नावली : मूत्रकृच्छ्राधिकार : ५१]

Śatāvarī Ghṛta and Kṣīra

Intake of the ghee or milk boiled with *śatāvarī*, *kāśa*, *kuśa*, *śvadaṃṣṭrā*, *vidārī*, *ikṣu* and *āmalakī* added with sugar is useful in *paittika* type of dysuria.

"त्रिकण्टकैरण्डकुशाद्यभीरुकर्कारुकेक्षुस्वरसेन सिद्धम् ।
सर्पिर्गुडार्द्धांशयुतं प्रपेयं कृच्छ्राश्मरीमूत्रविघातहेतोः ॥४२॥"
॥ इति त्रिकण्टकाद्यं घृतम् ॥

[भैषज्यरत्नावली : मूत्रकृच्छ्राधिकार : ४२]

Trikaṇṭakādya Ghṛta

Ghee cooked with *trikaṇṭaka*, *eraṇḍa*, *kuśa*, *abhīru*, *karkāru* and juice of *ikṣu* should be taken by adding half the quantity of jaggery. It cures dysuria, *aśmarī* (stone) and anuria.

"पुनर्नवामूलतुला दशमूलं शतावरी ।
बला तुरगगन्धा च तृणमूलं त्रिकण्टकम् ॥४३॥
विदारीगन्धा नागाह्वा गुडूच्यतिबला तथा ।
पृथग्दशपलान् भागानपां[3]द्रोणे विपाचयेत् ॥४४॥

1. ०कास० इति प्रथमपंचमपुस्तकयोः पाठः ।
2. शतावर्यादिसर्पिः इति आकरे पाठः ।
3. भागान् जलद्रोणे इति आकरे पाठः ।

तेन पादावशेषेण घृतस्यार्द्धाढकं पचेत् ।
मधूकं शृङ्गवेरञ्च द्राक्षासैन्धवपिप्पलीः ॥४५॥
द्विपलानि पृथग्दद्यात् यमान्याः कुडवं तथा ।
त्रिंशद् गुडपलान्यत्र रसस्यैरण्डजस्य[1] च ॥४६॥
प्रस्थं दत्त्वा समालोड्य सम्यग्मृद्वाग्निना पचेत् ।
एतदीश्वरपुत्राणां प्राग्भोजनमनिन्दितम् ॥४७॥
राज्ञां राजसमानाञ्च बहुस्त्रीपतयश्च ये ।
मूत्रकृच्छ्रे कटीस्तम्भे तथा गाढपुरीषिणाम् ॥४८॥
मेढ्रवंक्षणशूले च योनिशूले च शस्यते ।
यथोक्तानाञ्च गुल्मानां वातशोणितकाश्च ये ॥४९॥
बल्यं रसायनं शीतं सुकुमारकुमारकम् ।
पुनर्नवा शते द्रोणे देयोऽन्येषु तथापरः ॥५०॥

॥ इति सुकुमारकं घृतम् ॥"

[भैषज्यरत्नावली : मूत्रकृच्छ्राधिकार : ४३-५०]

Sukumāraka Ghṛta

In one *droṇa* of water, one *tulā* of the root of *punarnavā* and ten *palas* of each of *daśa mūla*, *śatāvarī*, *balā*, *turaga gandhā*, *tṛṇa pañca mūla*, *trikaṇṭaka*, *vidārī gandhā*, *nāgāhva*, *guḍūcī* and *ati balā* should be added and boiled till one fourth remains. To this decoction, half *āḍhaka* of ghee, two *palas* of each of *madhūka*, *śṛṅgavera*, *drākṣā*, *saindhava* and *pippalī*, one *kuḍava*

---

1. तैलस्यैरण्डजस्य इति आकरे पाठः ।

of *yamānī*, thirty *palas* of jaggery and one *prastha* of the oil of *eraṇḍa* should be added and cooked over mild fire. It is an excellent recipe to be administered before food to wealthy persons, kings and similar other persons who have many wives. It is useful in dysuria, stiffness of lumber region, costive bowels, pain in male genital organ and pelvic region, pain in female genital tract, all types of *gulma* (phantom tumour) and gout. It promotes strength. It is rejuvenating, cooling and useful to young people with tender health. [The meaning of the last line is not clear].

"रसबल्लं यवक्षारसितातक्रयुतं पिबेत् ।

मूत्रकृच्छ्राण्यशेषाणि लभन्तेऽनित्यतां[1] जवात् ॥५१॥"

[योगरत्नाकर : मूत्रकृच्छ्रचिकित्सा : (उत्तरार्द्ध) पृष्ठ ६]

One *valla* of the *bhasma* of *pārada* should be taken along with *yava kṣāra*, sugar and butter-milk which instantaneously cures all types of dysuria.

"रसभस्माच्च[2] भागैकं चत्वारः[3] शुद्धगन्धकम्[4] ।

पिष्ट्वा वराटकान्कुर्याद्रसपादं[5] च टंकणम् ॥५२॥

क्षीरेण पिष्ट्वा रुध्वास्यं भाण्डे रुध्वा पुटे पचेत् ।

स्वांगशीतं विचूर्ण्याथ लघुलोकेश्वरो रसः ॥५३॥

चतुर्गुञ्जो धृतैर्देयो मरिचैकोनविंशतिः ।

जातीमूलपलैकं[6] तु अजाक्षीरेण पाययेत् ॥

1. हन्यन्ते पानतो इति आकरे पाठः ।
2. रसभस्म च इति आकरे पाठः ।
3. चतुरः इति आदर्शपुस्तकेषु पाठः ।
4. ०गंधकात् इति आदर्शपुस्तकेषु पाठः ।
5. वराटकाः पूर्य्याः रसपादेन टंकणम् इति आदर्शपुस्तकेषु पाठः ।
6. जातिमूलपलं चैकमजाक्षीरेण पाचयेत् । इति आकरे पाठः ।

शर्कराभावितं चानुपीतं कृच्छ्रहरं ध्रुवम्[1] ॥५४॥"

॥ लघुलोकेश्वरः[2] रसः ॥

[योगरत्नाकर : मूत्रकृच्छ्रचिकित्सा : (उत्तरार्द्ध) पृष्ठ ६०]

Laghu Lokeśvara Rasa

Pārada bhasma (one part) purified *gandhaka* (four parts) and *ṭaṅkaṇa bhasma* (¼th part) should be triturated with milk and kept inside cowri shells. These shells should be kept in a sealed jar and cooked in *puṭa*. When it becomes cool of its own, these cakes should be removed and triturated. This is called *laghu lokeśvara rasa*. It should be given in the dose of 4 *guñjās* (500 mg) along with ghee. Thereafter, goat's milk added with ninteen seeds of *marica*, one *pala* of the root of *jāti* and sugar should be given as post-prandial drink (*anupāna*) which certainly cures dysuria.

इति श्रीमहाराजाधिराजटोडरमल्लविरचिते टोडरानन्दे आयुर्वेदसौख्ये मूत्रकृच्छ्रनिदानचिकित्साकथनं नाम एकचत्वारिंशत्तमो हर्षः ॥५५॥

Thus, ends the 41st Chapter dealing with the diagnosis and treatment of dysuria in *Āyurveda saukhya* of *Ṭoḍarānanda* composed by the great king Ṭoḍara Malla.

---

1. परम् इति आकरे चतुर्थपुस्तके च पाठः ।
2. पाठोऽयं प्रथमपंचमषष्ठपुस्तकेषु नोपलभ्यते ।

CHAPTER VII

अथ मूत्राघातनिदानं चिकित्सा च ।

Diagnosis and Treatment of Mūtrāghāta (Anuria)

"जायन्ते[1] कुपितैर्दोषैर्मूत्राघातास्त्रयोदश[2]: ।
प्रायो मूत्रविघाताद्यैर्वातकुण्डलिकादय: ॥१॥

[योगरत्नाकर: मूत्राघातनिदान: (उत्तरार्द्ध) पृष्ठ ६१]

Varieties

Because of the aggravated *doṣas*, thirteen varieties of

---

1. This is the begninning of 46th Chapter of *Āyurveda saukhya* in *Ṭoḍarānanda* and the invocation reads as follows:
गवेंद्रकाभ्यां प्रणुतोभिषिक्तो गोविंदनाम्ना हि गवां प्रभुत्वे ।
प्रभुत्वमापदयतां व्रजेशो रमास्यदं टोडरमल्ल भूपे ॥
2. ०दश इति आकरे पाठ: ।

mūtrāghāta, viz. *vāta kuṇḍalikā*, etc. are caused. Generally, in all these varieties, there is suppression of urination.

"रौक्ष्याद्वेगविघाताद्वा[1] वायुर्बस्तौ सवेदनः ।
मूत्रमाविश्य चरति विगुणः कुण्डलीकृतः ॥२॥"

[सुश्रुत : उत्तरतन्त्र ५८ : ५]

मूत्रमल्पाल्पमथवा सरुजं संप्रवर्त्तते ।
वातकुण्डलिकां तां तु व्याधिं विद्यात्सुदारुणम् ॥३॥

Vāta Kuṇḍalikā

Because of ununctuous food as well as regimens and suppression of natural urges, the *vāyu*, located in the urinary bladder, gets vitiated and remains like a whirl while afflicting the urine. The patient passes extremely small quantity of urine with pain. This is called *vāta kuṇḍalikā* which is a serious ailment.

आध्मापयन्बस्तिगुदं रुद्ध्वा वायुश्चलोन्नताम् ।
कुर्यात्तीव्रार्तिमष्ठीलां मूत्रविण्मार्गरोधिनीम् ॥४॥

Aṣṭhīlā

The aggravated *vāyu* causes obstruction and sensation like blowing in the urinary bladder and anus as a result of which mobile and elevated hard tumour (*aṣṭhīlā*) is produced. This causes excruciating pain and obstruction in the passage of urination.

---

1. क. रौक्षाद्वे ०इति आदर्शपुस्तकेषु पाठः ।
ख. "रौक्षा.........कुण्डलीकृतः" पाठोऽयं षष्ठपुस्तके नोपलभ्यते ।

"वेगं विधारयेद्यस्तु मूत्रस्याकुशलो नरः ।
निरुणद्धि मुखं तस्य बस्तेर्बस्तिगतोऽनिलः ॥५॥"

[सुश्रुतः उत्तरतन्त्र ५८:९]

"मूत्रसङ्गो[1] भवेत्तेन बस्तिकुक्षौ निपीडितः ।
वातबस्तिः स विज्ञेयो व्याधिः कृच्छ्रप्रसाधनः ॥६॥"

[सुश्रुत : उत्तरतन्त्र ५८:१०]

Vāta Basti

If the unwise person suppresses the urge for urination, the *vāyu* located in the urinary bladder, obstructs the mouth of this bladder as a result of which no urine will come out and there will be pain in the region of urinary bladder and pelvic regions. This is called *vāta basti* which is difficult of cure.

चिरं धारयतो मूत्रं त्वरया न प्रवर्त्तते ।
मेहमानस्य मन्दं वा मूत्रातीतः स उच्यते ॥७॥

Mūtrātīta

If a person suppresses the urge for micturation for a long time, then he becomes incapable of passing urine whenever he feels i.e. he passes urine only after waiting for some time. His urination also becomes slow. This condition is called ***mūtrātīta.***

"मूत्रस्य वेगेऽभिहते तदुदावर्त्तहेतुकः ।
अपानः कुपितो वायुरुदरं पूरयेद् भृशम् ॥८॥

---

1. बस्तिकुक्षिनिपीडितः इति आकरे पाठः ।

नाभेरधस्तादाध्मानं जनयेत्तीव्रवेदनम् ।
तन्मूत्रजठरं विद्यादधोबस्तिनिरोधनम् ॥९॥

Mūtra Jaṭhara

By the suppression of the urge for urination, *udāvarta* (upward movement of the wind) is caused as a result of which *apāna* type of *vāyu* gets aggravated and the whole abdomen gets further filled up with wind. There will be distension below the umbilicus and excruciating pain. This is called *mūtra jaṭhara* which causes obstruction at the lower part of the urinary bladder.

बस्तौ वाऽप्यथवा नाले[1] मणौ वा यस्य देहिनः ।
मूत्रं प्रवृत्तं सज्येत सरक्तं वा प्रवाहतः ॥१०॥
स्रवेच्छनैरल्पमल्पं[2] सरुजं वाऽथ नीरुजम् ।
विगुणानिलजो व्याधिः स मूत्रसंगसंज्ञितः[3] ॥११॥

Mūtra Saṅga

If the flow of urine gets obstructed in the urinary bladder or urethra or *maṇi* (glans penis or external urethral sphincter) or if the flow of urine is accompanied with blood, then the passage of urine will be slow, in small quantities and very frequently with or without any pain. This ailment caused by vitiated *vāyu* is called *ūmtra saṅga.*

---

1. नीडे इति प्रथमपंचमषष्ठपुस्तकेषु पाठः ।
2. क. श्रवेष्थ० इति प्रथमपुस्तके पाठः ।
   ख. श्रवेत्श० इति पंचमपुस्तके पाठः ।
3. स मूत्रोत्सर्गं संज्ञितः इति आदर्शपुस्तकेषु पाठः ।

रूक्षस्य क्लान्तदेहस्य[1] बस्तिस्थौ पित्तमारुतौ ।'

[सुश्रुत : उत्तरतन्त्र ५८ : १३-१७]

मूत्रक्षयं सरुग्दाहं[2] जनयेतां तदाह्वयम् ॥१२॥

Mūtra Kṣaya

In a patient, who is ununctuous and who is physically fatigued, *pitta* and *vāyu* located in the urinary bladder cause suppression of urine along with pain and burning sensation. This is called *mūtra kṣaya.*

अन्तर्बस्तिमुखे वृत्तः स्थिरोऽल्पः सहसा भवेत् ।

अश्मरीतुल्य रुग्ग्रन्थिर्मूत्रग्रन्थिः स उच्यते ॥१३॥

Mūtra Granthi

Sudden appearance of a round, immobile and small stony hard tumour with pain in the internal opening of the urinary bladder is called *mūtra granthi.*

मूत्रितस्य स्त्रियं यातो वायुना शुक्रमुद्धतम् ।

स्थानाच्युतं मूत्रयतः प्राक् पश्चाद्वा प्रवर्तते ।

भस्मोदकप्रतीकाशं मूत्रशुक्रं तदुच्यते ॥१४॥

Mūtra Śukra

If a person, having the urge for urination but without voiding urine, indulges in sexual intercourse with a woman, then the semen during the process of ejaculation gets displaced by *vāyu* and it comes out before or after the urination. The

---

1. क्लिन्नदेहस्य इति प्रथमषष्ठपुस्तकयोः पाठः ।
2. बस्तिदाहं इति षष्ठपुस्तके पाठः ।

urine, therefore, appears like water mixed with ash. This is called *mūtra śukra.*

व्यायामाध्वातपैः पित्तं बस्तिं प्राप्यानिलान्वितम् ।
बस्तिं मेढ्रं गुदं चैव प्रदहेत्स्रावयेदधः ॥१५॥
मूत्रं हारिद्रमथवा सरक्तं रक्तमेव वा ।
कृच्छ्रात्पुनः पुनर्जन्तोरुष्णवातं वदन्ति[1] तम् ॥१६॥

Uṣṇa Vāta

Because of excessive exercise, long walk and exposure to hot sun, aggravated *pitta* along with *vāyu* enters into the urinary bladder and comes out through the urine while causing burning sensation in the urinary bladder, male genital organ and anus. The urine is yellow or reddish in colour or only blood comes out as urine. The patient frequently voids urine in small quantities and with pain. This is called *uṣṇa vāta.*

पित्तं कफो द्वावपि वा संहन्येतेऽनिलेन चेत् ।
कृच्छ्रान्मूत्रं तदा पीतं रक्तं श्वेतं घनं सृजेत् ॥१७॥
सदाहं रोचना शङ्खचूर्णवर्णं भवेच्च[2] तत् ।
शुक्लं[3] समस्तं वर्णं वा मूत्रसादं वदन्ति तम् ॥१८॥

Mūtra Sāda

If either *pitta* or *kapha* or both of them get afflicted (lit. condensed) by *vāyu,* then with difficulty the patient passes urine which is yellow, red or white and thick. There will be burning

---

1. ब्रुवन्ति इति आकरे पाठः ।
2. तु इति आकरे पाठः ।
3. शुष्कं इति आकरे पाठः ।

sensation during micturation and the colour of the urine will be like that of *gorocana* (cow's bile) or powder of conch-shell. The urine and the whole body may even become white in colour. This is called *mūtra sāda*.

रूक्षदुर्बलयोर्वातेनोदावर्त्तं शकृद्यदा ।
मूत्रस्रोतो[ऽ]नुपद्येत विट्संसृष्टं तदा नरः ॥
विड्गन्ध[1]ं मूत्रयेत् कृच्छ्राद्विड्विघातं विनिर्दिशेत् ॥१६॥

Viḍ Vighāta

If, in an ununctuous and weak person, *vāyu* causes *udāvarta* (upward movement of wind), then the stool reaches the urinary channel. The patient passes urine with difficulty and the urine is mixed with fecal material and smells like feces. This is called *viḍ vighāta*.

द्रुताध्वलङ्घनायासैरभिघातात्प्रपीडनात् ।
स्वस्थानाद्बस्तिरुद्वृत्तः स्थूल[2]स्तिष्ठति गर्भवत् ॥२०॥
शूलस्पन्दनदाहार्त्तो बिन्दुं बिन्दुं स्रवत्यपि[3] ।
पीडितस्तु सृजेद्धारां स्तम्भोद्वेष्टनार्तिवान्[4] ॥२१॥
बस्तिकुण्डल[5]माहुस्तं घोरं शस्त्रविषोपमम्[6] ।
पवनप्रबलं प्रायो दुर्निवार[7]मबुद्धिभिः ॥२२॥

---

1. विडं इति आदर्शपुस्तकेषु पाठः ।
2. शूलस्तिष्ठति० इति आदर्शपुस्तकेषु पाठः ।
3. श्रवत्यपि इति आदर्शपुस्तकेषु पाठः ।
4. संस्तम्भोद्वेष्टनार्तिमान् इति आकरे पाठः ।
5. ०कुण्डलि० इति पंचमपुस्तके पाठः ।
6. शस्त्रविषेणमाम् इति प्रथमपुस्तके पाठः ।
7. दुर्न्निवारोह्य० इति प्रथमपुस्तके पाठः ।

Basti Kuṇḍalikā

Because of the exhaustion caused by fast walking over a long distance, and because of injury, the urinary bladder gets displaced and becomes a compact mass like a foetus in the uterus. The patient passes urine in drops while suffering from colic pain, uncomfortable movements in the urinary bladder and burning sensation. His urine flows only when pressure is applied over the bladder and he suffers from stiffness, *udveṣṭana* (upward movement of the bladder) and pain. This is called *basti kuṇḍala.* It is a dangerous condition like a weapon or a poison. It is generally associated with extremely aggravated *vāyu* and extremely difficult of cure.

तस्मिन्पित्तान्विते दाहः[1] शूलं मूत्रविवर्णता ।
श्लेष्मणा गौरवं शोथः[2] स्निग्धं मूत्रं घनं सितम्[3] ॥२३॥

If *basti kuṇḍalikā* is associated with aggravated *pitta*, then, there will be burning sensation, colic pain and discoloration of the urine. If it is associated with *kapha*, then there will be heaviness, oedema and the urine will be unctuous, thick and white.

श्लेष्मरुद्धविलो बस्ति पित्तोदीर्णो न सिध्यति ।
अविभ्रान्तविलः साध्यो न च[4] यः कुण्डलीकृतः ॥
स्याद् बस्तौ कुण्डलीभूते[5] तृण्मोहः श्वास एव च ॥२४॥"

॥ मूत्राघातनिदानम् ॥२५॥

[योगरत्नाकर : मूत्राघातचिकित्सा : (उत्तरार्द्ध) पृष्ठ ६१-६४]

[माधवनिदान : मूत्राघातनिदान : १-२६]

---

1. दाहशूलविवर्णता इति प्रथमपंचमपुस्तकयोः पाठः ।
2. शोफः इति आदर्शपुस्तकेषु पाठः ।
3. सितां इति प्रथमपंचमपुस्तकयोः पाठः ।
4. तु इति आकरे पाठः ।
5. कुण्डलीमूत्रे हृत्मोहः इति प्रथमपंचमपुस्तकयोः पाठः ।

Prognosis

If the passage of the bladder is obstructed by *kapha* and if there is aggravation of *pitta*, then the patient is not curable. If the passage of the bladder is intact and not obstructed, then the patient is curable. If the passage of the bladder is twisted, then there will be thirst, unconsciousness and dyspnoea and such a patient is not curable.

Thus ends the description of the diagnosis of *mūtrāghāta* (anuria).

[मूत्राघाते क्रियाक्रमः]

"मूत्राघातान् यथादोषं मूत्रकृच्छ्रहरैर्जयेत् ।
बस्तिमुत्तरबस्तिञ्च दद्यात्स्निग्धं विरेचनम् ॥२६॥"

[भैषज्यरत्नावली : मूत्राघाताधिकार : १]

Line of Treatment

Depending upon the *doṣas* involved, the patient suffering from *mūtrāghāta* should be treated with the therapies prescribed for *mūtra kṛcchra* (dysuria). The patient should be given medicated enema, *uttara basti* (application of douche through the genital tract) and unctuous purgation.

"कल्कमेर्वारुबीजानामक्षमात्रं ससैन्धवम् ।
धान्याम्लयुक्तं पीत्वा च मूत्राघाताद्विमुच्यते ॥२७॥"

[सुश्रुत : उत्तरतन्त्र ५८ : २६]

[भैषज्यरत्नावली : मूत्राघाताधिकार : २]

One *akṣa* of the paste of the seeds of *ervāru* should be mixed with rock salt and administered along with *dhānyāmla* (a sour drink) which cures *mūtrāghāta*.

"पाटल्या यावशूकं[1] च पारिभद्रात्तिलादपि[2] ।
क्षारोदकेन[3] मदिरां[4] त्वगेलोषणसंयुतम् ॥
पिबेद्[5] गुडोपदंशान् वा लिह्यादेतान् पृथक् पृथक् ॥२८॥"

[सुश्रुत : उत्तरतन्त्र ५८ : ४८-४९]

Alkali preparations of *pāṭalī*, *yava*, *pāribhadra* or *tila* should be added with water. Along with this alkali water, jaggery pieces should be taken in a linctus form by adding *madirā* (alcoholic preparation), *tvak*, *elā* and *uṣaṇa*.

त्रिफलाकल्कसंयुक्तं लवणं वा[6] पिपाययेत् ।
"निदिग्धिकायाः स्वरसं पिबेत् कुडवसंमितम् ॥२९॥"

[सुश्रुत : उत्तरतन्त्र ५८ : ३९]

One *kuḍava* of the juice of *nidigdhikā* should be given by adding the paste of *triphalā* or rock salt.

"बलान् पिबेत्कुडवदुग्धेन मुहुर्मूत्रस्य शान्तये ॥३०॥

Balā should be boiled with one *kuḍava* of milk and given for the cure of polyuria.

---

1. यावशूकाच्च इति पंचमपुस्तके पाठः ।
2. पारिभद्रान्तिलादपि इति प्रथमपुस्तके पाठः ।
3. क. क्षीरोदकेन इति प्रथमपुस्तके पाठः ।
   ख. क्षीयदकेन इति प्रथमपुस्तके पाठः ।
4. मतिमान् इति आकरे पाठः ।
5. पिबेद्गुडेन मिश्रं वा लिह्याल्लेहान् इति आकरे पाठः ।
6. इति षष्ठपुस्तके अधिकः पाठः ।

पथ्याविभीतधात्रीणां चूर्णं चूर्णं मृतायसः ।
मधुना सह संलीढं मुहुर्मूत्रस्य शान्तिकृत् ॥३१॥

Powder of *harītakī*, *bibhitakī* and *āmalakī*, and the *bhasma* of *lauha* should be mixed with honey and taken for the treatment of polyuria.

अष्टाविंशत्संख्यकानि पलान्यानीय गोक्षुरः ।
पचेदष्टगुणे नीरे क्वाथो ग्राह्योर्द्धशेषतः ॥३२॥
ततः पुनः पचेत्तत्र पुरं सप्तपलं क्षिपेत् ।
गुडपाकसमाकारं ज्ञात्वा तत्र विनिक्षिपेत् ॥३३॥
त्रिकटुत्रिफलामुस्तं चूर्णितं पलसप्तकम् ।
ततः पिण्डीकृतस्यास्य गुटिकामुपयोजयेत् ॥३४॥
हन्यात्प्रमेहकृच्छ्रं च प्रदरं मूत्राघातकम् ।
वातास्रं वातरोगांश्च शुक्रदोषं तथाश्मरिम् ॥३५॥"[1]

॥ इति गोक्षुरादि गुग्गुलुः ॥

Gokṣurādi Guggulu

Twenty eight *palas* of *gokṣura* should be boiled with eight times of water and reduced to half. In this decoction, seven *palas* of *guggulu* should be boiled till the stage of *guḍa pāka* is attained. To this, seven *palas* in total of the powder of *triphalā*,

---

1. पाठोऽयं पंचमपुस्तके अधिकमुपलभ्यते ।

trikaṭu and *musta* should be added. From out of this paste, pills should be prepared. Administration of this cures *prameha* (obstinate urinary disorders including diabetes), dysuria, menorrhagea, anuria, *vāta rakta* (gout), diseases caused by *vāyu*, seminal ailments and stone in the urinary tract.

जले कुंकुमकल्कं वा सक्षौद्रमुषितं निशि[1] ॥३६॥"

[योगरत्नाकर : मूत्राघातचिकित्सा : (उत्तरार्द्ध) पृष्ठ ६५]

Alternatively, the paste of *kuṅkuma* mixed with honey should be kept overnight and then administered along with water.

सतैलं पाटलाभस्मक्षारबद्धं परिस्रुतम् ।

"सुरां सौवर्चलवतीं मूत्राघाती पिबेन्नरः ॥३७॥"

[सुश्रुत : उत्तरतन्त्र ५८ : ३०]

"दाडिमाम्लयुतं[2] मुख्यमेलाबीजं[3] सनागरम्[4] ।

पीत्वा सुरां सलवणां मूत्राघाताद्विमुच्यते ॥३८॥"

[भैषज्यरत्नावली : मूत्राघाताधिकार : १२]

[सुश्रुत : उत्तरतन्त्र ५८ : ३२]

The *kṣāra* (alkali preparation) of *pāṭalā* should be mixed with water, tied in a piece of cloth and kept hanging. The water

1. निशां इति प्रथमपंचमपुस्तकयोः पाठः ।
2. दाडिमाम्लां युतां इति आकरे पाठः ।
3. ०जीरकनागरैः इति आकरे पाठः ।
4. सानागरम् इति प्रथमपुस्तके पाठः ।

which comes out of it should be added with gingili oil and given. Intake of *surā* (alcoholic preparation) added with *sauvarcala* cures *mūtrāghāta*.

"पिबेत्छिलाजतुक्वाथे गणे वीरतरादिके ।
रसं दुरालभायाः वा[1] कषायं वासकस्य च ॥३९॥"

[योगरत्नाकर : मूत्राघातचिकित्सा : (उत्तरार्द्ध) पृष्ठ ६४]

Śilājatu along with the decoction of drugs belonging to *vīratarvādi* group or juice of *durālabhā* or decoction of *vāsaka* is useful for patients suffering from *mūtrāghāta*.

"त्रिकण्टकैरण्डशतावरीभिः सिद्धं पयो वातभवे[2] च शूले ।
गुडप्रगाढं सघृतं पयो वा रोगेषु कृच्छ्रादिषु शस्तमेतत् ॥४०॥"

[योगरत्नाकर : मूत्राघातचिकित्सा : (उत्तरार्द्ध) पृष्ठ ६५]

Milk boiled with *trikaṇṭaka*, *eraṇḍa* and *śatāvarī* is useful in *vātika* type of colic pain. Jaggery along with ghee or milk is useful in diseases like *mūtra kṛcchra*.

"नलकाशकुशेक्षुशिफां क्वथितां प्रातः[3] सुशीतां ससिताम् ।
पिबतः प्रयाति नियतं मूत्रग्रह[4] इत्युवाच चरकः ॥४१॥"

[योगरत्नाकर : मूत्राघातचिकित्सा : पृष्ठ ६४ (उत्तरार्द्धम्)]

[भैषज्यरत्नावली : मूत्राघाताधिकार : ५]

1. वा इति प्रथमपंचमपुस्तकयोः पाठः ।
2. तृणपञ्चमूलैः इति आदर्शपुस्तकेषु पाठः ।
3. पीतः इति आकरे पाठः ।
4. मूत्रग्रह इवाम्बुवाच रेचेकः इति प्रथमपुस्तके पाठः ।

The decoction of the root of *nala*, *kāśa*, *kuśa* and *ikṣu* should be cooled and given along with sugar early in the morning. This, according to Caraka, certainly cures *mūtragraha* (obstruction to the passage of urine).

"गोधावत्या मूलं क्वथितं घृततैलगोरसोन्मिश्रम् ।
पीतं निरुद्धमचिराद् भिनत्ति मूत्रस्य[1] संघातम् ॥४२॥"

[योगरत्नाकर : मूत्राघातचिकित्सा : (उत्तरार्द्ध) पृष्ठ ६४]

[भैषज्यरत्नावली : मूत्राघाताधिकार : १०]

Intake of the decoction of the root of *godhāvatī* along with ghee, oil or cow's milk instantaneously helps in the passage of the obstructed urine.

"जलेन खदिरीबीजं मूत्राघाताश्मरीहरम् ।
मूलं रुद्रजटायाश्च तक्रपीतं तदर्थकृत्[2] ॥४३॥"

[भैषज्यरत्नावली : मूत्राघातचिकित्सा : ८]

Intake of the seeds of *khadirī* along with water cures *mūtrāghāta* and *aśmarī* (stone in urinary tract). These ailments are also cured by the intake of the root of *rudra jaṭā* along with butter-milk.

"मूत्रे विबद्धे कर्पूरचूर्णं लिङ्गे प्रवेशयेत् ॥४४॥"

[भैषज्यरत्नावली : मूत्राघातचिकित्सा : ७]

If there is obstruction to the passage of urine, then the powder of camphor should be inserted into the urethra.

1. मूलस्य संरोधम् इति आकरे पाठः ।
2. तदर्थहृत् इति प्रथमपुस्तके पाठः ।

"शृतशीतपयोऽन्नाशी चन्दनं तण्डुलाम्बुना ।
पिबेत्सशर्करं श्रेष्ठमुष्णवाते[1] सशोणिते[2] ॥४५॥"

[योगरत्नाकर : मूत्राघातचिकित्सा : (उत्तरार्द्ध) पृष्ठ ६५]

[भैषज्यरत्नावली : मूत्राघाताधिकार : ६]

For the treatment of *uṣṇa vāta* associated with bleeding, sandal wood powder should be given along with rice-wash and sugar. The patient should take boiled and cooled milk as diet.

शीतावगाहश्च बस्तिश्चोष्मवातनिवारणः ।
"कूष्माण्डकरसश्चापि पीतः सक्षारशर्करः[3] ॥४६॥"

Cold bath and medicated enema with cooling drugs cure *uṣṇa vāta*. Intake of the juice of *kūṣmāṇḍa* along with *kṣāra* (alkali preparation) and sugar is also useful in this condition.

"स्त्रीणामतिप्रसङ्गेन शोणितं यस्य सिच्यते ।
मैथुनोपरमश्चास्य बृंहणीयो हितो[4] विधिः ॥
[5]ताम्रचूडवसातैलं हितं चोत्तरबस्तिषु ॥४७॥

---

1. ०वात विनाशनम् इति आकरे पाठः ।
2. सशोणितम् इति षष्ठपुस्तके पाठः ।
3. द्रष्टव्यम्—भैषज्यरत्नावली : मूत्राघाताधिकार : ७ ।
4. विधिर्मतः इति आकरे पाठः ।
5. क. "ताम्र०.........०वस्तिषु" पाठोऽयं प्रथमपंचमषष्ठपुस्तकेषु नोपलभ्यते ।
   ख. "पिष्टाखुवर्चकोष्णेन कांजिकेन प्रलेपयेत् ।
   बृहन्मूत्रान् निहन्त्याशु रंभाकन्दं तथैव च ।
   सीपचूडरसातैलं हितं चोत्तरबस्तिषु ।"
   पाठोऽयं पंचमषष्ठपुस्तकयोः अधिकमुपलभ्यते ।

If there is bleeding through urethra because of excessive indulgence in sex, the patient should be given nourishing therapy, and thereafter, he should go for sexual intercourse. Such a patient should be administered *uttara basti* (douche through genital tract) with the help of the oil collected from the fat of cock.

स्वगु[1]प्ताफलमृद्वीकाकृष्णेक्षुरसितारजः ।
समां[2] समर्द्धभागानि क्षीरक्षौद्रघृतानि च ॥४८॥
सर्वं[3] सम्यग्विमर्द्याक्ष[4]मात्रां लीढ्वा पयः पिबेत् ।
हन्ति शुक्रक्षवोत्थाश्च दोषान् वंध्यासुतप्रदम् ॥४९॥"

[योगरत्नाकर : मूत्राघातचिकित्सा : (उत्तरार्द्ध) पृष्ठ ६५-६६]

The powder of the fruit of *svayaṃ guptā*, *mṛdvikā*, *kṛṣṇā ikṣuraka* and *sitā*, taken in equal quantities should be added with half the quantity of each of milk, honey and ghee. All these should be triturated properly. This linctus should be administered in a dose of one *akṣa* followed by milk. This cures all diseases caused by diminution of semen. This also cures sterility in women.

"चित्रकं सारिवा चैव बला कालानुसारिवा ।
द्राक्षा विशाला पिप्पल्यस्तथा च त्रिफला भवेत् ॥५०॥
तथैव मधुकं दद्यात् दद्यादामलकानि च ।
घृताढकं पचेदेभिः कल्कैरक्षसमन्वितैः ॥५१॥

---

1. सुगुप्ताः इति प्रथमपंचमपुस्तकयोः पाठः ।
2. समानमर्धभागानि इति आकरे पाठः ।
3. सर्वं इति आकरे पाठः ।
4. ०मथ्याक्षमानं इति आदर्शपुस्तकेषु पाठः ।

क्षीरद्रोणे जलद्रोणे तत्सिद्धमवतारयेत् ।
शीतं परिस्रुत[1]तञ्चैव शर्कराप्रस्थसंयुतम्[2] ॥५२॥
तुगाक्षीर्याश्च तत्सर्वं मतिमान् प्रतिमिश्रयेत् ।
ततो मितं पिबेत् काले यथादोषं यथाबलम् ॥५३॥
वातरेताः पित्तरेताः श्लेष्मरेताश्च यो भवेत् ।
रक्तरेताः ग्रन्थिरेताः पिबेदिच्छन्नरोगताम्[1] ॥५४॥
जीवनीयश्च वृष्यश्च सर्पिरेतन्महागुणम् ।
प्रजाहितश्च धन्यश्च सर्वरोगहरं[2] परम् ॥५५॥
सर्पिरेतत्प्रयुञ्जाना स्त्री गर्भं लभते ध्रुवम्[3] ।
असृग्दोषान् जयेच्चापि योनिदोषांश्च संहतान् ॥
मूत्रदोषेषु सर्वेषु कुर्यादेतच्चिकित्सितम् ॥५६॥"

॥ इति चित्रकाद्यं घृतम् ॥

[भैषज्यरत्नावली : मूत्राघाताधिकार : १७-२३]

Citrakādya Ghṛta

One *āḍhaka* of ghee should be added with the paste of one *akṣa* of each of *citraka*, *sārivā*, *balā*, *kālānusarī*, *drākṣā*, *viśālā*, *pippālī*, *triphalā*, *madhuka* and *āmalakī*, and one *droṇa* of each of milk as well as water. After cooking, the ghee should be cooled, and to this, one *prastha* of each of sugar and *tugā kṣīrī* should be added and mixed well. Depending upon the strength

1. ०रोगिताम् इति आकरे पाठः ।
2. सर्वरोगापहं शिवम् इति आकरे पाठः ।
3. लभतेऽचिरात् इति आकरे पाठः ।

of the patient and the nature of the aggravated *doṣas*, this recipe should be administered in appropriate time in appropriate dose. This cures affliction of semen by *vāyu*, *pitta*, *kapha* and *rakta*. This is useful for patients suffering from *granthi retas* (semen with nodules). It promotes longevity and virility. It promotes progeny and fame and cures all types of diseases. It helps in the conception of women. It cures menorrhagea, diseases of female genital tract and all types of urinary disorders.

लवणांबु वरायुक्तं ससूतं यः पिबेन्नरः ।
तस्य नश्यन्ति वेगेन मूत्राघातास्त्रयोदशः[1] ॥५७॥

The patient, who takes salt water mixed with decoction of *triphalā* and purified *pārada*, gets instantaneously cured of 13 types of *mūtrāghāta*.

तिलनिंबपटोलानां क्षारनीरेण[2] यः पिबेत्
मदिरां तेन तेन स्युः त्वगेलोषणसंयुताम्[3] ॥५८॥

Kṣāras (alkali preparations) of *tila*, *nimba* and *paṭola* should be added with water. Along with this alkaline water, *madirā* (a type of alcoholic drink) should be taken by adding *tvak*, *elā* and *uṣaṇa* which cures *mūtrāghāta*,

[4]ओदनं रक्तशालीनां शर्करा च पयस्तथा ।
मूत्रकृच्छ्रे सदा योज्यं पिष्टान्नं च विवर्जयेत् ॥५९॥

---

1. मूत्राघातस्त्रयोदशः इति षष्ठपुस्तके पाठः ।
2. क. क्षरानीरेण यः पिबेत् इति पंचमपुस्तके पाठः ।
   ख. क्षरनीरेण यः पिबेत् इति प्रथमपुस्तके पाठः ।
3. ०संयुतम् इति षष्ठपुस्तके पाठः ।
4. "ओदनं ...... विवर्जयेत्" पाठोऽयं पंचमपुस्तके अधिकमुपलभ्यते ।

Diet

Red variety of *śāli* rice, sugar and milk are always useful for a patient suffering from dysuria. The patient should avoid *piṣṭānna* (pastries).

इति श्रीमहाराजाधिराजटोडरमल्लविरचिते टोडरानन्दे आयुर्वेदसौख्ये मूत्राघातनिदानचिकित्साकथनं नाम द्विचत्वारिंशत्तमो हर्षः ॥६०॥

Thus, ends the 42nd Chapter dealing with diagnosis and treatment of *mūtrāghāta* in *Āyurveda saukhya* of *Taḍarānanda* composed by the great king Ṭoḍara Malla.

CHAPTER VIII

अथ अश्मरीनिदानं चिकित्सा च ।

Diagnosis and Treatment of Aśmarī (Stone in Urinary Tract)

[1]वातपित्तकफैस्तिस्रश्चतुर्थी शुक्रजाऽपरा ।
प्रायः श्लेष्माश्रयाः सर्वा अश्मर्यः स्युर्यमोपमाः ॥१॥

Varieties

Aśmarī (stone) is of four types, viz. *vātika*, *paittika*, *kaphaja* and *śukraja* (seminal). All the varieties of *aśmarī* are dominated by *kapha* and these are like *yama* (the god of death).

---

1. This is the beginning of the 47th Chapter of *Āyurveda saukhya* in *Ṭoḍarānanda* and the invocation reads as follows :—
शिलोवायोच्छानामवेक्ष्यविस्मितान्व्रजौकसोवोधयदच्छितं पिता ।
यंगग्रंवाक्यैः सददा तु भूमिये हरिः शिवं विप्रविहं गपादये ॥

"विशोषयेद्बस्तिगतं सशुक्रं मूत्रं सपित्तं पवनः कफं वा ।
यदा तदाऽश्मर्युपजायते तु क्रमेण पित्तेष्विव रोचना गोः ॥२॥"

[चरक : चिकित्सा २६:३६]

Pathogenesis

When *vāyu* dries up urine along with semen, *pitta* and *kapha* located in the urinary bladder [the term *basti* generally refers to urinary bladder, but in the present context it includes kidneys and ureters], then *aśmarīs* (stones) are formed gradually as *gorocanā* (solidified cattle bile or biliary stone in the cattle) is gradually formed in the cattle.

"नैकदोषाश्रयाः सर्वाः[1] अथासां पूर्वलक्षणम् ।
बस्त्याध्मानं तदासन्नदेशेषु परितोऽतिरुक् ।
मूत्रे बस्तसगन्धत्वं मूत्रकृच्छ्रं ज्वरोऽरुचिः ॥३॥

Premonitory Signs and Symptoms

All these varieties of stone are not based exclusively upon a single *doṣa*. Its premonitory signs and symptoms are distension in the region of urinary bladder, excruciating pain around the urinary bladder region, smell of urine like that of the goat, dysuria, fever and anorexia.

सामान्यलिङ्गं रुङ्नाभिसेवनीबस्तिमूर्धसु ।
विशीर्णधारं मूत्रं स्यात्तया मार्गे[2] निरोधिते ॥४॥

---

1. अश्मर्याः इति पचमपुस्तके पाठः ।
2. मार्गनिरेषने इति म्राकरे पाठः ।

तद्व्यपायात्सुखं मेहेदच्छं गोमेदकोपमम् ।

तत्सङ्क्षोभात्क्षते[1] सास्रमायासाच्चातिरुग्भवेत् ॥५॥

General Signs and Symptoms

The signs and symptoms of *aśmarī* (stone) in general are as follows :

1. Pain in umbilicus, suture which connects the umbilicus with the pelvis and above the region of urinary bladder ;
2. If the stone obstructs the urinary passage, the urinary flow will be in several lines ;
3. When the obstruction is over, the patient passes urine with ease. The urine may be transparent or cloudy like *gomedaka* (cat's eye) ; and
4. If there is injury because of the impact of the stone, then blood passes along with urine and there is excruciating pain.

तत्र वाताद्भृशं त्वार्तो[2] दन्तान् वादति[3] वेपते ।

मृद्गाति मेहनं नाभिं पीडयत्यनिशं क्वणन्[4] ॥६॥

सानिलं मुञ्चति शकृन्मुहुर्मेहति बिन्दुशः ।

श्यावारुणाश्मरी चास्य स्याच्चिता कण्टकैरिव ॥७॥

---

1. तत् संक्षोभात् कृते इति प्रथमपंचमपुस्तकयोः पाठः ।
2. क. व्याप्तो इति पंचमपुस्तके पाठः ।
   ख. ०भृशात्यर्तो इति आकरे पाठः ।
3. खादति इति आकरे पाठः ।
4. क. क्वणत इति प्रथमपुस्तके पाठः ।
   ख. ०क्वणान् इति पंचमपुस्तके पाठः ।

Signs and Symptoms of Vātika Stone

If stone is formed because of excessive aggravation of *vāyu*, then the following special signs and symptoms are manifested :

1. Excruciating pain ;
2. Trembling of both the jaws as a result of which teeth of the one jaw strike against the teeth of the other jaw to produce sound ;
3. The patient rubs his genital organ and umbilicus and always presses these areas ;
4. He passes stool with lot of flatus and frequently passes urine in drops ;
5. The colour of the stone is grayish-pink with sharp projections.

पित्तेन दह्यते बस्तिः पच्यमान इवोष्मवान् ॥
भल्लातकास्थिसंस्थाना रक्तपीताऽसिताऽश्मरी[1] ॥८॥

Signs and Symptoms of Paittika Stone

If the stone is caused by aggravation of *pitta*, then the following special signs and symptoms are manifested :

1. Burning sensation in the urinary bladder ;
2. The patient feels as if the bladder is getting suppurated and there is heating sensation ; and
3. The stone is red, yellow or black in colour and it looks like a seed of *bhallātaka*.

1, रक्तपित्ताशिताश्मरी इति आदर्शपुस्तकेषु पाठः ।

बस्तिर्निस्तुद्यत इव श्लेष्मणा शीतलो गुरुः ॥
अश्मरी महती श्लक्ष्णा मधुवर्णाऽथवा सिता[1] ॥९॥

Signs and Symptoms of Kaphaja Stone

If the stone is caused by the aggravation of *kapha*, then the following special signs and symptoms are manifested.

1. Pain in the region of urinary bladder with cooling sensation and heaviness; and

2. The stone is of big size and smooth and it's colour is like that of honey or white.

एता भवन्ति बालानां तेषामेव च भूयसा ॥
आश्रयोपचयाल्पत्वाद्ग्रहणाहरणे[2] सुखाः ॥१०॥

Generally, young people get afflicted by the above mentioned three types of stones. It is easy to hold and bring out these stones because these are smaller in size and less of *doṣas* are involved in their causation.

शुक्राश्मरी तु महतां जायते शुक्रधारणात् ।
स्थानाच्युतममुक्तं हि मुष्कयोरन्तरेऽनिलः ।
शोषयत्युपसङ्गृह्य शुक्रं तच्छुक्राश्मरी[3] ॥११॥
बस्तिरुक्कृच्छ्रमूत्रत्वं मुष्कश्वयथुकारिणी ।
तस्यामुत्पन्नमात्रायां शुक्रमेति विलीयते ॥१२॥

---

1. शिता इति प्रथमपंचमपुस्तकयोः पाठः ।
2. क. ग्रहणीहरणे इति प्रथमपुस्तके पाठः ।
   ख. ग्रहणीहरणो इति पंचमपुस्तके पाठः ।
3. तच्छुष्कमश्मरी इति आकरे पाठः ।

Signs and Symptoms of Śukrāśmarī

Suppression of the urge for the ejaculation of semen is cause for the manifestation of stone by the semen in adults. If the semen is out from its own place i.e. testicles but could not be ejaculated then *vāyu* located between the two testicles afflicts the semen and makes it compact as a result of which *śukrāśmarī* (seminal stone) is formed. In such cases, there will be pain in urinary bladder, dysuria and oedema in testicles. When these seminal stones are formed, the semen which is subsequently ejaculated does not come out but get mixed up with the urine.

पीडिते त्ववकाशेऽस्मिन् अश्मर्येव च शर्करा ।
अणुशो[1] वायुना भिन्ना सा तस्मिन्ननुलोमगे[2] ।
निरेति[3] सह मूत्रेण प्रतिलोमे विबध्यते ॥१३॥"

[अष्टाङ्गहृदय : निदान ६:७-१६]

Śarkarā (Gravels)

When the space between the particles of the stone is pressurised, small gravels are formed. This pressure is brought about by *vāyu* which breaks stones into small particles. If these particles move downwards, then they come out through the urine. If, however, these particles move upwards, then they obstruct the passage of urine.

"मूत्रस्रोतःप्रवृत्ता[4] सा सक्ता कुर्यादुपद्रवात् ॥
दौर्बल्यं सदनं कार्श्यं कुक्षिशूलमथारुचिम् ॥१४॥

1. अतुशो इति प्रथमपुस्तके पाठः ।
2. त्वस्मिन्ननुलोमगे इति आकरे पाठः ।
3. निरोति इति प्रथमपुस्तके पाठः ।
4. मूत्रस्रोतः श्रिता सा तु सक्ता इति आकरे पाठः

पाडुत्वमुष्णवातं च तृष्णां हृत्पीडनं वमिम्[1] ।
प्रसूननाभिवृषणं रुद्धमूत्र[2]रुजान्वितम् ।
अश्मरी क्षपयत्याशु सिकता शर्करान्विताः ॥१५॥"

॥अश्मरीनिदानम् ॥१६॥

[योगरत्नाकर : अश्मरीनिदान : पृष्ठ ६९-७०]

Complications

When the stone, while passing down through the urinary channel, gets obstructed it causes several complications like weakness, prostration, pain in the pelvic region, anorexia, anemia, *uṣṇa vāta* (burning micturation), thirst, pressure in the cardiac region, vomiting, oedema in umbilicus and scrotum, obstruction to the passage of urine and painful micturation. The stone, in due course of time gets broken into small particles, viz. gravels and sands.

Thus, ends the diagnosis of *aśmarī* (stone).

"अथ सुश्रुतः—

चतस्रोऽश्मर्यो भवन्ति; श्लेष्माधिष्ठानाः; तद्यथाश्लेष्मणा, पित्तेन, वातेन, शुक्रेण चेति ॥१७॥

According to Suśruta

There are four types of *aśmari* (stone) all of which are based on *kapha*. These four varieties are *kaphaja, pittaja, vāta ja* and *śukraja* (seminal).

तत्रासंशोधनशीलस्यापथ्यकारिणः प्रकुपितः श्लेष्मा मूत्रसंपृक्तोऽनुप्रविश्य बस्तिमश्मरीं जनयति ॥१८॥

1. वमिः इति आकरे पाठः ।
2. बद्धमूत्रं इति आकरे पाठः ।

In a person who does not cleanse his body and who indulges in unwholesome diet, *kapha* gets aggravated. This aggravated *kapha* mixed with urine comes to the bladder to cause stone.

तासां पूर्वरूपाणि—ज्वरो बस्तिपीडारोचकौ मूत्रकृच्छ्रं बस्तिशिरोमुष्कशेफसां[1] वेदना कृच्छ्रावसादो बस्तगंधित्वं मूत्रस्येति ॥१९॥

Its premonitory signs and symptoms are fever, pain in urinary bladder, anorexia, dysuria, pain in *basti śiras* (kindneys), scrotum and male genital organ, extreme prostration and smell of the urine like that of goat.

यथास्ववेदनावर्णं दुष्टं सान्द्रमथाविलम् ।
पूर्वरूपे ततः[2] कृच्छ्रान्मूत्रं सृजति मानवः ॥२०॥

During the premonitory stage, depending upon the nature of the *doṣas* involved, different types of pain appear and the colour of the urine varies. The urine becomes thick and cloudy. The patient passes urine with difficulty.

अथ जातासु नाभिबस्तिसेवनीमेहनेष्वन्यतमस्मिन् मेहतो वेदना मूत्रधारासङ्गः सरुधिरमूत्रता मूत्रविकरणं गोमेदकप्रकाशमत्याविलं ससिकतं विसृजति; [धावनलङ्घनप्लवनपृष्ठयानोष्णाध्वगमनैश्च[3] वेदना भवन्ति] ॥२१॥

---

1. ०शोफसां इति प्रथमपुस्तके पाठः ।
2. पूर्वरूपेऽश्मनः इति आकरे पाठः ।
3. "धावन०——भवन्ति" पाठोऽयं आदर्शपुस्तकेषु नोपलभ्यते ।

After the stone in manifested, there is excruciating pain in umbilicus, urinary bladder, *sevanī* (suture between umbilicus and pelvic region) or male genital organ, sudden obstruction to the flow of urine, passing of blood along with urine, change in the colour of the urine, passing of excessively cloudy urine like *gomedaka* along with small gravels and pain during running, jumping, swimming, travelling by riding over an animal, *uṣṇa* (exhaustion ?) and walking a long distance.

तत्र श्लेष्माश्मरी श्लेष्मलमन्नमभ्यवहरतोऽत्यर्थमुपलिप्य[1] परिवृद्धिं प्राप्य बस्तिमुखमधिष्ठाय स्रोतो निरुणद्धि, तस्य मूत्रप्रतिघातात् दाल्यते भिद्यते निस्तुद्यत इव च बस्तिर्गुरुः[2] शीतश्च भवति; अश्मरी चात्र श्वेता स्निग्धा महती कुक्कुटाण्ड-प्रतीकाशा मधूकपुष्पवर्णा [वा][3] भवति, तां श्लैष्मिकीमिति विद्यात् ॥२२॥

Kaphaja type of stone in a patient indulging in *kapha* aggravating diet gets more of layers deposited over it as a result o- which its size gets enlarged. This stone gets lodged in the mouth (opening) of the urinary bladder and obstructs the passage of urine because of which there is pain as if the urinary bladder is getting twisted, ruptured and punctured. The urinary bladder becomes heavy and cool. The stone is white in colour, unctuous, large in size like the egg of hen in shape or like the flower of *madhūka*. This should be diagnosed as *kaphaja* type of *aśmari* (stone).

---

1. ०मुपलिप्याध: इति आकरे पाठ: ।
2. बस्तिर्गुरुश्च भवति इति आदर्शपुस्तकेषु पाठ: ।
3. पाठोऽयं आदर्शपुस्तकेषु नोपलभ्यते ।

पित्तयुतस्तु श्लेष्मा संघातमुपगम्य यथोक्तां परिवृद्धिं प्राप्य बस्तिमुखमधिष्ठाय स्रोतो निरुणद्धि, तस्य मूत्रप्रतिघाताद्दूष्यते चूष्यते दह्यते पच्यते[1] प्रमुष्यते इव बस्तिरुष्णवातश्च भवति; अश्मरी वा[2] सरक्ता पीतावभासा कृष्णा भल्लातकास्थिप्रतिमा मधुवर्णा वा भवति, तां पैत्तिकीमिति विद्यात् ॥२३॥

Kapha associated with *pitta* enters into the compact mass of the stone and causes enlargement of its size. This stone gets lodged in the mouth (opening) of the urinary bladder and obstructs the passage of urine. Because of the obstruction to the passage of urine, there will be sensations as if getting heated, absorbed, burnt, suppurated and dribbling. There will be burning sensation during micturation. The stone is either red or yellowish or black in colour like a fruit of marking-nu (*bhallātaka*). The stone may also have the colour of honey. This should be diagnosed as *paittika* type of stone.

वातयुष्ठस्तु[3] श्लेष्मा संघातमुपगम्य यथोक्तां परिवृद्धिं प्राप्य बस्तिमुखमधिष्ठाय स्रोतो[4] निरुणद्धि, तस्य मूत्रप्रतिघातात्तीव्रा वेदना भवति, तदाऽत्यर्थं[5] पीड्यमानो दन्तान् खादयति,[6] नाभिं पीडयति, मेढ्रं मृद्नाति,[7] पायुं स्पृशति, विवर्त्तते,[8] विदहति,

1. पच्यत इव इति आकरे पाठः ।
2. चात्र इति आकरे पाठः ।
3. वातयुतस्तु इति आकरे पाठः ।
4. श्रोतो इति आदर्शपुस्तकेषु पाठः ।
5. तदाऽत्यर्थं इति प्रथम द्वितीय पुस्तक योः पाठः ।
6. खादति इति आकरे पाठः ।
7. प्रमृद्नाति इति आकरे पाठः ।
8. विशर्धते इति आकरे पाठः ।

वातमूत्रपुरीषाणि कृच्छ्रेण चास्य महता[1] निश्चरति; अश्मरी चात्र श्यावा परुषा विषमा खरा कदम्बपुष्पवत्कण्टकाचिता भवति; तां वातिकीमिति विद्यात् ॥२४॥

The aggravated *vāyu* along with *kapha* enters into the mass of stone and increases its size. When this stone gets lodged in the mouth of the bladder, it obstructs the urinary flow and causes excruciating pain. Because of excruciating pain, the patient presses his teeth, applies pressure on his umbilicus, rubs his genital organ, touches his anus, gets twisted and feels burning sensation. His flatus, urine and stool come out with considerable difficulty. The stone of this type is grayish, dry, uneven and rough. It is covered with sharp projections like the flower of *kadamba*. This should be diagnosed as *vātika* type of stone.

प्रायेणैतास्तिस्रोऽश्मर्यो[2] दिवास्वप्नासमशनाध्यशनशीत[3]स्निग्ध-गुरुमधुराहारप्रियत्वाद्विशेषेण बालानां भवन्ति; तेषामेवाल्पबस्ति-कायत्वादनुपचितमांसत्वाच्च बस्तेः सुखग्रहणाहरणा भवन्ति । [[4]महतां तु शुक्राश्मरी शुक्रनिमित्ता भवति] ॥२५॥"

[सुश्रुत : निदान ३ : ३-११]

1. मेहतो निःसरन्ति इति आकरे पाठः ।
2. क. प्रायशो एतास्तिस्रोशमर्या इति षष्ठपुस्तके पाठः ।
   ख. प्रायशोष्टतास्तिस्तोऽश्मुर्य्यो इति चतुर्थपुस्तके पाठः ।
3. ०सनसीत० इति आदर्शपुस्तकेषु पाठः ।
4. "महतां——भवति" पाठोऽयं आकरे अधिकमुपलभ्यते ।

All these three varieties of stone generally occur by sleep during day time, irregular diet, intake of food before the previous meal is digested and by habitually taking cooling, unctuous, heavy and sweet food. These types of stone specially occur in young persons. In view of the smaller size of their urinary bladder and fleshy bladder, stones in these patients could be gripped and removed with ease. In adults *śukrāśmarī* (seminal stone) is caused because of the affliction of their semen.

आत्रेयात्—

मूत्राविष्टः[1] चयति[2] सुरतं कुरुते यदि
मूत्रेण सहितं शुक्रं च्यवते गर्भसंभवे ।
यस्य यस्य च देहस्य तच्च तत्र प्रवर्त्तते ॥२६॥
मूत्रं मूत्रस्य संस्थाने करोति त्रिकचं[3] धनम् ।
सोऽप्यसाध्यो मूत्रगदो बाल्याद् भवति मानुषे ॥२७॥

According to Ātreya

If a person having the urge for urination enters into sexual intercourse then semen comes out along with urine. If conception takes place by such semen, then, with the part of the semen which is afflicted in this process, the offspring gets afflicted. The urinary bladder and *trika* (lumbo-sacral joint) of the child is specially affected and the child passes thick urine. This ailment, even in children, is incurable. [There are several mistakes in these verses].

---

1. मूत्रविष्टोसरे इति षष्ठपुस्तके पाठः ।
2. पयति इति चतुर्थपुस्तके पाठः ।
3. क. तृकचं इति प्रथमपंचमपुस्तकयोः पाठः ।
   ख. वृकत्वं इति चतुर्थपुस्तके पाठः ।

तारुण्येऽपि[1] प्रजायते विपरीतरते[2] कृते
शुक्रं प्रचलितं यच्च स्त्री शुक्रं यच्च मुंचति ॥२८॥
पुनर्मेहने प्रविशति वातेनाशोषितं च तत् ।
दृषत्वं प्रतिपद्येत मूत्रद्वारं प्ररुंध्यते[3] ॥२९॥
इति तेन मूत्रप्ररोधं वा जायते तीव्रवेदना ।
अण्डसंधिस्थिता सा[4] च शर्करा[5] शस्त्रसाधिनी ॥३०॥

Stone is also formed in adults because of *viparīta rati* (having sexual intercourse with the man sleeping below and woman above him). The semen of the man and the *strī śukra* (vaginal discharge of the woman) enter into the urinary bladder of the man. This semen gets dried up by *vāyu* to form a stone which obstructs the urinary passage as a result of which urination gets obstructed. The patient gets excruciating pain. The stone in this case is lodged at joint between the scrotum and urethra. It might break into small gravels. This is curable by surgery.

सुश्रुतात्

"महतां तु शुक्राश्मरी शुक्रनिमित्ता भवति ॥
मैथुनाभिघातादतिमैथुनाद्वा शुक्रं चलितमनिर्गच्छद्विमार्ग-
गमनादनिलोऽभिहितः[6] संगृह्य मेढ्रवृषणयोरन्तरे संहरति, संहृष्य[7]

---

1. तरुण्यपि इति षष्ठपुस्तके पाठः ।
2. रेते इति चतुर्थपुस्तके पाठः ।
3. प्ररुंध्यतिति तेन इति पंचमपुस्तके पाठः ।
4. ०मा इति पंचमेतरपुस्तकेषु पाठः ।
5. सर्क्करा इति पंचमपुस्तके पाठ : ।
6. ०भिहतः इति आकरे पाठः ।
7 संहृत्य इति आकरे पाठः ।

चोपशोषयति, सा मूत्रमार्गमावृणोति[1] मूत्रकृच्छ्रं बस्तिवेदनां वृषणयोश्च श्वयथुमापादयति[2], पीडितमात्रे च तस्मिन्नेव प्रविलयमापद्यते ॥३१॥"

[सुश्रुत : निदान ३ : १२]

According to Suśruta

In adults *Sukrāśmarī* (seminal stone) is produced as a result of the affliction of the semen.

Because of the injury during intercourse or because of excessive intercourse, the semen which is already exudated from the testicles does not get ejaculated through the normal channel but goes astray into the urinary bladder where it gets afflicted by *vāyu*. This afflicted semen gets accumulated between the *meḍhra* (male genital organ) and scrotum and then gets dried up. This stone obstructs the urinary channel, causing thereby dysuria, pain in urinary bladder and oedema in the scrotum. If pressure is applied, the stone gets broken in that place.

खरनादः

पूर्वं वामे कटिदेशे वेदना समुदीर्यते[3] ।
सफेनं शर्कराचूर्णं[4] मूत्रं सृजति शर्करा ॥३२॥

"तां शुक्राश्मरीमिति विद्यात् ॥३३॥"

[सुश्रुत : निदान ३ : १२]

---

1. मूत्रमार्गं मान्तृणेति इति प्रथमपुस्तके पाठः ।
2. ०माप्सदयति इति प्रथमषष्ठपुस्तकयोः पाठः ।
3. ०दीर्यतौ इति चतुर्थपुस्तके पाठः ।
4. चूर्णमूत्रीं इति प्रथमपुस्तके पाठः ।

धावनलंघनप्लवनपृष्ठयानोष्णाध्वगमनैश्चास्य[1] वेदना भवति ॥३४॥

According to Kharanāda

In the beginning, pain starts in the left lumber region and the patient passes foamy urine along with gravels. This condition is called *śukrāśmarī* (seminal stone). The patient gets pain by running, jumping, swimming, riding on the back of aniꟺals ezposure to heat and walking a long distance.

"भवन्ति चात्र

शर्करासिकतामेहो भस्माख्योऽश्मरिवैकृतम् ।
अश्मर्या शर्करा ज्ञेया तुल्यव्यञ्जनवेदना ॥३५॥
पवनेऽनुगुणे सा तु निरेत्यल्पा विशेषतः ।
सा भिन्नमूर्तिर्वातेन शर्करेत्यभिधीयते ॥३६॥

Thus, it is said :

Śarkarā meha, *sikatā meha* and *bhasma meha* are the different forms of *aśmarī* (stone in the urinary bladder). *Aśmari* (stone) and *śarkarā* (gravel) have similar signs, symptoms and pain. If there is downward movement of wind, then this stone or gravel comes out through the urine particularly if this is smaller in size. Because of *vāyu*, the stone gets broken into small pieces and this condition is called *śarkarā* (gravel).

---

1. क. ०नोष्णधूगमनै० इति प्रथमपुस्तके पाठः ।
   ख. धावनलंघनप्लवनतीक्ष्णपानोष्णाध्व० इति षष्ठपुस्तके पाठः ।
2. च वेपथु इति आकरे पाठः ।

हृत्पीडा सक्थिसदनं कुक्षिशूलं सवेपथुः ।
तृष्णोर्ध्वगोऽनिलः[1] कार्ष्ण्यं[2] दौर्बल्यं पाण्डुगात्रता ।
अरोचकाविपाकौ च[3] शर्करार्त्तो[4] भवन्ति हि[5] ॥३७॥

Signs and Symptoms of Śarkarā

Pain in the cardiac region, weakness in thighs, pain in pelvic region, trembling, thirst, upward movement of the *vāyu*, grayish coloration, weakness, pale body, anorexia and indigestion—these are the signs and symptoms of *śarkarā* (gravel in the urinary tract).

मूत्रमार्गप्रवृत्ता[6] सा सक्ता कुर्यादुपद्रवान्[7] ।
दौर्बल्यं सदनं कार्श्यं कुक्षिशूलमरोचकम् ॥३८॥

Complications

When these gravels come into the channel of urine and cause obstruction, then this gives rise to several complications like weakness, prostration, emaciation, pain in the pelvic regions, anorexia, anemia, burning micturation, thirst, pressure in the cardiac region and vomiting.

---

1. कृष्णोर्ध्वगोनिलः इति प्रथमपंचमपुस्तकयोः पाठः ।
2. कार्ष्ण्यं इति पंचमपुस्तके पाठः ।
3. तु इति आकरे पाठः ।
4. क. शर्करार्त्त इति आकरे पाठः ।
   ख. शर्करार्त्त इति षष्ठपुस्तके पाठः ।
5. च इति आकरे पाठः ।
6. मूत्रमार्गे प्रवृत्ता इति प्रथमपंचमपुस्तकयोः पाठः ।
7. कुर्यादुपद्रवात् इति प्रथमपंचमपुस्तकयोः पाठः ।

पाण्डुत्वमुष्णवातं च तृष्णां हृत्पीडनं वमीम् ।
नाभिपृष्ठकटीमुष्कगुदवंक्षणशेफसाम्[1] ॥३९॥
एकद्वारस्तनुत्वक्को[2] मध्ये बस्तिरधोमुखः ।
अलाब्वा इव रूपेण शिरास्नायुपरिग्रहः[3] ॥४०॥

Urinary Bladder

The urinary bladder is located in the centre of umiblicus, back, lumber region, testicles, anus, pelvic regions and *śephas* (pudendum). It has a thin covering and it faces downwards with one opening. In shape, it is like a gourd (*alābu*). It is full of vessels and ligaments (or it is fastened to the other abdominal viscera with the help of vessels and ligaments).

बस्तिर्बस्तिशिरश्चैव पौरुषं वृषणौ गुदं[4] ।
एकसंबंधना[5] ह्येते गुदास्थिविवराश्रिताः ॥४१॥
मूत्राशयो[6] मलाधारः[7] प्राणायतनमुत्तमम् ॥४२॥

Basti (urinary bladder), *basti śiras* (kidneys), *pauruṣa* (prostrate gland), two *vṛṣaṇas* (testicles) and *guda* (anus) are inter-connected and all these are located in the pelvic region. The urinary bladder is a receptacle of waste products and it is one of the important vital organs.

---

1. क. माभि० इति षष्ठपुस्तके पाठः ।
   ख. ०कटी मुधुगुदवक्षण० इति प्रथमपुस्तके पाठः ।
2. द्वास्तनुत्वक्को इति आदर्शपुस्तकेषु पाठः ।
3. सिरा० इति आकरे पाठः ।
4. गुदः इति आकरे पाठः ।
5. एकसंबन्धिनो इति आकरे पाठः ।
6. मूत्राश्रयो इति प्रथमपंचमपुस्तकयोः पाठः ।
7. मलाधारा इति प्रथमपंचमपुस्तकयोः पाठः ।

पक्वाशयगतास्तत्र नाड्यो मूत्रबहास्तु याः ।
तर्पयन्ति तु ता मूत्रं सरितः[1] सागरं यथा ॥४३॥
सूक्ष्मत्वान्नोपलभ्यन्ते मुखान्यासां सहस्रशः ।
नाडीभिरुपनीतस्य मूत्रस्यामाशयान्तरात् ॥४४॥

Urine Formation

As the sea is supplied with water by rivers, similarly various fine channels coming from the colon and carrying urine supply this urine to the bladder. Since these channels are very subtle, the openings of thousands of these channels are not visible while they carry urine from the *āmāśaya* (intestines).

जाग्रतः स्वपतश्चैव[2] स निःस्यन्देन पूर्यते ।
आमुखात्सलिले न्यस्तः पार्श्वेभ्यः पूर्यते नवः[3] ॥
घटो यथा तथा विद्धि बस्ति मूत्रेण पूर्यते ॥४५॥

As a new jar kept floated in water gets filled up with water from its sides through its numerous pores, similarly, the urinary bladder gets filled up with urine through these innumerable channels by the process of exudation while the person is awake and sleeping.

एवमेव प्रवेशेन वातः पित्तं कफोऽपि वा ।
मूत्रयुक्तमुपस्नेहात्[4] प्रविश्य कुरुतेऽश्मरीम्[5] ॥४६॥

1. सरिताः इति प्रथमपंचमपुस्तकयोः पाठः।
2. स्वपतस्यैव इति पंचमपुस्तकयोः पाठः ।
3. नरः इति आदर्शपुस्तकेषु पाठः ।
4. मूत्रयुक्त उपस्नोहा प्रविश्य इति प्रथम पंचमपुस्तकयोः पाठः ।
5. कुरुतेऽस्मरीन् इति आदर्शपुस्तकेषु पाठः ।

Similarly, *vāyu, pitta* and *kapha* enter into the bladder along with urine because of *upasneha* (exudation) to produce *aśmari* (stone).

अप्सु स्वच्छास्वपि यथा निषिक्तासु नवे घटे ।
कालान्तरेण पङ्कः स्यादश्मरीसंभवस्तथा ॥४७॥

As clear water collected in a new jar gets muddy after the passage of time, similarly, stones are formed in the urinary bladder.

संहन्त्यापो यथा दिव्या मारुतोऽग्निश्च वैद्युतः ।
तद्वद्बलासं बस्तिस्थमूष्मा संहन्ति[1] सानिलः ॥४८॥

As the water vapour in the sky gets condensed to form hail stones because of wind, fire and lightening, similarly, the *kapha* in the urinary bladder gets condensed to form stone by the impact of *pitta* (heat) and *vāyu* (wind).

मारुते प्रगुणे बस्तौ मूत्रं सम्यक् प्रवर्तते ।
विकारा विविधाश्चापि शुक्रदोषास्तथैव च ।
मूत्रदोषाश्च ये केचित्बस्तावेव भवन्ति ते[2] ॥४९॥"

॥ अश्मरीनिदानम् ॥५०॥

[सुश्रुत : निदान ३ : १३-२८]

If *vāyu* is in normal state, then urination takes place properly. In its abnormal condition, it produces various types of urinary and seminal disorders in the urinary bladder.

1. सहति सानिलः इति प्रथमपचमपुस्तकयोः पाठः ।
2. हि इति आकरे पाठः ।

Thus, ends the diagnosis of *aśmari* (stone in the urinary tract).

"अश्मरी दारुणो व्याधिरन्तकप्रतिमो मतः ।
औषधैस्तरुणः साध्यः प्रवृद्धो[1] छेदमर्हति ॥५१॥

[भैषज्यरत्नावली : अश्मर्यधिकार : १]

Line of Treatment

Aśmarī is a serious disease like *yama* (the god of death). The freshly occurring disease is curable by the administration of drugs but the chronic condition needs surgical intervention.

तस्य पूर्वेषु रूपेषु स्नेहादि क्रम इष्यते[2] ।
तेनास्यापचयं यान्ति व्याधेर्मूलान्यशेषतः ॥५२॥"

[सुश्रुत : चिकित्सा ७ : ३-४]

During its premonitory stage, the patient should be administered oleation therapy, etc. by which the stone gets reduced in size and disease gets completely uprooted.

"[3]शुण्ठ्याग्निमंथपाषाणशिग्रुवरुणगोक्षुरैः ।
[4]अभयारग्वधफलैः क्वाथं कुर्याद्विचक्षणः ॥५३॥
रामठक्षारलवणचूर्णं दत्त्वा पिबेन्नरः ।
अश्मरीमूत्रकृच्छ्रघ्नं दीपनं पाचनं परम् ॥

1. प्रवृद्धश्छेदमर्हति इति आकरे पाठः ।
2. इत्यते इति द्वितीयपुस्तके पाठः ।
3. "शुण्ठ्यग्नि०——मेढ्रगम्" पाठोऽयं षष्ठपुस्तके अधिकमुपलभ्यते ।
4. काश्मर्यारग्वधफलैः क्वाथं कृत्वा विचक्षणः इति आकरे पाठः ।

हन्यात्कोष्ठाश्रितं वातं कट्यूरुगुदमेढ्रगम् ॥५४॥"

[भैषज्यरत्नावली : अश्मर्यधिकार : ११-१२]

Intake of the decoction of *śuṇṭhī*, *agni mantha*, *pāṣāṇa bheda*, *śigru*, *varuṇa*, *gokṣura*, *abhayā* and fruit of *āragvadha* along with the powder of *rāmaṭha* (*hiṅgu*), *kṣāra* (alkali preparation) and *lavaṇa* (rock-salt) cures *aśmarī* and dysuria. It stimulates the power of digestion and promotes *pācana* (cooking of uncooked food). It cures aggravated *vāyu* located in the gastro-intestinal tract, lumber region, thighs, anus and pudendum.

"पाषाणभेदो वसुको वशिरास्मांतकौ तथा ॥
शतावरी स्वदंष्ट्रा च बृहती कंटकारिका ॥५५॥
कपोतवक्राऽर्त्तगलः[1] कच्चकोशीरकुंथकः ।
वृक्षादनी भल्लूकश्च वरुणः शाकजं फलम् ॥५६॥
यवाः कुलत्थाः कोलानि कतकस्य फलानि च ।
ऊषकादि प्रतीवापमेषां क्वाथैर्घृतं कृतम् ॥
भिनत्ति वातसंभूतामश्मरीं क्षिप्रमेव तु ॥५७॥
क्षारान् यवागू यूषांश्च कषायाणि पयांसि च ।
भोजनानि च कुर्वीत वर्गोऽस्मिन् वातनाशने ॥५८॥"

[सुश्रुत : चिकित्सा ७ : ५-९]

Treatment of Vātika Stone

Ghee cooked with *pāṣāṇa bheda*, *vasuka*, *vaśira*, *asmāntaka*, *śatāvarī*, *śvadaṃṣṭrā*, *bṛhatī*, *kaṇṭakārikā*, *kapota vakrā*, *ārtagala*,

---

1 कपोतकतिगलः कव्वकोशीरकुंथकः इति पंचमपुस्तके पाठः ।

kaccaka, *uśīra*, *kunthaka*, *vṛkṣādanī*, *bhallūka*, *varuṇa*, fruit of *śāka*, *yava*, *kulattha*, *kola*, fruit of *kataka* and drugs belonging to *ūṣakādi* group quickly breaks the stone (*aśmarī*) caused by aggravated *vāyu*. The patient should take *kṣārās* (alkali preparations), *yavāgū* (thick gruel), vegetable soups, decoctions and milk prepared of the above mentioned *vāyu*-alleviating drugs.

"ऊषकं सैंधवं मृद्वी[1] कासीसद्वयगुग्गुलुः ।
शिलाजतु कुलत्थं[2] च ऊषकादिरुदाहृतः ॥५९॥
ऊषकादिः कफं हन्ति गणो मेदविनाशनः[3] ।
अश्मरीशर्करामूत्रकृच्छ्रघ्नः[4] कफमूत्रनुत् ॥६०॥"
॥ ऊषकादिः ॥

[भैषज्यरत्नावली : अश्मर्यधिकार : १४-१५]

Uṣakādi Group of Drugs

Uṣaka, *saindhava*, *mṛdvīkā*, both the varieties of *kāsisa*, *guggulu*, *śilā jatu* and *kulattha*—these drugs taken together are called *uṣakādi gaṇa* or group. These drugs alleviate *kapha*, reduces fat, cures stone as well as gravel in urine, dysuria and affliction of urine by *kapha*.

"वरुणस्य त्वचं श्रेष्ठां शुण्ठीगोक्षुरसंयुताम् ।
यवक्षारगुडं दत्त्वा क्वाथयित्वाऽपि वर्द्धितम् ॥
अश्मरीं वातजां हन्ति चिरकालानुबन्धिनाम् ॥६१॥"

[भैषज्यरत्नावली : अश्मर्यधिकार : ४]

1. हिंगु इति आकरे पाठः ।
2. तुत्थकञ्च इति आकरे पाठः ।
3. मेदोविशोधनः इति आकरे पाठः ।
4. ०मूत्रशूलघ्नं इति आकरे पाठः ।

The decoction of the bark of *varuṇa*, *śuṇṭhī* and *gokṣura* should be given by adding *yava kṣāra* and jaggery which cures *vātika* type of *aśmarī* even if it is there since a long time.

रुद्राक्षसकलं पिष्ट्वा कदलीकंदवारिणा ।
पीतं मधुकसंयुक्तं अचिरान्मूत्ररोधनुत् ॥६२॥

The paste of *rudrākṣa* should be taken along with the juice of the rhizome of *kadalī* by adding honey (or powder of *madhuka*) which instantaneously cures the obstruction to the passage of urine.

"कुशः काशः सरो[1] गुंद्रा इत्कटो मोरटोऽश्मभित्[2] ।
दर्भो विदारी वाराही शालिमूलं त्रिकंटकः[3] ॥६३॥
भल्लूकः पाटला पाठा पत्तूरोऽथ कुरण्टिका ।
पुनर्नवे[4] शिरीषश्च क्वथितास्तेषु साधितम् ।
घृतं शिलाजं मधुकं बीजैरिन्दीवरस्य च ॥६४।
त्रपुषैर्वारुकादीनां[5] बीजैश्चावापितं शुभम् ॥
भिनत्ति पित्तसम्भूतामश्मरीं क्षिप्रमेव तु ॥६५॥

Treatment of Paittika Stone

Ghee cooked with the decoction of *kuśa*, *kāśa*, *sara*, *gundrā*, *itkaṭa*, *moraṭa*, *aśma bheda*, *darbha*, *vidārī*, *vārāhi*, root of *śāli*,

1. शरो गुल्म उत्करो इति आकरे पाठः ।
2. ०स्मभित् इति प्रथमपुस्तके पाठः ।
3. शिकंटकः इति प्रथमपुस्तके पाठः ।
4. पुनर्नवा इति प्रथमपुस्तके पाठः ।
5. त्रपुषैर्वारुकाणां वा इति आकरे पाठः ।

tri kaṇṭaka, bhallūka, pāṭalā, pāṭhā, pattūra, kuraṇṭikā, śveta punarnavā, rakta punarnavā and *śirīṣa* and the paste of *śilāja, madhuka* and seed of *indīvara, trapuṣa, ervāruka*, etc. instantaneously cures *paittika* type of stone (*aśmarī*).

क्षारान् यवागूर्[1] यूषाश्च कषायाणि पयांसि च ।
भोजनानि च[2] कुर्वीत वर्गेऽस्मिन्पित्तनाशने[3] ॥६६॥

The patient suffering from *paittika* type of stone should take food, viz. *kṣārās* (alkali preparations), *yavāgū* (thick gruel), vegetable soup, decoctions and milk preparations boiled with the above mentioned *pitta*-alleviating drugs.

गणे[4] वरुणकादौ तु गुग्गुल्वेलहरेणुभिः ।
कुष्ठभद्रादिमरिचचित्रकैः[5] ससुराह्वयैः ॥६७॥
एतैः सिद्धमजासर्पिरूषकादिगणेन च ।
भिनत्ति कफसम्भूतामश्मरीं क्षिप्रमेव तु ॥६८॥

Treatment of Kaphaja Stone

Ghee prepared of goat's milk should be cooked with drugs belonging to *varuṇādi gaṇa, guggulu, elā, hareṇu, kuṣṭha, bhadra*, etc., *marica, citraka, surāhvā*, and drugs belonging to *paruṣakādi gaṇa*. This instantaneously cures *aśmarī* (stone) caused by *kapha*.

---

1. यवागूः पेयाश्च इति आकरे पाठः ।
2. प्रकुर्वीत इति आकरे पाठः ।
3. वर्गेऽस्मिन् पित्तनाशने इति आकरे पाठः ।
4. गणो इति प्रथमपुस्तके सुश्रुते च पाठः ।
5. कुष्ठमुस्ताह्व० इति आकरे पाठः ।

क्षारान् यवागूर्यूषाश्च[1] कषायाणि पयांसि च ।

भोजनानि च कुर्वीत वर्गेऽस्मिन् कफनाशने ॥६९॥"

[सुश्रुत : चिकित्सा ७ : ६-१६]

[भैषज्यरत्नावली : अश्मर्यधिकार : ३५-४१]

Kṣārās (alkali preparations), *yavāgū* (thick gruel), *yūṣa* (vegetable soup), decoctions and milk preparations added with the above mentioned *kapha*-alleviating drugs should be given as food to the patient suffering from *kaphaja* type of *aśmarī* (stone).

कफाश्मरीचिकित्सतमभिधाय शुक्राश्मरी चिकित्सतं न पृथगुक्तवान् आचार्यः[2] ॥ ७० ॥

Having described the treatment of *kaphaja aśmarī* the author (*ācārya*) has not described the treatment of *śukrāśmarī* (seminal stone) separately.

---

1. यवागूः पेयाश्च इति आकरे पाठः ।
2. 'वरुणांकुरं टकाशिग्रु । बृहतीद्वय । वरी । ककुभ । करंज बिल्व । अरणी । ऋषिभिः द्वि पवलयाग्निमंथयुत यासमोरप्या भवति गणः सकर्कटक मेषविषाणिकया गुल्मेषु विद्रधिषु वात- बलासजेषु कोष्ठान्तरास्थितेषु शूलरुगातरेत्सु प्रायः कफानिला विकारिरिति पीडितानामुक्तो नृणां वरुणादिरयं भिषग्भि ॥ वरुणकादिः ॥"
—पाठोऽयं चतुर्थपंचमषष्ठपुस्तकेषु अधिकमुपलभ्यते ।

भोजाचार्यस्तु पृथगुक्तवान्—

स्नेहाभ्यंगस्वेदनं तप्ततोयैः

सेको नृणां देहसंवाहनानि ।

तिक्तैः क्वाथैरूषणैः स्यान्निरूहः[1]

शुक्राश्मर्यां सेवनं योषितां च ॥७१॥

According to Bhoja

Bhoja has described the treatment of *śukrāśmarī* separately. According to him, the patient suffering from *śukrāśmarī* should take oleation, massage and fomentation therapies, sprinkling of hot water over the body, *saṃvāhana* (gentle massage) of the body and *nirūha* type of medicated enema with the decoction of bitter drugs added with *uṣaṇa*. The patient should have sexual intercourse with ladies.

"पिचुकङ्कोलकतकशाकेन्दीवरजैः[2] फलैः[3] ।

चूर्णितैः सगुडं[4] तोयं शर्कराशमनं पिबेत् ॥७२॥

Treatment of Śarkarā (Gravels)

The powder of *picu*, *kaṅkola*, *kataka*, *śāka*, fruit of *indīvara* should be taken along with jaggery and water which cures *śarkarā* (gravels) in urine.

क्रौश्चोष्ट्[5]रासभास्थीनि श्वदंष्ट्रा तालपत्रिका ।

---

1. ०निरूहैः इति षष्ठपुस्तके पाठः ।
2. ये चकंक्षालवणा केन्दीवरजैः इति षष्ठपुस्तके पाठः ।
3. पलैः इति षष्ठपुस्तके पाठः ।
4. क. सकलं इति षष्ठपुस्तके पाठः ।
   ख. सगुणं इति पंचमपुस्तके पाठः ।
5. क्रौष्ट्रोष्ट्र० इति पंचमपुस्तके पाठः ।

अजमोदा कदम्बस्य मूलं नागरमेव च ।
पीतानि शर्करां भिन्द्युः[1] सुरयोष्णोदकेन वा ॥७३॥

Intake of the powder of the bones of *krauñca*, *uṣṭra* and *rāsabha*, *śvadaṃṣṭrā*, *tālapatrikā*, *ajamodā*, root of *kadamba* and *nāgara* along with *surā* (alcoholic drink) or hot water cures *śarkarā* (gravels) in the urine.

त्रिकण्टकस्य बीजानां चूर्णं माक्षिकसंयुतम् ।
आविक्षीरेण सप्ताहमश्मरीभेदनं पिबेत् ॥७४॥"

[सुश्रुत : चिकित्सा ७ : १७-२०]

Intake of the powder of the seeds of *trikaṇṭaka* along with honey and milk of sheep for one week cures *aśmarī* (stone).

केतकीपत्रनिःक्वाथो हिंगुक्रौंचास्थिसंयुतः ।
अश्मरीं पातयेत् क्षिप्रमेलाहिंगुघृताविलः ॥७५॥

The decoction of the petals of *ketakī* should be added with ***hiṅgu*** and bone of *krauñca*. Intake of this decoction along with *elā*, ***hiṅgu*** and ghee instantaneously cures *aśmarī* (stone).

"द्रव्याणां तु घृतोक्तानां क्षारोऽविमूत्रगालितः[2] ।
ग्राम्यसत्त्वशकृत्क्षारैः संयुक्तः[3] साधितः शनैः ॥७६॥

---

1. सिन्धुः इति प्रथमपंचमपुस्तकयोः पाठः ।
2. क. ०वीमूत्रगालितः इति प्रथमपुस्तके पाठः
   ख. क्षारावीमूत्रगालितः इति पंचमपुस्तके पाठः ।
   ग. क्षारोवमूत्रगास्थितः इति षष्ठपुस्तके पाठः ।
3. संयुतः इति पंचमपुस्तके पाठः ।

तत्रोषकादिरावापः कार्यस्त्रिकटुकान्वितः ।
एष क्षारोऽश्मरीं गुल्मं शर्करां च भिनत्त्यपि[1] ॥७७॥

Drugs described above for the preparation of medicated ghee should be burnt to prepare *kṣāra* (alkali preparation). This *kṣāra* added with the *kṣāra* of cow-dung should be slowly boiled by adding sheep urine. To this, the powder of drugs belonging to *uṣakādi gaṇa* and *trikaṭu* should be added. This *kṣāra* (alkali preparation) cures *aśmarī* (stone), *gulma* (phantom tumour) and *śarkarā* (gravel) in the urine.

तिलापामार्गकदलीपलाशयवबिल्वजः[2] ।
क्षारः पेयोऽविमूत्रेण शर्करानाशनः परः ॥७८॥

Intake of the *kṣāra* (alkali preparation) of *tila*, *apāmārga*, *kadalī*, *palāśa*, *yava* and *bilva* along with sheep urine cures *śarkarā* (gravel) in the urine.

पाटलाकरवीराणां क्षारमेवं समाचरेत् ।
श्वदंष्ट्रायष्टिकाब्राह्मीकल्कं वाऽक्षसमं पिबेत् ॥७९॥
सहेलका[3]ख्यौ[?]पेयौ वा तथा शौभाञ्जनकमार्कवौ[4] ॥८०॥
कपोतवङ्कामूलं वा पिबेदम्लसुरादिभिः ।
तत्सिद्धं वा पिबेत्क्षीरं वेदनाभिरुपद्रुतः[5] ॥

1. विनित्यपि इति पंचमपुस्तके पाठः।
2. तिल्वजः इति षष्ठपुस्तके पाठः ।
3. क. सहैडकाख्यौ इति आकरे पाठः ।
   ख. सहैलकामयौ इति षष्ठपुस्तके पाठः ।
4. सौभंजनकमार्कवौ: इति आदर्शपुस्तकेषु पाठः ।
5. वेदनाभिरुपद्रवः इति प्रथमपंचमपुस्तकयोः पाठः ।

हरीतक्यादिसिद्धं वा वर्षाभूसिद्धमेव वा ॥८१॥"

[सुश्रुत : चिकित्सा ७ : २०-२६]

For the cure of *aśmari*, the patient may use the following :

1. *Kṣāra* (alkali preparation) of *pāṭalā and karavīra* ;
2. One *akṣa*, of the paste of *śvadaṃṣṭrā, madhu yaṣṭi* and *brāhmi* ;
3. Decoction of *śobhāñjana* and *mārkava* along with *elakākhya* [?];
4. Root of *kapota vaṅkā* along with sour juice, alcohol, etc.
5. Milk boiled with the root of *kapota vaṅkā* for pain ; and
6. Milk boiled with *harītakī*, etc. or *varṣābhū*.

वैद्यसुरद्रुमात्—

पत्रं कृष्णकुलत्थानां[1] वरुणां हृत्ववस्य[?]च ।
कूष्मांडमूलत्रपुसमूलं[2] च महती फलम् ॥८२॥
शतपुष्पा व[3] निर्गुंडी त्रिफलानगभिद्बला[4] ।
वृंत्तिकात्रिककर्णं च कासकुशरजं[5] तथा ॥८३॥
गुंद्रातरुणचित्रा[6] च चित्रकं तरुणा[7] तथा ।
पृथक् पृथक् शरावं[8] च प्रत्येकं ग्राहयेद्बुधः ॥८४॥

---

1. कृष्णकुलच्छानां इति प्रथमपुस्तके पाठः ।
2. ०त्रपुषमूलं च बृहती इति षष्ठपुस्तके पाठः ।
3. च इति चतुर्थषष्ठपुस्तकयोः पाठः ।
4. ०नगभिद्व्या इति चतुर्थपुस्तके पाठः ।
5. काशकाश इति षष्ठपुस्तके पाठः ।
6. गुंद्रारातरुण० इति पंचमपुस्तके पाठः ।
7. तरूणामजिष्ठा इति पंचमपुस्तके पाठः ।
8. सरावं इति प्रथमपंचमपुस्तकयोः पाठः ।

गोनीभीतजलेनैव क्वाथयेत् द्रोणशेषितम् ।
विमृद्य वस्त्रपूतं च ताम्रपात्रे नियोजयेत् ॥८५॥
घृतमौरभ्रजं पात्रं तक्षीरं चाक्षकं क्षिपेत् ।
कूष्मांडमूलं बीजं च तथा त्रपुससंभवम् ॥८६॥
अलाबुनालिकां वाऽपि शिलाभेदं शिलाग्रजम् ।
पाच्यं सकाकिनीमूलं दूर्वामूलं सगोक्षुरम् ॥८७॥
द्राविडींकर्निकारां च रुद्राक्षां कच्यकं तथा ।
पृथक् पृथक् शुक्तिसमं कल्कार्थं संप्रदापयेत् ॥८८॥
मृद्वग्निना घृतं पक्वं पिबेन्नित्यं हिताशिनः ।
शुक्रदोषविशुद्धयर्थं शर्कराश्मरीनाशनम्[1] ॥८९॥
[2]मूत्राघातेषु सर्वेषु मूत्रकृच्छ्रेऽतिदारुणे ।
प्रमेहे सोमरोगे च रक्तपित्ते विशेषतः ॥९०॥
रजोदोषेषु नारीणां जेतायं सर्पिरुत्तमः ।
नातः परतरं किंचिदेषु रोगेषु निश्चतम् ॥९१॥

According to Vaidya Sura Druma

Leaf of black variety of *kulattha*, bark of *varuṇa*, root of *kūṣmāṇḍa*, *trapusa* and *mahā phala*, *śata puṣpā*, *nirguṇḍi*, *triphalā*, *pāṣāṇa bheda*, *balā*, *vṛntāka*, *trika karṇa*, powder of *kāsa* and *kuśa*, *gundrā*, *taruṇa*, *citrā*, *citraka* and *taruṇā* (*mañjiṣṭhā*)—all these drugs taken separately in the quantity of one *śarāva* each should be boiled in one *goni* of water till one *droṇa* remains.

---

1. शर्करोऽश्मरिभेदनम् इति चतुर्थपुस्तके पाठः ।
2. 'मूत्राघातेषु ·········भेदनम्' पाठोऽयं चपुर्थषष्ठपुस्तकयोः नोपलभ्यते ।

It should be squeezed, strained through a cloth and stored in a copper vessel. To this, one *pātra* of the ghee prepared of the milk of sheep, one *akṣa* of sheep milk and the paste of one *śukti* of each of root and seed of *kūṣmāṇḍā*, seed of *trapusa*, stem of *alābu*, *śilā bheda*, *śilāgraja*, *pācya*, root of *kākini* and *dūrvā*, *gokṣura*, *drāviḍi*, *karnikāra*, *rudrākṣa* and *kataka* should be added and cooked over mild fire. This should be taken daily along with wholesome food. It cleanses the vitiated semen and cures *śarkarā* (gravel) and *aśmari* (stone). It is an excellent recipe for all types of *mūtrāghāta* (anuria), serious types of dysuria, *prameha* (obstinate urinary disorders including diabetes), *soma roga* (polyuria or diabetes insipidus), *rakta pitta* (an ailment characterised by bleeding from different parts of the body) and menstrual disorders in ladies. There is certainly no other recipe better than this for the cure of the above mentioned diseases.

आत्रेयात्—

पाके लघ्वादिकं [?] सर्पि सर्वरोगविनाशनम् ।

वृद्धि करोति चास्थीनां शर्कराश्मरिभेदनम्' ॥६२॥

According to Ātreya

The ghee is light for digestion and it cures all diseases. It promotes growth of bones disintegrates *śarkarā* (gravel) and *aśmari* (stone) in the urinary tract. [The meaning of the first of the verse is not clear].

स्निग्धं[1] घनं वरुणजं वल्कलं[2] कंससम्मितम् ।

---

1. "पाषाणरोगभीतः सौवर्च्चलयुतां सुरां पिबेत् ।
शुक्राश्मर्य्यास्तु सामान्ये शुक्राश्मरि विनाशनम् ।
तद्वन्मधुदुग्धयुतां त्रिरातं तिलनालभूतिं च ।
॥एलोपल्येति योगः ॥
पाषाणभेदवृषकश्वदंष्ट्रा पाठाभया व्योषसठीनिकुंभाः ।
हिंस्रावराह्वासितिवारकानामेर्वारुकाणी त्रपुषाद्यवीजम् ।
उपकुचिकाहिंगुसवेतसाम्लं स्याद्वे वृहत्यौंहपुषा वचा च ।
चूर्णं पिवेदश्मरि भेदपक्वं सर्पिश्च गोमूत्र चतुर्गुणं तैः ।"
—पाठोऽयं षष्ठपुस्तके अधिकमुपलभ्यते ।

2. वल्कल इति प्रथमपुस्तके पाठः ।

मधूकजं तदर्धं च यूथीमूलं तदर्द्धतः ॥९३॥
गुडूचीसारिवावासापृथक्पर्णीशतावरी— ।
कूष्मांडनाडीसूक्ष्मैलानगभिच्च[1] पृथक् पृथक् ॥९४॥
प्रत्येकमष्टपलिकं चंदनं कुडवत्रयम् ।
जलं चतुर्गुणं दत्त्वा कुर्यादर्द्धावशोषितम् ॥९५॥
वस्त्रपूतं कृतं पश्चात्प्रपुराणं तुलासमम् ।
गुडं संभिश्रयेत् क्षौद्रं प्रस्थार्द्धं निक्षिपेत्तथा ॥९६॥
गौरांगी गोक्षुरफलं भार्गवीमर्कट्यस्थि च ।
रुद्राक्षशर्करीगोपेवरावरुणवल्कलम् ।
पृथक् पलद्वयं नीत्वा चूर्णयित्वा भिषक्तमः ॥९७॥
पाषाणभेदकुडवं चूर्णितं वाऽपि निक्षिपेत् ।
एतत् सर्वसमालोड्य नवे कुंभे विनिक्षिपेत् ॥९८॥
सुखोषितं द्वादशाहमेतच्चोर्ध्वं पिबेत् वरम् ।
मूत्राघातं मूत्रकृच्छ्रमश्मरीं शर्कराश्मरी ॥९९॥
बस्तेगुरुत्वं दुर्न्नामं प्रमेहं च जयेत् ध्रुवम् ।
वरुणासवसंज्ञोऽयं प्रोवाच कपिलो मुनिः ॥१००॥
॥ वरुणासवः ॥

Varuṇāsava

One *kaṁsa* of the unctuous and compact barks of *varuṇa*, half *kaṁsa* of the bark of *madhūka*, one fourth *kaṁsa* of the

---

1. ०धूत्रैं इति चतुर्थपुस्तके पाठः ।

root of *yūthikā*, eight *palas* of each *of guḍūcī, sarivā, vāsā,, pṛthak parṇi, śatāvarī, stalk* of *kuṣmāṇḍa, sūkṣmailā* as well as *pāṣāṇa bheda* and one *kuḍava of candana* should be boiled by adding four times of water and reduced to half. This should be strained through a cloth. To this decoction, one *tulā* of very old jaggery, half *prastha* of honey and the two *palas* of the powder of each of *gourāṅgī*, fruit of *gokṣura, bhārgavi, markaṭāsthi, rudrākṣa, śarkari, gope* [?], *varā* and bark of *varuṇa* should be added. In addition, one *kuḍava* of the powder of *pāṣāṇa bheda* should be added to it. All these ingredients should be mixed properly and kept in a new jar covered all around with paddy husk for twelve days. Thereafter, this should be administered which cures *mūtrāghāta* (anuria), dysuria, *aśmarī* (stone), *śarkarā* (gravel) in the urinary tract, heaviness of the urinary tract, piles and *prameha* (obstinate urinary disorders including diabetes). This is called *varuṇāsava* and it was propounded by sage Kapila.

नमेरुगोक्षंटदुरालभा च सशृंगवेरांघ्रि[1] हरीतकी च ।
हारामृतारग्वधकिकिरातसु[2]कंदशुण्ठीवरुणादिभिश्च ॥१०१॥

[द्वि[3]श्रामा]पाषाणभित्कृष्णकुलत्थकं[4] च ।
कु[5]लत्थिका संहृतक्षत्तिकाभिः[?] ।
कृत्वा कषायोऽष्टगुणजलेन ।
पि[6]बेत सामुद्रिकशर्क[7]राद्यः ॥१०२॥

1. ०म० इति षष्ठपुस्तके पाठः ।
2. किरातरक्तकं इति षष्ठपुस्तके पाठः ।
3. ह्निरा० इति पंचमपुस्तके पाठः ।
4. कुलच्छकं इति प्रथमपुस्तके पाठः ।
5. ०कुलच्छिकासं हृतच्छत्तिकाभिः इति प्रथमपुस्तके पाठः ।
6. क. पिबेतसामुद्रिक० इति प्रथमपुस्तके पाठः ।
7. शर्कराढ्यः इति पंचमपुस्तके पाठः ।

मूत्राघातं मूत्रकृच्छ्राश्मरीं च ।
मूत्रग्रंथिं शर्करां कष्टसाध्यां ।
बस्त्याध्मानं कुक्षिशूलं ज्वरं च ।
हन्यादेतत्क्वाथराजो न चित्रम्[1] ॥१०३॥

Nameru, gokaṇṭaka, durālabhā, śṛṅgavera, harītakī, hārā [?], *amṛtā, āragvadha, kiṃ kirāta, sukanda, śuṇṭhī*, drugs belonging to *varuṇādi gaṇa, pāṣāṇa bheda*, black variety of *kulattha* and *kulatthikā* should be boiled in eight times of water. This decoction should be taken by adding salt, sugar, etc. It cures *mūtrāghāta* (anuria), dysuria, *aśmarī* (stone), *mūtra granthi* (nodular growth in the urinary tract), incurable type of *śarkarā* (gravel) in the urinary tract, distension of urinary bladder, pain in the pelvic region and fever. This is the best among the decoctions for the undoubtedly cure of the above mentioned ailments.

गोपुरात्—

नित्यं सेवेत मतिमान् कृतं कूष्मांडनालिकाम्[2] ।
कूष्मांडसुकृतं[3] सेवेत्पुराणपक्वमेव वा ॥१०४॥
पित्तनुत्तेषु[4] कूष्मांडं बालं मध्यं कफापहम् ।
पक्वं लघूष्णं सक्षारं दीपनं बस्तिशोधनमिति[5] ॥१०५॥

According to Gopura

A wise person should take daily *Kūṣmāṇḍa* which may be either tender or matured or ripe. The tender *kūṣmāṇḍa* alleviates

1. ०राजोनचि चा इति पंचमपुस्तके पाठः ।
2. ०नालिकां इति षष्ठपुस्तके पाठः ।
3. शकृतं इति पंचमपुस्तके पाठः ।
4. पित्ततुत्तेषु इति प्रथमपुस्तके पाठः ।
5. शोधनं । ॥इति सुश्रुतः॥ इति षष्ठपुस्तके पाठः ।

pitta, the moderately matured one alleviates *kapha* and the fully matured or ripe one is light, hot, *sakṣāra* (having action of the alkalis) and stimulant of digestion. The matured one also cleanses the urinary bladder.

"सुश्रुतः

"सर्वथैवोपयोज्यः[1] स्याद्गणो वीरतर्वादिकः ।
घृतैः क्षारैः कषायैश्च क्षीरैः सोत्तरबस्तिभिः[2] ॥१०६॥
यदि नोपशमं गच्छेच्छेद्स्तत्रोत्तरो[3] विधिः ।
कुशलस्यापि वैद्यस्य यतः सिद्धिरिहाध्रुवा ॥१०७॥
उपक्रमो जघन्योऽयं संमतः परिकीर्त्तितः ।
अक्रियायां[4] ध्रुवो मृत्युः क्रियायां संशयो भवेत् ।
तस्मादापृच्छ्य कर्त्तव्यमीश्वरं साधुकारिणा[5] ॥१०८॥

According to Suśruta

For the treatment of *aśmarī* (stone), drugs belonging to *Vīratarvādi* group should always be used in the preparation of medicated ghee, *kṣāra* (alkali preparation), decoction, milk preparation and *uttara basti* (medicated douche through the genital tract). If the disease does not subside by these therapies

---

1. सर्वथैवोपयोज्यगः इति षष्ठपुस्तके पाठः ।
2. सोन्पृखवस्तिभिः इति प्रथमपंचमपुस्तकयोः पाठः ।
3. गच्छेदुच्छ्रस्तनूत्तारो इति षष्ठपुस्तके पाठः ।
4. क. अकृपायां इति पंचमपुस्तके पाठः ।
   ख. अकृयायां इति प्रथमपुस्तके पाठः ।
   ग. अत्रियायां इति षष्ठपुस्तके पाठः ।
5. साधुवारिणा इति प्रथमपंचमपुस्तकयोः पाठः ।

then surgical measures should be adopted. Even an expert physician (surgeon) cannot guarantee success in these operations. Therefore, surgical methods are considered to be extreme measures. Without treatment (surgical) the patient is certain to die; if these surgical measures are adopted, there is a possibility of survival. Therefore, surgery should be performed with good intentions after taking permission of the authorities.

अथ रोगान्वितमुपस्निग्धमपकृष्टदोषमीषत्कर्शितमभ्यक्तस्विन्न-
शरीरं भुक्तवंतं कृतबलिमङ्गलस्वस्तिवाचनमग्रोपहरणीयोक्तेन
विधानेनोपकल्पितसम्भारमाश्वास्य, ततो बलवन्तमविक्लवमा-
जानुसमे फलके प्रागुपवेश्य पुरुषं तस्योत्संगे निषण्णपूर्वकायमुत्तान-
मुत्तरकटीकं वस्त्राधारकोपविष्टं संकुचितजानुकूर्परमितरेण
सहावबद्धं[1] सूत्रेण शाटकैर्वा[2] ततः स्वभ्यक्तनाभिप्रदेशस्य वामपार्श्वं
विमृद्य मुष्टिनाऽवपीडयेदधोनाभेर्यावदश्मर्यधःप्रपन्नेति[3], ततः
स्नेहाभ्यक्ते कृत्तनखे[4] वामहस्तप्रदेशिनीमध्यमे[5] पायौ प्रणिधायानु-
सेवनीमासाद्य[6] प्रयत्नबलाभ्यां पायुमेढ्रान्तरमानीय, निर्बलायमना-[7]

---

1. क. सहावधं इति प्रथमपञ्चमपुस्तकयोः पाठः ।
   ख. सदावधं इति षष्ठपुस्तके पाठः ।
2. साकटैर्वा इति आदर्शपुस्तकेषु पाठः ।
3. प्रवर्तति इति प्रथमपंचमपुस्तकयोः पाठः ।
4. क्लृप्तनखे इति आकरे पाठः ।
5. क. ०मध्ये इति आदर्शपुस्तकेषु पाठः ।
   ख. मध्यमे अंगुल्यौ इति आकरे पाठः ।
6. च पाठोऽयं आदर्शपुस्तकेषु अधिकमुपलभ्यते ।
7. निर्व्यलीकमनायतमविषमं इति आकरे पाठः ।

यतमविषमं च बस्तिं सन्निवेश्य, भृशमुत्पीड्येदंगुलीभ्यां[1] यथा ग्रंथिरिवोन्नतं शल्यं भवति ॥१०९॥

स चेद्गृहीते[2] शल्ये तु विवृताक्षो विचेतनः ।
हतवर्णं[3] च मूर्च्छा च निर्विकारो मृतोपमः ॥११०॥
न तस्य निर्हरेच्छल्यं निर्हरेत्तु[4] म्रियेत सः ।
विना त्वेतेषु रूपेषु निर्हर्तुं समुपाचरेत् ॥१११॥

ततः सव्ये पार्श्वे सेवनीं यवमात्रेण मुक्त्वाऽवचारयेच्छस्त्रमश्मरीप्रमाणं, दक्षिणतो वा[5] क्रियासौकर्यहेतोरित्येके, यथा सा न भिद्यते चूर्ण्यते तां[6] तथा प्रयतेत[7], चूर्णमल्पमल्पमप्यव[8]स्थितं हि पुनः परिवृद्धिमेति, तस्मात् समस्तामग्रवक्रेणाददीत ॥११२॥"

[सुश्रुत : चिकित्सा ७ : २६-३३]

The patient should first of all be given oleation therapy and his body should be cleansed of waste products. By these measures his body will be slightly emaciated. He should be massaged,

---

1. भृशमुत्पीडयेदङ्गुलिभ्यां इति आकरे पाठः ।
2. चेद्गृहीतशल्ये इति आकरे पाठः ।
3. हतवल्लम्बशीर्षश्च इति आकरे पाठः ।
4. निर्हर्तेत्तु इति आदर्शपुस्तकेषु पाठः ।
5. व इति प्रथमपंचमपुस्तकयोः पाठः ।
6. वा इति आकरे पाठः ।
7. क. प्रजयेत् इति प्रथमपंचमपुस्तकयोः पाठः ।
   ख. प्रयोज्येत् इति षष्ठपुस्तके पाठः ।
8. क. चूर्णमल्पमप्यवस्थितं इति आकरे पाठः ।
   ख. चर्णमल्पस्थितं इति षष्ठपुस्तके पाठः ।

given fomention therapy and food to eat. After performing *bali* (sacred offerings), *maṅgala* (auspicious invocation) and *svasti vācana* (recitation of incantations for the welfare of the patient) and after collecting all drugs and equipments as described in the *agropaharaṇiya* section, the patient, prepared as stated above, should be consoled with assuring words. The patient, who is physically strong and who is not mentally disturbed, should be made to sit over a chair having the height of his knees. His lower limbs should then be raised; he should be made to rest his lumber region over a pad of clothes. Then his bent elbo joints should be tied to his raised knees with the help of ropes or a piece of cloth. Oil should be applied to his umbilical region and downward pressure should be applied in the left side of his umbilical region till the stone comes down. The physician should have his nails properly clipped and fingers greased with oil. Then he should insert his ring and middle fingers of the left hand into the anus of the patient, pass them deep into it on the line of the suture (*sevanī*) and bring these fingers with efforts to the space between the anus and pudendum. Without twisting, stretching and uneven movement, he should make these fingers to enter into wall of the urinary bladder and apply more pressure with these fingers so that the stone projects with the skin of the urethra like a tumour. If the patient, while handling the stone in the above mentioned manner bears a wild look with retracted eyelids, becomes unconscious and cynosed, faints, becomes non-responsive and like a dead person, then the stone should not be removed because in that case he is sure to die. If such signs are absent, then efforts should be made to remove the stone. Then, with the scalpel, an incision should be made in the left side of the urethral suture leaving the space of the size of one *yava* (thickness of a barley grain). According to some authorities, this incision can also be made in the right side of the suture depending upon the convenience of the surgeon. The size of the incision should be such as would allow the stone to come out through it. While removing the stone through this incision it should be ensured that the stone does not break or become powder because if a small quantity of the powder remains, then stone may be formed again. Theretore, the entire stone should be removed with the help of the equipment called *agra vakra* (a metallic rod with a curved top).

अथ वैतरणा: –

गर्भस्याधः[1] स्त्रियां बस्तिरुर्ध्वं[2] गर्भाशयाश्रितः ।
गर्भाशयश्च बस्तिश्च महास्रोतः समाश्रितौ ॥११३॥
बस्तिभागं समुन्नस्य[3] प्रवजस्याश्मरीं[4] बुधः ।
स्फिगग्रे भेदनं तासां हितमन्यत्र दोषकृदिति ॥११४॥

According to Vaitaraṇa

The urinary bladder in ladies is located at level lower than the uterus and the bladder rests over the uterus. Both the uterus and the urinary bladder are located above the *mahā srotas* (alimentary tract). Having pressed the appropriate portion of the bladder, the incision should be made over the pelvic bone (not near the suture in the perenium) failing which this may lead to complications.

---

1. "गुडां कृत्वा शल्य विद्धामशाम्यतीं प्रत्याख्याय समुद्धरेत् पायुस्थांद्धंगुलीतुमद्रोत्तरी कृताम् । सेवन्याः सक पार्श्वे च यवमात्रां विमुच्यते । गुडां कृत्वाश्मरी त्रकर्षेता शस्त्रकर्मकृत् । छिन्नेतवस्त्री व्रणवत्तलान्मृत्युस्थावरी विनानिशेषाश्मरीकुर्य्या बस्तौ रक्तं च निर्हरेत् । हृताश्मरीकमुष्णां भोगहयेत्सकृतं तथा । शुष्कमूलविशुद्धं च मध्वात्युक्तं व्रणं ततः । दद्यात्साज्यां त्र्यहं पेयां साधितां मूत्रशोधिभिः । आदशहततो दद्यात्पयसामृदुभोजनम् । स्वेदयेद्दधिमध्वाज्यैः कषायैः क्षालयेद्व्रणंम् । प्रपौंडरीक मंजिष्ठा यष्ठीलौढ्रैश्चलेपयेत् । एतैश्चसनिसैः सिद्धघृतं त्र्यञ्जनं हितम् । त्र्यहां दतेपि सप्ताहद्व्रणे दाहेपि वेष्यते । दहेन्मेढ्र तु लग्नां तां विपाद्याथ च कर्षयेत् ।" पाठोऽयं षष्ठपुस्तके अधिकमुपलभ्यते ।
2. ०रुर्ध्वं० इति षष्ठपुस्वके पाठः ।
3. समुन्नम्य इति चतुर्थपुस्तके पाठः ।
4. प्रवल० इति षष्ठपुस्तके पाठः ।

"तथा च सुश्रुतः

स्त्रीणां तु बस्तिपार्श्वगतो गर्भाशयः सन्निकृष्टः, तस्मात्तासामुत्सङ्गवच्छस्त्रं पातयेत्, अतोऽन्यथा खल्वासां मूत्रस्रावी व्रणो भवेत्, पुरुषस्य वा मूत्रप्रसेकक्षणनान्मूत्रक्षरणम्[1]; अश्मरीव्रणादृते भिन्नबस्तिरेक[2] भवति, द्विधा भिन्नबस्तिराश्मरिको न सिध्यति, अश्मरीव्रणनिमित्तमेकधाभिन्नबस्तिर्जीवति, क्रियाभ्यासाच्छास्त्रविहितच्छेदान्निःस्यदपरिवृद्धत्वाच्च[3] शल्यस्येति। उद्धृतशल्यं तूष्णोदकद्रोण्यामवगाह्य[4] स्वेदयेत्, तथा हि बस्तिरसृजा न पूर्यते; पूर्णे वा क्षीरवृक्षकषायं पुष्पनेत्रेण विदध्यात् ॥११५॥

According to Suśruta

In ladies, the uterus is located near the urinary bladder. Therefore, incision in them should be given on the pelvic surface failing which there will be passage of urine through this ulcer. Even in males, urine will pass through the ulcer if the urethral passage is injured during the operation. Apart from the ulcer of the passage through which the stone is removed, during the operation, the urinary bladder may also get incised. If this incision of the bladder affects two sides of the bladder, then the patient does not survive. If the incision is only on one side through which the stone is removed then the patient survives. This happens if the surgeon is well experienced, if the incision is done as per the description in the text and if the exudation

---

1. मूत्रप्रसेकक्षतान्मूत्रकरण इति आदर्शपुस्तकेषु पाठः।
2. भिन्नबस्तिरेकधाऽपि न इति आकरे पाठः।
3. ०न्निःस्यन्दपरिवृद्धत्वाच्च इति आकरे पाठः।
4. क. ०द्रोणे ऽवगाह्य इति चतुर्थपुस्तके पाठः।
   ख. द्रोवगाह्य इति प्रथमपंचमषष्ठपुस्तकेषु पाठः।

takes place appropriately in sufficient quantity. After the stone is removed, the patient should be made to sit in a tub containing warm water and the operated part should be fomented by which the bladder does not get filled up with blood. If, however, the bladder gets filled up with blood, the patient should be given douche prepared with the decoction of drugs belonging to *kṣiri vṛkṣa* group through a *puṣpa netra* (catheter).

भवति चात्र—

क्षीरवृक्ष[कषायस्तु][1] पुष्पनेत्रेण योजितम् ।
निर्हरेदश्मरीचूर्णं[2] रक्तं बस्तिगतं च यत् ॥११६॥

Thus, it is said

If the decoction of drugs belonging to *kṣiri vṛkṣa* group is given as a douche through a *puṣpa netra* (catheter), then it helps in the removal of the broken particles of stone (*aśmarī*) and blood from the urinary bladder.

मूत्रमार्गविशोधनार्थं चास्मै गुडसौहित्यं वितरेत्; उद्धृत्य चैनं मधुघृताभ्यक्तव्रणं मूत्रविशोधनद्रव्यसिद्धामुष्णां सघृतां यवागूं पाययेत् उभयकालं त्रिरात्रं; त्रिरात्रादूर्ध्वं गुडप्रगाढेन पयसा मृद्वोदनमल्पं भोजयेद्दशरात्रं, दशरात्रादूर्ध्वं फलाम्लैर्जाङ्गलरसै-[रुपाचरेत् ततो][3] दशरात्रं चैनमप्रमत्तः स्वेदयेत्[स्नेहेन द्रवस्वेदेन वा;][4]क्षीरवृक्षकषायेण चास्य व्रणं प्रक्षालयेत्; रोध्रमधुकमञ्जिष्ठा-

1. पाठोऽयं आदर्शपुस्तकेषु नोपलभ्यते ।
2. निर्हरेदश्मरीं तूर्णं इति आकरे पाठः ।
3. पाठोऽयं आदर्शपुस्तकेषु नोपलभ्यते ।
4. पाठोऽयं आदर्शपुस्तकेषु नोपलभ्यते ।

प्रपौण्डरीककल्कैर्व्रणं प्रतिग्राहयेत्; एतेष्वेव हरिद्रायुतेषु तैलं घृतं वा[1] विपक्वं व्रणाभ्यञ्जनमिति; स्त्यानशोणितं चोत्तरबस्तिभिरुपाचरेत्; [सप्तरात्राच्च[2] स्वमार्गप्रतिपद्यमा मूत्रे व्रणं यथोक्तेन विधिना दहेदग्निना, स्वमार्गप्रतिपन्ने चोत्तरबस्त्यास्थापनानुवासनैरुपाचरेन्मधुरकषायैरिति; यदृच्छया वा मूत्रमार्गप्रतिपन्नामन्तरासक्ता शुक्राश्मरीं शर्करां वा स्रोतसाऽपहरेत्, एवं चाशक्ये विदार्य नाडीं[3]]शस्त्रेण बडिशेनोद्धरेत् ॥११७॥

Post-operative Management

For the cleansing of the urinary channel, the patient should be given enough quantity of jaggery daily. After the removal of the stone, the ulcer should be anointed with honey and ghee and the patient should be given hot *yavāgū* (thick gruel) along with ghee to take both the times for three days. Thereafter, the patient should be given milk boiled with soft rice and mixed with adequate quantity of jaggery for ten days. For the next ten days, the patient should be given rice mixed with sour fruits and soup of the meat of animals inhabiting arid land. The patient should be given fomentation therapy over the operated part for ten days with the help of warm ghee or hot water without fail. The ulcer should be washed with the decoction of drugs belonging to *kṣīrī vṛkṣa* group. Over the ulcer, the paste of *rodhra*, *mañjiṣṭhā* and *prapauṇḍarīka* should be applied. Along with these drugs and by adding *haridrā*, oil or ghee should be cooked. With this medicated oil or ghee, gentle massage should be employed over the ulcer. If the blood becomes clotted, then the

---

1. व इति आदर्शपुस्तकेषु पाठः ।
2. पाठोऽयं आदर्शपुस्तकेषु नोपलभ्यते ।
3. 'सप्त रात्राच्च.........नाडीं' पाठोऽयं आदर्शपुस्तकेषु नोपलभ्यते ।

patient should be treated with *uttara basti* (medicated douche employed through the urethra). After seven days, when the urine starts passing through its normal passage, the ulcer should be cauterized. After the urine passes through its normal passage, the patient should be given *uttara basti* (medicated douche) and *āsthāpana* as well as *anuvāsana* types of medicated enema with the decoction of drugs belonging to *madhura* and *kaṣāya* groups. If the seminal stone or gravel comes to the urethra of its own and gets lodged, it should be taken out through the urethra. If it is not possible, then the urethra should be incised and the stone or gravel should be removed with the help of the equipment called *baḍiśa*.

रूढव्रणश्चाङ्गनाश्व नगनागरथद्रुमान् नारोहेत् वर्षं, नाप्सु प्लवेत, भुञ्जीत वा गुरु ॥११८॥

Diet and Regimens

After the ulcer is healed, the patient is forbidden to have sexual intercourse, to climb mountains, to ride on elephants and *ratha* (carts) and to climb trees for one year. He should not swim in the water and should not take heavy food.

मूत्रवहशुक्रवहमुष्कस्रोतो[1]मूत्रप्रसेकसे[2]वनीयोनिगुदबस्तिनष्टौ परिहरेत् । तत्र मूत्रवहच्छेदान्मरणं मूत्रपूर्णबस्तेः, शु[3]क्रवहच्छेदान्मरणं क्लैब्यं वा, मुष्कस्रोत उ[4]पघाताद् ध्वजभङ्गः, मूत्रप्रसेकक्षणनान्मूत्रप्रक्षरणं, सेवनीयोनिच्छेदाद्रुजः प्रादुर्भावः[5], बस्तिगुदविद्धलक्षणं प्रागुक्तमिति ॥११९॥

1. ०श्रागतमूत्र० इति षष्ठपुस्तके पाठः ।
2. ०सीवनीया० इति षष्ठपुस्तके पाठः ।
3. शुक्ल० इति षष्ठपुस्तके पाठः ।
4. ०नुपघाताद् इति पंचमपुस्तके पाठः ।
5. प्रादुर्भावो इति चतुर्थषष्ठपुस्तकयोः पाठः ।

Complications

During surgical operation, the surgeon should not touch eight organs, viz. *mutra vaha srotas* (urinary channel), *śukra vaha srotas* (seminal channel), *muṣka srotas* (vas deferns) *mūtra praseka* (urethra), *sevanī* (suture in the perenium), *yoni* (female genital tract), *guda* (anus) and *basti* (urinary bladder). If the urinary channel is incised by mistake then the bladder becomes filled up with urine (without an outlet); if the seminal channel is incised by mistake, then this leads to death or impotency; if the vas deferns gets incised then it leads to non erection of the penis; if the urethra gets incised, then urine will flow continuously (absence of sphincter action); if the perenial suture or the female genital tract is incised by mistake, this leads to pain; and if urinary bladder or anus is cut, then symptoms as mentioned before will appear.

भवतश्चात्र—

मर्माण्यष्टावसंबुध्य स्रोतोजानि[1] शरीरिणाम् ।
व्यापादयेद्बहून्मर्त्यान् शस्त्रकर्मापटुर्भिषक् ॥१२०॥"

[सुश्रुत : चिकित्सा ७ : ३३-३७]

Thus, it is said :

A physician, who is not experienced in surgical methods, kills several persons by his ignorance about eight vital organs and their channels.

अष्टाङ्गकांड:[2]—

मूत्रे ह्यागच्छति दहेदश्मरीव्रणमग्निना ।
स्वमार्गप्रतिपत्तौ तु स्वादु प्रायैरुपाचरेत् ॥१२१॥

---

1. ०यानि इति प्रथमपंचमपुस्तकयो: पाठ: ।
2. अष्टाङ्गकाण्डे इति पंचमषष्ठपुस्तकयो: पाठ: ।

मूत्रशुक्रवहे बस्तिं वृषणं सीवनीं गुदम् ।
मूत्रप्रसेकं योनिं च शस्त्रेनाष्टौ विवर्जयेत् ॥१२२॥

According to Aṣṭāṅga Kāṇḍa

When urine starts passing, the surgeon should cauterize the ulcer, and after the passing of urine, the patient should be treated by drugs having mostly sweet taste. The surgeon should not touch with his instruments eight vital parts, viz. *mūtra vaha srotas* (urinary channel), *śukra vaha srotas* (seminal channel), urinary bladder, testicles, *sīvanī* (sutures in perenium), anus, urethra and female genital tract including uterus.

'निर्गुण्डिकाद्रिर्वलिसूततताम्रं विमर्द्य गोलं सिकताख्ययन्त्रे ।
पक्त्वास्य वल्लः किल मातुलंगीजलैर्निहंत्यश्मरिरोगमुग्रम् ॥
॥ त्रिविक्रमरसः[1] ॥१२३॥"

Trivikrama Rasa

Purified *gandhaka* and *pārada*, *tāmra bhasma* and *śilā jatu* should be triturated with the juice of *nirguṇḍī* and cooked in *vālukā yantra*. This should be administered in a dose of one *valla* along with the juice of *mātuluṅga* which cures even serious types of *aśmarī* (stone in the urinary tract).

इति श्रीमहाराजाधिराजटोडरमल्लविरचिते टोडरानन्दे आयुर्वेदसौख्ये अश्मरीनिदानचिकित्साकथनं नाम त्रिचत्वारिंशत्तमो हर्षः ॥१२४॥

Thus, ends the 43rd Chapter dealing with the diagnosis and treatment of *aśmarī* (stone in urinary tract) in the *Āyurveda saukhya* of *Ṭoḍarānanda* composed by the great king Ṭoḍara Malla.

---

1. 'निर्गुण्डिका ....त्रिविक्रमरसः' पाठोऽयं चतुर्थषष्ठपुस्तकयोः अधिकमुपलभ्यते ।

CHAPTER IX

अथ प्रमेहप्रमेहपिडकानिदानं चिकित्सा च ।

Diagnosis and Treatment of Prameha and Prameha Piḍakā

"प्रमेहाः[1] विंशतिस्तत्र श्लेष्मजा[2] दश, पित्ततः ।
षट्, चत्वारोऽनिलात्, तेषां मेदोमूत्रकफावहम् ॥१॥"

॥ अष्टाङ्गहृदय : निदान १० : १॥

Varieties

Prameha is of twenty types, ten of them are caused by

---

1. This is the beginning of 48th Chapter of *Āyurveda saukhya* in *Ṭoḍarānanda* and the invocation reads as follows :
जलेशमजित्यत्दालयं गतं समानयद्योजनकं व्रतस्तिथम् । ऋद्धि सपुत्रां प्रददातु भूपेमिस्थिरां सदा टोडरमल संज्ञके ॥
2. श्लेष्मतो इति आकरे पाठः ।

kapha, six by *pitta* and four by *vāyu*. These *pramehas* are caused by the vitiation of *medas* (adipose tissues), urine and *kapha*.

आस्यासुखं स्वप्नसुखं दधीनि ग्राम्यौदकानूपरसाः पयांसि ।
नवान्नपानं गुडवैकृतं च प्रमेहहेतुः कफकृच्च सर्वम् ॥२॥

Etiology

Leisurely living and indulgence in long sleep, various curd preparations, soup of the meat of domestic, aquatic and marshy land inhabiting animals, milk preparations, freshly harvested cereals as well as corns, freshly prepared wines as well as other alcoholic drinks, various preparations of sugar cane juice and such other foods as well as regimens which aggravate *kapha* cause *prameha* (obstinate urinary disorders including diabetes).

मेदश्च मांसं च शरीरजं च क्लेदं कफो बस्तिगतं[1] प्रदूष्य ।
करोति मेहान् समुदीर्णमुष्णैस्तानेव पित्तं परिदूष्य चापि ॥
क्षीणेषु दोषेष्ववकृष्य धातून्
संदूष्य मेहान् कुरुतेऽनिलश्च ॥३॥

Pathogenesis

Kapha, located in the urinary bladder, vitiates the *meda* (fat tissue), *māṃsa* (muscle tissue) and *kleda* (sticky metabolic by products) of the body to produce *kaphaja pramehas*. *Pitta* also afflicts the above mentioned tissue elements with its increased heat to cause *paittika pramehas*. Similarly, aggravated *vāyu*, because of diminished *doṣas*, reduces and afflicts the above mentioned tissue elements to cause *vātika prameha*.

---

1. ०गत: इति आकरे पाठः ।

[1] साध्याः कफोत्था दश, पित्तजाः षड्
याप्या, न साध्याः पवनाच्चतुष्कः ।
समक्रियत्वाद् विषमक्रियत्वा-
न्महात्ययत्वाच्च यथाक्रमं ते ॥४॥

Prognosis

Ten varieties of *prameha* caused by *kapha* are curable, six varieties of *prameha* caused by *pitta* are palliable and four varieties of *prameha* caused by *vāyu* are incurable. In *kaphaja prameha*, the *doṣa* involved (i.e. *kapha*) and the tissue elements afflicted are all amenable to similar type of treatment (*sama kriyā*) ; therefore, these are curable. In *paittika* types of *prameha*, the *doṣa* involved (i.e. *pitta*) and the tissues afflicted need dissimilar (opposite) types of treatment (*viṣama kriyā*) for which these are only palliable i.e. the patient remains free from these ailments as long as he is taking medicines but becomes victim to these ailments again after he gives up medicines. *Vātika* types of *prameha* are by nature very serious ailments (*mahātyaya*), and therefore, these are incurable.

कफः सपित्तः पवनश्च दोषा
मेदोऽस्रशुक्राम्बुवसालसीका- :
मज्जारसौजः पिशितं च दूष्यं
प्रमेहिणां विंशतिरेव मेहाः ॥५॥

Three *doṣas*, viz. *kapha*, *pitta* and *vāyu* and tissue elements like *medas* (fat tissue), *asra* (blood), *śukra* (semen), *ambu* (watery

1. "दोषो हि बस्तिसमपेत्य मूत्रं संदूष्य मेहान् कुरुते यथा" पाठोऽयं चतुर्थषष्ठपुस्तकयोः अधिकमुपलभ्यते ।

elements), *vasā* (muscle fat), *lasīkā* (lymph), ***majjā*** (***bone marrow***), ***rasa*** (plasma), *ojas* (essence of all tissue elements) and ***piśita*** (muscle tissue)—all these are afflicted in the twenty types of *prameha*.

दन्तादीनां मलाढ्यत्वं प्राग्रूपं पाणिपादयोः ।
दाहश्चिक्कणता देहे तृट् स्वाद्वास्यं च जायते ॥६॥

Premonitory Signs and Symptoms

Premonitory signs and symptoms of ***prameha*** are appearance of profuse quantity of sticky material in the joints of teeth, etc., burning sensation in hands and feet, smoothness of the skin in the body, thirst and appearance of sweet taste in the mouth.

"सामान्यं लक्षणं तेषां प्रभूताविलमूत्रता ।
दोषदूष्यविशेषेण[1] तत्संयोगविशेषतः ॥
मूत्रवर्णादिभेदेन भेदो मेहेषु कल्प्यते ॥७॥

Common Signs and Symptoms

Voiding large quantity of muddy urine is the characteristic of feature of all types of *prameha*. Depending upon the *doṣas* and *dūṣyas* involved in the manifestation of the disease and their permutation as well as combination, the colour etc. of the urine varies in different types of *prameha*.

अच्छं बहु सितं शीतं निर्गन्धमुदकोपमम् ।
मेहत्युदकमेहेन, किंचिच्च[2]ाविलपिच्छिलम् ॥८॥

---

1. विशेषेऽपि इति आकरे पाठः ।
2. किंचिदाविलपिच्छिलम् इति आदर्शपुस्तकेषु पाठः ।

Udaka Meha

In *udaka meha*, the patient passes transparent, white, cold and smellless urine like water (*udaka*) in large quantity.

इक्षो रसमिवात्यर्थं मधुरं चेक्षुमेहतः ॥९॥

Ikṣu Meha

In *ikṣu meha*, the urine of the patient is slightly muddy and slimy. The urine is extremely sweet like sugar-cane juice (*ikṣu rasa*).

सान्द्रीभवेत्पर्युषितं सान्द्रमेहेन[1] मेहति ।

सुरामेही सुरातुल्यमुपर्यच्छमधो घनम् ॥

संहृष्टरोमा पिष्टेन पिष्टवद्बहुलं सितम् ॥१०॥

Sāndra Meha, Surā Meha and Piṣṭa Meha

In *sāndra meha*, the urine becomes thick (*sāndra*) if it is kept over night. In *surā meha*, the urine is transparent above and thick below like alcohol (*surā*). In *piṣṭa meha*, the patient gets horripilation and passes urine in large quantity which is thick and white like a paste of flour (*piṣṭa*).

शुक्राभं शुक्रमिश्रं वा शुक्रमेही प्रमेहति ।

मूत्रेण[2] सिकतामेही सिकतारूपिणो मलान् ॥११॥

Śukra Meha and Sikatā Meha

In *śukra meha*, the patient passes urine which is like *śukra* (semen) or which is mixed with semen. In *sikatā meha*, the

1. सान्द्रमेही इति आकरे पाठः ।
2. मूत्राणून् इति आकरे पाठः ।

patient passes urine along with waste products like ***sikatā*** (gravel or sand).

शीतमेही सुबहुशो मधुरं भृशशीतलम् ।
शनैः शनैः शनैर्मेही मन्दं मन्दं प्रमेहति ॥१२॥

Śīta Meha and Śanaiḥ Meha

In *śīta meha*, the patient passes extremely large quantity of urine which is sweet in taste and which is extremely cold (*śīta*) to touch. In *śanaiḥ meha*, the patient passes urine very slowly (*śanaiḥ śanaiḥ*) in very small quantities.

लालातन्तुयुतं मूत्रं लालामेहेन पिच्छिलम् ॥१३॥

Lālā Meha

In *lālā meha*, the urine of the patient is extremely slimy (*lālā yukta*) and string come out of it when touched.

गन्धवर्णरसस्पर्शैः क्षारेण क्षारतो भवेत्[1] ।
नीलमेहेन नीलाभं कालमेही मषीनिभम् ॥१४॥

Kṣāra Meha, Nīla Meha and Kāla Meha

In *kṣāra meha*, the smell, colour, taste and touch of the urine is like those of *kṣāra* (alkali preparation). In *ṇīla meha*, the colour of the urine like indigo or blue (*nīla*). In *kāla meha* the patient passes urine which is black (*kāla*) like ink.

[2]हारिद्रमेही कटुकं हरिद्रासन्निभं भवेत्[3] ।
विस्रं माञ्जिष्ठमेहेन मञ्जिष्ठासलिलोपमम् ।
विस्रमुष्णं सलवणं रक्ताभं रक्तमेहतः ॥१५॥

---

1. क्षारतोयवत् इति आकरे पाठः ।
2. हरिद्रमेही इति आदर्शपुस्तकेषु पाठः ।
3. दहत् इति आकरे पाठः ।

Hāridra Meha, Mañjiṣṭha Meha and Rakta Meha

In *hāridra meha,* the taste of the urine is pungent and the colour is yellow like turmeric (*haridrā*). In *mañjiṣṭhā meha,* the urine is foul-smelling and it is red in colour like the juice or decoction of *mañjīṣṭhā.* In *rakta meha,* the urine is foul smelling, hot, saline in taste and red in colour like blood (*rakta*).

वसामेही वसामिश्रं वसां वा मूत्रयेन्मुहुः ।

मज्जानं मज्जमिश्रं वा मज्जमेही मुहुर्मुहुः ॥१६॥"

[अष्टाङ्गहृदय : निदान १० : ७-१६]

Vasā Meha and Majjā Meha

In *vasā meha,* the urine is mixed with *vasā* (muscle fat) or the patient voids only *vasā* (muscle fat) while passing urine. The patient suffering from *majjā meha* passes urine very frequently and the urine is mixed with bone-marrow (*majjā*) like substance or he voids only bone-marrow (*majjā*) while passing urine.

कषायं मधुरं रूक्षं क्षौद्रमेहेन मेहति ॥१७॥

Madhu Meha

In *madhu meha,* the urine of the patient is astringent as well as sweet in taste and ununctuous.

"हस्ती मत्त इवाजस्रं मूत्रवेगाविवर्जितम् ॥

सलसीकं विबद्धं च हस्तिमेही प्रमेहति ॥१८॥"

[अष्टाङ्गहृदय : निदान १० : १७-१८]

Hasti Meha

In *hasti meha,* the patient passes urine in large quantity like a rogue elephant. He always has the urge for passing urine. The urine contains *lasīkā* (lymph) and nodule like substance.

'इक्षुमेहः सुरामेहः पिष्टमेहश्च सांद्रकः ।
शुक्रमेहोदकाख्यौ च लालामेहश्च शीतकः ।
सिकताह्वः शनैर्मेही दशैते कफसंभवाः ॥१६॥

Classification

Ikṣu meha, surā meha, piṣṭa meha, sāndra meha, śukra meha, udaka meha, lālā meha, śīta meha, sikatā meha and *śanair-meha* —these ten varieties are caused by *kapha.*

मंजिष्ठाख्योः हरिद्राख्यो नीलाख्यो रक्तमेहकः ।
कृष्णमेहः क्षारमेहः षडैते पित्तसंभवाः ॥२०॥

Mañjiṣṭhā meha, hāridra meha, nīla meha, rakta meha, kṛṣṇa meha and *kṣāra meha*—these six varieties of *prameha* are caused by *pitta.*

हस्तिमेहो वसामेहो मज्जामेहो मधुप्रभः ।
चत्वारो वातजा ज्ञेया इति मेहाश्च विंशतिः ॥२१॥

Hasti meha, vasā meha, majjā meha and *madhu meha*—these four varieties of *prameha* are caused by *vāyu.* These are twenty varieties of *prameha.*

अपरः खटिकामेहः खटिकोदकसंनिभः ।
वातश्लेष्मकृतत्वाच्च सुखसाध्यतमो मतः ॥२२॥

Additional Varieties

Another variety of *prameha* is called *khaṭikā meha*, in which the patient passes urine like chalk (*khaṭikā*) powder mixed with water. It is caused by *vāyu* and *kapha.* This ailment is very easily curable.

पूयमेहोऽपरः प्रोक्तः पूयस्रावः सवेदनः ।
त्रिदोषजकृतत्वाच्च कृच्छ्रसाध्यतमो मतः[1] ॥२३॥'

Pūya Meha

In *pūya meha*, the patient passes urine with pus (*pūya*) and pain. This is caused by the vitiation of all the three *doṣas* It is extremely difficult of cure.

"अविपाकोऽरुचिश्छर्दिनिद्राकासः सपीनसः ।
उपद्रवाः प्रमेहानां प्रजायन्ते कफात्मनाम्[2] ॥२४॥

Complications

Indigestion, anorexia, vomiting, excessive sleep, cough and *pīnasa* (chronic rhinitis)—these are the complications of *kaphaja* type of *prameha*.

बस्तिमेहनयोः शूलं[3] मुष्कावदरणं ज्वरः ।
दाहस्तृष्णा क्लमो[4] मूर्च्छा विड्भेदः पित्तजन्मनाम् ॥२५॥

Pain in the region of urinary bladder and pudendum, craking pain in the scrotum, fever, burning sensation, thirst, mental fatigue, fainting and diarrhoea—these are the complications of *paittika* type of *prameha*.

[5]वातजानामुदावर्तकण्ठहृद्ग्रहलोलताः ।
शूलमुन्निद्रता शोषः कासः श्वासश्च जायते ॥२६॥"

[अष्टाङ्गहृदय : निदान १० : २२-२४]

---

1. 'इक्षुमेहः..................मतः' पाठोऽयं चतुर्थषष्ठपुस्तकयोः अधिकमुपलभ्यते ।
2. कफजन्मनाम् इति आकरे पाठः ।
3. बस्तिमेहनयोस्तोदो इति आकरे पाठः ।
4. दाहस्तृष्णाम्लको इति आकरे पाठः ।
5. वातिका० इति आकरे पाठः ।

Udāvarta (upward movement of wind in the abdomen) obstruction and irritation in the throat and the heart, colic pain sleeplessness, consumption, cough and dyspnoea—these are the complications of *vātika* type of *prameha.*

"यथोक्तोपद्रवाविष्टमतिप्रस्रुतमेव[1] च ।
पिडिकापीडितं गाढं[2] प्रमेहो हंति मानवम् ॥२७॥

Bad Prognosis

Patients having the above mentioned complications or having dehydration because of excessive urination or having deep seated diabetic carbuncles do not survive.

जातः प्रमेही मधुमेहिनो वा न साध्यरोगः[3] स हि बीजदोषात् ।
ये चापि केचित्कुलजा विकारा
भवन्ति तांश्च[4] प्रवदन्त्यसाध्यान् ॥२८॥

Congenital Diabetes

The patient who is diabetic right from the birth or who is borne of diabetic parents is not curable because of defective genes (*bīja doṣa*). Similarly, other congenital or hereditary diseases (*kulajā*—lit. familial) are not curable.

सर्वं एव प्रमेहास्तु कालेनाप्रतिकुर्वताम्[5] ।
मधुमेहत्वमायान्ति तदाऽसाध्या भवन्ति हि ॥२९॥

---

1. ०प्रस्रुतमेवपि इति द्वितीयपुस्तके पाठः ।
2. गाढः इति आकरे पाठः ।
3. वा न साध्य उक्तः इति आकरे पाठः ।
4. तांस्तान् इति आकरे पाठः ।
5. कालेनाप्रतिकारिणः इति आकरे पाठः ।

Secondary Diabetes

All the types of *prameha*, if not treated in appropriate time, lead to *madhu meha* (diabetes mellitus) which then becomes incurable.

मधुमेहे मधुसमं जायते स किल द्विधा ।
क्रुद्धे धातुक्षयाद्वायौ दोषावृतपथेऽथवा ॥३०॥
आवृतो दोषलिङ्गानि सोऽनिमित्तं प्रदर्शयन्[1] ।
क्षीणः[2] क्षणात् क्षणात्पूर्णो भजते कृच्छ्रसाध्यताम् ॥३१॥

Pathogenesis of Madhu Meha (Diabetes Mellitus)

In *madhu meha*, the urine is like *madhu* (honey). It is of two types. One variety is caused by the diminution of *dhātus* (tissue elements) as a result of the aggravated *vāyu* and the second variety is caused by the diminution of tissue elements because of the obstruction in their channels of circulation by the *doṣas*. In the second variety, signs and symptoms of obstructed (*āvṛtta*) *doṣas* are manifested. At times, these tissue elements get reduced, and at times, these are replenished. Ultimately, *madhu meha* becomes incurable.

मधुरं यच्च सर्वेषु[3] प्रायो मध्विव मेहति ।
सर्वेऽपि मधुमेहाख्या माधुर्याच्च तनोरतः ॥३२॥"

[माधवनिदान : ३३ : २१-२६]

In all types of diabetes, the sweet elements in the body

1. प्रदर्शयेत् इति षष्ठपुस्तके पाठः ।
2. क्षणात्क्षीणः इति आकरे पाठः ।
3. मेहेषु इति आकरे पाठः ।

come out through the urine like honey. Because of excessive sweetness in the body, all such ailments are called *madhu meha.*

प्रमेहिणो यदा मूत्रमनाविलमपिच्छिलम् ।
विशदं तिक्तकटुकं तदारोग्यं प्रचक्षते ॥३३॥

Signs of Cure

When the *prameha* patient passes urine which is not cloudy or slimy, which is transparent and which is either bitter or pungent in taste, then he should be considered to be free from this ailment.

"शराविका[1] कच्छपिका जालिनी विनताऽलजी ।
मसूरिका सर्षपिका पुत्रिणी सविदारिका ॥३४॥
विद्रधिश्चेति पिडका:[2] प्रमेहोपेक्षया दश ।
सन्धिमर्मसु जायन्ते मांसलेषु च धामसु ॥३५॥"

[अष्टाङ्गहृदय : निदान १० : २५-२६]

Diabetic Carbuncles

When the treatment of *prameha* is ignored, ten types of carbuncle (*pīḍakā*) are produced, viz. *śarāvikā*, *kacchapikā*, *jālinī*, *vinatā*, *alajī*, *masūrikā*, *sarṣapikā*, *putriṇī*, *vidārikā* and *vidradhi*. These carbuncles occur in vital joints and in fleshy parts of the body.

"अन्तोन्नता च तद्रूपा निम्नमध्या शराविका ।
गौरसर्षपसंस्थाना तत्प्रमाणा च सर्षपी ॥३६॥

1. सराविका इति प्रथमपुस्तके पाठः ।
2. पिटिका: इति आकरे पाठः ।

Śarāvikā and Sarṣapikā

The *śarāvikā* type of carbuncle is characterised by raised borders and pit in the centre. The *sarṣapikā* type of carbuncle is like a white variety of mustard seed in size, shape and colour.

सदाहा कूर्मसंस्थाना ज्ञेया कच्छपिका बुधैः ।
जालिनी तीव्रदाहा तु मांसजालसमावृता ॥३७॥

Kacchapikā and Jālinī

The *kacchapikā* type of carbuncle is like the back of a tortoise and there is burning sensation. *Jālinī* type of carbuncle is associated with excessive burning sensation and it is surrounded with a net work of thin muscle tissues.

अवगाढरुजाक्लेदा पृष्ठे वाऽप्युदरेऽपि वा ।
महती पिडका नीला सा[1] बुधैर्विनता स्मृता ॥३८॥

Vinatā

Vinatā type of carbuncle is deep seated, painful and accompanied with sticky material. The carbuncle is of large size and it is blue in colour. These carbuncles are generally located either in the back or in the abdomen.

महत्युपचिता[2] ज्ञेया पिडका सा[3] च पुत्रिणी ।
मसूराकृतिसंस्थाना विज्ञेया तु मसूरिका ॥३९॥

Putriṇī and Masūrikā

Putriṇī type of carbuncle is big in size and elevated. The carbuncle which is like seed of *masūra* in size, shape and colour is called *masūrikā*.

---

1. विनता नाम सा स्मृता इति आकरे पाठः ।
2. महत्यल्पाचिता इति आकरे पाठः ।
3. चापि इति आकरे पाठः ।

रक्ता सिता स्फोटचिता दारुणा त्वलजी[1] भवेत् ।
विदारीकन्दवद्वृत्ता कठिना च विदारिका ॥४०॥

Alajī and Vidārikā

Alajī is a serious type of carbuncle which is red and white in colour and is surrounded by pustules. *Vidārikā* type of carbuncle is round and hard like the root of *vidārī.*

विद्रधेर्लक्षणैर्युक्ता ज्ञेया विद्रधिका तु सा ॥४१॥

Vidradhi

Vidradhi type of carbuncle is like an abscess.

ये यन्मयाः स्मृता मेहास्तेषामेतास्तु तन्मयाः ॥४२॥

The *doṣas* and tissue elements involved in the production of these carbuncles are similar to those which are affected in the type of *prameha* of which the patient is suffering.

विना प्रमेहमप्येता जायन्ते दुष्टमेदसः ।
तावच्चैनं न लक्ष्यन्ते यावद्वास्तुपरिग्रहः[2] ॥४३॥

These carbuncles may also occur because of vitiate d *medas* (fat tissue) even if the patient is not suffering from *prameha.* These are not visible as long as they do not get firmly located in the tissue (*vāstu parigraha*).

गुदे हृदि शिरस्यंशे पृष्ठे मर्म्मसु चोत्थिताः ।
सोपद्रवा दुर्बलाग्नेः पिडकाः परिवर्जयेत् ॥४४॥"

[माधवनिदान : ३३ : २७-३६]

1. ०त्वजलजी इति आदर्शपुस्तकेषु पाठः ।
2. यावद्वस्तु० इति आदर्शपुस्तकेषु पाठः ।

Prognosis of Carbuncles

If carbuncles are located in the anus, heart, head, shoulder back and vital organs, if these are associated with complications and if there is suppression of the digestive power of the patient, then such cases should not be treated.

"तृट्श्वासमांससंकोच[1]मोहहिक्कामदज्वराः ।
[2]विसर्पमर्मसंरोधाः पिडकानामुपद्रवाः ॥४५॥"

[चरक : सूत्रस्थान १७ : ११०]

Complications of Carbuncles

Thirst, dyspnoea, muscular contracture, unconsciousness, hiccup, intoxication, fever, erysipelas and obstruction to vital organs—these are the complications of carbuncles.

मूर्च्छाच्छर्दिज्वरश्वासकासवीसर्पगौरवैः ।
उपद्रवैरुपहतो [3]यः प्रमे[4]ही साप्रतिक्रियः ॥४६॥

If the patient of carbuncle suffers from complications like fainting, vomiting, fever, dyspnoea, cough, erysipelas and heaviness, then he becomes incurable.

रजः प्रसेकान्नारीणां मासि मासि विशुध्यति ।
कृत्स्नं शरीरं दोषाश्च न प्रमेहन्त्यतस्स्त्रियः ॥४७॥

Low incidence of Prameha in Ladies

The body of a woman gets cleansed of its impurities every

1. ०संकोथ० इति आकरे पाठः ।
2. वीसर्प० इति आकरे पाठः ।
3. ०तोतः इति चतुर्थपुस्तके पाठः ।
4. प्रमेहः इति षष्ठपुस्तके पाठः ।

month because of menstrual flow. Therefore, women generally do not suffer from *prameha.*

"[1]हरिद्रावर्णं रुधिरं च मूत्रं बिना प्रमेहस्य च पूर्वरूपैः ।
यो मेहयेत् तं न वदेत् प्रमेहं रक्तस्य पित्तस्य हि स प्रकोपः[2] ॥४८॥"

॥ प्रमेहमधुमेहपिडकानिदानम् ॥४९॥

Differential Diagnosis

If a patient passes urine which is yellow in colour and which contains blood without the premonitory signs and symptoms of *prameha*, then he should not be diagnosed as a case of *prameha.* He is actually suffering from *rakta pitta* (an ailment characterised by bleeding from different parts of the body).

Thus, ends the diagnosis of *prameha*, *madhu meha* and *prameha piḍakā*.

"श्यामाककोद्रवोद्दालगोधूमचणकाढकी ।
कुलत्थाश्च हिता भोज्ये पुराणा मेहिनां सदा ।
जाङ्गलं तिक्तशाकानि यवान्नञ्च श्रमो मधु ॥५०॥"

[भैषज्यरत्नावली : प्रमेहाधिकार : ४]

Diet and Regimens

For the patient suffering from *prameha* food ingredients containing *śyāmāka*, *kodrava*, *uddālaka*, *godhūma*, *caṇaka*, *āḍhakī* and *kulattha* which are stored for a long time after harvesting are always wholesome. He should take meat of *jāṅgala* animals (inhabiting arid land), vegetables having bitter taste, barley and honey. He should perform physical exercise.

---

1. द्रष्टव्यम्—अष्टाङ्गहृदयः निदान १०:३७ ।
2. कृत्स्नं शरीरं संपीड्य मेदो मज्जवसानुगः । अधः प्रक्रमते वायुर्ह्योताः साध्यास्तु वातजाः । पाठोऽयं चतुर्थषष्ठपुस्तकयोः अधिकमुपलभ्यते ।

"पारिजातजयानिंबवह्निगायत्रिणां पृथक् ।
पाठायाः सागुरोः पीताद्वयस्य शारदस्य च ॥५१॥
जलेक्षुमद्यसिकताशनैर्लवणपिष्टकान् ।
सान्द्रमेहान् क्रमाद्[1] घ्नन्ति अष्टौ क्वाथाः समाक्षिकाः ॥५२॥"

[भैषज्यरत्नावली : प्रमेहाधिकार : ३३-३४]

Eight types of decoctions prepared of 1. *pārijāta,* 2. *jayā,* 3. *nimba.* 4. *vahni,* 5. *gāyatrī,* 6. *pāṭhā,* 7. *aguru* and 8. *śārada,* when taken along with honey cure eight types of *prameha* viz. 1. *udaka meha,* 2. *ikṣu meha,* 3. *surā meha,* 4. *sikatā meha,* 5. *śanair-meha,* 6. *lavaṇa meha,* 7. *piṣṭa meha* and 8. *sāndra meha* respectively.

"दुर्वाकशेरुपूतीककुम्भीकप्लवशैवलम् ।
जलेन क्वथितं पीतं शुक्रमेहहरं परम् ॥५३॥

The decoction of *dūrvā, kaśeru, pūtīka, kumbhīka, plava* and *śaivala* prepared by boiling with water is excellent for the cure of *śukra meha.*

त्रिफलाऽऽरग्वधद्राक्षाकषायो मधुसंयुतः ।
पीतो निहंति फेनाख्यं प्रमेहं त्वरितं[2] नृणाम् ॥५४॥"

[भैषज्यरत्नावली : प्रमेहाधिकार : २९-३०]

---

1. क्रमाशघ्नन्ति इति प्रथमपुस्तके पाठः ।
2. नियतं इति आकरे पाठः ।

Intake of the decoction of *triphalā*, *āragvadha* and *drākṣā* along with honey cures *phena* [?] *meha* in human beings.

"लोध्राभयाकट्फलमुस्तकानां, विडङ्गपाठार्जुनधन्वनानाम् ।
कदम्बशालार्जुनदीपकानां, विडङ्गधात्री[1]धवशल्यकानाम् ।
चत्वार एते मधुना कषायाः, कफप्रमेहेषु निषेवणीयाः ॥५५॥"

[भैषज्यरत्नावली : प्रमेहाधिकार : २५-२६]

Intake of the four decoctions of either 1. *lodhra*, *abhayā*, *kaṭphala* and *mustā*, or 2. *viḍaṅga*, *pāṭhā*, *arjuna* and *dhanvana* or 3. *kadamba*, *śāla*, *arjuna* and *dīpaka* or 4. *viḍaṅga*, *dhātrī*, *dhava* and *śalyaka* along with honey cures *kaphaja* varieties of *prameha*.

"अश्वत्थाच्चतुरङ्गुल्यान्[2]न्यग्रोधादेः फलत्रयात् ।
सर्ज्जिका[3]रक्तसाराच्च क्वाथाः पञ्चसमाक्षिकाः ॥५६॥
नीलहारिद्रशुक्राख्यक्षारमञ्जिष्ठकाह्वयान् ।"

[भैषज्यरत्नावली : प्रमेहाधिकार : ३५]

मेहान् घ्नन्ति क्रमादेते सक्षौद्रो रक्तमेहनुत् ॥५७॥

Intake of the five decoctions of 1. fruit of *aśvattha*, 2. fruit of *caturaṅgula*, 3. fruit of *nyagrodha*, 4. *svarjikṣāra* and

---

1. ०दार्वी० इति आदर्शपुस्तकेषु पाठः ।
2. अश्वत्थाद्राजवृक्षाच्च न्यग्रोधाच्च इति आकरे पाठः ।
3. सचन्दनसमङ्गाया इति आकरे पाठः ।

5. *rakta sāra* along with honey cures five varieties of *prameha*, viz., 1. *nīla meha*, 2. *hāridra meha*, 3. *śukra meha*, 4. *kṣāra meha* and 5. *mañjiṣṭhā meha*, respectively. Taken along with honey, these decoctions also cure *rakta meha*.

"क्वाथः खर्जूरकाश्मर्यतिन्दुकाख्यामृताकृतः ।
'सुहिमः पीतमात्रस्तु सक्षौद्रो रक्तमेहनुत्'[1] ॥५८॥"

[योगरत्नाकर : प्रमेहचिकित्सा : पृष्ठ ८४]

Intake of the cooled decoction of *kharjūra*, *kāśmarya*, *tinduka* and *amṛtā* along with honey instantaneously cures *rakta meha*.

"लोध्रार्जुनोशीरकुचन्दनानामरिष्टसेव्यामलकाभयानाम् ।
धात्र्यर्जुनारिष्टकवत्सकानां नीलोत्पलानां तिनिशार्जुनानाम् ।
चत्वार एते विहिताः कषायाः पित्तप्रमेहे मधुसंप्रयुक्तः ॥५९॥"

[भैषज्यरत्नावली : प्रमेहाधिकार : २८]

Intake of the four decoctions of either 1. *lodhra*, *arjuna*, *uśīra* and *kucandana*, 2. *ariṣṭa*, *sevya*, *āmalaka* and *abhayā*, 3. *dhātri*, *arjuna*, *ariṣṭaka* and *vatsaka or* 4. *nīlotpala*, *tiniśa* and *arjuna* along with honey cures *paittika* varieties of *prameha*.

---

1. क. 'सुहिमः——रक्तमेहनुत्' पाठोऽयं प्रथमपंचमपुस्तकयोः नोपलभ्यते ।
   ख. रक्तमेहहा इति आकरे पाठः।

"छिन्नावह्निकषायेण पाठाकुटजरामठम् ।
तिक्तां कुष्ठं च संचूर्ण्य सर्पिर्मेहे[1] पिबेन्नरः ॥६०॥"

[भैषज्यरत्नावली : प्रमेहाधिकार : ३१]

Intake of the powder of *pāṭhā*, *kuṭaja*, *rāmaṭha*, *tiktā* and *kuṣṭha* along with the decoction of *chinnā* and *vahni* cures *sarpi meha.*

"कदरखदिरपूगक्वाथं[2] क्षौद्राह्वये पिबेत् ।
अग्निमंथकषायन्तु[3] वसामेहे प्रयोजयेत् ॥६१॥"

[भैषज्यरत्नावली : प्रमेहाधिकार : ३६]

The decoction of *kadara*, *khadira* and *pūga* is useful in *kṣaudra meha.* The decoction of *agni mantha* should be given to the patient suffering from *vasā meha.*

"पाठा शिरीषो[4] दुःस्पर्शा मूर्वा किंशुकतिन्दुकम् ।
कपित्थानां भिषक् क्वाथं हस्तिमेहे प्रयोजयेत् ॥६२॥"

[भैषज्यरत्नावली : प्रमेहाधिकार : ३७]

The decoction of *pāṭhā*, *śirīṣa*, *duḥsparśā*, *mūrvā*, *kīṃśuka*, *tinduka* and *kapittha* is useful in *hasti meha.*

---

1. सर्पिर्मेही इति आकरे पाठः ।
2. कदरः खदिरः पूगः क्वाथं इति आदर्शपुस्तकेषु पाठः ।
3. अग्निमंथकषायंबु इति पंचमपुस्तके पाठः ।
4. पाठाशीर्षकदुस्पर्शा इति प्रथमपंचमपुस्तकयोः पाठः ।

"सुश्रुतः[1]

तत्रोदकमेहिनं निम्बकषायं[2] पाययेत्,[3] इक्षुवालिकामेहिनं[4] वैजयन्तीकषायं, सुरामेहिनं निम्बकषायं, सिकतामेहिनं चित्रककषायं, शनैर्मेहिनं खदिरकषायं, लवणमेहिनं पाठाऽगुरुकषायं,[5] पिष्टमेहिनं हरिद्राद्वितयकषायं,[6] सांद्रमेहिनं सप्तपर्णकषायं, शुक्रमेहिनं दूर्वाशैवलप्लवहठकरञ्जकसेरुककषायं ककुभचन्दनकषायं वा, फेनमेहिनं त्रिफलारग्वधमृद्वीकाकषायं, मधुमधुरं,[7] पैत्तिकेषु प्रमेहेषु नीलमेहे[8] शालसारादिकषायमश्वत्थकषायं वा पाययेत्, हरिद्रामेहिनं राजवृक्षकषायम्, अम्लमेहिनं न्यग्रोधादिकषायं मधुमिश्रम्, क्षारमेहिनं त्रिफलाकषायं, मञ्जिष्ठामेहिनं मञ्जिष्ठाचन्दनकषायं, शोणितमेहिनं गुडूचीतिन्दुकास्थिकाश्मर्यखर्जूरकषायं मधुमिश्रं पाययेत् ।" ॥६३॥

[सुश्रुत : चिकित्सा ११:६]

According to Suśruta

The patient of *udaka meha* should be given the decoction of *nimba*. The patient of *ikṣu vālikā meha* should be

1. "सुश्रतः———पाययेत्" पाठोऽयं षष्ठपुस्तके अधिकमुपलभ्यते ।
2. पारिजातकषायं इति आकरे पाठः ।
3. पाठोऽयं आदर्शपुस्तकेषु नोपलभ्यते ।
4. इक्षुमेहिनं इति आकरे पाठः ।
5. पाठाऽगुरुहरिद्राकषायं इति आकरे पाठः ।
6. हरिद्रादारुहरिद्राकषायं इति आकरे पाठः ।
7. मधुमधुरमिति इति आकरे पाठः ।
8. पैत्तिकेषु नीलमेहिनं इति आकरे पाठः ।

given the decoction of *vaijayantī*. The patient of *surā meha* should be given the decoction of *nimba*. The patient of *sikatā meha* should be given the decoction of *citraka*. The patient of *śanair-meha* should be given the decoction of *khadira*. The patient of *lavaṇa meha* should be given the decoction of *pāṭhā* and *aguru*. The patient of *piṣṭa meha* should be given the decoction of *haridrā* and *dāru haridrā*. The patient of *sāndra meha* should be given the decoction of *sapta parṇa*. The patient of *śukra meha* should be given the decoction of *dūrvā*, *śaivāla*, *plava*, *haṭha*, *karañja* and *kaseru* or the decoction of *kakubha* and *candana*. The patient of *phena meha* should be given the decoction of *triphalā*, *āragvadha* and *mṛdvikā*. All these decoctions should be given along with honey. Among *paittika pramehas*, the patient of *nīla meha* should be given the decoction prepared of drugs belonging to *śālasārādi gaṇa* or the decoction of *aśvattha*. The patient of *hāridra meha* should be given the decoction of *rāja vṛkṣa*. The patient of *amla meha* should be given the decoction of drugs belonging to *nyagrodhādī gaṇa* by adding honey. The patient of *kṣāra meha* should be given the decoction of *triphalā*. The patient of *mañjiṣṭhā meha* should be given the decoction of *mañjiṣṭhā* and *candana*. The patient of *rakta meha* should be given the decoction of *guḍūcī*, *tinduka* seeds, *kāśmarya* and *kharjūra* along with honey.

"कम्पिल्लसप्तच्छदशालजानि बिभीतरोहीतककौटजानि ।"

पुष्पाणि[1] दध्नश्च[2] विचूर्णितानि[3] क्षौद्रेण लिह्यात् कफपित्तमेहे[4] ॥६४॥

[योगरत्नाकरः प्रमेहचिकित्साः पृष्ठ ८४]

Flowers of *kampillaka*, *saptacchada*, *śāla*, *bibhītaka*, *rohītaka* and *kuṭaja* should be burnt and made to a powder. Intake of

1. कपित्थपुष्पाणि इति आदर्शपुस्तकेषु पाठः ।
2. पाठोऽयं आदर्शपुस्तकेषु नोपलभ्यते ।
3. च चूर्णितानि इति आदर्शपुस्तकेषु पाठः ।
4. कफपित्तमेही इति आदर्शपुस्तकेषु पाठः ।

this powder along with honey is useful in the *prameha* caused by *kapha* and *pitta*.

"सर्वमेहहरो धात्र्या रसः क्षौद्रनिशायुतः ।

कषायस्त्रिफलादारुमुस्तकैरथवा कृतः ॥६५॥"

[भैषज्यरत्नावली : प्रमेहाधिकार : ६]

The juice of *dhātrī* along with honey and *niśā* cures all types of *prameha*. Similarly, the decoction of *triphalā*, *deva dāru* and *mustā* mixed with honey and *niśā* cures all types of *prameha*.

"फलत्रिकं दारुनिशां विशालां मुस्तां च निःक्वाथ्य निशांशकल्कम् ।

पिबेत्कषायं मधुसंप्रयुक्तं सर्वप्रमेहेषु समुच्छ्रितेषु ॥६६॥"

[भैषज्यरत्नावली : प्रमेहाधिकार : ६]

In all serious types of *prameha*, the patient should take the decoction of *triphalā*, *dāru niśā*, *viśālā* and *mustā* by adding the paste of *niśā* and honey.

कटंकटेरीमधुकत्रिफलाचित्रकैः समैः ।

सिद्धः कषायः पातव्यः प्रमेहानां[1] विनाशनः ॥६७॥

Intake of the decoction of *kaṭaṅkaṭerī*, *madhuka*, *triphalā* and *citraka*—all taken in equal quantities, cures different types of *prameha*.

"त्रिफला दारुदार्व्यब्दक्वाथः क्षौद्रेण मेहहा ।"

[भैषज्यरत्नावली : प्रमेहाधिकार : ७]

कुटजासनदार्व्यब्दफलत्रयभवोऽथवा ॥६८॥

[योगरत्नाकर : प्रमेहचिकित्सा : पृष्ठ ८५]

---

1. प्रमेहानं इति पंचमपुस्तके पाठः ।

The decoction of either *triphalā*, *deva dāru* and *dārvi* or *kuṭaja*, *asana*, *dārvī*, *abda* and *triphalā*, taken along with honey cures *prameha*.

"त्रिफलालौहशिलाजतुपथ्याचूर्णञ्च लीढमेकैकम् ।
मधुना मुरास्वरस[1] इव सर्वान्मेहान्निवारयति ॥६९॥"

[भैषज्यरत्नावली : प्रमेहाधिकार : ८]

Intake of the powder of *triphalā* or *lauha bhasma* or *śilā jatu* or *pathyā* along with honey cures all types of *prameha* as the gods destroyed all the demons. [mistakes in second line; translation based on note in fifth mss].

"सालमुस्तककम्पिल्लककल्कमक्षसमं पिबेत् ।
धात्रीरसेन सक्षौद्रं सर्वमेहहरं परम् ॥७०॥"

[योगरत्नाकरः प्रमेहचिकित्साः पृष्ठ ८६]

One *akṣa* of the paste of *sāla*, *mustaka* and *kampillaka* should be taken along with the juice of *dhātrī* and honey which cures all types of *prameha*.

"न्यग्रोधोदुम्बराश्वत्थश्योनाकारग्वधासनम् ।
आम्रजम्बूकपित्थं च प्रियालं ककुभं धवम् ॥७१॥
मधूको[2] मधुकं लोध्रं वरुणं पारिभद्रकम् ।
पटोलं मेषशृङ्गीं च दन्तीचित्रकमाढकीम्[3] ॥७२॥

---

1. क. मधुताऽमरासुरारु इति प्रथमपुस्तके पाठः ।
   ख. मधुनामरासुरारु इति पंचमषष्ठपुस्तकयोः पाठः ।
2. मधुकं इति आकरे पाठः ।
3. ०चित्रकपाटली इति आकरे पाठः ।

करञ्जत्रिफलाशक्रभल्लातकफलानि च ।
एतानि समभागानि श्लक्ष्णचूर्णानि[1] कारयेत् ॥७३॥
न्यग्रोधाद्यमिदं चूर्णं मधुना सह लेहयेत् ।
फलत्रयरसं चानु पिबन्मूत्रं विशुद्ध्यति ॥७४॥

[योगरत्नाकर : प्रमेहचिकित्सा : पृ० ८६]

एतेन विंशतिर्मेहाः मूत्रकृच्छ्राणि यानि च ।
प्रशमं यांति योगेन पिडका च न जायते ॥

[योगरत्नाकर : प्रमेहचिकित्सा : पृष्ठ ८६]

न्यग्रोधाद्यमिदं चूर्णमाम्रजम्बवस्थि गृह्यते ॥७५॥"

॥ न्यग्रोधाद्यं चूर्णम् ॥

[भैषज्यरत्नावली : प्रमेहाधिकार : ५३-५७]

Nyagrodhādya Cūrṇa

Nyagrodha, *udumbara*, *aśvattha*, *śyonāka*, *āragvadha*, *asana*, *āmra*, *jambū*, *kapittha*, *priyāla*, *kakubha*, *dhava*, *madhūka*, *madhuka*, *lodhra*, *varuṇa*, *pāribhadraka*, *paṭola*, *meṣa śṛṅgī*, *dantī*, *citraka*, *āḍhakī*, *karañja*, *triphalā*, *śakra* and fruits (nuts) of *bhallātaka*—all taken in equal quantities, should be made to a fine powder. This is called *nyagrodhādya cūrṇa*. It should be taken along with honey. Thereafter, the patient should take the juice or decoction of *triphalā*. This cleanses the urine. It cures twenty types of *prameha* and dysuria. It prevents the occurrence of carbuncles. In this *nyagrodhādya cūrṇa*, seed-pulp of *āmra* and *jambū* should be used.

"त्रिकण्टकाश्मन्तकसोमवल्कैर्भल्लातकैः सातिविषैः सलोध्रैः ।
वचापटोलार्जुननिम्बमुस्तैर्हरिद्रया पद्मकदीप्यकैश्च ॥७६॥

1. सूक्ष्मचूर्णानि इति आकरे पाठः ।

मञ्जिष्ठया चागुरुचन्दनैश्च सर्वैः समस्तैः कफवातजेषु ।
मेहेषु तैलं विपचेद्घृतन्तु[1] पैत्तेषु मिश्रं त्रिषु लक्षणेषु ॥७७॥"

[भारतभैषज्यरत्नाकर : द्वितीयभाग : पृष्ठ ३६७]

॥ त्रिकण्टकादिघृतम्[2] ॥

Trikaṇṭakādya Ghṛta and Taila

Trikaṇṭaka, *aśmantaka*, *somavalka*, *bhallātaka*, *ativiṣā*, *lodhra*, *vacā*, *paṭola*, *arjuna*, *nimba*, *musta*, *haridrā*, *padmaka*, *dīpyaka*, *mañjiṣṭhā*, *aguru* and *candana* should be boiled with sesame oil. This medicated oil is useful in *pramehas* caused by *kapha* and *vāyu*. Ghee boiled along with the above mentioned drugs is useful in the treatment of *pramehas* caused by *pitta* and *sannipāta* (simultaneous vitiation of all the three *doṣas*).

कफमेहहरक्वाथसिद्धं सर्पिः कफे हितम् ।
पित्तमेहघ्नं निर्यूहसिद्धं पित्ते हितं घृतम् ॥७८॥

Decoctions of drugs have been described above for the cure for *kaphaja pramehas* and *paittika pramehas*. If the ghee is cooked with the decoction of the former category, then this medicated ghee also cures *kaphaja pramehas* and if the ghee is cooked with the decoction of the later category, then this medicated ghee cures *paittika pramehas*.

"दशमूलं करञ्जौ द्वौ देवदारु हरीतकी ।
वर्षाभूर्वरुणो दन्ती चित्रकं सपुनर्नवम् ॥७९॥
सुधानिम्बकदम्बाश्च बिल्वं भल्लातकानि च ।
शटीपुष्करमूलञ्च पिप्पलीमूलमेव च ॥८०॥

---

1. घृतञ्च इति आदर्शपुस्तकेषु पाठः ।
2. त्रिकण्टकाद्यं घृतं तैलञ्च [यमकं च] इति आदर्शपुस्तकेषु पाठः ।

पृथग् दशपलानेतान् भागांस्तोयार्मणे पचेत् ।
यवकोलकुलत्थानां प्रस्थं प्रस्थञ्च दापयेत् ॥८१॥
तेन पादावशेषेण घृतप्रस्थं विपाचयेत् ।
निचुलं त्रिफला भार्ङ्गी[1] रोहिषं गजपिप्पली ॥८२॥
शृङ्गवेरं विडङ्गानि वचा कम्पिल्लकं तथा ।
गर्भेणानेन तत्सिद्धं पाययेच्च यथाबलम् ॥८३॥
एतद्धान्वन्तरं नाम विख्यातं सर्पिरुत्तमम् ।
[2]'कुष्ठगुल्मप्रमेहांश्च श्वयथुं वातशोणितम् ॥८४॥
प्लीहोदरं तथार्शांसि विद्रधिं पिडकाश्च याः ।'
अपस्मारं तथोन्मादं सर्पिरेतन्नियच्छति ॥८५॥
पृथक् तोयार्मणे तत्र पचेद् द्रव्याच्छतं शतम् ।
शतत्रयाधिके तोयमुत्सर्गक्रमतो मतम्[3] ॥८६॥"

॥ धान्वन्तरं[4] घृतम् ॥

[भैषज्यरत्नावली : प्रमेहाधिकार : ७८-८५]

---

1. भार्गी इति आदर्शपुस्तकेषु पाठः ।
2. 'कुष्ठ———याः' पाठोऽयं चतुर्थषष्ठपुस्तकयोः नोपलभ्यते ।
3. भवेत् इति आकरे पाठः ।
4. दंतीदारुशटीशिलाह्वदहनैर्भल्लातकार्काभयाः युक् वर्षाभुकरंज-युग्मवरणैयुक्पंचमूलीयुतैः । इत्येभिर्द्दशपालिकैः शृतमयां द्रोणं पृथक् प्रास्थिकैः । एभिश्चापि कुलत्थकोलकयूषैः पादावशेषीकृतं । अस्मिन्नीयकिराततरोहिषकणार्कपिल्लविश्वौषधैः । भार्ङ्गी चव्य-गजाह्वपिप्पलियुतैरेभिश्च सिद्धं घृतं एतत्मेहहरं क्षयं क्षयकरं हिक्कापहं गुल्मजित् पांडुत्वं प्रतिहृद्गदरुजः प्रध्वंसि धान्वन्तरम् । ॥धान्वंतरि घृतम्॥" पाठोऽयं चतुर्थषष्ठपुस्तकयोः अधिकमुपलभ्यते ।

Dhānvantara Ghṛta

In one *armaṇa* of water, ten *palas* of each of *daśa mūla*, *karañja*, *latā karañja*, *deva dāru*, *harītakī*, *varṣābhū*, *varuṇa*, *dantī*, *citraka*, *punarnavā*, *sudhā*, *nimba*, *kadamba*, *bilva*, *bhallātaka*, *śaṭī*, *puṣkara mūla* and *pippali mūla* and one *prastha* of each of *yava*, *kola* as well as *kulattha* should be added and boiled till one fourth remains. To this decoction, one *prastha* of ghee and the paste of *nicula*, *triphalā*, *bhārṅgī*, *rohiṣa*, *gaja pippalī*, *śṛṅgavera*, *viḍaṅga*, *vacā* and *kampillaka* should be added and cooked. This medicated ghee should be administered to the patient in a suitable dose depending upon his power of digestion. This is called *dhānvantara ghṛta*. It cures *kuṣṭha* (obstinate skin diseases including leprosy), *gulma* (phantom tumour), *pramehas* of different types, oedema, gout, splenic disorder, piles, abscess, carbuncle, epilepsy and insanity. In one *armaṇa* of water one hundred *palas* of the drugs of each category should be boiled for the preparation of the decoction. If, however, the quantity of drugs exceeds three hundred *palas*, then the quantity of water should be determined according to the general rule of *paribhāṣā*.

"दाडिमस्य तु बीजानि कृमिघ्नस्य च तण्डुलाः ।
रजनी चविकाजाजी नागरं त्रिफला कणा ॥८७॥
त्रिकण्टकस्य च फलं[1] यमानी धान्यकं तथा ।
वृक्षाम्लं चपला कोलं सिंधूद्भवसमायुतैः[2] ॥८८॥
कल्कैरक्षसमैरेभिर्घृतप्रस्थं विपाचयेत् ।
भोज्ये पाने प्रदातव्यं[3] सर्वर्त्तुषु च मात्रया ॥८९॥

1. क. तु फलं इति षष्ठपुस्तके पाठः ।
   ख. बीजानि इति आकरे पाठः ।
2. ०समायुतम् इति चतुर्थषष्ठपुस्तकयोः आकरे च पाठः ।
3. च दातव्यं इति आकरे पाठः ।

प्रमेहान् विंशतिविधान् मूत्राघातं तथाश्मरीम् ।
कृच्छ्रं सुदारुणं चैव हन्यादेतान्न संशयः ॥६०॥
विबन्धानाहशूलघ्नं कामलाज्वरनाशनम् ।
[1]'दाडिमाद्यं घृतं नाम्ना ह्यश्विभ्यां निर्मितं पुरा ॥६१॥'

॥ दाडिमाद्यं घृतम् ॥"

[भैषज्यरत्नावली : प्रमेहाधिकार : ५८-६२]

Dāḍimādya Ghṛta

One *prastha* of ghee should be cooked with the paste of one *akṣa* of each of *dāḍima* (seeds), *viḍaṅga* (pulp of the dehusked seed), *rajanī*, *cavikā*, *ajājī*, *nāgara*, *triphalā*, *kaṇā*, *trikaṇṭaka* (fruit), *yamānī*, *dhānyaka*, *vṛkṣāmla*, *capalā*, *kola* and rock-salt. This medicated ghee should be administered along with food and drinks in all seasons in appropriate dose. It undoubtedly cures twenty varieties of *prameha*, *mūtrāghāta* (anuria), *aśmarī* (stone) and serious type of dysuria. It also cures constipation, *ānāha* (abdominal distension), colic pain, jaundice and fever. This is called *dāḍimādya ghṛta*. In the days of yore, it was propounded by the Aśvins.

पौष्करं सोत्पलं चैव मृद्वीकां च पचंपचम् ।
त्वग्रसांजनयष्ट्याह्वशिलाजत्वम्लवेतसम् ॥६२॥
पुष्करमूलउत्पलफूलद्राक्षादारुहलदिगुडत्वक्रसाञ्जनशिलाजतु
अम्लवेतस तदेव घृतमेतान्यौषधानि दत्त्वा यदा पचेत्तदा-
बृहद्दाडिमादिः ॥६३॥

॥ बृहद्दाडिमाद्यं घृतम् ॥

---

1. 'दाडिमाद्यं———पुरा' पाठोऽयं आदर्शपुस्तकेषु नोपलभ्यते ।

Bṛhat Dāḍimādya Ghṛta

If, to the above mentioned recipe, the paste of *puṣkara mūla*, *utpala*, *mṛdvīkā*, *pacampacā*, *tvak*, *rasāñjana*, *madhu yaṣṭi*, *śilā jatu* and *amla vetasa* are added and cooked, the preparation is called *bṛhat dāḍimādya ghṛta*. [The prose paragraph is the explanation of the two line verse. This appears to be an interpolation]

"त्रिकटुत्रिफलाचूर्णतुल्यं युक्तन्तु[1] गुग्गुलुः ।
गोक्षुरक्वाथसंयुक्तं[2] गुटिकां कारयेद्भिषक्[3] ॥९४॥
दोषकालबलापेक्षी[4] भक्षयेच्चानुलोमिकाम् ।
न चात्र परिहारोऽस्ति कर्मकुर्याद्यथेप्सितम् ।
प्रमेहान्मूत्राघातांश्च[5] वातरोगोदरान् जयेत् ॥९५॥"

॥ त्र्यूषणाद्यगुटिका[6] ॥

[योगरत्नाकर : प्रमेहचिकित्सा : (उत्तरार्द्ध) पृष्ठ ८७]

Tryūṣaṇādya Guṭikā

The powder of *trikaṭu* and *triphalā* (one part each) and *guggulu* (six parts) should be triturated by adding the decoction of *gokṣura*. Pills should be prepared out of this paste and

---

1. गुग्गुलुं च समांशकम् इति आकरे पाठः ।
2. ०संयुक्तां इति आकरे पाठः ।
3. ०बुधः इति आकरे पाठः ।
4. देश० इति आकरे पाठः ।
5. "प्रमेहान्वातरोगांश्च वातशोणितमेव च । मूत्राघातं मूत्रदोषं प्रदरं ! चानु नाशयेत्" इति आकरे पाठः ।
6. गोक्षुरादि गुटी इति आकरे पाठः ।

administered in appropriate dose depending upon the *doṣas* involved and the nature of the season. This helps in the downward movement of *vāyu*. There is no dietatic restriction and the patient can do his work as he desires. It cures various types of *prameha*, *mūtrāghāta* (anuria), diseases caused by *vāyu* and *udara* (abstinate abdominal diseases including ascites).

"शालसारादितोयेन भावितं यच्छिलाजतु ।
पिबेत्तेनैव संशुद्धदेहः पिष्टं यथाबलम् ॥६६॥
जाङ्गलानां रसैः सार्द्धं तस्मिन् जीर्णे च भोजनम् ।
कुर्यादेवं[1] तुलां यावदुपयुञ्जीत मानवः ॥६७॥
मधुमेहं विहायासौ शर्करामश्मरीं तथा ।
वपुर्वर्णबलोपेतं शतं जीवत्यनामयः ॥६८॥"

॥ [शिलाजतुप्रयोगः] ॥

[भैषज्यरत्नावली : प्रमेहाधिकार : ४५-४७]

Administration of Śilā Jatu

Śilā jatu (an exudate from stone) should be impregnated with decoction of drugs belonging to *śālasārādi gaṇa*. The patient, who has got his body cleansed, should take this paste in a suitable dose depending upon his strength. After the medicine is digested, he should take food along with the soup of the meat of animals inhabiting arid land. In total, upto one *tulā* of *śilā jatu* should be administered to him. This cures *madhu meha* (diabetes mellitus), *śarkarā* (graveluria) and *aśmarī* (stone in the urinary tract). The patient being free from these diseases live for one hundred years with complexion and strength of the body.

1. एवं च कुडवं इति श्राकरे पाठः ।

"चन्द्रप्रभा-वचा-मुस्ताभूनिम्बामरदारवः[1] ।
हरिद्रातिविषा दार्वी पिप्पलीमूलचित्रकाः[2] ॥९९॥
धान्यकं त्रिफला चव्यं विडंगं गजपिप्पली ।
व्योषं[3] माक्षिकधातुश्च द्वौ क्षारौ लवणत्रयम् ॥१००॥
एतानि शाणमात्राणि[4] प्रत्येकं कारयेद्बुधः ।
त्रिवृद्दन्तीपत्रकञ्च त्वगेला वंशलोचना[5] ॥१०१॥
प्रत्येकं कर्षमात्राणि कुर्यादेतानि बुद्धिमान् ।
द्विकर्षं हृतलोहं स्याच्चतुःकर्षा सिता भवेत् ॥१०२॥
शिलाजत्वष्टकर्षं स्यादष्टौ कर्षाश्च गुग्गुलोः[6] ।
एभिरेकत्र[7] संसूक्ष्मं कर्त्तव्या गुटिका[8] शुभा ॥१०३॥
चन्द्रप्रभेति[9] विख्याता सर्वरोगप्रणाशिनी ।
प्रमेहान्[10] विंशति कृच्छ्रान् मूत्राघातं तथाश्मरीम् ॥१०४॥

---

1. ०सुरदारवः इति आकरे पाठः ।
2. चित्रकम् इति आकरे पाठः ।
3. सुवर्णमाक्षिकं व्योषं इति आकरे पाठः ।
4. टङ्कमात्राणि सङ्गृह्णीयात्पृथक् पृथक् इति आकरे पाठः ।
5. वंशरोचना इति प्रथमचतुर्थपुस्तकयोः पाठः ।
6. गुग्गुलाः इति पंचमपुस्तके पाठः ।
7. विधिना योजितैरेतैः इति आकरे पाठः ।
8. गुटिकाः शुभाः इति प्रथमपुस्तके पाठः ।
9. चन्द्रप्रभाति इति आदर्शपुस्तकेषु पाठः ।
10. निहान्त विंशतिं मेहान् कृच्छ्रमष्टविधं तथा इति आकरे पाठः ।

विबंधानाहशूलानि[1] मेदग्रन्थिमथार्बुदम् ।
अंत्रवृद्धि[2] तथा पांडुं कामलाञ्च हलीमकम् ॥१०५॥
अण्डवृद्धि[3] कटीशूलं श्वासं कासं विचर्चिचकाम् ।
कुष्ठानि रकसा [?] कण्डूप्लीहोदरभगंदरम् ॥१०६॥
नेत्ररोगं दन्तरोगं स्त्रीणामार्त्तवजां रुजम् ।
पुसां शुक्रगतान्दोषान्मन्दाग्निमरुचिं तथा ॥१०७॥
वायुपित्तकफं हन्याद्बल्या वृष्या रसायनी ।
चन्द्रप्रभायाः कर्षस्तु चतुःशाणो विधीयते ॥१०८॥"

॥चन्द्रप्रभा गुटिका ॥

[भैषज्यरत्नावली : प्रमेहाधिकार : २१३-२२०]

Candra Prabhā Guṭikā

One *śāṇa* of each of *candra prabhā, vacā, mustā, bhūnimba, deva dāru, haridrā, ativiṣā, dārvī, pippalī mūla, citraka, dhānyaka, triphalā, cavya, viḍaṅga, gaja pippalī, vyoṣa, bhasma* of *mākṣika* (copper pyrite), *svarji kṣāra, yava kṣāra, sāmudra lavaṇa, saindhava lavaṇa* and *viḍa lavaṇa*, one *karṣa* of each of *trivṛt, dantī, patra, tvak, elā* and *vaṃśa locanā*, two *karṣas* of *lauha bhasma*, four *karṣas* of sugar and eight *karṣas* of each of *śilā jatu* as well as *guggulu* should be made to a powder (sticky material to be

---

1. चतस्रश्चाश्मरीस्तद्वन्मूत्राघातांस्त्रयोदश इति आकरे पाठः ।
2. अण्डवृद्धिं इति आकरे पाठः ।
3. कासं श्वासं तथाकुष्ठमग्निमान्द्यमरोचकम् । वातपित्तकफव्याधीन् बल्या वृष्या रसायनी । समाराध्य शिवं यस्मात्प्रयत्नाद् गुडिकामिमाम् । प्राप्तवांश्चन्द्रमास्तस्मादियं चन्द्रप्रभा स्मृता । इति आकरे पाठः ।

added separately) and mixed well. From out of this, pills are to be prepared. This is well known as *candra prabhā* and it cures all diseases. It cures twenty varieties of *prameha*, dysuria, *mūtrāghāta* (anuria), *aśmarī* (stone in the urinary tract), constipation, abdominal distension, colic pain, *meda granthi* (lipoma), *arbuda* (tumour), *antra vṛddhi* (inguinal hernia), anemia, jaundice, *halīmaka* (a serious type of jaundice), *aṇḍa vṛddhi* (scrotal tumour), lumbago, dyspnoea, cough, eczema, *kuṣṭha* (obstinate skin diseases including leprosy), itching, splenomegaly, fistula-in-ano, eye diseases, diseases of teeth, menstrual disorders (pain) in females, seminal disorders in males, suppression of the power of digestion and anorexia. It alleviates *vāyu*, *pitta* as well as *kapha* and promotes strength as well as virility. It rejuvenates the body. In this recipe, *candra prabhā* is described to be taken in the quantity of one *karṣa* which should be treated as equivalent to four *śāṇas*.

"श्रीखण्डं त्रिसुगन्धिकेसरकणाशुण्ठीमरीचाम्बुदम् ।
श्रृङ्गारं जलजं प्रियालबदरीधात्र्यब्जबीजं तुगा ॥१०९॥
द्राक्षा जीरकधान्यकं ससुमनः पुष्पं च जातीदलम् ।
शुद्धारं बदरं[1] पलार्द्धकमिदं सन्नारिकेलात्[2]त्रयम् ॥११०॥
पूगं चाष्टपलं च सौरभपयः प्रस्थत्रये सम्पचेत् ।
पश्चादामलकीवरीजलशरावार्द्धेऽथ पिष्टीकृतम् ॥१११॥
शुष्कीकृत्य कटाहके च सघृते मन्दाग्निना चूर्णयुक्[3] ।
वङ्गव्योमपलार्द्धमर्द्धतुलया खण्डेन पाकीकृतम् ॥११२॥
भुक्तं प्रातरिदं प्रमेहसहिताध्मानानि शूलानि च ।
क्षैण्यं[4] दैन्यमसृक्स्रुतिं मुखगुदश्रोत्राक्षिलोमोद्भवाम् ॥११३॥

1. दरदं इति आकरे पाठः ।
2. ०केलाश्मवत् इति षष्ठपुस्तके पाठः ।
3. चूर्णयुग् इति आकरे पाठः ।
4. चक्ष्यं इति षष्ठपुस्तके पाठः ।

हन्याद्रोगजराविपत्तिशमनं मन्दाग्निजित्[1] बृंहणम् ।
बल्यं वृद्धिकरं प्रमोदजनकं पूगं न किं सेव्यते ॥११४॥"

॥ इति पूगपाकः[2] ॥

[भारतभैषज्यरत्नाकर : तृतीयभाग : पृष्ठ ३३६-३३७]

Pūga Pāka

Half *palas* of each of *śrī khaṇḍa*, *tri sugandhi*, *kesara*, *kaṇā śuṇṭhī*, *marica*, *ambuda*, *śṛṅgāṭa*, *jalaja*, *priyāla*, *badarī*, *dhātrī*,, seeds of lotus, *tugā*, *drākṣā*, *jīraka*, *dhānyaka*, jasmin flower (*jāti puṣpa*), mace (*jāti dala*) and purified *hiṅgula*, pulp of three coconuts and eight *palas* of *pūga* should be cooked in three *prasthas* of cow's milk. Thereafter, this should be added with half *śarāva* of the paste of each of *āmalakī*, *śatāvari* and *jala* and dried. All these should be fried in a pan with mild heat by adding ghee. To this half *pala* of *vaṅga bhasma* should be added and mixed. This should be cooked by adding water and half *tulā* of sugar. This recipe should be administered to the patient in the morning. It cures *prameha*, abdominal distension, colic pain, consumption, weakness and bleeding from the mouth, anus, ear, eyes and hair roots. It prevents aging process and stimulates the power of digestion. It is nourishing. It promotes strength and tissue elements and it gives physical as well as psychic comforts. This recipe should, therefore, be used regularly.

"माक्षिकं धातुमप्येवं युञ्ज्यादस्याप्ययं गुणः ।
शालसारादिवर्गस्य क्वाथे तु लघुतां[3] गते ॥११५॥

1. मन्दाग्निहृद्बृंहणम् इति आकरे पाठः ।
2. पूगीपाकः इति आकरे पाठ : ।
3. घनतां इति आकरे पाठः ।

दन्तीलोध्रशिवाकान्तलौहताम्ररजः क्षिपेत् ।
घनीभूतमदग्धञ्च प्राश्य मेहान् व्यपोहति ॥११६॥"

[भैषज्यरत्नावली : प्रमेहाधिकार : ४८-४९]

The *bhasma* of *mākṣika* (copper pyrite) should be boiled with the decoction of drugs belonging to *śāla sārādi gaṇa*. When it becomes semi-solid, the powder of *dantī*, *lodhra*, *kānta lauha bhasma* and *tāmra bhasma* should be added to it and cooked till the preparation becomes more dense but it does not get burnt. Intake of this linctus cures different varieties of *prameha*.

"[1]व्यायामजातमखिलं जयेत् मेहान्व्यपोहति ।
पादत्रच्छत्ररहितो भैक्ष्याशी मुनीवद्यतः ॥११७॥
योजनानां शतं गच्छेदधिकं वा निरन्तरम् ।
मेहान् जेतुं व[2]ने वापि नीवारामलकाशनः ॥११८॥"

[भैषज्यरत्नावली : प्रमेहाधिकार : १७-१८]

Exercise

All types of exercise cure *pramehas*. The patient should continuously walk for one hundred *yojanas* without using shoes and umbrella, and by begging for his food like a saint. Alternatively, he should reside in a forest by eating *nīvāra* and *āmalaka* which will make him free from *pramehas*.

शराविकाद्याः पिडकाः साधयेच्छोथवद्भिषक् ।
पक्वाश्चिकित्सेत् व्रणवत् तासां पाने प्रशस्यते ॥११९॥

---

1. 'व्यायाम———मेहान्व्यपोहति' पाठोऽयं प्रथमपंचमपुस्तकयोः नोपलभ्यते ।
2. वले इति प्रथमपुस्तके पाठः ।

क्वाथो वनस्पतेर्वाऽपि मूत्रं च व्रणशोधनम् ।
एलादिकेन कुर्वीत तैलं च व्रणरोपणम् ॥१२०॥
आरग्वधादिनां कुर्यात् क्वाथमुद्वर्त्तनानि च ।
शालसारादिसेक च भोज्यादिं वरुणादिना ॥१२१॥

Treatment of Carbuncles

Carbuncles like *śarāvikā*, etc. should be treated on the lines suggested for *śotha* (oedema). When suppurated, these carbuncles should be treated on the lines suggested for the treatment of *vraṇa* (ulcers). These patients should take decoctions of herbs and use cow's urine for cleansing ulcers. The oil cooked with drugs belonging to *elādi gaṇa* helps in the healing of ulcers. He should use the decoction of drugs belonging to *āragvadhādi gaṇa*. The powder of these drugs should be used by him for unction. He should take bath by boiling water with drugs belonging to *śālasārādi gaṇa* and his food should be prepared by boiling with drugs belonging to *Varuṇādi gaṇa.*

"सौविरकं सुरा शुक्तं तैलं क्षीरं[1] गुडं घृतम् ।
अम्लेक्षुरसपिष्टान्नानूपमांसानि वर्जयेत् ॥१२२॥"
[भैषज्यरत्नावली : प्रमेहाधिकार : २४६]

Prohibitions

The patient, suffering from *prameha*, should avoid *sauvīraka* (a type of vinegar), *surā* (alcoholic drinks), *śukta* (another type of vinegar), oil, milk, jaggery, ghee, sour juice, sugar cane juice, pastries and aquatic meat.

मारितं त्रपुसीसं वा दग्धं हरिणश्रृंगकम् ।
कर्पासबीजमज्जा च तुल्यमकोल्हबीजकम् ॥१२३॥

1. क्षारं इति आकरे पाठः ।

पेषयेत्माहिषे तक्रे दिनैकं वटकीकृतम् ।
माषद्वयं सदा खादेन्सुरानाम प्रमेहजित् ॥
अक्षपाठाभयादार्वीकषायमनुपाययेत् ॥१२४॥

Vaṅga bhasma, *nāga bhasma*, *bhasma* of deer horn, pulp of cotton-seed and seed of *akolha* [?] should be taken in equal quantities and triturated by adding the butter-milk prepared of buffalo-milk. This should always be taken for the cure of *surā meha*. The patient should use the decoction of *akṣa*, *pāṭhā*, *abhayā* and *dārvī* as *anupāna* (post-prandial drink).

गंधकं गुडसंयुक्तं कर्षभुक्तं प्रमेहजित्[1] ॥१२५॥

Intake of purified *gandhaka* along with jaggery in a dose of one *karṣa* cures *prameha*.

"रसं गंधं विषं लोहं जातीपत्रं च तत्फलम् ।
अब्धिशोषाहिफेनं च खुरासानं च चित्रकम् ॥१२६॥

---

1. 'किंशुकं गजकणा द्वयं गंधा गोपयस्यभिनिवेश्य सुमेधाः पाचयेदिह तु दोलकयन्त्रोत्तोलितम् । विशदगंधकचूर्ण तुलसी सह देविका रसाभ्यामपि । भृंगस्य रसेन जिह्विकायाः । मुनिभावनया सुसाधितं करहारेण च नागरेण चापि शतपुत्रिकया सहादनात् क्षयपत्येव फिरंगमारुतम् । किंशुकपुष्प सेर १, गजपिप्पली टांक १८, अश्वगन्धा टांक १८, चूर्णकरुन आवासरोद्‌बधा मध्ये कालवून त्यामध्ये दोलायन्त्री यथेच्छ गंधकशोधि ज्योति पर्यंत दूधजले मगकाटन तुलसी रस सहदेवी भृंगराज गोजिह्वायां वी प्रत्येके पुट देइन्योत्ति छायाशुष्ठ करिजे । आकरकल शुंठि शतावरी यांच्चै अनुपाने एकमासाभक्षिजे फिरंग जाई । शाल्मली व्येमूलांच्चेरसा मध्ये गंधक पाताल यंत्रें शोधिज्येष्ठ कविसवेला भाव नाष्टक-विसछाया शुष्क करिज्ये गोघृतें सीभक्षिजे मासाष्टकपोषकहोय । पाठोऽयं चतुर्थषष्ठपुस्तकयोः अधिकमुपलम्यते ।

देवपुष्पं समं सर्वं सर्वैस्तुल्यं मृताभ्रकम् ।
भावयेत्सप्तधा सर्वं चित्रमूलकषायकैः ॥
यथा सात्म्येन संयोज्यं सर्वमेहानुपात्तये ॥१२७॥
अर्शांसि ग्रहणीशोथपांडुशुक्रक्षये नृणाम् ।
यथानुपानतो योज्यः[1] सिद्धः श्रीमेहभैरवः ॥१२८॥"

॥ मेहभैरवरसः[2] ॥

[भारतभैषज्यरत्नाकर : चतुर्थभाग : पृष्ठ २६५]

Meha Bhairava Rasa

Purified *pārada*, purified *gandhaka*, purified *viṣa* (aconite), *lauha bhasma*, *jātī patra*, *jātī phala*, *abdhi śoṣa*, *ahi phena*, *khurāsāna*, *citraka*, *deva puṣpa*—all taken one part each and eleven parts of *abhraka bhasma* should be impregnated and triturated for seven times with the decoction of the root of *citraka*. This should be administered to the patient in an appropriate dose for the cure of all types of *prameha*, piles, *grahaṇī* (sprue syndrome), oedema, anemia and diminution of semen. This should be taken along with suitable *anupāna* (post-prandial drink). This is experienced to be effective in these ailments. It is called *śrī meha bhairava*.

"मृतसूतं[3] मृतगंधं मृतलोहाभ्रकं समम् ।
मर्दयेन्मधुना वह्निरसोऽयं[4] तालकेश्वरः[5] ॥१२९॥

1. भोज्यं इति पंचमपुस्तके पाठः ।
2. 'रसं———मेहभैरवरसः" पाठोऽयं प्रथमपुस्तके नोपलभ्यते ।
3. मृतं सूतं मृतं लौहं मृतवङ्गाभ्रकं समम् इति आकरे पाठः ।
4. चाह्नो इति आकरे पाठः ।
5. तारकेश्वरः इति आकरे पाठः ।

माषमात्रं[1] लिहेत्क्षौद्रैर्बहुमूत्रापनुत्तये ।
औदुम्बरं[2] फलं पक्वं चूर्णितं कर्षमात्रकम्[3] ।
'संलेह्य[4] मधुना सार्द्धमनुपानं सुखावहम् ॥१३०॥''

॥ तारकेश्वरः[5] ॥

[भैषज्यरत्नावली : प्रमेहाधिकार : ११५-११६]

Tārakeśvara Rasa

Bhasma of *pārada* (*rasa sindūra*), purified *gandhaka*, *lauha bhasma* and *abhraka bhasma*—all these drugs taken in equal quantities should be triturated by adding honey. This powerful recipe is called *tārakeśvara rasa*. This should be administered in the dose of one *māṣā* along with honey for the cure of *vahu mūtra* (diabetes insipidus). One *karṣa* of the powder of ripe *udumbara* fruit and honey should be given as *anupāna* (post-prandial potion).

सूतं कान्तं गंधस्तीक्ष्णो ताप्यं व्योषं फलत्रिकम् ।
शिलाजतु शिलां कोलहबीजं रात्रिः कपित्थजम्[6] ॥१३१॥
त्रिःसप्तकृत्वो भृंगाद्भिः भावयेन्निष्कसंज्ञिकः ।
मेघनादाख्य सूतस्यात् सर्वमेहान्प्रणाशयेत् ॥१३२॥

॥ मेघनादो[7] रसः ॥

---

1. गुञ्जाद्वयं इति आकरे पाठः ।
2. औडुम्बरं इति आकरे पाठः ।
3. मधुना लिहेत् इति आकरे पाठः ।
4. 'सं० ——सुखावहं' पाठोऽयं आकरे नोपलभ्यते ।
5. तालकेश्वरः इति चतुर्थपुस्तके पाठः ।
6. कपिच्छजम् इति प्रथमपुस्तके पाठः ।
7. मेघनादीय रसः इति षष्ठपुस्तके पाठः ।

Megha Nāda Rasa

Purified *pārada*, *kānta lauha bhasma*, purified *gandhaka*, *tīkṣṇa lauha bhasma*, *mākṣika bhasma*, *trikaṭu*, *triphalā*, *śilā jatu*, purified *manaḥ śilā*, seed of *kolha*, *haridrā* and pulp of *kapittha* —all these drugs should be impregnated and triturated for twenty one times by adding the juice of *bhṛṅga rāja*. This should be administered in a dose of one *niṣka* which cures all types of *prameha*. This is called *megha nāda rasa*.

महानिम्बस्य मूलानि[1] पेषयेत्तण्डुलाम्बुना ।
सघृतान्यचिराद्धन्युः पानान्[2]मेहांश्चिरोच्छ्रितान् ॥१३३॥

The root of *mahā nimba* should be made to a paste by adding *taṇḍulāmbu* (rice-wash). Intake of this paste along with ghee cures chronic type of *prameha*.

सूता[3]भ्रमामलजलैः सप्ताहं भावयेद्रसः ।
हरिशंकरसंज्ञः स्याद्[4] रक्तपित्तप्रमेहनुत् ॥१३४॥

॥ हरिशंकरः ॥

---

1. बीजा० इति चतुर्थषष्ठपुस्तकयोः पाठः ।
2. वातान्मेहाश्चिरोत्थिताम् इति चतुर्थपंचमपुस्तकयोः पाठः ।
3. क. सुतोभयामलजलैः इति षष्ठपुस्तके पाठः ।
   ख. "षट्पलं सूतराजस्य तदर्द्धं गंधकं मतम ।
   नागं गन्धसम योज्यं शिलातालकसीसकम् ॥
   दरदं वत्सनाभं च पर्पटं धूर्त्तबीजकम् ।
   प्रत्येकार्द्धपलं दद्यात्छुभे खल्वे भिषगवरः ॥
   संमर्द्य कज्जलीं कृत्वा कन्यानीरेण भावयेत् ।
   काचमाचीशिफातोये हस्तिशुण्डी जले ततः ॥
   हंसपादी रसे सम्यक् अष्टधा परिभावयेत् ।

(continued on next page

Hari Śaṅkara Rasa

Pārada bhasma and *abhraka bhasma* should be impregnated and triturated with the juice or decoction of *āmalakī* for seven days. This is called *Hari śaṅkara.* It cures *rakta pitta* (an ailment characterised by bleeding from different parts of the body) and *prameha.*

(*continued*)

ततः काचपटे देयं घटी सिकतयंत्रगाम् ।।
कृत्वाद्वादशयामं वै ज्वालयेतदधोनलम् ।
स्वागंशीतं समुत्तार्य खल्वे दत्त्वा विचूर्णयेत् ।।
पुनः शिलादिकं योज्यं भावयेत्कन्यकादिभिः ।
सिकताख्ये पुनर्देयो वह्निर्यामार्द्धमानतः ।।
स्वांगशीतं समुत्तार्य मेघनादो रसोत्तमः ।
करोति वह्निबलपुष्टिकांतिं हन्याच्च वातम् ।।
कफपित्तामुग्रं श्वासं च कासं च परिणामशूलम् ।
मेहात्रि हन्यात्किल मेघनादः ।।

।। वृहन्मेघनादो रसः ।।

शुद्धसूतसमं गंधं तदर्द्धं सितसोमलम् ।
स्नुह्यर्क्कपयसा मर्द्यं दिनमेकं पृथक् पृथक् ।।
खेचरी पयसार्द्यं फलतोयेन त्रिदिनं सुविमर्द्दयेत् ।
कांचकुप्युदरे क्षिप्त्वा वालुकायंत्रगं पचेत् ।
दिनमेकं क्रमादग्नौ पारंपर्य्योपदेशतः ।
शीतलं स्वांगसंजातं बल्लमात्रं प्रदापयेत् ।।
यथानुपानयोगेन सर्वरोगान्विनाशयेत् ।
अशीतिन्वातजान्रोगान्विंशतिं श्लेष्मजां तथा ।
सेवनादस्य नश्यंति सर्वेरोगाः सुदारुणाः ।
रसोयं मेघनादाख्यो स्वेदशैत्यं विनाशयेत् ।
जारणदिक्रमेणैव सप्तवारं विपाचयेत् ।
दुर्लभोयं रमादेवि ज्वालानलसमं प्रभः ।
शुक्रवृद्धिं करोत्याशु वाजिवेगसमं भवेत् ।
सन्निपातशूलिकायां शस्तमेतन्न संशयः ।

।।इति मेघनादाख्यो रसं ।।"

पाठोऽयं चतुर्थषष्ठपुस्तकयोः अधिकमुपलभ्यते ।

4. त्वात् इति षष्ठपुस्तके पाठः ।

"रसस्य भस्मना तुल्यं वङ्गभस्म प्रकल्पयेत्[1] ।
अस्य रक्तिकैकं[2] हंति मेहान् क्षौद्रसमन्वितम्[3] ॥१३५॥"

॥ वंगेश्वरः ॥

[भैषज्यरत्नावली : प्रमेहाधिकार : ६०]

Vaṅgeśvara

Pārada bhasma and *vaṅga bhasma* should be taken in equal quantities and triturated. This should be administered in a dose of one *ratti* (125 mg.) along with honey which cures *pramehas.*

"[4]एला सकर्पूरसिता सधात्री जातीफलं गोक्षुरशाल्मलीत्वक् ।
सूताभ्रवंगायसभस्म[5] सर्वमेतत्समानं परिमर्दनीयम्[6] ॥
निष्कार्धमात्रं[7] मधुना विलिह्य निहंति सर्वामयमेहजातान् ॥१३६॥"

॥ प्रमेहकुठारः[8] ॥

[भारतभैषज्यरत्नाकर : द्वितीयभाग : पृष्ठ २०८]

---

1. प्रयोज्येत् इति आकरे पाठः ।
2. क. अस्यमाषद्वयं इति प्रथमपुस्तके पाठः ।
   ख. अस्यगुंजात्रयं इति चतुर्थषष्ठपुस्तकयोः पाठः ।
3. क्षौद्रसमीक्षकम् इति प्रथमपंचमपुस्तकयोः पाठः ।
4. 'एला———प्रमेहकुठारः' पाठोऽयं प्रथमपुस्तके नोपलभ्यते ।
5. क. सूतागंधायस० इति षष्ठपुस्तके पाठः ।
   ख. सूतेन्द्रवङ्गायसभस्म इति आकरे पाठः ।
6. परिभावयेच्च इति आकरे पाठः ।
7. गुडूचिकाशाल्मलिकाकषायैर्निष्कार्धमाना मधुना ततश्च । बद्धा वटी चन्द्रकलेति संज्ञा सर्वं प्रमेहेषु नियोज्येत्ताम् । इति आकरे पाठः ।
8. चन्द्रकलावटी इति आकरे पंचमपुस्तके च पाठः ।

Prameha Kuthāra

Elā, *karpūra*, sugar, *dhātri*, *jāti phala*, *gokṣura*, bark of *śālmalī*, *pārada bhasma*, *abhraka bhasma* and *lauha bhasma*—all these taken in equal quantities should be triturated. This should be administered in a dose of half *niṣka* along with honey which cures all types of *prameha*.

कुलत्थ[1]चणकोद्दालश्यामाकाढकि[2]कोद्रवाः

पुराणाः मेहिनां पथ्याः अस्निग्धाः[3] जांगलाः रसाः ॥१३७॥

---

1. क. कुलित्थचनको इति षष्ठपुस्तके पाठः ।
   ख. एकविंशति वारं तु तैले वंगं विशोधयेत् ।
   अत्यम्ले महिषीतक्रे निशाचूर्णं नियोजयेत् ॥
   तद्वङ्गं शोधयेत्तस्मिन्येकविंशतिवारतः ।
   निक्षिप्य खर्परे वंगं लोहदर्व्या प्रचालयेत् ॥
   यामद्वयाद्भवेद्भस्म तद्भस्मं चैक सेरकम् ।
   सूतं तत्कर्षभागेन सूततुल्या शिला क्षिपेत् ॥
   संमर्द्य कन्यकातोये शाल्यलीवारिणा तथा ।
   धत्तूरकाकमाची वचिविनीरसमर्दितम् ॥
   काचकूप्यां क्षिपन् दद्यात् वह्निं यामचतुष्टयम् ॥
   स्वांगशीतं समुत्तार्य सर्वयोगेषु योजयेत् ।
   वंगेश्वरमिति ख्यातो प्रमेहान् हंति विंशतिः ।
   ॥ वंगेश्वरो बृहत् टीकी ॥
   वंग तेलांतुवेला २१ ताकमैप्ती चेदि सातींवें आवट सेर ४ त्यात हलदि टांक ६ वाट्निद्यालावोत्पातुवेला २१ मगखापरी छालून-चूली वरिठे वापो पत्नी करुनुघाटणें प्रहरां दौ मध्ये भस्म होइल केवल घाटो वेमंगवंग सेरु १ तरिपारा पाऊ सेरु मनसील पाऊसेरु काजली करावीवंगुमेल वा कुमारी पुट १ शल्मली पोस्तक्वाथ धोतरारस करडकांगरणी चिंचेबी अंतर सालि पाणी घनून रसुत्पांची पुटे प्रति पुटी शुष्क कीजे वालुका यंत्री च ठविजे अग्निप्रहर ४ शुद्धवंगेश्वर होय । पाठोऽयं द्वितीयषष्ठपुस्तकयोः अधिकमुपलभ्यते ।
2. ०काढद्दकिको इति षष्ठपुस्तके पाठः ।
3. अस्निग्धो जांगलो इति षष्ठपुस्तके पाठः ।

Wholesome Diet

Kulattha, *caṇaka*, *uddālaka*, *śyāmāka* *āḍhakī* and *kodrava*—all these stored for some time after harvesting (*purāṇa*) are useful for patients suffering from *prameha*. Similarly, soup of the meat of arid-land animals without adding ghee or oil is useful for these patients

इति श्रीमहाराजाधिराजटोडरमल्लविरचिते टोडरानंदे आयुर्वेदसौख्ये प्रमेहमधुमेहपिडकानिदानचिकित्साकथनं नाम चतुश्चत्वारिंशत्तमो हर्षः ॥१३८॥

Thus, ends the 44th Chapter dealing with the diagnosis and treatment of *prameha*, *madhu meha* and *piḍakā* in *Āyurveda saukhya* of *Ṭoḍarānanda* composed by the great king Ṭoḍara Malla.

CHAPTER X

अथ मेदोरोगनिदानं चिकित्सा च ।

(*Diagnosis and Treatment of Obesity*)

[1]अव्यायामदिवास्वप्नश्लेष्मलाहारसेविनः ।
मधुरोऽन्नरसः प्रायः स्नेहान्मेदो[2] विवर्द्धयेत् ॥१॥
मेदसा[3]ऽऽवृतमार्गत्वात् पुष्यन्त्यन्ये[4] न धातवः ।
मेदस्तु चीयते तस्मादशक्तः सर्वकर्मसु ॥२॥

---

1. This is the beginning of 49th Chapter of *Āyurveda saukhya* in *Ṭoḍarānanda* and the invocation reads as follows:
गोविंद गानेन ब्रजांगनागताः वनेद्धं कृत्यानि पृयं समाहृताः । कृत्वा प्रचक्रेसकृपां नरेन्द्रके कुर्यावतां (कुर्याच्च) टोडरमल संज्ञके ॥ पाठोऽयं चतुर्थषष्ठपुस्तकयोः नोपलभ्यते ।
2. स्नेहान्मेदः प्रवर्धयेत् इति आकरे पाठः ।
3. मेदस्या० इति षष्ठपुस्तके पाठः ।
4. ०न्नेनधावतः इति षष्ठपुस्तके पाठः ।

Etiology and Pathogenesis

In persons who do not perform any exercise, who sleep during the day time and who habitually take *kapha*-aggravating food, the end-product of food after digestion is generally sweet in taste. Because of its unctuousness, it produces more of fat which obstructs the channels circulating nourishments to other tissue elements. As a result of this obstruction, other tissue elements do not get nourished. Therefore, along with the excessive accumulation of fat, the man becomes weak and incapable of any activity.

क्षुद्रश्वासतृषामोहस्वप्नक्रथनसादनैः[1] ।
युक्तः क्षुत्स्वेददौर्गन्ध्यैरल्पप्राणोऽल्पमैथुनः[2] ॥३॥

Signs and Symptoms

The patient of obesity suffers from *kṣudra śvāsa* (minor form of dyspnoea), thirst, unconsciousness, prolonged sleep, trembling, prostration and foul smell of mouth as well as sweat. He is of low vitality and he is less capable of performing sexual intercourse.

मेदस्तु सर्वभूतानामुदरेष्वस्थिषु स्थितम् ।
अत एवोदरे वृद्धिः प्रायो मेदस्विनो भवेत् ॥४॥

Fat is primarily located in the abdomen and bones of all living beings. Therefore, the abdomen bulges out generally in all patients suffering from obesity.

मेदसाऽऽवृतमार्गत्वाद्वायुः कोष्ठे विशेषतः ।
चरन् सन्धुक्षयत्यग्निमाहारं शोषयत्यपि ॥५॥

---

1. ०सादने इति प्रथमपुस्तके पाठः ।
2. ०मैथुनैः इति प्रथमपञ्चमपुस्तकयोः आकरे च पाठः ।

तस्मात् स शीघ्रं जरयत्याहारं[1] चापि काङ्क्षति ।
विकारान्[2] सोऽश्नुते घोरान् कांश्चित्कालव्यतिक्रमात् ॥६॥

Fat obstructs the channel of circulation of *vāyu*. Therefore, *vāyu* specially moves in the *koṣṭha* (alimentary tract), stimulates the digestive enzymes and absorbs the end product of food. Thus, the patient having obesity digests his food very quickly and desires for more and more of food. As a result of this, after the passage of some time, he succumbs to several serious diseases.

एतावुपद्रवकरौ विशेषादग्निमारुतौ ।
एतौ तु दहतः स्थूलं वनदावो वनं यथा ॥७॥

In obesity, complications are caused by *agni* (digestive enzymes) and *vāyu*. Both of them burn (afflict) the patient of obesity as the fire originating in the forest destroys the forest itself.

मेदस्यतीव संवृद्धे सहसैवानिलादयः ।
विकारान् दारुणान्कृत्वा नाशयन्त्याशु जीवितम्[3] ॥८॥

When the fat of the body is increased very much in excess, *agni* (digestive enzymes), etc. all of a sudden give rise to several diseases leading to the death of the patient.

मेदोमांसातिवृद्धत्वाच्चलस्फिगुदरस्तनः ।
अयथोपचयोत्साहो नरोऽतिस्थूल उच्यते[4] ॥९॥

॥ मेदोनिदानम् ॥१०॥

---

1. जरयत्याहारमभिकाङ्क्षति इति आकरे पाठः ।
2. विकारांश्चाप्नुते इति आकरे पाठः ।
3. जीविताम् इति प्रथमपुस्तके पाठः ।
4. स्थूलेषु दुष्टास्तराकुष्ठविसर्पा सभगन्दराः ।
   ज्वरातिसर मेहार्शः श्लीपदोपचिकामलाः ॥
   मेदसः स्वेददौर्गन्ध्याज्जायन्ते जन्तवोणवः ॥
   पाठोऽयं प्रथमेपुस्तकेषु अधिकमुपलभ्यते ।

By the excessive increase of fat and muscle tissue, buttocks, abdomen and breasts of the patient becomes loose and mobile. There is increase in body weight and decrease in activities. Such a person is called *ati-sthūla* (excessively fatty or suffering from obesity).

Thus, ends the diagnosis of obesity.

"श्रमचिन्ताव्यवायाध्व[1]क्षौद्रजागरणप्रियः ।
हन्त्यवश्यमतिस्थौल्यं यवश्यामाकभोजनम्[2] ॥११॥

Persons indulging in physical exercise, worry, sexual intercourse, long walk, intake of honey, remaining awake at night and taking *yava* and *śyāmāka* as food get rid of obesity.

अस्वप्नञ्च व्यवायञ्च व्यायामं चिन्तनानि च ।
स्थौल्यमिच्छन् परित्यक्तुं क्रमेणातिप्रवर्द्धयेत् ॥१२॥

If the patient wants to be free from obesity, then he should gradually increase *asvapna* (remaining awake at night) sexual intercourse, physical exercise and mental activities.

प्रातर्मधुयुतं वारि सेवितं स्थौल्यनाशनम् ॥१३॥

Intake of water mixed with honey in the morning cures obesity.

उष्णमन्नस्य मण्डं[3] वा पिबन्[4] कृशतनुर्भवेत् ।
सचव्यजीरकव्योषहिंगुसौवर्चलानलाः ॥१४॥

1. ०वायाशू इति प्रथमपुस्तके पाठः ।
2. ०भोजनैः इति आकरे पाठः ।
3. मंत्रं इति षष्ठपुस्तके पाठः ।
4. पिबेत् इति चतुर्थषष्ठपुस्कयोः पाठः ।

If a person takes hot *maṇḍa* (scum) of the rice which comes out during boiling along with *cavya*, *jīraka*, *vyoṣa*, *hiṅgu*, *sauvarcala* and *citraka*, then he becomes thin (free from obesity).

मस्तुना शक्तवः[1] पीता मेदोघ्ना वह्निदीपनाः[2] ॥१५॥

Intake of *śaktu* (roasted corn-flour) along with butter-milk reduces obesity and stimulates the power of digestion.

'त्रिडङ्गं नागरं क्षारः काललोहरजो मधु ।
यवामलकचूर्णश्च प्रयोगः स्थौल्यनाशनः ॥१६॥'

॥ विडङ्गाद्यं लोहम्[3] ॥

Viḍaṅgādya Lauha

The powder of *viḍaṅga*, *nāgara* and *kṣāra* (alkali preparation), *kāla lauha bhasma* honey and the powder of *yava* and *āmalaka* cure obesity.

'व्योषं विडङ्गशिग्रूणि त्रिफलां कटुरोहिणीम् ।
बृहत्यौ द्वे हरिद्रे द्वे पाठामतिविषां स्थिराम् ॥१७॥
हिंगुकेबुकमूलानि[4] यमानीं धान्यचित्रकम् ।
सौवर्चलमजाजीश्च हवुषाञ्चेति[5] चूर्णयेत् ॥१८॥
चूर्णतैलघृतक्षौद्रभागाः स्युर्मानतः समाः ।
शक्तूनां षोडशगुणो भागः सन्तर्पणं[6] पिबेत् ॥१९॥

1. शक्तवी इति चतुर्थषष्ठपुस्तकयोः पाठः ।
2. वस्तिदीपनाः इति षष्ठपुस्तके पाठः ।
3. चूर्णम् इति आकरे पाठः ।
4. ०केयुकमूलानि इति प्रथमपुस्तके पाठः ।
5. पुष्करं० इति षष्ठपुस्तके पाठः ।
6. सन्तर्पणो पियेत् इति षष्ठपुस्तके पाठः ।

प्रयोगात्तस्य शाम्यन्ति रोगाः सन्तर्पणोत्थिताः ।
प्रमेहा मूढवाताश्च कुष्ठान्यर्शांसि कामलाः ॥२०॥
प्लीहापाण्ड्वामयः शोथो मूत्रकृच्छ्रमरोचकः ।
हृद्रोगो राजयक्ष्मा च कासश्वासगलग्रहाः ॥२१॥
कृमयो ग्रहणीदोषाः शैत्यं स्थौल्यमतीव च ।
नराणां दीप्यते चाग्निः स्मृतिर्बुद्धिश्च वर्द्धते ॥२२॥'

॥ व्योषाद्यशक्तुप्रयोगः ॥

Vyoṣādya Śaktu

Vyoṣa, viḍaṅga, śigrū, triphalā, kaṭu rohiṇi, bṛhatī, kaṇṭakārī, haridrā, dāru haridrā, pāṭhā, ativiṣā, sthirā, hiṅgu, root of *kebuka, yamānī, dhānya, citraka, sauvarcala, ajājī* and *havuṣā*—all these drugs should be made to a powder. To this powder, equal quantities of oil, ghee and honey should be added. All these should be mixed with sixteen parts of *śaktu* (roasted corn flour) and adequate quantity of water. Administration of this refreshing drink (*santarpaṇa*) cures diseases caused by excessive nourishment, *prameha* (obstinate urinary disorders including diabetes), *mūḍha vāta, kuṣṭha* (obstinate skin diseases including leprosy), piles, jaundice, splenic disorder, anemia, oedema, dysuria, anorexia, heart disease, tuberculosis, cough, dyspnoea, obstruction in throat, parasitic infestation, *grahaṇī doṣa* (sprue syndrome), feeling cold in the body and excessive obesity. It promotes the digestive power, memory as well as intellects of human beings.

बदरीपत्रकल्केन पेया काञ्जिकसाधिता ।
स्थौल्यनुत्स्यात्साग्निमन्थरसं वापि शिलाजतु ॥२३॥

Peyā (thin gruel) cooked with the paste of the leaves of *badarī* and *kāñji* (a type of vinegar) cures obesity. Similarly, the juice of *agni mantha* and *śilā jatu* cures obesity.

अमृतात्रुटिबिल्ववत्सकं[1] कलिङ्गपथ्यामलकानि गुग्गुलुः ।
क्रमवृद्धमिदं मधुप्लुतं पिडकास्थौल्यभगन्दरं जयेत् ॥२४॥

॥ अमृताद्यो गुग्गुलुः ॥

Amṛtādya Guggulu

Amṛtā (one part), *truṭi* (two parts), *bilva* (three parts), *vatsaka* (four parts), *kaliṅga* (five parts), *pathyā* (six parts), *āmalakī* (seven parts) and *guggulu* (eight parts) should be triturated. Intake of this with honey cures carbuncles, obesity and anal fistula.

व्योषाग्नित्रिफलामुस्ताविडङ्गैर्गुग्गुलुं समम् ।
खादन्सर्वाञ्जयेद् व्याधीन् मेदःश्लेष्मामवातजान्[2] ॥२५॥

॥ नवकगुग्गुलुः[3] ॥

Navaka Guggulu

One part of each of *trikaṭu*, *triphalā* and *trimada* and nine parts of *guggulu* should be triturated. Intake of this potion. cures diseases caused by obesity, *kapha* and *āma vāta* (rheumatism).

"गुग्गुलुस्तालमूली च त्रिफला खदिरं वृषम् ।
त्रिवृतालम्बुषा चैव निर्गुण्डी चित्रकं स्नुही ॥२६॥
एषां दशपलान् भागान् तोये पञ्चाढके पचेत् ।
पादशेषं ततः कृत्वा कषायमवतारयेत् ॥२७॥

---

1. ०वेल्लवत्सकं इति आकरे पाठः ।
2. ०वातजित् इति षष्ठपुस्तके पाठः ।
3. नककार्षिकं इति पंचमपुस्तके पाठः ।

पलं द्वादशकं देयं तीक्ष्णलोहस्य चूर्णितम् ।
पचेत्ताम्रमये पात्रे सुशीते चावतारिते ॥२८॥
प्रस्थार्द्धं माक्षिकं देयं शिलाजतु पलद्वयम् ।
एलत्वचः[1] पलार्द्धञ्च विडङ्गानि पलद्वयम् ॥२९॥
मरिचञ्चाञ्जनं कृष्णा द्विपलं त्रिफलान्वितम् ।
पलद्वयन्तु काशीशं श्लक्ष्णचूर्णीकृतं बुधैः ॥३०॥
चूर्णं कृत्वा[2] सुमथितं स्निग्धे भाण्डे निधापयेत् ।
ततः संशुद्धदेहस्तु भक्षयेदक्षमात्रकम्[3] ॥३१॥
अनुपानं पिबेत् क्षीरं जाङ्गलानां रसस्तथा ।
वातश्लेष्महरं श्रेष्ठं कुष्ठमेहोदरापहम्[4] ॥३२॥
कामलां पाण्डुरोगञ्च श्वयथुं सभगन्दरम् ।
मूर्छामोहविषोन्मादं गराणि विविधानि च ॥३३॥
स्थूलानां कर्षणं श्रेष्ठं मेदुरे[5] परमौषधम् ।
कर्षयेच्चतिमात्रेण कुक्षिं पातालसन्निभम् ॥३४॥
बल्यं रसायनं मेध्यं बाजीकरणमुत्तमम् ।
श्रीकरं प्रीतिजननं[6] वलीपलितनाशनम् ॥३५॥

---

1. एलात्वचो इति आकरे पाठः ।
2. दत्वाथमथितं इति आकरे पाठः ।
3. भक्षयेन्माषमात्रकम् इति आकरे पाठः ।
4. कुष्ठमेहज्वरापहम् इति आकरे पाठः ।
5. मेदुरोगे इति पंचमपुस्तके पाठः ।
6. पुत्रजननं इति आकरे पाठः ।

नाश्नीयात् कदलीं कन्दं[1] काञ्जिकं करमर्दकम्[2] ।
करीरं कारवेल्लञ्च षट ककारादिन्[3] विवर्जयेत्[4] ॥३६॥'

॥ लोहरसायनम् ॥"

[भैषज्यरत्नावली : स्थौल्याधिकार : १-२५]

Loha Rasāyana

Guggulu, *tāla mūlī*, *triphalā*, *khadira*, *vṛṣa*, *trivṛt*, *alambuṣā*, *nirguṇḍī*, *citraka* and *snūhī*—all these drugs should be taken ten *palas* each and boiled in five *ādhakas* of water till one fourth remains. In a copper vessel, this decoction should be further cooked by adding twelve *palas* of *tīkṣṇa lauha bhasma*. It should then be removed from the oven and after it is cooled down, half *prastha* of honey, two *palas* of *śilā jatu*, half *palas* of each of *elā* and *tvak*, two *palas* of each of *viḍaṅga*, *marica*, *añjana*, *kṛṣṇā*, *triphalā* and *kāśīśa bhasma* should be added to it and made to a fine powder. This should be kept in a jar smeared with ghee. The patient, having his body cleansed, should take this potion in a dose of one *akṣa* along with the *anupāna* (post-prandial drink) of milk and soup of animals inhabiting arid land. It alleviates *vāyu* as well as *kapha* and cures *kuṣṭha* (obstinate skin diseases including leprosy), *meha* (obstinate urinary disorders including diabetes), *udara* (obstinate abdominal diseases including ascites), jaundice, anemia, oedema, anal fistula, fainting, unconsciousness, poisoning, insanity and poisoning by artificially prepared things (*gara viṣa*). It is an excellent recipe for reducing obesity and diseases caused by excessive fat in the

---

1. कदलीस्कंदं इति प्रथमपुस्तके पाठः ।
2. करमर्दनम् इति प्रथमपुस्तके पाठः ।
3. ककाराणि इति आदर्शपुस्तकेषु पाठः ।
4. त्र्युषणादिमिदं लोहं रसायनमुत्तमम् पाठोऽयं षष्ठपुस्तके अधिकमुपलभ्यते ।

body. It exceedingly reduces the bulged abdomen. It promotes strength, rejuvenation, intellect and virility. It endows auspiciousness, as well as love and removes wrinkles as well as gray hair from the body. While taking this recipe, the patient should avoid six things that begin with the Sanskrit alphabet '*ka*' like *kadalī*, *kanda*, *kāñjī* (a type of vinegar), *kara mardaka*, *karīra* and *kāra vellaka*.

"त्रिफलातिविषामूर्वात्रिवृच्चित्रकवासकैः[1] ।
निम्बारग्वधषड्ग्रन्थासप्तपर्णनिशाद्वयैः ॥३७॥
गुडूचीन्द्रसुरीकृष्णाकुष्ठसर्षपनागरैः[2] ।
तैलमेभिः समैः पक्वं सुरसादिरसाप्लुतम् ॥३८॥
पानाभ्यञ्जनगण्डूषनस्यवस्तिषु योजितम् ।
स्थूलतालस्यकण्ड्वादीन्[3] जयेत्कफकृतान् गदान् ॥३९॥"

॥ त्रिफलाद्यं तैलम्[4] ॥

Triphalādya Taila

Oil should be cooked with the paste of *triphalā*, *ativiṣā*, *mūrvā*, *trivṛt*, *citraka*, *vāsaka*, *nimba*, *āragvadha*, *ṣaḍgranthā*,

---

1. सूतः सतारः सरविः सवोलः । सूर्याबुघृष्टोऽस्य त्र वल्लषट्कान्क्षौद्रेणहंत्युद्ध तमेदुरत्वं मध्ववुतस्यानुपिवेत्पिपासाम् । ॥ वडवाग्निरसः ॥ पाठोऽयं चतुर्थपुस्तके अधिकमुपलभ्यते ।
2. क. सुरा इति प्रथमपुस्तके पाठः ।
   ख. मुरो इति षष्ठपुस्तके पाठः ।
3. शूलता० इति षष्ठपुस्तके पाठः ।
4. क. त्रिकतैलाद्यं इति षष्ठपुस्तके पाठः ।
   ख. त्रिफलादितैलम् इति पंचमपुस्तके पाठः ।

sapta parṇa, niśā, dāru niśā. gudūcī. indra surī, kṛṣṇā, kuṣṭha, sarṣapa and *nāgara*—all these drugs taken in equal quantities and with the juice or decoction of drugs belonging to *surasādi gaṇa*. This medicated oil should be used in drinks, massage, gargle, inhalation therapy and *uttara basti* (medicated douche administered through the genital tract). It cures obesity indolence, itching, etc., and diseases caused by *kapha*.

"शिरीषलामज्जकहेमलोध्रैस्त्वग्दोष[1]संस्वेदहरः प्रघर्षः[2] ।
पत्राम्बु[3]लोहाभयाचन्दनानि शरीरदौर्गन्ध्यहरः प्रदेहः[4] ॥४०॥

The patient suffering from skin diseases and excess of sweating should use over his body, the unction prepared of the powder of *śirīṣa, lāmajjaka, hema* (*nāga kesara*) and *lodhra*. He should also use the *pradeha* (thick ointment) of *patra, ambu, lauha bhasma, abhayā* and *candana*.

वासादलरसो लेपात्[5] शङ्खचूर्णेन संयुतः ।
बिल्वपत्ररसो वापि गात्रदौर्गन्ध्यनाशनः[6] ॥४१॥

Application of the ointment of *śaṅkha bhasma* and the juice of *vāsaka* leaves or the juice of *bilva* leaves removes foul smell of the body.

हरीतकी लोध्रमरिष्टपत्रं त्रिवृत्त्वचो[7] दाडिमवल्कलं च ।
एषो[8]ऽङ्गरागः कथितोऽङ्गनानां जङ्घाकषायश्च नराधिपाणाम् ॥४२॥

1. ०द्दोष० इति आकरे पाठः ।
2. प्रहर्षः इति षष्ठपुस्तके पाठः ।
3. पत्राम्ल० इति प्रथमपंचमपुस्तकयोः पाठः ।
4. प्रघर्षः इति आदर्शपुस्तकेषु पाठः ।
5. लेपां इति चतुर्थषष्ठपुस्तकयोः पाठः ।
6. ०नाशनम् इति षष्ठपुस्तके पाठः ।
7. चूतत्वचो इति आकरे पाठः ।
8. एषे० इति प्रथमपुस्तके पाठः ।

गोमूत्रपिष्टं विनिहन्ति कुष्ठं वर्णोज्ज्वलं[1] गोपयसा च युक्तम् ।
कक्षादिदौर्गन्ध्यहरं पयोभिः शस्तं वशीकृद्रजनीद्वयेन ॥४३॥

The paste of *harītakī*, *lodhra*, leaves of *ariṣṭa* and the bark of *trivṛt* as well as *dāḍima* should be used as a cosmetic over the thighs of ladies and kings which reduces the accumulated fat in this part. If the above mentioned drugs are made to a paste by adding cow's urine, then it cures *kuṣṭha* (obstinate skin diseases including leprosy). If the paste is prepared by adding cow's milk, then it promotes complexion. If the paste is prepared by adding water, then it removes foul smell from axilla, etc. It becomes more effective, if *niśā* and *dāru niśā* are added to the paste.

चिञ्चापत्रस्वरसम्रक्षितकल्कादियोजितं जयति ।
मुण्डरीदुग्धहरिद्रोद्वर्त्तनमचिराद्देहस्य[2] दौर्गन्ध्यम् ॥४४॥

The paste of *haridrā* added with the milky latex of *muṇḍirī* and the juice or paste of the leaves of *ciñcā* should be used as unction (*udvartana*) all over the body. It instantaneously removes the foul smell of the body.

जलदलजलमलयाभयलेपतो हरति देहदौर्गन्ध्यम् ।
विमलारनालसहितं पीतमिवालम्बुषाचूर्णम् ॥४५॥"

[भैषज्यरत्नावली : स्थौल्याधिकार : २८-३६]

हस्तपादश्रुतौ योज्यो गुग्गुलुः पञ्चतिक्तकः ।
अशक्तौ पञ्चतिक्ताख्यं घृतं खादेदतान्द्रतः ॥४६॥

1. ०क्कलं इति षष्ठपुस्तके पाठः ।
2. ०दग्धहरिद्रो० इति आदर्शपुस्तकेषु पाठः ।

Application of the paste of *jalada lajala* (*lajjālu*), *malaya* (*candana*) and *abhayā* removes foul smell of the body. Intake of the powder of *alambuṣā* along with pure *āranāla* (a type of vinegar) also removes foul smell of the body

इति श्रीमहाराजाधिराजटोडरमल्लविरचिते टोडरानन्दे आयुर्वेदसौख्ये मेदोनिदानचिकित्साकथनं नाम पंचचत्वारिंशत्तमो हर्षः ॥४७॥

Thus, ends the 45th Chapter, dealing with the diagnosis and treatment of obesity in the *Āyurveda saukhya* of *Ṭoḍarānanda* composed by the great king Ṭoḍara Malla.

CHAPTER XI

अथ कृशरोगनिदानं चिकित्सा च ।

Diagnosis and Treatment of Kṛśa Roga (Excessive Emaciation)

"सेवा[1] रूक्षान्नपानानां लङ्घनं प्रमिताशनम् ।
क्रियातियोगः[2] शोकश्च वेगनिद्राविनिग्रहः ॥१॥
रूक्षस्योद्वर्तनं स्नानस्याभ्यासः प्रकृतिर्ज्जरा ।
विकारानुशयः क्रोधः कुर्वन्त्यतिकृशं नरम् ॥२॥

---

1. This is the beginning of the 50th Chapter of *Āyurveda saukhya* in *Ṭoḍarānanda* and the invocation reads as follows :—
यंवल्लवी वृंदमपृच्छदातुरं सुशाखिल्ली सुमनांसिनिर्गतम् ।
प्राणप्रियं टोडरमल्ल भूमिपं कृष्णोपरोक्षोविदधातु मंगलम् ॥
2. कृयाति इति प्रथमपंचमपुस्तकयोः पाठः ।

Etiology

Intake of ununctuous diet and drinks, fasting, intake of food in small quantity, excessive administration of purificatory therapies, worry, suppression of natural urges, suppression of sleep, unction of ununctuous drugs, more of bath, natural old age, suffering continuously of diseases and anger make the person excessively emaciated.

व्यायाममतिसौहित्यं क्षुत्पिपासामयौषधम् ।
कृशो न सहते तद्वदतिशीतोष्णमैथुनम् ॥३॥

Signs and Symptoms

An emaciated person cannot tolerate exercise, excessive intake of food, hunger, thirst, invasion of any disease, administration of any strong medicine, excessive cold, excessive heat and excessive sexual intercourse.

प्लीहा कासः क्षयः श्वासो गुल्ममेहोदराणि[1] च ।
कृशं प्रायोऽभिधावन्ति रोगाश्च ग्रहणीगताः ॥४॥

Susceptibility to Diseases

An emaciated person is susceptible to diseases like splenic disorder, cough, consumption, asthma, *gulma* (phantom tumour), *meha* (obstinate urinary disorders including diabetes), *udara* (obstinate abdominal diseases including ascites) and diseases afflicting *grahaṇī* (small intestine including duodenum).

शुष्कस्फिगुदरग्रीवो धमनीजालसंततिः[2] ।
त्वगस्थिशेषोऽतिकृशः स्थूलपर्वा नरो मतः ॥५॥"

[चरक : सूत्र २१ : ११-१५]

1. गुल्मोऽर्शांस्युदराणि इति भ्राकरे पाठः ।
2. धमनीजालसन्ततः इति भ्राकरे पाठः ।

Description of the Patient

An excessively emaciated person is characterised by emaciation of buttocks, abdomen and neck, having a vascular net work over the body, the body having only skin and bone and prominence of joints specially those of the fingers.

स्वेदक्षयाद्भवेद्ग्रीष्मे सदा सक्षीरभोजनम् ।
मेदःसिद्धानि मांसानि ग्राम्यानूपौदकानि च ॥
मेदःक्षीणाः कांक्षन्ते[1] च निर्वातशयनं सदा ॥६॥

Emaciated persons desire always to take milk with food in summer because of excessive sweating. In other seasons they desire to eat meat of domesticated, marshy and aquatic animals cooked with oil or ghee. They like to sleep in a house free from wind.

यथा पिपीलिका स्वल्पा[2] यथा वा वरटी बलाः ।
स्वतश्चतुर्गुणं[3] भारं नीत्वा[4] गच्छति संसुखम्[5] ॥७॥

---

1. कांछते इति प्रथमपुस्तके पाठः ।
2. स्वल्या इति प्रथमपुस्तके पाठः ।
3. तश्चतुर्गुणं इति प्रथमपुस्तके पाठः ।
4. नीतं चतुर्थपुस्तके पाठः ।
5. क. सत्सुखम् प्रथमपुस्तके पाठः ।
   ख. तत्सुखम् इति चतुर्थषष्ठपुस्तकयोः पाठः ।

तथातपाध्वव्यायामैः प्रकृत्या क्षीणमानवः ।
पीड्यते व्यसनैः[1] भारै[2] स्त्रीगतैश्च सुखं तथा ।
[3]'स्वभावदुर्बले देहे भेषजं नैव कारयेत्' ॥८॥

॥ इति कृशनिदानम् ॥६॥

Naturally Emaciated Persons

As an ant or *varaṭi* can carry weight four times of its own and move easily with this weight, similarly, persons who are naturally emaciated because of exposure to hot sun, long walk and exercise can easily stand hardships and sexual intercourse. These naturally emaciated persons should not be treated with medicines.

Thus, ends the description of diagnosis of emaciation.

"स्वप्नो हर्षः सुखा शय्या मनसो निर्वृतिः समः ।
चिन्ताव्यवायव्यायामविरतिः प्रियदर्शनम् ॥१०॥
नवान्नानि नवं मद्यं ग्राम्यानूपौदका रसाः ।
संस्कृतानि च मांसानि दधि सर्पिः पयांसि च ॥११॥
[4]इक्षव शालयो माषा गोधूमा गुडवैकृतम् ।
बस्तयः स्निग्धमधुरास्तैलाभ्यङ्गश्च[5] सर्वदा ॥१२॥

---

1. व्यसनैः शूरैः स्त्रीगतैश्च इति षष्ठपुस्तके पाठः ।
2. भारैस्त्रीगतेश्च इति प्रथमपुस्तके पाठः ।
3. 'स्वभाव——कारयेत्' । पाठोऽयं चतुर्थषष्ठपुस्तकयोः नोपलभ्यते ।
4. एक्षवः इति षष्ठपुस्तके पाठः ।
5. ०भ्यङ्गाश्च सर्वशः इति आदर्शपुस्तकेषु पाठः ।

'स्निग्धमुद्वर्तनं[1] स्नानं गंधमाल्यनिषेवणम् ।
शुक्लवासो यथाकालं दोषाणामवसेचनम् ॥१३॥'
रसायनानां वृष्याणां योगानां चोपसेवनम्[2] ।
हत्वाभिकार्श्यमाधत्ते नृणामुपचयम् परम् ॥१४॥
अचिन्तनाच्च कार्याणां ध्रुवं सन्तर्पणेन च ।
स्वप्नप्रसङ्गाच्च[3] नरो वराह इव पुष्यति ॥
'क्षयरोगोक्तमखिलां क्रियां कुर्यात् भिषक्तमः[4]' ॥१५॥"
॥ अग्निवेश[5] ॥

[चरक : सूत्र २१ : २९-३४]

According to Agniveśa

Sleep, happiness, comfortable bed, non-attachment, equanimity, absence of worry, sexual intercourse as well as physical exertion, pleasant sight-seeing, freshly harvested cereals and pulses, freshly prepared wine, soup of the meat of domesticated, marshy and aquatic animals, meat cooked with oil and ghee, curd, ghee, milk preparations, preparations of sugar cane juice, *śāli* rice, *māṣa*, wheat, jaggery preparations, medicated enema prepared of unctuous and sweet drugs, habitual oil massage, unctuous unction, bath, application of perfumes, wearing garlands, white cloth, elimination of *doṣas* in appropri-

---

1. 'स्निग्ध——सेचनम्' पाठोऽयं षष्ठपुस्तके नोपलभ्यते ।
2. योगानामुपसेवनम् इति आकरे पाठः ।
3. स्वप्नसंस्वरो वराह इति प्रथमपुस्तके पाठः ।
4. 'क्षय——भिषक्तमः' पाठोऽयं आकरे नोपलभ्यते ।
5. पाठोऽयं प्रथमपुस्तके नोपलभ्यते ।

ate time and intake of rejuvenating as well as aphrodisiac recipes corrects emaciation and promotes plumpness of the body. Absence of worry about work, intake of nourishing therapies and the habit of continuous sleep for a long time make a person plumpy like a boar. To a patient suffering from emaciation, all the therapies prescribed for the treatment of *kṣaya* (consumption) should be administered.

अग्निवेशः—

सद्यः क्षीणो हि सद्यो वै तर्पणेनोपचीयते ।
नित्यसंतर्पणाभ्यासाच्चिरक्षीणस्तु पुष्यति ॥१६॥

According to Agniveśa

If a person has become suddenly emaciated, then he will instantaneously recover from it and become plumpy by the administration of nourishing therapies. Habitual use of nourishing therapies makes even a chronic emaciated person plumpy.

देहाग्निदोषभैषज्यमात्राकालानुवर्त्तिना[1] ।
कार्यं [2]सत्वरमानेन भेषजं चिरदुर्बलैः[3] ॥१७॥

Keeping in view the nature of the body, digestive power, condition of *doṣas* and the dose as well as the time of administration of drugs, the patient, who is emaciated since a long time, should take medicine without any delay.

[4]'अश्वगन्धातिबलानागबलामाषगुडयवाः ।
बलं कुर्वन्ति भुक्तं मत्तवारणवारणानाम्' ॥१८॥

---

1. ०वर्त्तिनम् इति षष्ठपुस्तके पाठः ।
2. कार्यमत्वरमाने इति प्रथमपुस्तके पाठः ।
3. चिरदुर्बले इति पंचमपुस्तके पाठः ।
4. 'अश्वगन्धाति——वारणाम्' पाठोऽयं पंचमपुस्तके अधिकमुपलभ्यते ।

Intake of *aśvagandhā*, *atibalā*, *nāga balā*, *māṣa*, jaggery and barley produces strength of a rogue elephant.

इति श्रीमहाराजाधिराजटोडरमल्लविरचिते टोडरानंदे आयुर्वेदसौख्ये कृशरोगनिदानचिकित्साकथनं नाम षट्चत्वारिंशत्तमो हर्षः ॥१६॥

Thus, ends the 46th Chapter dealing with the diagnosis and treatment of emaciation in the *Āyurveda saukhya* of *Ṭoḍarānanda* composed by the great king Ṭoḍara Malla.

CHAPTER XII

अथ उदरनिदानं चिकित्सा च ।

Diagnosis and Treatment of Udara (Obstinate Abdominal Diseases including Ascites)

"[1]रोगाः सर्वेऽपि मन्देऽग्नौ सुतरामुदराणि च ।

अजीर्णान्मलिनैश्चान्नैर्जायन्ते मलसंचयात् ॥१॥

Etiology

Mandāgni (suppression of the power of digestion and metabolism) is the cause of the manifestation of all diseases.

---

1. This is the beginning of 51st Chapter of *Āyurveda saukhya* in *Ṭoḍarānanda* and the invocation reads as follows:—
   तरंगिणी तीरगताः प्रशक्ताज गूरमेश जगतां निधानम् ।
   गोपांगनायं सनिधिं विदध्याद् दामोदरष्टोडरमल्लभूपे ॥

Therefore, various types of *udara roga* are manifested by th accumulation of waste products as a result of indigestion an intake of polluted food.

रुध्वा स्वेदाम्बुवाहिनी दोषाः स्रोतांसि संचिताः ।
प्राणाग्न्यपानान् संदूष्य जनयन्त्युदरं नृणाम् ॥२॥"

[माधवनिदान : उदर ३५ : १-२]

Pathogenesis

Aggravated *doṣas* obstruct the channels of circulation of sweat and *ambu* (aqueous elements of the body) and vitiate *prāṇa vāyu, agni* (enzymes responsible for digestion and metabolism) as well as *apāna vāyu* to produce *udara roga*.

"तत्पूर्वरूपं बलवर्णकाङ्क्षा वलीविनाशो जठरे व[1] राज्यः ।
जीर्णापरिज्ञानविदाहवत्यो बस्तौ रुजः पादगतश्च शोफः ॥३॥"

[सुश्रुत : निदान ७ : ७-८]

Premonitory Signs and Symptoms

Diminution of strength and complexion, disappearance of wrinkles, appearance of vascular net work over the abdomen, uncertainty about digestion of food, burning sensation in the abdomen and chest, pain in the region of urinary bladder and oedema in feet—these are the premonitory signs and symptoms of *udara roga*.

अतिसंचितदोषाणां म[2]लिनान्ननिषेविणाम् ।
उदराण्युपजायन्ते मंदाग्नीनां विशेषतः ॥४॥

1. हि इति आकरे पाठः ।
2. मनिलान्न० इति आदर्शपुस्तकेषु पाठः ।

By the intake of polluted food, *doṣas* get excessively accumulated to cause various types of *udara roga* specially in those persons whose power of digestion is suppressed (*mandāgni*).

"आध्मानं गमनेऽशक्तिर्दौर्बल्यं दुर्बलाग्निता ।
शोथः सदनमङ्गानां सङ्गो वातपुरीषयोः ॥
दाहस्तन्द्रा च[1] सर्वेषु जठरेषु भवन्ति हि ॥५॥

Common Signs and Symptoms

Ādhmāna (abdominal distension), inability to walk, weakness, weak digestive power, oedema, prostration in the limbs, obstruction to the passage of flatus and stool, burning sensation and drowsiness—these signs and symptoms are commonly manifested in all types of *udara roga*.

पृथग्दोषैः समस्तैश्च प्लीहबद्धक्षतोदकैः ।
संभवन्त्युदराण्यष्टौ तेषां लिङ्गं पृथक् शृणु ॥६॥

Varieties

Udara roga is of eight types, viz. *vātika*, *paittika*, *kaphaja*, *sānnipātika*, *plīhodara*, *baddhodara*, *kṣatodara* and *udakodara*. Signs and symptoms of each of these varieties are described below.

'तत्र वातोदरे शोफः पाणिपान्नाभिकुक्षिषु ।
कुक्षिपार्श्वोदरकटीपृष्ठरुक् पर्वभेदनम् ॥७॥
शुष्ककासोऽङ्गमर्दोऽधोगुरुता मलसंग्रहः ।
श्यावारुणत्वगादित्वमकस्माद् वृद्धिह्रासवत् ॥८॥

1. व इति प्रथमपुस्तके पाठः ।

सतोदभेदमुदरं तनुकृष्णसिराततम् ।
आध्मातदृतिवच्छब्दमाहतं[1] प्रकरोति च ॥
वायुश्चात्र सरुक्शब्दो विचरेत्सर्वतो गतिः ॥९॥

Vātodara

Following are the signs and symptoms of *vātodara* :

1. Oedema in hands, legs, umbilicus and sides of the abdomen ;
2. Pain in the sides of the abdomen, sides of the chest, abdomen, lumber region and back ;
3. Cracking pain in the finger joints ;
4. Dry cough, malaise, heaviness in the lower abdomen and accumulation of waste products ;
5. Grayish and reddish colouration of the skin, etc., and sudden increase as well as decrease of these colours ;
6. Stabbing and cracking types of pain in the abdomen ;
7. Appearance of thin and black vessels all over the abdo men ;
8. In percussion, resonant sound comes out of the abdomen as if it is done over a distended leather blower ; and
9. Movement of *vāyu* all over the abdomen with pain and gurgling sound.

पित्तोदरे ज्वरो मूर्च्छा दाहस्तृट्[2] कटुकास्यता ।
भ्रमोऽतिसारः पीतत्वं त्वगादाबुदरं हरित् ॥१०॥
पीतताम्रसिरानद्धं सस्वेदं सोष्मदह्यते ।
धूमायते मृदुस्पर्शं क्षिप्रपाकं प्रदूयते ॥११॥

---

1. आध्मानं हृति० इति प्रथमपंचमपुस्तकयोः पाठः ।
2. दाहस्त्रिक्कटुकास्यता इति प्रथमपंचमपुस्तकयोः पाठः ।

Pittodara

Following are the signs and symptoms of *pittodara* :

1. Fever, fainting, burning sensation, thirst, pungent taste in the mouth, giddiness and diarrhoea ;
2. Yellow colour of the skin all over the body and green colour of the skin over the abdomen ;
3. Appearance of yellow and copper-coloured vessels all over the abdomen ;
4. Sweating and heating sensation ;
5. A feeling as if smoke is coming out of the abdomen ;
6. The abdomen is soft to touch ;
7. It gets quickly suppurated ; and
8. Feeling of discomfort over the abdomen.

श्लेष्मोदरेऽङ्गसदनं स्वापश्वयथुगौरवम्[1] ।
निद्रोत्क्लेशोऽरुचिः श्वासः कास शुक्लत्वगादिता ॥१२॥
उदरं स्तिमितं स्निग्धं[2] शुक्लराजीततं महत् ।
चिराभिवृद्धि कठिनं शीतस्पर्शं गुरु स्थिरम् ॥१३॥'

[अष्टाङ्गहृदय : निदान १२ : १२-१६]

Kaphodara

Following are the signs and symptoms of *kaphodara* :

1. Prostration in limbs, numbness, oedema, heaviness, excessive sleep, nausea, anorexia, dyspnoea, cough and pale white colour of the skin, etc. ;

1. स्वासः स्वयथुगौरवम् इति प्रथमपंचमपुस्तकयोः पाठः ।
2. श्लक्ष्णं इति आकरे पाठः ।

2. Abdomen is numb, unctuous and covered with net work of white vessels in excess ; and
3. The abdomen gets enlarged slowly and it is hard, cold to touch, heavy and stable.

स्त्रियोऽन्नपानं नखरोममूत्रविडार्त्तवैर्युक्तमसाधुवृत्ताः ।
यस्मै प्रयच्छन्त्यरयो गरांश्च दुष्टाम्बुदूषीविषसेवनाद् वा ।
तेनाशु रक्तं कुपिताश्च दोषाः कुर्युः सुघोरं जठरं त्रिलिङ्गम् ॥१४॥
तच्छीतवाते भृशदुर्दिने च विशेषतः कुप्यति दह्यते च ।
स चतुरो मूर्च्छति संप्रसक्तं पाण्डुः कृशः शुष्यति तृष्णया च ॥१५॥
दूष्योदरं कीर्तितमेतदेव प्लीहोदरं कीर्तयतो निबोध ॥१६॥

Sānnipātika Udara

Sānnipāka type of *udara roga* is caused by the following factors :

1. Intake of food and drinks mixed with nail, hair, urine, stool and menstrual blood given by ladies of bad character ;
2. Intake of *gara* type poison given by enemies ; or
3. Intake of polluted water or *dūṣī* type of poison.

Because of the above mentioned factors, the vitiated *rakta* (blood) and aggravated *doṣas* produce serious type of *udara roga* in which the above mentioned symptoms of all the three *doṣas* are manifested. This ailment gets aggravated when the patient is exposed to cold wind and in cloudy weather. He gets burning sensation, fainting, anemia, emaciation and dryness as a result of thirst. This is called *dūṣyodara*. Hereafter, *plīhodara* will be described.

विदाह्यभिष्यन्दिरतस्य जन्तोः प्रदुष्टमत्यर्थमसृक् कफश्च ।
प्लीहाभिवृद्धिं कुरुतः प्रवृद्धौ प्लीहोत्थमेतज्जठरं वदन्ति ॥
तद्वामपार्श्वे परिवृद्धिमेति विशेषतः सीदति चातुरोऽत्र ॥१७॥

Plīhodara

In a person, indulging in *vidāhī* (which causes burning sensation) and *abhiṣyandi* (which causes obstruction to the channels of circulation) types of food, *rakta* (blood) and *kapha* get excessively vitiated which cause splenic enlargement. This is called *Plīhodara*. Spleen is located in the left side of the abdomen. Therefore, the left side of the abdomen bulges out. The patient becomes very weak.

'यस्यप्लीहानमुद्धूयक्रूरस्तिष्ठति मारुतः ।
शूलैः परिरुदत्पार्श्वं तस्य प्लीहाभिवर्द्धते ॥१८॥'

If the extremely aggravated *vāyu* afflicts the spleen, then splenic enlargement takes place in association with pain in the left side.

मन्दज्वराग्निः कफपित्तलिङ्गैरुपद्रुतः क्षीणबलोऽतिपाण्डुः ।
सव्यान्यपार्श्वे यकृति प्रदुष्टे ज्ञेयं यकृद्दाल्युदरं तदेव ॥१९॥
उदावर्त्तरुजानाहैर्मोहतृट्[1]दहनज्वरैः ।
गौरवारुचिकाठिन्यैर्विद्यात्तत्र मलान् क्रमात् ॥२०॥

Yakṛddālyudara

If the liver located in right side is afflicted, if there is mild fever, if the power of digestion is sluggish, if signs and symptoms of aggravated *kapha* and *pitta* are manifested and if there is diminution of strength as well as anemia, then the condition is called *yakṛddālyudara*. *Udāvarta* (upward movement of wind), pain, abdominal distension, unconsciousness, thirst, burning sensation, fever, heaviness, anorexia and hardness—these signs and symptoms of *doṣas* are manifested in *yakṛddālyudara*.

1. तृड् इति आकरे पाठः ।

यस्यान्त्रमन्नैरुपलेपिभिर्वा बालाश्मभिर्वा पिहितं यथावत् ।
संचीयते तस्य मलः सदोषः शनैः शनैः संकरवच्च नाड्याम् ॥२१॥
निरुध्यते तस्य गुदे पुरीषं
निरेति कृच्छ्रादपि चाल्पमल्पम् ।
हृन्नाभिमध्ये परिवृद्धिमेति
तस्योदरं बद्धगुदं वदन्ति ॥२२॥

Baddha Gudodara

If the intestines of a person get obstructed by the intake of sticky material, hair or stone, then waste products along with *doṣas* get gradually accumulated in it as waste products get accumulated in the tube used in *śaṅkara sveda* (a type of fomentation by medicated steam). There is obstruction to the passage of stool in the rectum. The patient voids stool with difficulty and in small quantities. The abdomen between the heart and umbilicus bulges out. This is called *baddha gudodara.*

शल्यं तथाऽन्नोपहितं[1] यदन्त्रं भुक्तं भिनत्त्यागतमन्यथा वा ।
तस्मात्स्रुतोऽन्त्रात्सलिलप्रकाशः[2] स्रावः स्रवेद्वै गुदतस्तु भूयः ॥२३॥
नाभेरधश्चोदरमेति वृद्धिं निस्तुद्यते दाल्यति चातिमात्रम् ।
एतत्परिस्राव्युदरं प्रदिष्टं दकोदरं कीर्तयतो निबोध ॥२४॥

Kṣatodara

If by mistake a patient swallows a sharp edged substance along with food or if there is injury to the intestinal tract from outside, then watery exudation takes place from the intestines

1. ०पहृतं इति प्रथमपुस्तके पाठः ।
2. तस्माच्छ्रुतेन्त्रात्० इति प्रथमपुस्तके पाठः ।

and this watery exudation comes out through the anus. The abdomen below the umbilicus bulges out with excruciating pain and discomfort. This is called *parisrāvyudara. Dakodara* is being described below.

यः स्नेहपीतोऽप्यनुवासितो वा वान्तो विरिक्तोऽप्यथवा निरूढः ।

पिबेज्जलं शीतलमाशु तस्य स्रोतांसि दुष्टयन्ति[1] (हि) तद्वहानि ॥२५॥

स्नेहोपलिप्तेष्वथवाऽपि तेषु दकोदरं पूर्ववदभ्युपैति[2] ।

स्निग्धं महत्तत्परिवृत्तनाभि[3] समाततं पूर्णमिवाम्बुना च ॥

यथा दृतिः क्षुभ्यति कम्पते च शब्दायते चापि दकोदरं तत् ॥२६॥

Dakodara

If a person, after taking oleation therapy, *anuvāsana* type of medicated enema, emetic therapy, purgation therapy or *nirūha* type of medicated enema, drinks cold water immediately, then his *udaka vaha srotas* (channel carrying water) get vitiated. This vitiation of *udaka vaha srotas* can also take place if these channels get smeared with *sneha* (fat). The umbilicus of the patient becomes unctuous, enlarged in size and round in shape. By percussion, there will be resonant sound, irritation and trembling as if it is being done over a leather bag filled with water. This is called *dakodara.*

जन्मनैवोदरं सर्वं प्रायः कष्टतमं मतम् ।

बलिनः[4] तवजाताम्बु यत्नसाध्यं नवोत्थितम् ॥२७॥

---

1. संदुष्ट्य इति षष्ठपुस्तके पाठः ।
2. पूर्ववदत्युपैति इति प्रथमपंचमपुस्तकयोः पाठः ।
3. ०वृत्त० इति आदर्शपुस्तकेषु पाठः ।
4. बलिनस्तद० इति आकरे पाठः ।

Prognosis

All types of *udara roga*, right from the time of their onset are difficult of cure. However, if the patient is strong, if water accumulation has not taken place and if the disease is of recent origin, then the patient is curable with great deal of effort.

पक्षाद्बद्धगुदं तूर्ध्वं[1] सर्वं जातोदकं तथा ।
प्रायो भवन्त्यभावाय छिद्रान्त्रं चोदरं[2] नृणाम् ॥२८॥

The patient of *baddha gudodara* dies in a fortnight. All other varieties of *udara roga* become incurable after a fortnight if water accumulation takes place (*jātodaka*). *Kṣatodara* also leads to the death of the patient.

[3]शूनाक्षं कुटिलोपस्थमुपक्लिन्नतनुत्वचम् ।
बलशोणितमांसाग्निपरिक्षीणं विवर्जयेत्[4] ॥२९॥

The physician should avoid treatment of a patient of *udara roga* if he has oedema over the eyes, if his penis is twisted, if his skin has become very thin as well as sticky, and if he is diminished of strength, blood, muscle tissue and digestive power.

पार्श्वभङ्गान्नविद्वेषशोफा[5]तीसारपीडितम् ।
विरिक्तं चाप्युदरिणं[6] पूर्यमाणं विवर्जयेत् ॥३०॥"

[माधवनिदान : उदररोग ३५ : ३-२८]

॥ उदरनिदानम् ॥३१॥

1. रुद्धं इति प्रथमपुस्तके पाठः ।
2. छिद्रांततूदरं इति प्रथमपंचमपुस्तकयोः पाठः ।
3. सूनाक्षं इति प्रथमचतुर्थषष्ठपुस्तकेषु पाठः ।
4. च वर्जयेत् इति आकरे पाठः ।
5. ०शोथा० इति आकरे पाठः ।
6. चाशुदरिणं इति प्रथमपुस्तके पाठः ।

If the patient is bent to one side, if he dislikes food, if he gets oedema as well as diarrhoea and if his abdomen gets filled up with water after being emptied by purgation therapy, then such a patient should not be treated.

Thus, ends the diagnosis of *udara roga.*

"उदरे दोषसम्पूर्णे कुक्षौ मन्दानलो[1] यतः ।
तस्माद् भोज्यानि योज्यानि दीपनानि लघूनि च ॥३२॥
रक्तशालीन्[2] यवान् मुद्गान् जाङ्गलान् मृगपक्षिणः ।
पयो मूत्रासवारिष्टमधुसीधु[3] तथा पिबेत् ॥३३॥"

[भैषज्यरत्नावली : उदररोगाधिकार : २-३]

Diet and Drinks

In *udara roga*, the abdomen gets completely afflicted with *doṣas* as a result of which the power of digestion gets suppressed. Therefore, in such a condition, food ingredients, which stimulate the power of digestion and which are light for digestion, are given to the patient. The patient should take red variety of rice, barley, *mudga*, meat of animals and birds inhabiting arid land, milk, cow's urine and *āsava, ariṣṭa, madhu* as well as *sīdhu* types of alcoholic drink.

"वातोदरं बलवतः पूर्वं[4] स्नेहैरुपाचरेत् ।
स्निग्धाय स्वेदिताङ्गाय दद्यात् स्नेह[5]विरेचनम् ॥३४॥

1. मन्दो यतोऽनलः इति आकरे पाठः ।
2. क. रक्तशालिर्यवामुद्गाजाङ्गलाश्च रसा हिताः इति प्रथमपंचमपुस्तकयोः पाठः ।
   ख. रक्तशालिगोधूम यवनीवारभोजनम् । मुद्गास्तिक्तकशाकाश्च जांगलाश्च मृगाद्विजाः । इति चतुर्थषष्ठपुस्तकयोः पाठः ।
3. ०शीधु इति आकरे पाठः ।
4. स्नेहस्वेदैरुपाचरेत् इति आकरे पाठः ।
5. स्निग्धं विरेचनम् इति आकरे पाठः ।

हृते दोषे परिम्लानं वेष्टयेद्वाससोदरम् ।
[1] यथास्यानवकाशत्वाद् वायुर्नाध्मापयेत्पुनः ॥३५॥"

[भैषज्यरत्नावली : उदररोगाधिकार : ५-६]

Treatment of Vātodara

A strong patient of *vātodara* should first of all be given oleation and fomentation therapies. Thereafter, purgation therapy containing unctuous drugs should be administered. When the *doṣas* are removed, the abdomen shrinks, and then, it should be tightly wrapped with a piece of cloth so that *vāyu*, finding empty space in abdomen may not cause distension again.

"दोषातिमात्रोपचयात् स्रोतोमार्गनिरोधनात् ।
सम्भवत्युदरं तस्मान्नित्यमेनं विरेचयेत्[2] ॥३६॥"

[भैषज्यरत्नावली : उदररोगाधिकार : ४]

Need for Purgation

Udara rogas are caused by excessive accumulation of *doṣas* and obstruction to the channels of circulation. Therefore, such patients should be given purgation therapy every day.

"विरिक्ते च यथादोषहरैः पेया शृता हिता ॥३७॥

---

1. तथा० इति प्रथमपंचमपुस्तकयोः पाठः ।
2. क. पाययेत्तैलमैरण्डं समूत्रं सपयोऽपि वा । पाठोऽयं आकरे अधिकमुपलभ्यते ।
   ख. क्षारेणैरण्डजं तैलं पिबेन्मूत्रेण वासकृत् । ज्योतिष्मत्याः पिबेत्तैलं पयसा च विरेचनम् । सर्वेभ्यो जठरेभ्यस्तु शीघ्रं मुच्येत मानवः । पाठोऽयं चतुर्थषष्ठपुस्तकयोः अधिकमुपलभ्यते ।

Peyā

After purgation therapy, the patient should be given *peyā* (thin gruel) prepared by boiling with such drugs as would alleviate the concerned aggravated *doṣas*.

वातोदरी पिबेत्तक्रं पिप्पलीलवणान्वितम् ।
शर्करामरिचोपेतं स्वादु पित्तोदरी पिबेत् ॥
यमानीसैन्धवजाजीव्योषयुक्तं कफोदरी ॥३८॥"

[भैषज्यरत्नावली : उदररोगाधिकार : ७-८]

"मधुतैलवचाशुण्ठीशताह्वाकुष्ठसैन्धवैः ।
युक्तं प्लीहोदरी जातं सव्योषन्तूदकोदरी ॥३९॥
बद्धोदरी तु हवुषादीप्यकाजाजिसैन्धवैः ।
पिबेच्छिद्रोदरी तक्रं पिप्पलीक्षौद्रसंयुतम् ॥
त्र्यूषणक्षार[1]लवणैर्युक्तन्तु निचयोदरी ॥४०॥

Administration of Butter-Milk.

The patient of *vātodara* can take butter-milk mixed with *pippalī* and rock-salt. The patient of *pittodara* can take butter-milk added with sugar and *marica*. The patient of *kaphodara* can take butter-milk with *yavānī*, *saindhava*, *ajājī* and *vyoṣa*. The patient of *plīhodara* can take butter-milk added with honey, oil, *vacā*, *śuṇṭhī śatāhvā*, *kuṣṭha* and rock-salt. The patient of *dakodara* should take butter-milk mixed with *vyoṣa*. The patient of *baddhodara* should take butter-milk with *havuṣā*, *dīpyaka*, *ajājī* and rock-salt. The patient of *chidrodara* should take butter-milk mixed with *pippalī* and

---

1. ०क्षारनि० इति प्रथमपुस्तके पाठः ।

honey. The patient of *sānnipātika udara* should take butter-milk mixed with *tryūṣaṇa*, *kṣāra* (alkali preparation) and rock-salt.

गौरवारोचकार्त्तानां समन्दाग्न्यतिसारिणाम् ।
तक्रं वातकफार्त्तानाममृतत्वाय कल्पते ॥४१॥"

[भैषज्यरत्नावली : उदररोगाधिकार : ६-११]

Butter-Milk in Other Diseases

Butter-milk works as ambrosia (*amṛta*) in patients suffering from heaviness, anorexia, suppressed power of digestion, diarrhoea and diseases caused by *vāyu* as well as *kapha*.

वातोदरे पयोभ्यासो निरूहो दशमूलकः ।
सोदावर्त्ते वातघ्नाम्लशृतैरण्डानुवासनः ॥४२॥

Medicated Enema

In *vātodara*, habitual intake of milk and administration of *nirūha* type of medicated enema with the decoction of *daśa mūla* are useful. If the disease is associated with *udāvarta* (upward movement of wind) then *anuvāsana* type of medicated enema prepared of *eraṇḍa* boiled with *vāyu*-alleviating and sour drugs is useful.

"सामुद्रसौवर्चलसैन्धवानि क्षारं यवानीमजमोदकञ्च[1] ।
सपिप्पली चित्रकशृंगवेरं हिङ्गु विडञ्चेति समानि कुर्यात् ॥४३॥

1. सैन्धवाना क्षारोषणानामजमोदकं च इति षष्ठपुस्तके पाठः ।

एतानि चूर्णानि घृतप्लुतानि भुञ्जीत पूर्वं कवलं प्रशस्तम् ।
वातोदरं गुल्ममजीर्णभक्तं
वायुप्रकोपं ग्रहणीं प्रदुष्यम् ।
अर्शांसि दुष्टानि च पाण्डुरोगं
भगन्दरं चापि[1] निहन्ति सद्यः ॥४४॥"

॥ सामुद्राद्यं चूर्णम् ॥

[भैषज्यरत्नावली : उदररोगाधिकार : १४-१६]

Sāmudrādya Cūrṇa

Sāmudra lavaṇa, *sauvarcala lavaṇa*, *saindhava lavaṇa*, *kṣāra* (*yava kṣāra*), *yavānī*, *ajamodā*, *pippalī*, *citraka*, *śṛṅgavera*, *hiṅgu* and *viḍa lavaṇa*– all these drugs should be taken in equal quantities. To this, the powder of *elā* and ghee should be added and taken along with the first morsel of food. This instantaneously cures *vātodara*, *gulma* (phantom tumour), indigestion of food, aggravation of *vāyu*, *grahaṇī* (sprue syndrome), serious type of piles, anemia and anal fistula.

रोहितकत्वक्त्रिफलाद्रवन्तीदन्तीकषायसकटु[2]त्रिकश्च ।
[3]सयावशूकः सकलोदरघ्नः स्नुक्पिप्पली वा सकलोदरघ्नी ॥४५॥

The decoction of the bark of *rohitaka*, *triphalā*, *dravantī* and *dantī* should be taken along with *trikaṭu* and *yava kṣāra* which cures all types of *udara rogas*.

---

1. चेति इति आदर्शपुस्तकेषु पाठः ।
2. ०सकथुजिकश्च इति प्रथमपुस्तके पाठः ।
3. सपावशूकः इति प्रथमपुस्तके पाठः ।

"पित्तोदरेषु[1] बलिनं पूर्वमेव विरेचयेत् ।
अनुवास्याबलं क्षीणं[2] बस्तिशुद्धं विरेचयेत् ॥४६॥

Treatment of Pittodara

A strong patient of *pittodara* should be given purgation therapy in the beginning. If the patient is weak, then in the beginning, he should be given *anuvāsana* type of medicated enema, and after his body is cleansed, he should be given purgation therapy.

पयसा सत्रिवृत्कल्केनोरुबूकशृतेन वा ।
सातला[3]त्रायमाणाक्षं शृतेनारग्वधेन वा ॥४७॥

Purgation Therapy

For the purpose of purgation the following recipes should be used :

1. Paste of *trivṛt* with milk ;
2. Milk boiled with *urubūka* ;
3. Milk boiled with *śātalā* and *trāyamāṇā.* ; and
4. Milk boiled with *āragvadha.*

कफादुदरिणं शुद्धं कटुक्षारान्नभोजिनम्[4] ।
मूत्रारिष्टायस्कृतिभिर्योजयेच्च कफापहैः[5] ॥४८॥

---

1. ०तु इति प्रथमपञ्चमपुस्तकयोः पाठः ।
2. क्षीरबस्तिशुद्धं इति आकरे पाठः ।
3. शातलात्रायमाणाभ्यां श्रृतमारग्वधेन इति आकरे पाठः ।
4. क. ०मोजितम् इति प्रथमपंचमपुस्तकयोः पाठः ।
   ख. ०योजितम् इति षष्ठपुस्तके पाठः ।
5. कफापह इति आकरे पाठः ।

Treatment of Kaphodara

The patient of *kaphodara* should be given purgation therapy to cleanse his body, and thereafter, along with food mixed with pungent drug and *kṣāra* (alkali preparation), he should be given cow's urine, *ariṣṭa* (a type of alcoholic preparation) and *ayaskṛti* (specially processed iron) for the alleviation of *kapha*.

सन्निपातोदरे सर्वा यथोक्ताः कारयेत्क्रियाः ॥४६॥

Treatment of Sannipātodara

In the treatment of *sannipātodara*, all therapies described above should be employed.

प्लीहोदरे प्लीहहरं कर्मोदरहरं[1] तथा ॥५०॥

Treatment of Plīhodara

In *plīhodara*, the patient should be administered therapies which cure splenic disorder and which cure *udara roga* simultaneously.

स्विन्नाय बद्धोदरिणे मूत्रतीक्ष्णौषधान्वितम्[2] ।
सतैललवणं दद्यात् निरूहं सानुवासनम् ।
परिस्रंसीनि चान्नानि तीक्ष्णञ्चैव विरेचनम् ॥५१॥

Treatment of Baddhodara

The patient of *baddhodara* should first of all be given fomentation therapy, and thereafter, *nirūha* as well as *anuvāsana* types

---

1. कर्म्मोदरहरत्तथा इति प्रथमपुस्तके पाठः ।
2. मूत्रं तीक्ष्णोषधान्वितं इति प्रथमपुस्तके पाठः ।

of medicated enema should be administered along with cow's urine, drugs having *tīkṣṇa guṇa* (sharp attribute), oil and rock-salt. He should be given such food which causes purgation. In addition, strong purgative therapy should be administered to him.

छिद्रोदरमृते स्वेदाच्छ्लेष्मोदरवदाचरेत् ॥५२॥

Treatment of Chidrodara

The patient of *chidrodara* should be treated with all therapies prescribed for the treatment of *kaphodara* except fomentation therapy.

जातं जातं जलं स्राव्यं शास्त्रोक्तं शस्त्रकर्म च ।
जलोदरे विशेषेण द्रवसेवां विवर्जयेत् ॥५३॥"

[भैषज्यरत्नावली : उदररोगाधिकार : १८-२३]

Treatment of Jalodara

The ascitic fluid in the abdomen of the patient suffering from *jalodara* should be frequently removed immediately after it gets accumulated by surgical measures prescribed in the text. In this condition, intake of water (or any liquid) is specially prohibited.

"देवदारुपलाशार्कहस्तिपिप्पलिशिग्रुकैः ।
साश्वगन्धै सगोमूत्रैः प्रविष्टादुदरं[1] शनैः ।
मूत्राण्यष्टावुदरिणां सेके पाने[2] च योजयेत् ॥५४॥"

[भैषज्यरत्नावली : उदररोगाधिकार : २७]

1. प्रदिह्यादुदरं इति श्राकरे पाठः ।
2. पानं इति श्राकरे पाठः ।

The paste of *deva dāru, palāśa, arka, hasti pippalī, śigru* and *aśvagandhā* prepared by triturating with cow's urine should be applied and gently rubbed over the abdomen of the patient. Cow's urine should be used in *seka* (sprinkling) and *pāna* (drink) of patients suffering from all the eight types of *udara roga*.

"स्नुहीपयो भावितानां पिप्पलीनां शनैः[1] शनैः ।
सहस्रं च[2] प्रयुञ्जीत शक्तितो जठरामयी ॥५५॥"

[भैषज्यरत्नावली : उदररोगाधिकार : ३७]

Administration of Pippalī

One thousand fruits of *pippalī* impregnated with the milky latex of *snuhī* should be gradually administered (in small doses) to the patient suffering from *udara roga* depending upon his strength.

"शिलाजतूनां[3] मूत्राणां गुग्गुलोस्त्रैफलस्य[4] च ।
स्नुहीक्षीरप्रयोगश्च शमयत्युदरामयम् ॥५६॥"

[भैषज्यरत्नावली : उदररोगाधिकार : ४२]

Administration of Snuhī

The milky latex of *snuhī* should be administered along with various preparations of *śilā jatu*, cow's urine, *guggulu* and *triphalā* which cures *udara roga*.

---

1. पयोऽशनः इति आकरे पाठः ।
2. चेह भुञ्जीत इति आकरे पाठः ।
3. मुक्तरोगश्चिरंजीवेद् घलवर्णसमन्वितः । पाठोऽयं षष्ठपुस्तके अधिकमुपलभ्यते ।
4. ०श्रीफलस्य इति पंचमपुस्तके पाठः ।

"स्नुक्पयसा परिभाविततण्डुलचूर्णै[1] विनिर्मितः पूपः ।
उदरमुदारं हिंस्याद्[2]योगोऽयं सप्तरात्रेण ॥५७॥"

[भैषज्यरत्नावली : उदररोगाधिकार : २४]

If pastries (*pūpa*) are prepared with rice flour impregnated with the milky latex of *snuhī* and taken, then it cures *udara roga* within seven nights.

"पिप्पलीबर्द्धमानं च[3] कल्पदृष्टं प्रयोजयेत् ।
जठरामयनाशाय नास्ति तेन समं भुवि ॥५८॥"

[भैषज्यरत्नावली : उदररोगाधिकार : ३८]

Pippali vardhamāna kalpa (i.e. intake of *pippalis* in gradually increased quantities and then decreased gradually which is generally done for the purpose of rejuvenation) should be administered for the cure of *udara rogas* and there is no other therapy comparable to it.

"पटोलमूलं रजनी विडङ्गं त्रिफलात्वचम् ।
कंपिल्लकं नीलिनीश्च त्रिवृ[4]ताञ्चेति चूर्णयेत् ॥५९॥
षडाद्यान्[5] कार्षिकान[6]न्त्यांस्त्रींश्च द्वित्रिचतुर्गुणान् ।
कृत्वा चूर्णं ततो माषं[7] गवां मूत्रेण वा[8] पिबेत् ॥६०॥

1. क. ०चूर्णेन निर्मित: इति आकरे पाठ: ।
   ख. ०विनिर्मितो इति षष्ठपुस्तके पाठः ।
2. हन्यात् इति षष्ठपुस्तके पाठ: ।
3. वा इति आकरे पाठ: ।
4. तृवृताञ्चति इति प्रथमपुस्तके पाठ: ।
5. षटाद्यात् कार्षिकानन्यात्त्रींश्च इति प्रथमपंचमपुस्तकयो: पाठ: ।
6. कार्षिकान्भागांस्त्रिश इति षष्ठपुस्तके पाठ: ।
7. मुष्टिं इति आदर्शपुस्तकेषु पाठ: ।
8. सम्पिबेत् इति आकरे पाठ: ।

विरिक्तो[1] जाङ्गलरसैर्भुञ्जीत मृदु[2] ओदनम्[3] ।
मण्डं पेयां च पीत्वा वा[4] सव्योषं षडहं पयः ॥६१॥
शृतं पिबेत्तु तच्चूर्णं पिबेदेवं[5] पुनः पुनः ।
हन्ति सर्वोदराण्येतच्चूर्णं जातोदकान्यपि ॥
कामलां पाण्डुरोगश्च श्वयथुं चापकर्षति ॥६२॥
॥ पटोलाद्यं[6] चूर्णम् ॥"
[भैषज्यरत्नावली : उदररोगाधिकार : ५३-५६]

Paṭolādya Cūrṇa

Paṭola root (one *karṣa*), *rajanī* (one *karṣa*) *viḍaṅga* (one *karṣa*), pulp of *harītakī* (one *karṣa*), pulp of *bibhītakī* (one *karṣa*), pulp of *āmalakī* (one *karṣa*), *kampillaka* (two *karṣaṣ*), *nīlinī* (three *karṣas*) and *trivṛt* (four *karṣas*) should be made to a powder. This powder should be administered in a dose of one *karṣa* along with cow's urine. Prior to this, the patient should have been given purgation therapy. The patient, using this recipe, should take soft boiled-rice along with the soup of the meat of animals inhabiting arid land. The patient can also take the milk boiled with this powder along with *maṇḍa* (thin gruel) or *peyā* (another type of thin gruel) mixed with the powder of *vyoṣa*. Intake of this for six days cures all types of *udara roga* even if there is water accumulation (*jātodaka*), jaundice, anemia and oedema.

---

1. विविक्तो इति प्रथमपंचमपुस्तकयोः पाठः ।
2. मृदुः मोदतः इति प्रथमपुस्तके पाठः ।
3. नोदरं इति षष्ठपुस्तके पाठः ।
4. तु इति आकरे पाठः ।
5. ह्री वेदेवं इति प्रथमपुस्तके पाठः ।
6. पटोलादि चूर्ण इति पंचमपुस्तके पाठः ।

"यमानी हवुषा धान्यं त्रिफला सोपकुञ्चिका[1] ।
कारवी पिप्पलीमूलमजगन्धा शटी[2] वचा ॥६३॥
शताह्वा जीरकं व्योषं स्वर्णक्षीरी सचित्रका ।
द्वौ क्षारौ पौष्करं मूलं कुष्ठं लवणपञ्चकम् ॥६४॥
विडङ्गञ्च समांशानि दन्त्याः भागत्रयं तथा ।
त्रिवृद्विशाले द्विगुणे सातला[3] स्याच्चतुर्गुणा ॥६५॥
एष नारायणो नाम चूर्णो रोगगणापहः ।
नैनं प्राप्याभिवर्द्धन्ते[4] रोगा विष्णुमिवासुराः ॥६६॥
तक्रेणोदरिभिः पेयो गुल्मिभिर्बदराम्बुना ।
आनद्धवाते सुरया वातरोगे प्रसन्नया ॥६७॥
दधिमण्डेन विट्सङ्गे दाडिमाम्बुभिरर्शसे[5] ।
परिकर्त्ते च वृक्षाम्लैरुष्णाम्बुभिरजीर्णके[6] ॥६८॥
भगन्दरे पाण्डुरोगे श्वासे कासे[7] गलग्रहे ।
हृद्रोगे ग्रहणीदोषे कुष्ठे मन्देऽनले[8] ज्वरे ॥६९॥

---

1. त्रिफलाचोपकुञ्चिका इति आकरे पाठः ।
2. शठी इति पंचमपुस्तके पाठः ।
3. शातला स्याच्चतुर्गुणाम् इति पंचमपुस्तके पाठः ।
4. क. प्राप्यानिवर्त्तते इति प्रथमपुस्तके पाठः ।
   ख. ०निवर्त्तन्ते इति पंचमपुस्तके पाठः ।
5. क. ०भिरर्शसा इति प्रथमपुस्तके पाठः ।
   ख. ०भिरर्शसाम् इति पंचमपुस्तके पाठः ।
6. ०रुष्णाह्विरजीर्णके इति प्रथमपंचमपुस्तकयोः पाठः ।
7. पाठोऽयं षष्ठपुस्तके नोपलभ्यते ।
8. मन्दानले इति आकरे पाठः ।

दंष्ट्राविषे मूलविषे सगरे कृत्रिमे विषे ।

यथार्हं स्निग्धकोष्ठेन पेयमेतद्विरेचनम् ॥७०॥"

॥ नारायणं चूर्णम् ॥

[भैषज्यरत्नावली : उदररोगाधिकार : ४५-५२]

Nārāyaṇa Cūrṇa

One part of each of *yamānī*, *havuṣā*, *dhānya*, *triphalā*, *upakuñcikā*, *kāravī*, *pippalī mūla*, *ajagandhā*, *śaṭī*, *vacā*, *śatāhvā*, *jīraka*, *vyoṣa*, *svarṇa kṣīrī*, *citraka*, *yava kṣāra*, *svarji kṣāra*, *puṣkara mūla*, *kuṣṭha*, *pañca lavaṇa* and *viḍaṅga*, three parts of *dantī*, two parts of each of *trivṛt* and *viśāla* and four parts of *sātalā* should be made to a powder. This is called *nārāyaṇa cūrṇa* which cures all diseases. No disease will get aggravated if the patient is using this recipe as demons do not flourish in the presence of Lord *Viṣṇu*. Patients of *udara roga* should use this recipe along with butter-milk. Patients of *gulma* (phantom tumour) should use this recipe along with *badara* juice. In *ānaddha vāta* (a condition caused by the obstruction to the movement of *vāyu*), this recipe should be used along with *surā* (a type of alcoholic drink). In *vātika* diseases, this recipe should be used along with *prasannā* (another type of alcoholic drink). If there is constipation, then it should be taken, along with whey (*dadhi maṇḍa*). Along with the juice of *dāḍima*, it shuold be taken if the patient is suffering from piles. In *parikartikā* (sawing pain in the abdomen), it should be taken along with *vṛkṣāmla*. In indigestion it should be taken along with hot water. After oleation therapy this purgative recipe should be appropriately taken for the treatment of anal fistula, anemia, dyspnoea, cough, obstruction to the throat, heart disease, *grahaṇī* (sprue syndrome), *kuṣṭha* (obstinate skin diseases including leprosy), suppression of the digestive power, fever, tooth-poisoning, root poisoning, *gara* type of poisoning and affliction by artificially prepared poisons.

कंकुष्टसैन्धवफलत्रयरजनीभिः

कृष्णावचारुचक[1]तिक्तकरोहिणीभिः ।

सत्रायमाणहपुषायवतिक्तकाभि-

श्चूर्ण[2]त्रिवृद्युतमिदं सकलोदरघ्नम् ॥७१॥

The powder of *trivṛt* added with *kaṅkuṣṭha*, rock-salt, *triphalā*, *rajanī*, *kṛṣṇā*, *vacā*, *rucaka*, *tiktaka rohiṇī*, *trāyamāṇā*, *hapuṣā* and *yava tiktā* cures all types of *udara roga*.

[3]'सामुद्रं सैन्धवं काचं यवक्षारं सुवर्च्चलम् ।

टंकणं स्वर्जिकाक्षारं तुल्यं चूर्णं विभावयेत् ॥७२॥

अर्कक्षीरैः स्नुहीक्षीरैरातपे भावयेत्त्र्यहम् ।

अर्कपत्रप्रलेपेन रुध्वा चांतःपुटे पचेत् ॥७३॥

तत् क्षारं चूर्णयेत् पश्चात् त्र्यूषणं त्रिफलारजः ।

जीरकं रजनी वह्नि नवभागं समं समम् ॥७४॥

क्षारार्द्धमेतदर्द्धं च [4]एकीकृत्य प्रयोजयेत् ।

वज्रक्षारमिदं प्रोक्तं स्वयमुक्तं पिनाकिना ॥७५॥

सर्वोदरेषु गुल्मेषु शूले शोफे च योजयेत् ।

अग्निमांद्येप्पजीर्णे च भक्ष्यं निष्कद्वयं द्वयम् ॥७६॥

1. रुचका० इति प्रथमपुस्तके पाठः ।
2. शकलो० इति पंचमपुस्तके पाठः ।
3. 'सामुद्रं.........त्रिदोषजे ॥ ॥वज्रक्षारः ॥' पाठोऽयं चतुर्थषष्ठ-पुस्तकयोः नोपलभ्यते ।
4. चक्रीकृत्य इति प्रथमपुस्तके पाठः ।

वाताधिके जले कोष्णे घृते पित्ताधिके हितम् ।
कफे गोमूत्रसंयुक्तमारनाले त्रिदोषजे ॥७७॥

॥ वज्रक्षारः ॥[1]

Vajra Kṣāra

Sāmudra lavaṇa, *saindhava lavaṇa*, *kāca lavaṇa*, *yava kṣāra*, *sauvarcala lavaṇa*, *ṭaṅkaṇa* and *svarji kṣāra* should be taken in equal quantities and made to a powder. This powder should be impregnated with the milky latex of *arka* as well as *snuhī* and dried in the sun for three days. Leaves of *arka* should be smeared with the powder, kept in a sealed jar and cooked in *puṭa*. This *kṣāra* (alkali preparation) should be made to a powder. Nine parts of this *kṣāra* should be added with the powder of one part of each of *śuṇṭhī*, *pippalī*, *marica*, *harītakī*, *bibhītakī*, *āmalakī*, *jīraka*, *rajani* and *citraka*. This is called *vajrī kṣāra*. This recipe is propounded by Lord Śiva himself. It should be used in all types of *udara roga*, *gulma* (phantom tumour), colic pain and oedema. In suppression of the digestive power and indigestion, it should be used in a dose of two *niṣkas*. In diseases caused by aggravated *vāyu*, it should be taken with hot water ; in diseases caused by aggravated *pitta*, it should be taken along with ghee ; in diseases caused by aggravated *kapha*, it should be taken along with cow's urine ; and in *sānnipātika* diseases, it should be taken along with *ārañāla* (a type of vinegar).

दन्ती वचा गवाक्षी च शंखिनी तिल्वकं[2] त्रिवृत् ।
गोमूत्रेण पिबेदेतत् कल्कं जठरनाशनम् ॥७८॥

Intake of the paste of *danti*, *vacā*, *gavākṣi*, *śaṅkhini*, *tilvaka* and *trivṛt* along with cow's urine cures abdominal diseases.

---

1. पाठोऽयं पंचमपुस्तके अधिकमुपलभ्यते ।
2. तिलुकं इति प्रथमपुस्तके पाठः ।

स[1]क्षारं माहिषं मूत्रं निराहारः पिबेन्नरः ।
शाम्यत्यनेन जठरं सप्ताहादिति निश्चयः ॥७९॥

Intake of buffalo's urine along with *kṣāra* (alkali preparation) in empty stomach certainly cures abdominal diseases within one week.

गवाक्षीशंखिनीद[2]न्तीनीलिनीकल्कसंयुतम् ।
सर्वोदरविनाशाय गोमूत्रं [3]पातुमाचरेत् ॥८०॥

For the cure of all types of *udara roga*, the patient should take the paste of *gavākṣī*, *śaṅkhinī*, *dantī* and *nīlinī* along with cow's urine.

अर्कपत्रं सलवणम[4]न्तर्धूमं दहेत्ततः ।
[5]मस्तुना तत्पिबेत् क्षारं गुल्मप्लीहोदरापहम् ॥८१॥

॥ व[6]ज्रक्षारः ॥

Vajra Kṣāra (second recipe)

Leaves of *arka* along with salt should be burnt in a sealed container. This *kṣāra* (alkali preparation) should be taken along with whey which cures *gulma* (phantom tumour) and *plīhodara*.

---

1. सक्षीरमाहिषं इति षष्ठपुस्तके पाठः ।
2. दन्तीनिलिनी इति षष्ठपुस्तके पाठः ।
3. पानमाचरेत् इति षष्ठपुस्तके पाठः ।
4. ०मंतर्धूमंदहेत्ततः इति षष्ठपुस्तके पाठः ।
5. मस्तूनातत्पिबेत् इति पंचमपुस्तके पाठः ।
6. पाठोऽयं षष्ठपुस्तके अधिकमुपलभ्यते ।

पीतः प्लीहोदरं हन्यात् पिप्पलीमरिचान्वितः ।
अम्लवेतससंयुक्तः शिग्रुक्वाथः ससैन्धवः ॥८२॥

Intake of the decoction of *śigru* along with *pippalī*, *marica*, *amla vetasa* and rock-salt cures *plīhodara*

यस्य गृहीत्वा संज्ञायां[1] पाटयित्वेन्द्रवारुणीमूलम्[2] ।
प्रक्षिप्यते सुदूरे[3] शाम्येत् प्लीहोदरस्तस्य ॥८३॥

Indra vāruṇi should be uprooted by reciting the name of the patient and thrown away at a long distance. This cures the named patient's *plīhodara.*

रौहितकाभयाक्षौद्रभावितं मूत्रमम्बु वा ।
पीतं सर्वोदरप्लीहमेहाऽर्शः[4]कृमिगुल्मनुत् ॥८४॥

Intake of *rohitaka*, *abhaya* and honey along with cow's urine or water cures all types of *udara roga*, splenic disorder, *meha* (obstinate urinary disorders including diabetes), piles, parasitic infestation and *gulma* (phantom tumour).

देवद्रुमं शिग्रुमयूरकञ्च गोमूत्रपिष्टामथवाश्वगन्धाम् ।
पीत्वाशु हन्यादुदरं प्रवृद्धं कृमीन्[5]सशोथानुदरञ्च दूष्यम् ॥८५॥

The paste of *deva druma*, *śigru* and *mayūraka* prepared by triturating with cow's urine or the paste of *aśva gandhā* prepared by triturating with cow's urine instantaneously cures serious type of *udara roga*, parasitic infestation, oedema and *dūṣyodara.*

1. संज्ञां इति प्रथमपुस्तके पाठः ।
2. पाटपित्वेन्द्र वारुणी इति षष्ठपुस्तके पाठः ।
3. सदरे शाम्ये प्लीहोदरं तस्य इति षष्ठपुस्तके पाठः ।
4. ०गुल्मार्शः इति षष्ठपुस्तके पाठः ।
5. कृमान्स० इति पंचमपुस्तके पाठः ।

दशमूलदारुनागरछिन्नरुहापुनर्नवाभयाक्वाथः ।

जयति जलोदरशोथश्लीपदगलगण्डवातरोगांश्च[1] ॥८६॥

The decoction of *daśa mūla*, *deva dāru*, *nāgara*. *chinna ruhā*, *punarnavā* and *abhayā* cures ascites, oedema, filariasis, *gala gaṇḍa* (goitre) and diseases caused by *vāyu*.

'[2]हरीतकीनागरदेवदारुपुनर्नवाछिन्नरुहाकषायः ।

सगुग्गुलुर्मूत्र[3]युतश्च पेयः शोथोदराणां प्रवलं[4] प्रयोगः ॥८७॥

Intake of the decoction of *haritakī*, *nāgara*, *deva dāru* *punarnavā* and *chinnaruhā* along with *guggulu* and cow's urine cures oedema and *udara roga*.

'[5]एरण्डतैलं दशमूलमिश्रं गोमूत्रयुक्तं त्रिफलारसैर्वा ।

निहन्ति पीतोदरशोथशूलं क्वाथः समूत्रो दशमूलजश्च ॥८८॥'

Eraṇḍa taila mixed with the decoction of *daśa mūla*, cow's urine or decoction of *triphalā* cures *udara roga*, oedema and colic pain. These diseases are cured also by the intake of the decoction of *daśa mūla* along with cow's urine.

पुनर्नवानिम्बपटोलशुण्ठीतिक्तामृतादार्व्यभयाकषायः[6] ।

सर्वाङ्गशोथोदरपार्श्वशूलश्वासान्वितं[7] पाण्डुगदं निहन्ति ॥८९॥

---

1. ०जान् रोगान् इति चतुर्थपुस्तके पाठः ।
2. 'हरीतकी——०कषायः' पाठोऽयं चतुर्थपुस्तके नोपलभ्यते ।
3. ०मुत्र० इति षष्ठपुस्तके पाठः ।
4. प्रवरः इति चतुर्थषष्ठपुस्तकयोः पाठः ।
5. 'एरण्डतैलं———दशमूलजश्च' पाठोऽयं षष्ठपुस्तके नोपलभ्यते ।
6. ०दार्वभया० इति षष्ठपुस्तके पाठः ।
7. ०कासशूलश्वास० इति षष्ठपुस्तके पाठः ।

The decoction of *punarnavā*, *nimba*, *paṭola*, *śuṇṭhī*, *tiktā*, *amṛtā*, *dārvī* and *abhayā* cures general anasarca, *udara roga*, pain in the sides of the chest, dyspnoea and anemia.

पुनर्नवादार्वभयां गुडूचीं पिबेत्समूत्रां महिषाक्षयुक्ताम् ।
त्वग्दोषशोथोदरपाण्डुरोगस्थौल्यप्रसेकोर्ध्वकफामयेषु ॥६०॥

The decoction of *punarnavā*, *dārvī*, *abhayā* and *guḍūci* should be taken along with cow's urine and *guggulu*. This cures skin diseases, oedema, *udara roga*, anemia, obesity, nausea and diseases of head as well as neck caused by *kapha*.

गोमूत्रयुक्तं महिषी पयो वा क्षीरं गवां वा[1] त्रिफलां विमिश्रम् ।
क्षीरान्नभुक्ते बलमेव गव्यं मूत्रं पिबेद्वा श्वयथूदरेषु ॥६१॥

The following recipes cure oedema and *udara roga* :

1. Buffalo milk along with cow's urine ;
2. *Triphalā* mixed with cow's milk ; and
3. Cow's urine along with milk preparations as food.

पुनर्नवादार्व्यमृतापाठाबिल्वं श्वदंष्ट्रका[2] ।
बृहत्यौ द्वे रजन्यौ द्वे पिप्पल्यग्निचित्रकं वृषम् ॥६२॥
समभागानि संचूर्ण्य गवां मूत्रेण वा पिबेत् ।
बहुप्रकारश्वयथुं सर्वगात्रविसर्पिणाम्[3] ।
हन्ति शूलोदराण्यष्टौ[4] नृणां श्चैवोद्धतानपि[5] ॥६३॥

---

1. पाठोऽयं चतुर्थपुस्तके नोपलभ्यते ।
2. क. सुदंष्ट्रका इति पंचमपुस्तके पाठः ।
 ख. श्वदंष्ट्रिका इति चतुर्थषष्ठपुस्तकयोः पाठः ।
3. ०विकारिणाम् इति चतुर्थषष्ठपुस्तकयोः पाठः ।
4. क. शूलोदराणि अष्टौनृणां० इति पंचमपुस्तके पाठः ।
 ख. शूलोदरान्यष्टौ० इति षष्ठपुस्तके पाठः ।
5. ०तान्यपि इति चतुर्थषष्ठपुस्तकयोः पाठः ।

The powder of *punarnavā*, *dārvī*, *amṛtā*, *pāṭhā*, *bilva*, *śvadaṃṣṭrā*, *bṛhatī*, *kaṇṭakārī*, *haridrā*, *dāru haridrā*, *pippalī*, *citraka* and *vṛṣa*—all taken in equal quantities should be taken along with cow's urine. This cures many types of general anasarca, colic pain, eight types of *udara roga* even in their acute stage.

पुराणं माणकं पिष्ट्वा द्विगुणीकृततन्दुलम्[1] ।
साधितं[2] क्षारतोयाभ्यामभ्यसेत्पायसं तु तम् ॥६४॥
हन्ति वातोदरं शोथं ग्रहणीं पाण्डुतामपि[3] ।
'सिद्धो[4] भिषग्भिराख्यातः प्रयोगोयं निरत्पयः ॥६५॥'

Pāyasa (a type of milk preparation) should be made out of the paste of old *māṇaka* and double the quantity of rice by cooking along with milk and water. Regular intake of this milk preparation cures *vātodara*, oedema, *grahaṇī* (sprue syndrome) and anemia. This recipe is absolutely harmless and its effectiveness is practically experienced.

'क्षारं[5] वज्रतरुद्भवं दशपलं तावत्पयोप्यर्कजम् ।
प्रत्यकं पलपंचकं च लवणं क्षारं च पंचात्मकम् ॥६६॥'

---

1. ०कृततन्डुलम् इति षग्ठपुस्तके पाठः ।
2. क्षीरतोयाभ्यामभ्यसेभ्याससंद्रुतम् इति षष्ठपुस्तके पाठः ।
3. पंचक लवणं क्षारं च पंचात्मकम् पाठोऽयं चतुर्थपुस्तके अधिकमुपलभ्यते ।
4. 'सिद्धो०........निरत्पयः' पाठोऽयं चतुर्थपुस्तके नोपलभ्यते ।
5. 'क्षारं........पंचात्मकम्' पाठोऽयं षष्ठपुस्तके अधिकमुपलभ्यते ।

विंशत्यर्कदलैर्युतं पचितरेभिस्तैश्चतुर्भिः[1] पलैः[?] ।
मृद्भांडे[2] गुरुमार्गतो गजपुटे वह्नौ[3] विपक्वीकृतम् ॥९७॥
संचूर्ण्याथ कटुत्रयं त्रिपलमप्येकं पलं रामठं ।
सर्वं वस्त्रपुनीतमेतदमले पात्रे सुसंस्थापयेत्[4] ॥९८॥
वज्रक्षारमिदं[5] निहन्ति सकलान्गुलमानुदग्रान्[6] नृणाम् ।
पीतं[7] तक्रयुतं प्रभातसमये[8] कर्षप्रमाणं क्रमात् ॥९९॥
मंदाग्निं सविसूचिकामरुचिताभापाण्डुतां[9] क्षीणताम् ।
श्वासं कासमजीर्णशैत्य[10]पवनव्याधीन्वलासो[11]द्भवात् ॥१००॥

---

1. चाति० इति षष्ठपुस्तके पाठः ।
2. क. भृद्भांडे इति पंचमपुस्तके पाठः ।
   ख. मृद्भांडे इति षष्ठपुस्तके पाठः ।
3. वक्तौ इति प्रथमपुस्तके पाठः ।
4. क. सुषंस्थापयेत् इति पंचमपुस्तके पाठः ।
   ख. सुखंस्थापयेत् इति चतुर्थषष्ठपुस्तकयोः पाठः ।
5. बज्रक्षारामद इति प्रथमपुस्तके पाठः ।
6. ०दग्जा इति प्रथमपुस्तके पाठः ।
7. पातं इति प्रथमपुस्तके पाठः ।
8. प्रभातस्य मयेकषंडामाणं इति प्रथमपुस्तके पाठः ।
9. ०तामा० इति प्रथमपुस्तके पाठः ।
10. ०शैभ्य इति पंचमपुस्तके पाठः ।
11. ०व्याधान्वला० इति प्रथमपुस्तके पाठः ।

वज्रक्षारमिदं निवार्य[1] भिषजां कीर्तिं प्रदत्ते[2] तराम् ।
आसंद्रावयति[3] स्फुटं घटिकयोर्द्धं द्वे किमन्यत्[4] पुनः ॥१०१॥

॥ वज्रक्षारः ॥

Vajra Kṣāra (*third recipe*)

Ten *palas* of the *kṣāra* of *vajra taru*, ten *palas* of the milky latex of *arka* and one *pala* of each of *pañca lavaṇa* and *pañca kṣāra* should be added with twenty leaves of *arka* and kept in an earthen jar. According to the instructions of teachers, this should be cooked in *gaja puṭa* and made to a powder. To this, the powder of *trikaṭu* (three *palas*) and *rāmaṭha* (one *pala*) should be added and strained through a piece of cloth. This should then be stored in a clean jar. It is called *vajra kṣāra* and it cures all types of *gulma* (phantom tumour). It is to be taken in a dose of one *karṣa* in the early morning along with butter-milk. It cures suppressed power of digestion, *visūcikā* (choleric diarrhoea), anorexia, anemia, emaciation, asthma, cough, indigestion, feeling of cold and diseases of *vāyu* as well as *kapha*. It endows fame to the physician by relieving abdominal disorders in two hours. [There are several mistakes in these verses].

"दशमूलतुलाऽर्द्धरसे सक्षारैः पंचकोलकैः पलिकैः ।
सिद्धं घृतार्द्धपात्रं[5] द्विर्मस्तुकमुदरगुल्मघ्नम्[6] ॥१०२॥"

॥ दशमूलषट्पलकं घृतम् ॥

[भैषज्यरत्नावली : उदररोगाधिकार : ७३]

---

1. सदार्य इति षष्ठपुस्तके पाठः ।
2. प्रदत्वेत० इति षष्ठपुस्तके पाठः ।
3. संद्रावयातस्युदर० इति प्रथमपुस्तके पाठः ।
4. किमन्भं इति प्रथमपुस्तके पाठः ।
5. ०मात्रं इति षष्ठपुस्तके पाठः ।
6. द्विर्मुस्तकं गुल्ममुदरघ्नम् इति प्रथमपुस्तके पाठः ।

Daśa Mūla Ṣaṭ Palaka Ghṛta

Half *pātra* of ghee should be boiled with half *tulā* of the decoction of *daśa mūla*, one *pala* of each of *kṣāra* and *pañca kola*, and two *pātras* of whey. Intake of this medicated ghee cures *udara roga* and *gulma* (phantom tumour).

"चतुर्गुणे जले मूत्रे द्विगुणे चित्रकात् पले[1] ।
कल्के सिद्धं घृतप्रस्थं सक्षारं जठरी पिबेत् ॥१०३॥"

॥ चित्रकं घृतम् ॥

[भैषज्यरत्नावली : उदररोगाधिकार : ७२]

Citraka Ghṛta

One *prastha* of ghee should be cooked by adding four *prasthas* of water, two *prasthas* of cow's urine and one *pala* of the paste of *citraka*. Intake of this medicated ghee along with *kṣāra* (alkali preparation) cures *udara roga*.

"अर्कक्षीरपले द्वे तु[2] स्नुहीक्षीरपलानि[3] षट् ।
पथ्या कम्पिल्लकं श्यामा शम्पाकं[4] गिरिकर्णिका[5] ॥१०४॥
नीलिनी त्रिवृता दन्ती शंखिनी चित्रकं तथा ।
एतेषां पलिकैर्भागैर्घृतप्रस्थं विपाचयेत् ॥१०५॥

---

1. पलो इति षष्ठपुस्तके पाठः ।
2. च इति आकरे पाठः ।
3. ०पलोनि इति आकरे पाठः ।
4. सम्पाकं इति प्रथमपंचमपुस्तकयोः पाठः ।
5. गिरिमल्लिका इति आकरे पाठः ।

अथास्य मलिने कोष्ठे बिन्दुमात्रं प्रदापयेत् ।

यावतोऽस्य पिबेद्बिन्दून् तावद्वेगान्विरिच्यते[1] ॥१०६॥

कुष्ठं गुल्ममुदावर्त्तं श्वयथुं सभगन्दरम् ।

शमयत्युदराण्यष्टौ वृक्षमिन्द्राशनिर्यथा ।

एतद्बिन्दुघृतनाम[2] येनाभ्यक्तो[3] विरिच्यतो[4] ॥१०७॥"

॥ बिन्दुघृतम् ॥

[भैषज्यरत्नावली : उदररोगाधिकार : ५७-६०]

Bindu Ghṛta

One *prastha* of cow's ghee should be cooked by adding two *palas* of the milky latex of *arka*, six *palas* of the milky latex of *snuhī*, and one *pala* of each of *pathyā*, *kampillaka*, *śyāmā*, *śampāka*, *giri karṇikā*, *nīlinī*, *trivṛt*, *dantī*, *śaṅkhinī* and *citraka*. This should be administered in the dose of one drop to a patient having vitiated gastro-intestinal tract. As soon as he takes the drop, he purges strongly. It cures *kuṣṭha* (obstinate skin diseases including leprosy), *gulma* (phantom tumour), *udāvarta* (upward movement of wind), oedema, anal fistula and eight types of *udara roga* as a tree is destroyed by the thunder bolt of Lord Indra. This is called *bindu ghrta*. Even a massage of this drug causes purgation.

---

1. तावद्वारान् विरिच्यते इति आकरे पाठः ।
2. ०घृतं नाम इति आकरे पाठः ।
3. नाभिलेपाद्वि इति पंचमपुस्तके पाठः ।
4. क. विरिच्यते इति चतुर्थपंचमषष्ठपुस्तकेषु पाठः ।
   ख. विरच्यते इति आकरे पाठः ।

"चित्रकः शङ्खिनी पथ्या कम्पिल्लस्त्रिवृतायुतः[1] ।
वृद्धदारुश्च[2] शम्पाको दन्ती कुम्भीफलं[3] तथा ॥१०८॥
कोशातकी देवदाली नीलिनी[4] गिरिकर्णिका ।
सातला पिप्पली चैव[5] विडङ्गं कटुकी तथा ॥१०९॥
हेमक्षीरी च विपचेत् कल्कैरेभिः[6] पिचून्मितैः ।
घृतप्रस्थं स्नुहीक्षीरे षट्पले[7] तु पलद्वये[8] ॥११०॥
अर्कक्षीरस्य मतिमांस्तत्सिद्धं कुष्ठगुल्मनुत् ।
हन्ति शूलमुदावर्त्तं शोथाध्मानं भगन्दरम् ॥१११॥
शमयत्युदराण्यष्टौ तत्पीतं[9] बिन्दुसङ्ख्यया[10] ।
गोदुग्धेनोष्ट्रदुग्धेन[11] कौलत्थेन शृतेन वा ॥११२॥

---

1. युगम् इति आकरे पाठः ।
2. वृद्धदारश्च इति आदर्शपुस्तकेषु पाठः ।
3. दन्तीफलं इति आकरे पाठः ।
4. नीली च इति आकरे पाठः ।
5. पिप्पलीमूलं इति आकरे पाठः ।
6. कल्कैरेतैः इति आकरे पाठः ।
7. व पले इति चतुर्थपुस्तके पाठः ।
8. पलंद्वये इति आदर्शपुस्तकेषु पाठः ।
9. निपीतं इति आकरे पाठः ।
10. सङ्खयम् इति चतुर्थपुस्तके पाठः ।
11. गोघृतेर्नाकदुग्धेन तथा कौलित्थकेन वा इति षष्ठपुस्तके पाठः ।

उष्णोदकेन वा पीत्वा बिन्दुवेगैर्विरिच्यते ।
एतद्बिन्दुघृतं नाम नाभिर्लेपाद्विरिच्यते[1] ॥११३॥
॥ महाबिन्दु[2] घृतम् ॥"
[भारतभैषज्यरत्नाकर : चतुर्थभाग : पृष्ठ ६४४]

Mahā Bindu Ghṛta

One *prastha* of ghee should be cooked with the paste of one *picu* of each of *citraka, śaṅkhinī, pathyā, kampillaka, trivṛt, vṛddha dāru, śampāka, danti*, fruit of *kumbhī, kośātakī, devadālī, nīlinī, giri karṇikā, sātalā, pippalī, viḍaṅga, kaṭuki* and *hemakṣīrī*, six *palas* of the milky latex of *snuhī* and two *palas* of the milky latex of *arka*. It cures *kuṣṭha* (obstinate skin diseases including leprosy), *gulma* (phantom tumour), colic pain, *udāvarta* (upward movement of wind in the abdomen), oedema, abdominal distension, anal fistul and eight types of *udara roga*. It is administered in a dose of only one drop. Intake of this drop of medicated ghee along with cow's milk, camel milk, decoction of *kulattha* or hot water causes strong purgation. This is called *bindu ghṛta*. It causes purgation even if applied over the umbilicus.

[3]त्रिवृत्पलं [4]स्नुक्पयसः पलं च कम्पिलकस्य पलं तृतीयं च ।
चतुःपलं चामलकीरसस्य शाणार्धमन्यलवणस्य चैव ॥११४॥

---

1. विरेचयेत् इति ग्राकरे पाठः ।
2. क. विन्दुघृतम् इति ग्राकरे पाठः ।
ख. "चित्रकः ———महाविन्दुघृतम्" पाठोऽयं प्रथमपुस्तके नोपलभ्यते ।
3. 'स्नुह्यर्कपयसोरत्र पाकार्थमुपर्यात्ततः ।
चतुर्गुणं जलं देयं पाकार्थं बिन्दुसर्पिषा ।' पाठोऽयं पंचमपुस्तके अधिकमुपलभ्यते ।
4. स्नुक्पयसपलं च कापलकंस्यापि इति प्रथमपुस्तके पाठः ।

प्रस्थार्द्धमेभिर्हविषो[1] विपक्वं जले[2] महाबिन्दुघृतं प्रशस्तम्[3] ।
निहन्ति[4] गुल्मं जठराणि चैव प्लीहानमप्याशुविरेकयोगात्[5] ॥

॥ बिन्दुघृतम् ॥११५॥

Bindu Ghṛta (*second recipe*)

Half *prastha* of ghee should be cooked with one *pala* of *trivṛt*, one *pala* of the milky latex of *snuhī*, one *pala* of *kampillaka*, four *palas* of the juice or decoction of *āmalakī*, half *śāṇa* of rock-salt and (two *prasthas* of) water. This is called *mahā* (?) *bindu ghṛta*. By its purgative action, it instantaneously cures *gulma* (phantom tumour), *udara roga* and splenic disorder.

दधिमण्डाढके[6] सिद्धं स्नुक्क्षीरपलकल्कितम् ।
घृतप्रस्थं पिबेन्मात्रां तद्वज्जठरशान्तये ॥११६॥

One *prastha* of ghee should be cooked with one *āḍhaka* of whey and one *pala* of the milky latex of *snuhī*. Intake of this medicated ghee in appropriate dose cures *udara roga*.

तथा सिद्धं घृतप्रस्थं पयस्यष्टगुणे[7] पिबेत् ।
स्नुक्क्षीरपत्रं[8] त्रिफला त्रिवृता षट्पलेन च ॥११७॥

1. ०मोमहवुषो इति प्रथमपुस्तके पाठः ।
2. नले महाविन्दुवृतं इति प्रथमपुस्तके पाठः ।
3. प्रसिद्धं इति षष्ठपुस्तके पाठः ।
4. निहात इति प्रथमपुस्तके पाठः ।
5. प्लीहानम घासु विरेक योगात्या इति प्रथमपुस्तके पाठः ।
6. दधिमण्डार्द्धके इति षष्ठपुस्तके पाठः ।
7. घृतस्याष्टगुणे पचेत् इति षष्ठपुस्तके पाठः ।
8. ०मत्र इति षष्ठपुस्तके पाठः ।

One *prastha* of ghee should be cooked by adding eight times of milk and six *palas* of each of the milky latex of *snuhī*, *patra*, *triphalā* and *trivṛt*. This also cures *udara roga*.

"स्नुक्क्षीरदन्तीत्रिफलाविडङ्गसिंहीत्रिवृत्चित्रककल्कयुक्तम् ।
घृतं विपक्वं कुडवप्रमाणं तोयेन तस्याक्षमथार्द्धकर्षम्[1] ॥११८॥
पीत्वोष्णमम्भोऽनुपिबेद्विरिक्ते[2] पेयां सुखोष्णां वितरेद्विधिज्ञः ।
नाराचमेतज्जठरामयानां युक्त्योपयुक्तं शमनं प्रदिष्टम् ॥११९॥

॥ नाराचघृतम् ॥"

[भैषज्यरत्नावली : उदररोगाधिकार : ६६-६७]

Nārāca Ghṛta

One *kuḍava* of ghee should be cooked by adding the paste of *snuhī* (milky latex), *dantī*, *triphalā*, *viḍaṅga*, *siṃhī*, *trivṛt* and *citraka* and water. This medicated ghee should be taken in the dose of one *akṣa* or half *karṣa* with warm water. After purgation, luke warm *peyā* (thin gruel) should be given as food. This is called *nārāca*. It cures *udara roga* when administered appropriately.

रसमन्यं प्रवक्ष्यामि सर्वोदरविनाशनम्[3] ।
पातितात्स्वेदितात्सूतात्पलद्वयमुपाहरेत् ॥१२०॥
शुद्धस्य दानवेन्द्रस्य ग्राह्यं पलचतुष्टयम् ।
निर्गुण्डीसलिलैर्मद्यो[4] दिनत्रयमतन्द्रितम्[5] ॥१२१॥

---

1. तस्यापि हि तोलकार्द्धम् इति आकरे पाठः ।
2. ०द्विरिक्तः इति आकरे पाठः ।
3. विनासनम् इति प्रथमपुस्तके पाठः ।
4. सस्थिलै० इति षष्ठपुस्तके पाठः ।
5. ०तन्द्रितः इति षष्ठपुस्तके पाठः ।

पश्चाद्गोलं समासाद्य दृढभाण्डे निवेशयेत् ।
वक्षमाणक्रमेणाथ शुल्वं संशोध्य बुद्धिमान् ॥१२२॥
पलद्वयप्रमाणेन ताम्रवाटीं[1] विधापयेत्[2] ।
अधोमुखीं ताम्रवाटीं[3] सूतगोलोपरि क्षिपेत् ॥१२३॥
संधिं निरोधयेद्यत्नात्[4] उपरिष्टात्परिक्षिपेत् ।
पुटो तु[5] परिसन्दद्यात्शरावं[6] सुदृढाव्रणम्[?] ॥१२४॥
संधिनिरोधयेद्भाण्डं बालुकभिः प्रपूरयेत्[7] ।
भाण्डेनान्येन संरुध्य सम्पुटं संधिलेपितः[8] ॥१२५॥
उपरिष्टाच्चुल्लिकायां[9] यत्नमारोपयेद्बुधः ।
अद्यस्तान् ज्वालयेद्वह्निं मध्यमानेन सर्वदा ॥१२६॥
दिनानि पंच यत्नेन[10] स्वतःशैत्यै विरोधयेत्[11] ।
म्रियते सह शुल्वेन रसेन्द्रो नात्र संशयः ॥१२७॥

---

1. ताम्रवांटी इति प्रथमपुस्तके पाठः ।
2. मिधामयेत् इति पष्ठपुस्तके पाठः ।
3. ताम्रवांटी इति प्रथमपुस्तके पाठः ।
4. क. ०द्यन्नात् इति प्रथमपुस्तके पाठः ।
   ख. ०द्यत्नात् बुपरिष्टान्नपरिक्षितेत् इति षष्ठपुस्तके पाठः ।
5. पुटैरुपरिसंद्दाद्यत्शरावं सुदृढव्रणं इति षष्ठपुस्तके पाठः ।
6. ०सरावं इति पंचमपुस्तके पाठः ।
7. बालुकभिन्यपूरयेत् इति प्रथमपुस्तके पाठः ।
8. संधिलेपतः इति प्रथमपुस्तके पाठः ।
9. ०चुल्हिकायां इति चतुर्थषष्ठपुस्तकयोः पाठः ।
10. पलेन स्वमः शैत्यैऽवरोधयेत् इति चतुर्थपुस्तके पाठः ।
11. वरोहयेत् इति षष्ठपुस्तके पाठः ।

Tri Mūrti Rasa (*Vāmania, Culuka Bheda and Kālāri Rasa*)

Hereafter, a mercurial preparation will be described for the cure of all *udara rogas*. Two *palas* of *pārada* purified by *pātana* and *svedana* and four *palas* of purified *gandhaka* should be triturated with the juice of *nirguṇḍī* for three days. The paste should be made to a bolus form and kept in a strong earthen jar. Similarly, two *palas* of *tāmra* should be purified according to the prescribed procedure and kept in a copper cup. This copper cup containing purified *tāmra* should be kept with face downwards over the bolus of mercury in the jar. The joint of the copper cup and the jar should be sealed properly. Over the mouth of the earthen jar, a strong earthen plate should then be placed and the joint of this jar and the plate should be sealed properly. This sealed jar should be kept in another earthen jar and the space between these two jars should be filled with sand. The outer jar should then be covered with an earthen plate and the joint should be sealed. This should be kept over oven and cooked in moderate heat for five days with care. Thereafter, when it is cooled of its own, medicines including the copper cup should be removed from the inner jar. By this, the *pārada* along with *tāmra* is undoubtedly reduced to a *bhasma* form.

विचूर्णयेत्ताम्रवाटीं तच्चूर्णं विभजेत् त्रिधा ।
एकं तु भागमादाय भावयेदौषधैरथ ॥१२८॥
मदनस्य फलोत्थेन वारिणादौ विभावयेत् ।
पुटयेच्छतवारं[1] तं अंकुल्लत्वग्भवै[2] रसैः ॥१२९॥
कुसुम्भनीरैः[3] पुटयेत्प्रत्येकं शतशस्ततः[4] ।

---

1. क. पुटयेत्शतवारं इति पंचमपुस्तके पाठः ।
   ख. पुटयेच्छनकंरं इति षष्ठपुस्तके पाठः ।
2. अंकोलत्वग्भवै इति चतुर्थषष्ठपुस्तकयोः पाठः ।
3. ०नीलै इति षष्ठपुस्तके पाठः ।
4. सत इति प्रथमपुस्तके पाठः ।

पञ्चकैश्छाणकैर्दद्यात्पुटमारण्यकोद्भवैः[1] ॥१३०॥

मदनस्य फलांभोभिः[2] त्रीन् वारान् भावयेद्रसम् ।

अंकुलमूलत्वक्क्वाथैर्देवदालीरसैस्तथा[3] ॥

एवं सिद्धं रसं पश्चाद्वल्लमानेन[4] योजयेत् ॥१३१॥

गोमूत्रजेन मण्डेन चुलुकत्रयमानतः ।

दत्त्वा धर्म्मे स्थापयेत्[5] तं क्षणमात्रमतंद्रितम्[6] ॥१३२॥

[7]आवाल्पात्संगृहीतं यन्मलं देहे व्यवस्थितम् ।

तत्सर्वं घटिकामध्ये वमत्येव न संशयः ॥१३३॥

वामनीयो रसोनाम्ना[8] जलोदरविनाशनः ॥१३४॥

Drugs along with the copper cup should then be reduced to a powder form and this powder should be divided into three parts. One part of it should be impregnated with the decoction of *madana* and cooked in *puṭa* for one hundred times. Similarly, one hundred *puṭas* should be given by impregnating this recipe with the juice (or decoction) of the bark of *aṅkola* and one hundred *puṭas* with the juice of *kusumbha*. For each

---

1. क. पंचकैः छाणकै० इति चतुर्थपुस्तके पाठः ।
   ख. पंचकैछ्राणकै० इति पंचमपुस्तके पाठः ।
2. फलांभोभिस्त्रीन् इति चतुर्थषष्ठपुस्तकयोः पाठः ।
3. अंकोल० इति चतुर्थषष्ठपुस्तकयोः पाठः ।
4. ०मान न इति षष्ठपुस्तके पाठः ।
5. स्थापयत् इति षष्ठपुस्तके पाठः ।
6. ०तन्द्रितः इति चतुर्थषष्ठपस्तकयोः पाठः ।
7. अवाल्पात् इति षष्ठपुस्तके पाठः ।
8. रसोताम्रा इति चतुर्थपुस्तके पाठः ।

puṭa, five cowdung cakes should be used as fuel. Thereafter, the recipe should be impregnated with the decoction of the fruit of *madana*, decoction of the root-bark of *aṅkola* and juice of *devadālī*, three times in each. This prepared recipe should be administered in the dose of one *valla* followed by three *culukas* (handfuls) of cow's urine and the patient should be exposed to sun for a brief period. By this, he vomits out all the accumulated waste products in the body within one hour. This is called *vāmanīya rasa* and it cures *jalodara*.

द्वितीयं भागमादाय पुटयेदौषधैस्ततः ।
त्रिवृद्दन्त्यर्कसेहुंडो रेचकी शंखिनी तथा ।
इन्द्रवारुणिका चैषां क्वाथं कुर्याद्विचक्षणः ॥१३५॥
तेन क्वाथेन पुटयेत् शतं वारान्[1] रसेश्वरं ।
ततश्च भावना देयास्तिस्रो लिंगीरसैः पुनः ॥१३६॥
कम्पिल्लक्वाथतस्तिस्रो दंतीनीरैश्च[2] भावना ।
त्रिवृत्क्वाथेन तिस्रः[3] स्यात् शंखिनीक्वाथतस्तथा ॥१३७॥
शम्पाकफलनीरेण मूलनीरेण वा ततः ।
अष्टादशैवं जायन्ते भावना रेचने[4] रसे ॥१३८॥
यत्नतः स्थापयेत्पश्चात्करण्डे तं[5] रसेश्वरम् ।
अर्द्धवल्लप्रमाणेन रसो[6] दद्याच्च रोगिणे[7] ॥१३९॥

1. वारात् इति प्रथमपुस्तके पाठः ।
2. ०दंतीनिरैश्च तावतीः इति षष्ठपुस्तके पाठः ।
3. तिह्मः इति चतुर्थपुस्तके पाठः ।
4. रेचनै इति षष्ठपुस्तके पाठः ।
5. च इति चतुर्थषष्ठपुस्तकयोः पाठः ।
6. रसं इति प्रथमपुस्तके पाठः ।
7. ०रोगिणा इति षष्ठपुस्तके पाठः ।

अनुपाने जलं देयं सुशीतं चुलुकावधि ।
यावंति[1] चुलुकान्यंबु पिबेत्तावंति रेचयेत् ॥१४०॥
अयं चुलुकभेदाख्यो रसो ह्युदररोगहृत्[2] ।
जलोदरादिरोगाणां मूलकर्त्तनदक्षिणः ॥१४१॥

The second part of this recipe should be impregnated, triturated and cooked in *puṭa* for one hundred times in each of the decoction of *trivṛt*, *dantī*, *arka*, *sehuṇḍa*, *recakī*, *śaṅkhinī* and *indra vāruṇī*. Then the recipe should again be impregnated for three times in each of the juice of *liṅgī* and decoction of *kampillaka*, *dantī*, *trivṛt*, *śaṅkhinī* as well as fruit or root of *śampāka*. Thus, in total, the recipe should be impregnated for eighteen times. Then carefully, the recipe should be stored in a clean jar. This should be administered in a dose of half *valla* followed by handful of cooled water. The number of motions he passes is similar to the number of handful of water he takes. This is called *culuka bheda rasa*. It cures *udara roga*. It is specially useful in rooting out ascites.

तृतीयं भागमादाय पुटयेत् त्रिफलोदकैः ।
शतवारात्र रसेन्द्रो सिद्धत्येवं न संशयः ॥१४२॥
रसेन्द्रस्य हि योज्यं स्यात् द्विवल्लं तु[3] रसायने ।
संसिद्ध्यात्[4] वृद्धाया[?] वक्ष्यमाण क्रमेण वै ॥१४३॥

---

1. जावंति इति षष्ठपुस्तके पाठः ।
2. ०रोगह्यात् इति चतुर्थपुस्तके पाठः ।
3. हि इति षष्ठपुस्तके पाठः ।
4. क. संसिद्धया तृवृद्धाया इति प्रथमपुस्तके पाठः ।
   ख. संसिद्धयात्रिवृतथा इति चतुर्थपुस्तके पाठः ।
   ग. संसिद्धयातृवृतया इति षष्ठपुस्तके पाठः ।

संवत्सरेण पलितं नाशयेत्पारदेश्वरः ।
द्वाभ्यां रोगान्[1] हरेत्सर्वान् सहस्रं जीवयेन्नरम्[2] ।
कालारिसंज्ञया सोऽयं रसेन्द्रः[3] परिकीर्त्तितः ॥१४४॥

The third part should be cooked in *puṭa* for one hundred times by impregnating with the decoction of *triphalā*. For the purpose of rejuvenation, it should be administered in a dose of two *vallas*. By using it for one year, the patient becomes free from gray hair. By using it for two years it cures all diseases and promotes longevity. This is called *kālāri rasa.*

एवं त्रिमूर्त्तिनामायं रसः शंकरनिर्मितः[4] ॥१४५॥

These three recipes, viz. *vāmanīya rasa*, *culuka bheda rasa* and *kālāri rasa*, taken together are called *trimūrti rasa*. It is propounded by Lord Śiva himself.

जीर्णशाल्योदनं[5] पथ्यं गोघृतं कृष्णमुद्गकाः ।
गौपयस्तद्भवं[6] तक्रं, यत्नादपि विवर्जयेत् ॥१४६॥
शाकं न किञ्चिद्योज्यं[7] स्याद्रसायनविधौ नरः ।
मद्यं मांसं मैथुनं च वर्जयेद्रससेवने ।
रसेन्द्रोऽयं त्रिमूर्त्याख्यः[8] स्वस्थै[9] सर्वैश्च सेव्यते ॥१४७॥

---

1. रोमान् इति प्रथमपंचमपुस्तकयोः पाठः ।
2. जीवयं नरम् इति षष्ठपुस्तके पाठः ।
3. सेरंद्रेः इति प्रथमपुस्तके पाठः ।
4. संकर निर्मितः इति प्रथमपुस्तके पाठः ।
5. जीर्णसाल्योदनं इति प्रथमपुस्तके पाठः ।
6. गोपयस्द्भवं इति चतुर्थषष्ठपुस्तकयोः पाठः ।
7. क. किं विद्योज्यं इति प्रथमपुस्तके पाठः ।
   ख. किंविद्योह्यं इति षष्ठपस्तके पाठः ।
8. त्रिमूत्याख्यः इति षष्ठपुस्तके पाठः ।
9. स्वस्थैः इति चतुर्थषष्ठपुस्तकयोः पाठः ।

Diet and Regimens

Old *śāli* rice, cow's ghee, black variety of *mudga*, cow's milk and butter-milk prepared of cow's milk are useful for the patient using *trimūrti rasa.* He should not use any vegetable if the intention is to get rejuvenating effect of this drug. The patient using mercurial compounds should avoid alcoholic drinks, meat and sexual intercourse. This *trīmūrti rasa* should be used even by all healthy persons [for the preservation and promotion of their positive health].

रसायनार्थिनः[1] कुर्युः दशभिर्दशभिर्दिनैः ।
वान्तिं विरेकं कालारिं नित्यं खादेत्पुरातनम् ॥१४८॥
गुल्मोदरी तु कालारिमिच्छया सेवते न वा ।
त्रिदिनात् त्रिदिनात्कुर्याद्वान्तिरेके[2] च बुद्धिमान् ॥१४९॥

Persons desirous of getting the rejuvenating effect of this recipe should take emetic and purgative therapies on every tenth day and use this old recipe of *kālāri rasa* every day. Patients suffering from *gulma* and *udara roga* may or may not use *kālāri rasa* but they should take emetic and purgation therapies every third day.

यमानिकाचित्रकयावशूकषड्ग्रंथदन्तीमगधोद्भवानाम् ।
प्लीहानमेतद्विनिहन्ति चूर्णमुष्णाम्बुना मस्तुसुरासवैर्वा[3] ॥१५०॥

Intake of the powder of *yamānikā*, *citraka*, *yava kṣāra*, *ṣaḍ-granthā*, *danti* and *pippali* along with warm water, *mastu* (thin whey), *surā* (an alcoholic drink) and *āsava* (a type of wine) cures splenic enlargement.

---

1. क. सेवनायार्थिनः इति चतुर्थपुस्तके पाठः ।
   ख. सादनायार्थिनः इति पंचमपुस्तके पाठः ।
   ग. सेवनापार्थित: कुर्य्याद्दशभि० इति षष्ठपुस्तके पाठ: ।
2. ०द्वान्तित्रिंशके इति षष्ठपुस्तके पाठः ।
3. मूत्रसुरा० इति चतुर्थपुस्तके पाठः ।

"पिप्पलीं किंशुकक्षारभावितां तां[1] प्रयोजयेत् ।
गुल्मप्लीहापहां वह्निदीपनीं परमं मताम् ॥१५१॥"

[भैषज्यरत्नावली : प्लीहयकृत्रोगाधिकार : १०]

Administration of *pippali* impregnated with the *kṣāra* (alkali preparation) of *kiṃśuka* cures *gulma* (phantom tumour) and splenic enlargement. It effectively stimulates the power of digestion.

"विडङ्गाग्निकार्किसिन्धूत्थशक्तून् दग्ध्वा वचान्वितान् ।
पिबेत् क्षीरेण संचूर्ण्य गुल्मप्लीहोदरापहम् ॥१५२॥"

[भैषज्यरत्नावली : प्लीहयकृत्रोगाधिकार : १६]

Viḍaṅga, arka, citraka, rock-salt, *śaktu* (roasted corn flour) and *vacā* should be burnt and made to a powder. Intake of this along with milk cures *gulma* (phantom tumour) and *plīhodara.*

"तालपुष्पभवः क्षारः सगुडः प्लीहनाशनः ॥१५३॥"

[भैषज्यरत्नावली : प्लीहयकृत्रोगाधिकार : ७]

Intake of the *kṣāra* (alkali preparation) of the infloresence of *tāla* along with jaggery cures splenic enlargement.

"क्षारं विडङ्गकृष्णाभ्यां[2] पूतीकस्याम्बुनिःश्रुतम्[3] ।
प्लीहायकृत्प्रशान्त्यर्थं पिबेत्प्रातर्यथाबलम् ॥१५४॥"

[भैषज्यरत्नावली : प्लीहयकृत्रोगाधिकार : ६]

---

1. संप्रयोजयेत् इति चतुर्थपुस्तके पाठः ।
2. कृष्णात्यां इति प्रथमपुस्तके पाठः ।
3. रोहितकाभयाक्वाथः कणाभ्यां क्षारसमन्वितः प्लुतम् इति षष्ठ-पुस्तके पाठः ।

The *kṣāra* (alkali preparation) of *viḍaṅga*, *kṛṣṇā* and *pūtīka* should be mixed with water and taken early in the morning depending upon the strength of the patient. It cures enlargement of spleen and liver.

"पातव्यो युक्तितः क्षारः क्षीरेणोदधिशुक्तिजः[1] ।
पयसा वा प्रयोक्तव्यः पिप्पल्यः प्लीहशान्तये ॥१५५॥"

[भैषज्यरत्नावली : प्लीहायकृत्रोगाधिकार : ११]

Intake of the *kṣāra* (alkali preparation) of *udadhi śukti* (sea shell) along with milk and intake of *pippalī* along with milk cures splenic enlargement.

"भल्लातकाभयाजाजी गुडेन सह मोदकः ।
सप्तरात्रान्निहन्त्येष प्लीहानमतिदारुणम् ॥१५६॥"

॥ भल्लातकमोदकः[2] ॥

[भारतभैषज्यरत्नाकर : तृतीयभाग : पृष्ठ ६३२]

Bhallātaka Modaka

Bhallātaka, *abhayā* and *ajājī* should be made to a powder and mixed with jaggery. Out of this, *modakas* (large size pills) should be prepared. Intake of this for seven nights cure serious type of splenic enlargement.

"सौभाञ्जनकनिर्यूहं सैन्धवाग्निकणान्वितम् ।
पलाशक्षारयुक्तं वा यवक्षारं प्रयोजयेत् ॥१५७॥"

[योगरत्नाकर : उदरचिकित्सा : ११२]

---

1. क. दधिशुक्तिजा इति पंचमपुस्तके पाठः ।
   ख. दधिसंयुतम् इति षष्ठपुस्तके पाठः ।
2. भल्लातकादिः इति प्रथमपंचमपुस्कयोः पाठः ।

Intake of the decoction or juice of *soubhāñjana* along with rock-salt, *citraka* and *pippalī* or *yava kṣāra* along with the *kṣāra* (alkali preparation) of *palāśa* cures splenic enlargement.

तिलान् सलवणांश्चैव घृतं षट्पलकं तथा ।
प्लीहोदिष्टां क्रियां सर्वां यकृतः संप्रयोजयेत् ॥१५८॥

For the treatment of liver disorders, *tila* along with rock-salt, *ṣaṭ palaka ghṛta* and recipes prescribed for splenic disorders should be administered.

लशुनं पिप्पलीमूलमभयां चैव भक्षयेत् ।
पिबेद्गोमूत्रगण्डूषं प्लीहरोगविमुक्तये ॥१५९॥

Intake of *laśuna*, *pippalī mūla* and *abhayā* along with cow's urine cures splenic enlargement.

'कार्षिकं पिप्पलीमूलं पंचैव लवणानि च ।
पिप्पली चित्रकं शुंठी त्रिफला त्रिवृता वचा ॥१६०॥
द्वौ क्षारौ सातला दंती स्वर्णक्षीरी विषाणिका ।
कोलप्रमाणां वटिकां पिबेत् सौवीरसंयुतम् ।
श्वयथावथ पक्वे च प्रवृद्धे च दकोदरे ॥१६१॥

॥ क्षारगुटिका ॥

Kṣāra Guṭikā

One *karṣa* of each of *pippalī mūla*, *pañca lavaṇa*, *pippalī*, *citraka*, *śuṇṭhī*, *triphalā*, *trivṛt*, *vacā*, *yava kṣāra*, *svarji kṣāra*, *sātalā*, *dantī*, *svarṇa kṣīrī* and *viṣāṇikā* should be triturated and pills of one *kola* each should be prepared. Intake of these pills with *sauvīra* (a type of vinegar) cures oedema and suppurated as well as serious type of *dakodara* (ascites).

सप्ताहं[1] महिषीमूत्रं पयसा चाम्बुर्वाजितम् ।
पीतमौष्ट्रं पयो मासं श्वयथूदरनाशनम्[2] ॥१६२॥'

Intake of buffalo-urine along with milk and without water for seven days cures oedema and *udara roga*. Similarly, intake, of camel milk for one month cures oedema and *udara roga*.

प्लीहजिच्छरपुंखायाः कल्कस्तक्रेण सेवितः ।
दृष्ट्वा प्रभावं सृष्टोत्र लोकोपकृतिहेतवे ।
एवं शास्त्रानुसारेण भट्टरामेश्वरेण हि ॥१६३॥

Intake of the paste of *śara puṅkhā* along with butter-milk cures enlarged spleen. Bhaṭṭa Rāma Miśra has propounded this recipe for the welfare of human beings after experiencing its therapeutic efficacy.

[3]शुद्धानां ताम्रपत्राणां पलानां विंशतिः स्मृता ।
पलानि पंच सूतस्य मर्दयेत् निम्बुकद्रवैः ॥१६४॥
तावत्संमर्दनं कुर्यात् यावत्संलगते रसः ।
तत्पात्रमध्ये निक्षिप्येत्तस्योर्ध्वाधश्च गन्धकम् ॥१६५॥
पूरयेच्चूर्णयित्वा तु शम्यक् दशपलोन्मितम् ।
चुल्हिकोग्नौ पचेत्सम्यक् निरुध्य घटिकात्रयम् ॥१६६॥

1. सप्ताह० इति प्रथमपुस्तके पाठः ।
2. 'कार्षिकं——— नाशनम्' । पाठोऽयं चतुर्थषष्ठपुस्तकयोः अधिकमुपलभ्यते ।
3. 'शुद्धा०———उदयभास्कररस' । पाठोऽयं पंचमपुस्तके अधिकमुपलभ्यते ।

स्वांगशीतलमादाय चूर्णयित्वा पुनश्च तत् ।
त्रिभागं कारयेत्तत्र भागमेकं पुनः पचेत् ॥१६७॥
गोमूत्रैर्विंशतिर्वारान् सभेदी जायते रसः ।
उदराणि कृमीन् हन्ति हरेच्च मलसंचयम् ॥१६८॥
शाम्येत् शीतोपचारेण तस्मादुष्णक्रिया पचेत् ।
पुनः द्वितीयं भागं तु गोक्षीरेण पचेत् शनैः ॥१६९॥
दशवारं तथा तोयैर्नारिकेरस्य वा पचेत् ।
अयं ग्रेल्पौरसो [?] नाम सर्वशूलविनाशनः ॥१७०॥
नाभिकुक्षिभवं शूलं शिरकर्णाक्षिगौरवम् ।
मुखपाकं पाण्डुरोगं मुखरोगं च दारुणम् ॥१७१॥
वातज्वरं पित्तभवं द्वंद्वजं सान्निपातिकम् ।
क्षयं कासं कृमिं चैव निहन्त्यादियनं [?] परम् ॥१७२॥
पुनस्तृतीयं भागं तु कटुवलरिकरसैः ।
भावयेद्विंशतिर्वारान् वामनो जायते रसः ॥१७३॥
देयोऽस्यवल्लमात्रं तु ताम्बूलरससंयुतम् ।
वमनं सर्वदोषघ्नमुपचारं तु पूर्ववत् ॥१७४॥
विसूचिकामम्लपित्तं शिरोजाड्यं विनाशयेत् ।
किं पुनर्बहुनोक्तेन सर्वशूलहरः परः ॥१७५॥

यस्मादुद्दीपयेदग्निं तस्मादुदयभास्करः ।
राजिकां लवणं नारीं कषायं कटुकं त्यजेत् ॥१७६॥

॥ उदयभास्कररसः ॥'

Udaya Bhāskara Rasa

Twenty *palas* of the purified *tāmra patra* (thin leaves of copper) and five *palas* of purified *pārada* should be added with lemon juice and triturated till fully amalgamated. It should be kept in a pot with ten *palas* of purified *gandhaka* above and below. This pot should be sealed and cooked over an oven for three hours. When it gets cooled of its own, it should be made to a powder. This powder should be divided into three parts. One part of it should be cooked by adding cow's urine for twenty times. It is called *bhedī rasa* which cures *udara roga*, parasitic infestation and constipation. Its effect diminishes by cooling therapy. Therefore, it should be given with hot things. The second part of the recipe should be gradually cooked by adding cow's urine or milky juice of coconut for ten times. This is called *grelpau rasa* [?] and it cures all types of colic pain, pain in umbilicus and pelvis, heaviness in head, ear and eyes, stomatitis, anemia, serious diseases of the mouth, fever caused by *vāyu*, *pitta*, two *doṣas* combined and all the three *doṣas* vitiated simultaneously, consumption, cough and parasitic infestation. The third part should be impregnated with the juice of *kaṭu vala rika* [?] for twenty times. This is called *vāmana rasa*. This should be administered in the dose of one *valla* along with the juice of *tambūla*. It causes emesis and alleviates all *doṣas*. The patient, after taking this recipe, should be managed as described before. It cures *visūcikā* (choleric diarrhoea), *amla pitta* (acidity in stomach) and stiffness of the head. What to speak of more; it cures all types of colic pain. Since it promotes the power of digestion, it is called *udaya bhāskara rasa*. While taking this recipe, the patient should avoid *rajikā*, salt, sexual intercourse, astringent and pungent things.

सम्मीरपनगस्यास्य द्विगुणं जयपालकाः ।
अजादुग्धेऽपि पक्वा तु[1] श्लक्ष्णो गुंजाद्वयं रसः ॥१७७॥
खण्डव्योषार्द्रकैर्दद्यात् पृथग्वा घृतसंप्लुतः ।
जयेद्गुल्मोदरप्लीहशूलामविषमज्वरान् ॥१७८॥
पथ्यं भुक्तं गवां तक्रं समीरं [?] च ज्वरादिषु ।
तापशेषे गुडूच्यंबु[2] व्याधिविध्वंसकारकः ॥१७९॥

॥ व्याधिविध्वंसनो रसः ॥

Vyādhi Vidhvaṁsana Rasa

Samīra pannaga should be added with double the quantity of purified *jaya pāla* and triturated by adding goat's milk till it becomes very soft. This should be administered in a dose of two *guñjās* (250 mg.) along with sugar, *vyoṣa* and *ārdraka* or ghee. It cures *gulma* (phantom tumour), *udara roga* splenic enlargement, colic pain, *āma jvara* (first stage of fever) and *viṣama jvara* (irregular fever). In fever, etc. the patient should take butter-milk prepared of cow's milk and after the fever is over, he should take juice of *guḍūci* by which the disease is completely destroyed.

'शीतलजलेन[3] विरेकः उष्णेन स्तम्भः ॥१८०॥

The above mentioned recipe causes purgation if taken along with cold water. If the patient takes hot water, then purgation stops.

---

1. पक्वास्तुम्लक्षणो इति प्रथमपुस्तके पाठः ।
2. गडूच्याम्बु व्याधिविध्वंसकारके इति पंचमपुस्तके पाठः ।
3. 'शीतल०———जलोदरम्' पाठोऽयं चतुर्थपुस्तके नोपलभ्यते ।

पिप्पली मरिचं ताम्रं कांचनीचूर्णसंयुतम् ।
स्नुहीक्षीरे दिनं मर्द्य तुल्यं जैपालबीजकम् ।
निष्कपादं विरेकोयं सत्यं हंति जलोदरम् ॥१८१॥'

One part of each of *pippalī*, *marica*, *tāmra bhasma* and *kāñcanī* should be added with four parts of purified *jayapāla* and triturated by adding with the milky latex of *snuhī*. This recipe should be administered in a dose of 1/4th *niṣka* which certainly cures ascites.

रेचनानां तु सर्वेषां दध्यन्नं स्तम्भने हितम् ।
आमांते च प्रदातव्यमन्यथा मुद्गयूषकम्[1] ॥१८२॥

Intake of curd and rice stops purgation. It should be given after purgation therapy only when *āma* (undigested product of food) is eliminated. Before that, the patient should be given soup of *mudga*.

वंगेश्वरं प्रवक्ष्यामि रसं प्लीहोदरापहम् ।
मंदाग्निघातने[2] शस्तं अन्त्रवृद्धिविकर्त्तनम् ॥१८३॥
अनूक्तेन प्रकारेण रसभस्मांतिकां: क्रियाम् ।
कृत्वा सूतं समादाय खल्वमध्ये[3] विनिक्षिपेत्[4] ॥१८४॥
साधारणोक्तमार्गेण कुट्टितं[5] भस्मयेद्बुधः ।
पश्चात्तस्य[6] प्रदेयानि पुटानि दशसंख्यया ॥१८५॥

---

1. मुद्गयूरवकं इति प्रथमपुस्तके पाठः ।
2. घातनशस्तं इति पंचमपुस्तके पाठः ।
3. षल्वमध्ये इति प्रथमपुस्तके पाठः ।
4. ०क्षिपेत् इति पंचमपुस्तके पाठः ।
5. कुट्टिलं इति चतुर्थपुस्तके पाठः ।
6. ०त्तस्यै इति चतुर्थपुस्तके पाठः ।

[1]क्षीरेण भानो संमर्द्य [2]कुकुट्टाख्यानि यत्नतः ।
पलमात्रे सूतभस्मन्येत्द्भूस्मवचं गजम् [?] ॥१८६॥
पलं द्वे च [3]पले ताम्रात्साधारणमृताद्भवेत् ।
[4]सामान्यशुद्धगंधं च द्वे पले सर्वमेकतः ॥१८७॥
मर्दयेद्भास्करभवैः पयोभिर्दिवस[5]त्रयम् ।
तं सूतं पुटयेत्पश्चाद्धटबीजैः [?] अथोपलैः ॥१८८॥
[6]मूषायां तं रसं [7]क्षिप्त्वा कुक्कुटाख्यं च मंदशः ।
एष वंगेश्वरो नाम रसेन्द्रः संप्रकाशितः ॥१८९॥
गुल्मप्लीहोदरच्छेदि[8] चतुराविष्कृतो भुवि ।
गुंजाद्वयप्रमाणेन [9]रसेन्द्रं संप्रयोजयेत् ॥१९०॥
वसुभट्टस्य चूर्णेन घृतेन सुरभी [10]भुवः ।

---

1. क्षारेण भानोः इति प्रथमपुस्तके पाठः ।
2. संमर्द्यन्तु कुट्टाख्यानि इति पंचमपुस्तके पाठः ।
3. भवे इति द्वितीय पुस्तके पाठः ।
4. सामान्ये इति पंचमपुस्तके पाठः ।
5. त्रयाम् इति चतुर्थपुस्तके पाठः ।
6. भूखायातां रसं इति चतुर्थपुस्तके पाठः ।
7. क्षित्वा इति पंचमपुस्तके पाठः ।
8. ०छेदचतुरो विश्रुतो भुवि इति चतुर्थपुस्तके पाठः ।
9. क. रसेन्द्रे प्रयोजयेत् इति चतुर्थपुस्तके पाठः ।
   ख. रसेन्द्रः इति पंचमपुस्तके पाठः ।
10. क. भुवा इति चतुर्थपुस्तके पाठः ।
    ख. भुवः इति पंचमपुस्तके पाठः ।

पथ्यं च पूर्ववत्कुर्यात्प्लीहगुल्मोदरं छिदेत् ॥१६१॥

॥ वंगेश्वरः ॥

Vaṅgeśvara Rasa

Now *vaṅgeśvara rasa* which cures splenic enlargement, *udara roga*, suppression of the power of digestion and *āntra vṛddhi* (inguinal hernia) will be described. *Bhasma* of *pārada* should be prepared according to the prescribed procedure and kept in a pestle and mortar. Separately, according to the prescribed procedure, *bhasma* of *vaṅga* should be prepared. This should be impregnated with the milky latex of *arka* and cooked in *kukkuṭa puṭa* for ten times. One *pala* of the *bhasma* of *pārada* (described earlier), one *pala* of *vaṅga bhasma*, two *palas* of *tāmra bhasma* and two *palas* of purified *gandhaka*—all should be mixed together and triturated for three days by adding the milky latex of *arka*. This should then be kept in a *mūṣā* (crucible) and cooked in *kukkuṭa puṭa* by the fire of cow-dung cakes. This is called *vaṅgeśvara rasa*. It cures *gulma* (phantom tumour) and *plīhodara* and it is discovered by a wise physician. It should be administered in a dose of two *guñjās* (250 mg) along with the powder of *vasu bhaṭṭa*, ghee or cow's urine. While using this recipe for the cure of splenic enlargement, *gulma* (phantom tumour) and *udara roga*, the patient should use wholesome diet as described before.

प्रकारांतरेण वंगेश्वरो लिख्यते[1] ॥१६२॥

सूतभस्मं वंगभस्मभागैकैकं प्रकल्पयेत् ।

गंधकं मृतताम्रं[2] च प्रत्येकं च चतुःपलम् ॥१६३॥

अर्कक्षीरैर्दिनं मर्द्यं सर्वं तद्गोलकीकृतम् ।

रुध्वाह्लं भूधरे पचयात् पुटैकेन समुद्धरेत् ॥१६४॥

1. ०लिष्यतो इति प्रथमपुस्तके पाठः ।

2. च भागैकैकं प्रकल्प प्रत्येकं च चतुः पलं इति प्रथमपुस्तके पाठः ।

एष वंगेश्वरो नाम्ना प्लीहगुल्मोदरं जयेत् ।
घृतं[1] गुंजाद्वयं लिह्येत् निष्कं श्वेतपुनर्नवाम्[2] ।
गवां मूत्रे पिवेच्यानु रजनीं वा गवां जलैः ॥१९५॥

॥ वंगेश्वरः ॥

Vaṅgeśvara Rasa (*second recipe*)

Now another recipe of *vaṅgeśvara rasa* is being described. *Bhasma* of *pārada* (one *pala*), *bhasma* of *vaṅga* (one *pala*), purified *gandhaka* (four *palas*) and *tāmra bhasma* (four *palas*) should be triturated by adding the milky latex of *arka* for one day. This paste should be made to a bolus form, kept in a sealed container and cooked in *puṭa* for one day. This is called *vaṅgeśvara rasa* which cures splenic enlargement and *gulma* (phantom tumour). It should be administered in a dose of two *guñjās* (250 mg.) with white variety of *punarnavā* or *rajanī* and cow's urine as *anupāna*.

पंचागं देवदाल्यास्तु[3] चूर्णं कर्षं शिवाम्बुना ।
मासमात्रं पिवेद्यस्तु प्लीहा तस्य करोति किम् ॥१९६॥

Intake of the powder of all the five parts of *devadālī* in a dose of one *karṣa* along with cow's urine (*śivāmbu* also means one's own urine) for one month cures splenic enlargement.

"यमानिकाचित्रकयावशूकं षड्ग्रंथ[4]दन्तीमगधोद्भवानाम्[5] ।
प्लीहानमेतद्विनिहन्ति चूर्णमुष्णाम्बुना मस्तुसुरासवैर्वा ॥१९७॥"

[भैषज्यरत्नावली : प्लीहयकृद्रोगाधिकार : १]

---

1. घृतं इति चतुर्थपुस्तके पाठः ।
2. स्वेतपुनर्णवां इति प्रथमपुस्तके पाठः ।
3. ०स्तू चूर्णं कर्षशिवाम्बु इति पंचमपुस्तके पाठः ।
4. ०षड्ग्रन्थि इति चतुर्थपुस्तके पाठः ।
5. ०मगधाद्भवानाम् इति प्रथमपुस्तके पाठः ।

Intake of the powder of *yamānikā*, *citraka*, *yava kṣāra*, *ṣaḍ granthā*, *dantī* and *pippalī* along with hot water, *mastu* (thin whey), *surā* (alcoholic preparation) or *āsava* (a type of wine) cures splenic enlargement.

[1]"रसेन जम्भीरफलस्य शंखनाभीरजः पीतमवश्यमेव ।

कर्षप्रमाणं शमयेदशेषं प्लीहामयं कूर्मसमानमाशु ॥१९८॥"

[भैषज्यरत्नावली : प्लीहयकृद्रोगाधिकारः १४]

Intake of the *bhasma* of *śaṅkha nābhi* (conch shell) in a dose of one *karṣa* along with the juice of *jambīra* cures instantaneously splenic enlargement which is as hard and smooth as the back of a tortoise.

[2]शार्ङ्गष्ठा काकणन्ति च काकमाच्यां करञ्जके ॥१९९॥

Intake of *śārṅgaṣṭhā* and *kākaṇanti* along with *kākamācī* and *karañja* [cures splenic enlargement].

"शार्ङ्गष्ठा(यांग)निर्यूहः सैन्धवः तिन्तिडीसंविमिश्रः ।

प्लीहव्युपरमो योगः पक्वाम्ररसोऽथवा समधुः ॥२००॥"

[भैषज्यरत्नावलीः प्लीहयकृद्रोगाधिकार : ३]

Decoction of *śārṅgaṣṭhā* mixed with rock-salt and *tintiḍī* or the juice of mango mixed with honey cures splenic enlargement.

[3]'सुस्विन्नशाल्मलीपुष्पं निशापर्युषितं नरः ।

राजिकाचूर्णसंयुक्तं सद्यः प्लीहोपशांतये ॥२०१॥'

---

1. 'रसेन——कूर्मसमानमाशु' । पाठोऽयं चतुर्थपुस्तके अधिकमुपलभ्यते ।
2. 'शार्ङ्गष्टा——करञ्जके' पाठोऽयं पंचमपुस्तके अधिकमुपलभ्यते ।
3. 'सुस्विन्न०———प्लीहोपशांत्तये' पाठोऽयं षष्ठपुस्तके अधिकमुपलभ्यते ।

Flower of *śālmalī* should be soaked in water and kept overnight. Intake of this along with the powder of *rājikā* instantaneously cures splenic enlargement.

"रोहीतकाभयाक्षोद[1]भावितं मूत्रमम्बुना ।
पीतं सर्वोदरप्लीहमेहार्शकृमिगुल्मनुत्[2] ॥२०२॥"

Intake of the powder of *rohitaka* and *abhayā* along with cow's urine and water cures all types of *udara roga*, splenic enlargement, *meha* (urinary disorders including diabetes), piles, parasitic infestation and *gulma* (phantom tumour).

दध्ना भुक्तवतोः वामबाहुमध्ये शिरां भिषक् ।
बिध्येत् प्लीहविनाशाय यकृत् नाशाय दक्षिणे[3] ॥२०३॥
प्लीहान मर्द्दयेद्गाढं दुष्टरक्तप्रवृत्तये ॥२०४॥

After the intake of curd along with food, venesection should be performed in the left arm of the patient for the cure of splenic enlargement and in the right arm for the cure of liver enlargement. During venesection the spleen should be massaged forcefully for the elimination of the polluted blood.

"माणमाह्वामृता वासा स्थिरा चित्रकसैन्धवम् ।
नागरं तालखण्डं च प्रत्येकं च त्रिकार्षिकम् ॥२०५॥
विडसौवर्च्चल[4]क्षारपिप्पल्यश्चापि कार्षिकाः ।
एतच्चूर्णीकृत सर्वं गोमूत्रस्याढके पचेत् ॥२०६॥

---

1. ०शुण्ठीः पिबेन्मूत्रण शक्तितः इति आकरे पाठः ।
2. दृष्टव्यम्———योगरत्नाकरः उदरचिकित्साः पृष्ठ ११५ ।
3. दधिणे इति चतुर्थपुस्तके पाठः ।
4. ०क्षीर० इति प्रथमपुस्तके पाठः ।

सान्द्रीभूते गुडीं[1] कुर्यात् दत्वा त्रिफलामाक्षिकम्[2] ।
यकृत्प्लीहोदरहरो गुल्मार्शोग्रहणीहरः ।
योगः परिकरो नाम्ना अग्निसन्दीपनः[3] परा ॥२०७॥"

॥ माणादिगुडिका[4] ॥

[भैषज्यरत्नावली : प्लीहयकृद्रोगाधिकार : २२-२४]

Māṇādi Guṭikā

Three *karṣas* of each of *māṇa*, *amṛtā*, *vāsā*, *sthirā*, *citraka* and *saindhava*, and one *karṣa* of each of *viḍa*, *sauvarcala*, *kṣāra* (alkali preparation) as well as *pippalī*—all these drugs should be triturated and cooked in one *āḍhaka* of cow's urine. When it becomes semisolid, powder of *triphalā* and honey should be added and pills should be prepared out of this paste. It cures *yakṛt-dālyudara*, *plīhodara*, *gulma* (phantom tumour), piles and *grahaṇī* (sprue syndrome). It is called *parikara yoga* and it stimulates the power of digestion.

"पिप्पली नागरं दन्तीं समांशं द्विगुणाभयाम् ।
चूर्णं पीतं विडार्द्धांशं प्लीहघ्नमुष्णवारिणा ॥२०८॥"

[भैषज्यरत्नावली : प्लीहयकृद्रोगाधिकार : ४]

Intake of the powder of *pippalī* (one part), *nāgara* (one part), *danti* (one part), *abhayā* (two parts) and *viḍa* (half part) along with hot water cures splenic enlargement.

---

1. क. गुटीं इति षष्ठपुस्तके पाठः ।
   ख. भूते इति चतुर्थपुस्तके पाठः ।
2. त्रिपला० इति आदर्शपुस्तकेषु पाठः ।
3. वह्नि इति चतुर्थषष्ठपुस्तकयोः पाठः ।
4. मानकादि गुडिका इति आकरे पाठः ।

"क्रमवृद्ध्या दशाहानि दशपैप्पलिक दिनम् ।
वर्द्धयेत्पयसा सार्द्धं तथैवापनयेत्पुनः ॥२०६॥
जीर्णे जीर्णे च भुञ्जीत षष्टिकं[1] क्षीरसर्पिषा ।
पिप्पलीनां सहस्रस्य प्रयोगोऽयं रसायनः ॥२१०॥
पिष्टास्ता[2] बलिभिः पेया शृता मध्यबलैर्नरैः ।
[3]चूर्णीकृता स्त्वल्पबलैर्देहदोषामयान् प्रति ॥२११॥
दशपैप्पलिकः श्रेष्ठो मध्यमे[4] षट् प्रकीर्तितः[5] ।
[6]षष्टिपिप्पलिपर्यन्तः प्रयोगः सोऽवरः[7] स्मृतः ॥२१२॥
बृंहणं वृष्यमायुष्यं प्लीहोदरविनाशनम् ।
वयसः स्थापनं मेध्यं पिप्पलीनां रसायनम्[8] ।
पञ्चपिप्पलिकश्चातो दृश्यते वर्द्धमानकः ॥२१३॥
॥ पिप्पलीवर्द्धमानानि ॥"

[भैषज्यरत्नावली: प्लीहयकृद्रोगाधिकार : ४६-५३]

---

1. प्रस्थैकं इति षष्ठपुस्तके पाठः ।
2. पिष्ट्वा च इति आकरे पाठः ।
3. शीतीकृता ह्रस्वबलैर्देह० इति आकरे पाठः ।
4. मध्यमः इति आकरे पाठः ।
5. प्रकीर्तिताः इति आदर्शपुस्तकेषु पाठः ।
6. यस्त्रि० इति आकरे पाठः ।
7. क. सोयमानिका इति प्रथमपुस्तके पाठः ।
   ख. सोधमानिका इति पंचमपुस्तके पाठः ।
8. रसोयनम् इति प्रथमपुस्तके पाठः ।

Vardhamāna Pippalī Prayoga

One thousand *pippalīs* should be administered by increasing ten *pippalīs* every day for ten days and similarly by decreasing ten *pippalīs* every day along with milk. After *pippalī* and milk are digested, the patient should be given *ṣaṣṭika* type of rice to eat along with milk and ghee. This is rejuvenating. To a strong patient it should be given in the form of a paste. To a patient of moderate strength, it should be given in the form of a decoction and to the patient with less of strength, it should be given in a powder form. However, the mode of administration should be determined on the basis of the nature of the physique, *doṣas* and the disease. Increasing and decreasing by ten *pippalīs* is the best and it is moderate to increase and decrease at the rate of six *pippalīs* per day. Administration of only sixty *pippalīs* in total is of inferior nature. It promotes nourishment, virility and longevity. It cures splenic enlargement. It restores youth and promotes intellect. Some physicians administer this therapy even by increasing five *pippalīs* per day.

"पिप्पलीचित्रकान्मूलं पिष्ट्वा सम्यग्विपाचयेत् ।
घृतं चतुर्गुणं क्षीरं यकृत्प्लीहोदरापहम् ॥२१४॥

॥ चित्रकपिप्पलीघृतम् ॥

Citraka Pippalī Ghṛta

Ghee should be cooked by adding the paste of the root of *pippalī* and *citraka* and four times of milk. This medicated ghee cures *yakṛt dālyudara* and *plīhodara*.

पिप्पलीकल्कसंयुक्तं घृतं क्षीरचतुर्गुणम् ।
पचेत्प्लीहाग्निसादादियकृद्रोगहरं परम् ॥२१५॥"

॥ पिप्पलीघृतम् ॥

[भैषज्यरत्नावली : प्लीहयकृद्रोगाधिकार : ६७-६८]

Pippalī Ghṛta

Ghee should be cooked by adding the paste of *pippali* and four times of milk. This medicated ghee cures splenic enlargement, suppression of the power of digestion and enlargement of liver.

"चित्रकस्य तुलाक्वाथे घृतप्रस्थं विपाचयेत् ।
आरनालं तद्[1] द्विगुणं दधिमण्डं चतुर्गुणम् ॥२१६॥
पञ्चकोलकतालीशक्षारैर्लवणसंयुतैः[2] ।
द्विजीरकनिशायुग्मैर्मरिचं तत्र दापयेत् ॥२१७॥
प्लीहगुल्मोदराध्मानपाण्डुरोगारुचिज्वरान् ।
बस्तिहृत्पार्श्वकट्यूरुशूलोदावर्त्तपीनसान्[3] ॥२१८॥
हन्यात्पीतं तदर्शोघ्नं शोथघ्नं वह्निदीपनम् ।
बलवर्णकरश्चापि भस्मकञ्च नियच्छति ॥२१९॥

॥ चित्रकघृतम् ॥

[भैषज्यरत्नावली : प्लीहयकृद्रोगाधिकार : ६९-७२]

Citraka Ghṛta

One *prastha* of ghee should be cooked along with one *tulā* of the decoction of *citraka*, two *prasthas* of *āranāla*, four *prasthas* of *dadhi maṇḍa* and the paste of *pañca kola*, *tāliśa*, *kṣāra* (alkali preparation), *lavaṇa*, *śveta jīraka*, *kṛṣṇa jīraka*, *niśā*, *dāru*

1. च इति षष्ठपुस्तके पाठः ।
2. ०संयुतः इति षष्ठपुस्तके पाठः ।
3. ०पीनसात् इति प्रथमपंचमपुस्तकयोः पाठः ।

niśā and *marica*. It cures splenic enlargement, *gulma* (phantom tumour), *udara roga*, abdominal distension, anemia, anorexia, fever, pain in urinary bladder, heart, sides of the chest, lumber region and thighs, *udāvarta* (upward movement of *vāyu* in the abdomen), *pīnasa* (chronic rhinitis), piles and oedema. It stimulates the power of digestion and promotes strength as well as complexion. It also cures *bhasmaka* (voraceous appetite).

"कदलीतिलनालानां क्षारेण क्षुरकस्य च ।
तैलं[1] पक्वं जयेत्पानात् प्लीहानं कफवातजम् ॥२२०॥"
॥ कदलीक्षारतैलम्[2] ॥

[भैषज्यरत्नावली : प्लीहयकृद्रोगाधिकार : ५]

Kadalī Kṣāra Taila

Til oil should be cooked with the *kṣāra* (alkali preparation) of *kadali* and stems of *tila* and *kṣuraka*. Intake of this oil cures splenic enlargement caused by *kapha* as well as *vāyu*.

"[3]रोहीतकत्वचः श्रेष्ठाः पलानां पञ्चविंशतिः ।"
कोलं द्विप्रस्थसंयुक्तं कषायमुपकल्पयेत् ॥२२१॥
[4]पलिकैः पञ्चकोलैश्च तैः सर्वैश्चापि तुल्यया ।
रोहीतकत्वचापिष्टैर्घृतप्रस्थं विपाचयेत् ॥२२२॥

1. पीतं तैलं जयेन्नृणां प्लीहानम् इति आकरे पाठः ।
2. कदल्यादि क्षारतैलम् इति आकरे पाठः ।
3. 'रोहीतकत्वचः——विंशति' पाठोऽयं षष्ठपुस्तके नोपलभ्यते ।
4. पालिकैः इति आदर्शपुस्तकेषु पाठः ।

प्लीहाभिवृद्धि[1] शमयेदेतदाशु प्रयोजितम् ।
तथा गुल्मज्वरश्वासं कृमिपाण्डुत्वकामलाम्[2] ॥२२३॥"

॥ रोहातकघृतम् ॥

[भैषज्यरत्नावली : प्लीहयकृद्रोगाधिकार : ७३-७५]

Rohītaka Ghṛta

Twenty five *palas* of *rohītaka* bark and two *prasthas* of *kola* should be boiled with water and a decoction should be prepared. To this decoction, one *prastha* of ghee and the paste of one *pala* of each of *pippali*, *pippali mūla*, *cavya*, *citraka*, *nāgara* and five *palas* of the bark of *rohītaka* should be added and cooked. Administration of this medicated ghee instantaneously cures splenic enlargement, *gulma* (phantom tumour), fever, asthma, parasitic infestation, anemia and jaundice.

[3]भागा रसस्य चत्वारो ह्यष्टौ गन्धकभागकाः ।
मनः शिलाद्विभागं स्यात् हरिद्रात्रिफला तथा ॥२२४॥
आग्नेयो जयपालश्च तृवृत्ता त्रयभागिका ।
कटुत्रयं च वन्ती च तुम्बुरुश्चाष्टभागकाः ॥२२५॥
ऐषां चूर्णं समादाय दापयेत्सप्तभावना ।
जयन्त्या वज्रदुग्धस्य वानरीभृंगराजयोः ॥२२६॥
जलोदरं नुदत्याशु दापयेत् निष्कमात्रकम् ।
विरेकं किल संजातं तक्रभक्तं ससैन्धवम् ॥२२७॥

---

1. प्लीहानिवृद्धि इति पंचमपुस्तके पाठः ।
2. कामला इति आदर्शपुस्तकेषु पाठः ।
3. 'भागा———प्रदापयेत्' पाठोऽयं पंचमपुस्तके अधिकमुपलभ्यते ।

दिनान्ते दापयेत्पथ्यं शीतं वारि न दापयेत् ।
अपामार्गक्षारजलमनुपानं प्रदापयेत् ॥२२८॥

A powder should be prepared of purified *pārada* (four parts), purified *gandhaka* (eight parts), purified *manaḥ śilā* (two parts), *haridrā* (three parts), *harītakī* (three parts), *bibhītakī* (three parts), *āmalakī* (three parts), *āgneya* (three parts), purified *jayapāla* (three parts), *śuṇṭhī* (eight parts), *pippalī* (eight parts), *marica* (eight parts), *dantī* (eight parts) and *tumburu* (eight parts). This powder should be impregnated with the juice of *jayantī*, milky latex of *vajra*, juice of *vānarī* and the juice of *bhṛṅga rāja*. It should be administered in a dose of one *niṣka*. It immediately cures *jalodara* (ascites). If there is more of purgation, then the patient should be given rice with butter-milk and rock-salt to eat. Wholesome diet should be given to the patient in the evening. Cold water should not be given to him. As *anupāna* (post-prandial drink), the water mixed with the *kṣāra* (alkali preparation) of *apāmārga* should be given along with this recipe.

"रोहितकात्पलशतं क्षोदयेद्बदराढकम् ।
साधयित्वा जलद्रोणे चतुर्भागावशेषितम्[1] ॥२२९॥
घृतप्रस्थं समावाप्य छागक्षीरं चतुर्गुणम् ।
तस्मिन् दद्यादिमान् कल्कान् सर्वांस्तानक्षसम्मितान् ॥२३०॥
व्योषं फलत्रिकं हिंगु यमानी तुम्बुरु विडम् ।
अजाजी कृष्णलवणं दाडिमं देवदारु च ॥२३१॥

---

1. क. ०वशेषिते इति प्रथमपुस्तके पाठः ।
ख. ०वशेषते इति पंचमपुस्तके पाठः ।
ग. ०वशेवितम् इति षष्ठपुस्तके पाठः ।

पुनर्नवा[1] विशाला च यवक्षारं सपौष्करम् ।
विडङ्गं[2] चित्रकञ्चैव हवुषा चविका वचा ॥२३२॥
एतैर्घृतं[3] विपक्वन्तु स्थापयेद्भाजने शुभे ।
पाययेत्[4] त्रिपलां मात्रां व्याधि बलमवेक्ष्य च ॥२३३॥
रसकेनाथ यूषेण पयसा वापि[5] भोजयेत् ।
उपयुक्ते[6] घृते तस्मिन्[7] व्याधीन् हन्यादिमान् बहून् ॥२३४॥
यकृत्प्लीहोदरञ्चैव प्लीहशूलं यकृत्तथा ।
कुक्षिशूलं हृदिशूलं पार्श्वशूलमरोचकम् ॥२३५॥
विबन्धशूलं शमयेत् पाण्डुरोगं सकामलाम्[8] ।
छर्द्द्यतीसारशूलघ्नं[9] तन्द्राज्वरविनाशनम् ।
महारोहीतकं नाम प्लीहानं[10] हन्ति दारुणम् ॥२३६॥

॥ महारोहीतकघृतम् ॥"

[भैषज्यरत्नावली : प्लीहयकृद्रोगाधिकार : ७६-८३]

1. पुनर्नवां विशालां इति आदर्शपुस्तकेषु पाठः ।
2. विडङ्गचित्रकञ्चैव हवुषा चविकां वचां इति आदर्शपुस्तकेषु पाठः ।
3. एभिर्घृतं इति आकरे पाठः ।
4. द्वितोलकमितां मात्रां इति आकरे पाठः ।
5. वाथभोजयेत् इति षष्ठपुस्तके पाठः ।
6. उपयुक्तं घृतम् इति आकरे पाठः ।
7. त्वेतद् इति आकरे पाठः ।
8. क. सकामलम् इति आकरे पाठः ।
   ख. च कामलाम् इति षष्ठपुस्तके पाठः ।
9. छर्द्यतीसारशमनम् इति आदर्शपुस्तकेषु पाठः ।
10. प्लीहघ्नन्तु विशेषतः इति आदर्शपुस्तकेषु पाठः ।

Mahā Rohītaka Ghṛta

Coarse powder of *rohītaka* (one hundred *palas*) and *badara* (one *āḍhaka*) should be boiled with one *droṇa* of water and reduced to one fourth. To this decoction, one *prastha* of ghee, four *prasthas* of goat's milk and the paste of one *akṣa* of each of *vyoṣa, triphalā, hiṅgu, yamānī, tumburu, viḍa, ajājī, kṛṣṇa lavaṇa, dāḍima, deva dāru, punarnavā, viśālā, yava kṣāra, puṣkara mūla, viḍaṅga, citraka, havuṣā, cavikā* and *vacā* should be added and cooked. This medicated ghee should be stored in a clean jar and administered in a dose of three *palas* depending upon the condition of the disease as well as strength of the patient along with meat-soup, vegetable soup or milk. It cures *yakṛd dālyudara, plīhodara,* pain in spleen, liver, pelvis, heart and sides of the chest, anorexia, pain caused by constipation, anemia, jaundice, vomiting, diarrhoea, colic pain, drowsiness and fever. It is called *mahā rohītaka ghṛta* which is specially effective in curing serious type of splenic enlargement.

"पारिभद्रपलाशार्कस्नुह्यपामार्गचित्रकान् ।
वरुणाग्निमन्थवसुकश्वदंष्ट्राबृहतीद्वयम् ॥२३७॥
'पूतीकाऽस्फोत[1]कुटजकोशातक्यः पुनर्नवा ।
समूलदल[2]शाखास्तु क्षोदयित्वा उदूखले ॥२३८॥
तिलनालप्रदीप्ताग्निदग्धं[3] भस्म सुशीतलम्[4] ।'
क्षारप्रस्थं गृहीत्वा तु न्यसेत्पात्रे दृढे नवे ॥२३९॥
जलद्रोणे विपक्तव्यं यावत्[5] पादावशेषितम् ।
पूर्ववत्क्षारकल्केन साधयेच्च[6] विचक्षणः ॥२४०॥

1. ०श्वेतकुटजकोषातक्य: ति आदर्शपुस्तकेषु पाठः ।
2. ०पत्रशाखाश्च इति आकरे पाठः ।
3. सुदग्धं भस्मशीतलम् इति आकरे पाठः ।
4. 'पूतीका— —सुशीतलम्' पाठोऽयं षष्ठपुस्तके नोपलभ्यते ।
5. ग्राह्यं इति आकरे पाठः ।
6. स्रावयीत इति आकरे पाठः ।

प्रस्थमेकञ्च लवणं तदर्द्धाञ्च हरीतकीम् ।
तुल्याम्बुभागं गोमूत्रं साधयेन्मृदुनाग्निना ॥२४१॥
किञ्चित्सवाष्पसान्द्रे[1] च सम्यक्सिद्धेऽवतारिते ।
'[2]अजाजी त्र्यूषणं हिङ्गु यमानी पौष्करं[3] शटी ॥२४२॥
एतैरर्द्धपलभागैश्चूर्णं कृत्वा प्रदापयेत् ।'
लवणं[4] चाभया नाम भक्षयेच्च यथाबलम् ॥२४३॥
व्याधिञ्चावेक्ष्य[5] मतिमाननुपानं यथोचितम्[6] ।
ये च कोष्ठगता रोगास्तान्निहन्ति न संशयः ॥२४४॥
यकृत्प्लीहोदरानाहगुल्माष्ठीलाग्निसादनुत्[7] ।
हन्याच्छिरोऽर्त्तिहृद्रोगं[8] शर्कराश्मरिनाशनम् ॥२४५॥

॥ अभयालवणम् ॥"

[भैषज्यरत्नावली : प्लीहयकृद्रोगाधिकार : ३५-४३]

Abhayā Lavaṇa

Pāribhadra, *palāśa*, *arka*, *snuhī*, *apāmārga*, *citraka*, *varuṇa*, *agni mantha*, *vasuka*, *śvadamṣṭrā*, *bṛhati*, *kaṇṭakārī*, *pūtika*,

---

1. क. किञ्चित्सवास्य सान्द्रेषु इति प्रथमपुस्तके पाठः ।
   ख. किञ्चित्सवास्य सान्द्रे तु इति चतुर्थपंचमषष्ठपुस्तकेषु पाठः ।
2. 'अजाजी———प्रदापयेत्' पाठोऽयं प्रथमपंचमपुस्तकयोः नोपलभ्यते ।
3. पुष्करं इति चतुर्थषष्ठपुस्तकयोः पाठः ।
4. अभयालवणं नाम इति आकरे पाठः ।
5. व्याधिञ्च वीक्ष्य इति आकरे पाठः ।
6. यथाहितम् इति आकरे पाठः ।
7. क. ०सादजित् इति आकरे पाठः ।
   ख. सादहृत् इति षष्ठपुस्तके आकरे पाठः ।
8. प्रति हन्याच्चहृद्रोगं सर्वाश्मरिविनाशनम् इति आदर्शपुस्तकेषु पाठः ।

āsphota, *kuṭaja*, *kośātakī* and *punarnavā* along with their roots, leaves and stems should be pounded and burnt with the fire of stems of *tila*. The *kṣāra* (alkali preparation), thus prepared, should be allowed to cool down. One *prastha* of this *kṣāra* should be boiled by adding one *droṇa* of water till one fourth remains. To this, one *prastha* of rock-salt, half *prastha* of *harītakī* and one *droṇa* of cow's urine should be added and further boiled over mild fire. When it has become semi-solid, the cooking vessel should be taken out of the oven, and to this, the powder of half *pala* of each of *ajājī*, *tryūṣaṇa*, *hiṅgu*, *yamānī*, *puṣkara mūla* and *śaṭī* should be added. This is called *abhayā lavaṇa*. It should be administered with appropriate vehicles and in appropriate dose depending upon the strength of the patient and seriousness of the disease. It undoubtedly cures all diseases of gastro-intestinal tract including *yakṛd dālyudara*, *plīhodara*, abdominal distension, *gulma* (phantom tumour), *aṣṭhīlā* (stoney growth in the abdomen), suppression of the power of digestion, *chidrodara*, heart disease, *śarkarā* (graveluria) and *aśmarī* (stone in the urinary tract).

[1]औदकानूपजं मांसं शाकं पिष्टकृतं तिलाः ।
व्यायामा[2]ध्वदिवास्वप्नपानाजीर्णं विवर्जयेत् ॥२४६॥

Prohibitions

The patient suffering from *udara roga* should avoid meat of marshy and aquatic animals, vegetables, pastries, *tila*, exercise, walking a long distance, sleep during the day time and excessive intake of alcohol.

---

1. क्षादकानूपजं इति षष्ठपुस्तके पाठः ।
2. ०माध्व० इति पंचमपुस्तके पाठः ।

इति श्रीमहाराजाधिराजश्रीटोडरमल्लविरचिते टोडरानन्दे आयुर्वेदसौख्ये उदरनिदानचिकित्साकथनं नाम सप्तचत्वारिंशत्तमो हर्षः ॥२४७॥

Thus, ends the 47th Chapter dealing with the diagnosis and the treatment of *udara roga* in *Āyurveda saukhya* of *Ṭoḍarānanda* composed by the great king Ṭoḍara Malla.

CHAPTER XIII

अथ शोथनिदानं चिकित्सा च ।

Diagnosis and Treatment of Oedema

"रक्तपित्तकफान्[1] वायुर्दुष्टो दुष्टान्बहिःशिराम्[2] ।
नीत्वा रुद्धगतिस्तैर्हि कुर्यात्त्वङ्मांससंश्रयम् ।
उत्सेधं संहतं शोथं तमाहुर्निचयादतः ॥१॥

Pathogenesis

The aggravated *vāyu* afflicts *rakta* (blood), *pitta* and *kapha* and carry these vitiated elements to vessels in the exterior of

---

1. This is the beginning of the 52nd Chapter of *Āyurveda saukhya* in *Ṭoḍarānanda* and the invocation reads as follows :—
बृजांगनवीक्ष्य पुनारमेशकं प्रोतस्थुरुर्व्या इव जीव आगते ।
अंगानिता सांप्रददौमहत्सुखं ददातु यस्तन्नृपतौ महत्तरम् ॥
2. सिरा इति प्रथमपंचमपुस्तकयोः पाठः ।

the body. In the skin and the muscles, *vāyu* itself gets obstructed by these vitiated elements as a result of which elevated and compact oedema is manifested. Because of this oedema is considered to be caused by all the three *doṣas*, viz. *vāyu*, *pitta* and *kapha*.

सर्वं हेतुविशेषैस्तु रूपभेदान्नवात्मकम् ।
दोषैः पृथग्द्वयैः सर्वैरभिघाताद्विषादपि ॥२॥

Varieties

Even though, in the general pathogenesis, all the three *dosas* are afflicted, still depending upon the causative factors and signs as well as symptoms, oedema is classified into nine varieties, viz. *vātika*, *paittika*, *kaphaja*, *vāta-pittaja*, *vāta-kaphaja*, *pitta-kaphaja*, *sānnipātika*, *abhighātaja* (caused by external injury) and *viṣaja* (caused by poisoning).

तत्पूर्वरूपं क्षवथुः शिरायामोऽङ्गगौरवम् ॥३॥

Premonitory Signs and Symptoms

Sneezing, vascular prominence and heaviness of limbs—these are the premonitory signs and symptoms of oedema.

शुद्ध्यामयाभुक्त[1]कृशाबलानां क्षाराम्लतीक्ष्णोष्णगुरू[2]पसेवा ।
दध्याममृच्छाकविरोधिदुष्टगरोपसृष्टान्ननिषेवणं च ॥४॥
अर्शांस्यचेष्टा न च देहशुद्धिर्मर्मोपघातो विषमा[3] प्रसूतिः ।
मिथ्योपचारः प्रतिकर्मणां[4] च निजस्य हेतुः श्वयथोः[5] प्रदिष्टः ॥५॥

---

1. ०यालक्त० इति प्रथमपुस्तके पाठः ।
2. ०गुरुत्व० इति षष्ठपुस्तके पाठः ।
3. विषमोपशुद्धिः इति षष्ठपुस्तके पाठः ।
4. प्रतिसारणा इति षष्ठपुस्तके पाठः ।
5. स्वयथो इति प्रथमपुस्तके पाठः ।

Etiology of Endogenous Oedema

Following are the causative factors of *nija* (endogenous) type of oedema.

(1) Intake of *kṣāra* (alkali preparation), sour things, ingredients having *tīkṣṇa* (sharp) property and hot things by an emaciated and weak patient immediately after the purificatory therapies or after recovery from a disease;

(2) Intake of curd, uncooked food, mud, vegetables, mutually contradictory ingredients of food and polluted as well as poisoned food;

(3) Affliction by piles, lack of exercise, not taking purificatory therapies, injury to vital organs and difficulty in delivery; and

(4) Resorting to wrong corrective measures.

सगौरवं स्यादनवस्थितत्वं सोत्सेधमूष्मा[1]ऽथ शिरातनुत्वम् ।
सलोमहर्षाङ्ग[2]विवर्णता च सामान्यलिङ्गं श्वयथोः[3] प्रदिष्टम् ॥६॥

General Signs and Symptoms

Signs and symptoms of *śotha roga* (oedema) in general are heaviness, unstability, swelling, heating sensation, vascular thinness, horripilation and discoloration of the skin.

---

1. ०सूक्ष्मा० इति चतुर्थषष्ठपुस्तकयो पाठः ।
2. सलोमहर्षोगविवर्णता इति आदर्शपुस्तकेषु पाठः ।
3. क. स्वयथोः इति प्रथमपुस्तके पाठः ।
   ख. श्चयथो इति चतुर्थपुस्तके पाठः ।
   ग. श्वथ्येः इति षष्ठपुस्तके पाठः ।

चलस्तनुत्वक्[1] परुषोऽरुणोऽसितः
समुप्ति[2]हर्षार्तियुतोऽनिमित्ततः[3] ।
प्रशाम्यति प्रोन्नमति प्रपीडितो
दिवाबली स्यात्श्वयथुः समीरणात् ॥७॥

Signs and Symptoms of Vātika Oedema

Signs and symptoms of *vātika* type of oedema are as follows:

1. Mobility and thinness of the skin;
2. Roughness, reddishness and whiteness of the skin;
3. Numbness and tingling sensation in excess without any appreciable causative factor;
4. When pressed the oedema gets depressed but becomes elevated thereafter; and
5. Aggravation of oedema during the day time.

मृदुः सगन्धोऽसितपीतरागवान् भ्रमज्वरस्वेदतृषामदान्वितः ।
य उष्यते स्पष्टरुगक्षिरागकृत् स पित्तशोफो[4] भृशदाहपाकवान् ॥८॥

Signs and Symptoms of Paittika Oedema

Signs and symptoms of *paittika* type of oedema are as follows:

1. Softness of the skin with a smell;
2. Black and yellow coloration of the skin;

---

1. चरस्तनुत्वक् इति आदर्शपुस्तकेषु पाठः ।
2. क. सुसुप्ति० इति आकरे पाठः ।
   ख. प्रसुप्ति० इति चतुर्थषष्ठपुस्तकयोः पाठः ।
3. क. निमित्तैः इति पंचमषष्ठपुस्तकयोः पाठः ।
   ख. निमिन्तैः इति प्रथमपुस्तके पाठः ।
4. क. ०शोथो इति आकरे पाठः ।
   ख. ०शोको इति षष्ठपुस्तके पाठः ।

3. Giddiness, fever, sweating, thirst and feeling of intoxication; and
4. Heating sensation, pain, reddish colour of the eyes and excessive burning sensation as well as suppuration.

गुरुः स्थिरः पाण्डुररोचकान्वितः प्रसेकनिद्रावमिवह्निमान्द्यकृत् ।

स कृच्छ्रजन्मप्रशमो निपीडितो न चोन्नमेद्रात्रिबली कफात्मकः ॥९॥

Signs and Symptoms of Kaphaja Oedema

Signs and symptoms of *kaphaja* oedema are as follows :

1. Affliction by heaviness, stability, anemia, anorexia, salivation, sleep, vomiting and suppression of the power of digestion;
2. Its application and alleviation take place very slowly;
3. There is no pitting by pressure; and
4. Aggravation of oedema during night.

निदानाकृतिसंसर्गाच्छ्वयथुः स्याद् द्विदोषजः ।

सर्वाकृतिः सन्निपाताच्छोथो[1] व्यामिश्रलक्षणः ॥१०॥

Dvandvaja and Sānnipātika Oedema

Combination of causative factors and signs as well as symptoms are the characteristic features of *dvandvaja*, viz. *vāta-paittika*, *vāta-kaphaja* and *pitta-kaphaja* types of oedema. Similarly, *sānnipātika* type of oedema is characterised by the combination of signs and symptoms of all the three *doṣas*.

अभिघातेन शस्त्रादिच्छेदभेदकृतादिभिः[2] ।

हिमानिलोदध्यनिलैर्भल्लातकपिकच्छुजैः[3] ॥११॥

---

1. क. सन्निपातात्सोफो० इति प्रथमपुस्तके पाठः ।
   ख. सन्निपातात्शोफो इति षष्ठपुस्तके पाठः ।
2. ०भेदक्षतादिभिः इति आकरे पाठः ।
3. ०सास्नातकपिकच्छुजैः इति प्रथमपुस्तके पाठः ।

रसैः शूकैश्च संस्पर्शाच्छ्वयथुः स्याद्विसर्पवान्[1] ।
भृशोष्मा लोहिताभासः[2] प्रायशः[3] पित्तलक्षणः ॥१२॥

Abhighātaja Oedema

Because of the injury by sharp edged weapons, exposure to cold wind and the wind coming from the sea and contact with the juice or bristles of *bhallātaka* and *kapi kacchu* oedema takes place. It is of spreading nature. The skin will be very hot to touch and red in colour. Generally, signs and symptoms of *paittika* oedema are manifested in this variety.

विषजः सविषप्राणिपरिसर्पणमूत्रणात् ।
दंष्ट्रादन्तनखाघातादविषप्राणिनामपि ।
विण्मूत्रशुक्रोपहतमलवद्वस्त्रसंकरात्[4] ।
विषवृक्षानिलस्पर्शाद् गरयोगावचूर्णनात् ॥१३॥

Viṣaja Oedema

Viṣaja type of oedema is caused by the following :

1. Crawling or urination by poisonous animals;
2. Injury by fangs, teeth or nails of even non-poisonous animals;
3. Use of dirty clothes polluted by stool, urine and semen;

---

1. ०सर्पवत् इति चतुर्थषष्ठपुस्तकयोः पाठः ।
2. भाशः इति पंचमपुस्तके पाठः ।
3. प्रायसः इति प्रथमपुस्तके पाठः ।
4. ०सर्करात् इति षष्ठपुस्तके पाठः ।

4. Contact with the wind blowing over a poisonous tree; and
5. Dusting of powder containing poisonous material.

मृदुश्चलोऽवलम्बी च शीघ्रो दाहरुजाकरः ॥१४॥

This variety of oedema is soft, mobile and slightly hanging down. This causes burning sensation and pain immediately.

दोषाः श्वयथुमूर्ध्वं हि कुर्वन्त्यामाशयस्थिताः ।
पक्वाशयस्था मध्ये तु वर्चः[1] स्थानगतास्त्वधः ।
कृत्स्नदेहमनुप्राप्ताः कुर्युः सर्वसरस्तथा[2] ॥१५॥

Oedema in Different Parts of Body

If the vitiated *doṣas* are located in the *āmāśaya* (stomach including small intestine), then oedema takes place in the upper part of the body. If these vitiated *doṣas* are located in the *pakvāśaya* (colon) then oedema takes place in the middle portion of the body. If these *doṣas* are located in the rectum, then oedema takes place in the lower part of the body. If, however, these vitiated *doṣas* are located all over the digestive tract, then oedema takes place all over the body.

यो मध्यदेशे[3] श्वयथुः स कष्टः सर्वगश्च यः ।
अर्धाङ्गे रिष्टभूतः स्याद्यश्चोर्ध्वं परिसर्पति ॥१६॥

1. भुवर्वस्थान् इति प्रथमपुस्तके पाठः ।
2. क. सर्वसरं तथा इति आकरे पाठः ।
   ख. ०रसं तथा इति षष्ठपुस्तके पाठः ।
3. ०देशः इति षष्ठपुस्तके पाठः ।

Prognosis

Oedema in the middle portion of the body and general anasarca all over the body are difficult of cure. If oedema takes place in half of the body and if it spreads upwards, then it is incurable.

श्वासः पिपासा छर्दिश्च दौर्बल्यं ज्वर एव च ।
यस्य चान्ने रुचिर्नास्ति श्वयथुं तं विवर्जयेत्[1] ॥१७॥"

[माधवनिदान : शोथ ३६ : १-१८]

The patient of oedema having dyspnoea, thirst, vomiting, weakness, fever and anorexia should not be treated.

"छर्दिः श्वासोऽरुचिस्तृष्णा ज्वरोऽतिसार एव च ।
सप्तकोऽयं सदौर्बल्यं[2] शोफोपद्रवसंग्रहः[3] ॥१८॥"

[चरक : सूत्रस्थान १८ : १८]

Complications

Vomiting, dyspnoea, anorexia, thirst, fever, diarrhoea and weakness—these are the seven complications of oedema.

"ऊर्ध्वगामी नरं पदभ्यामधोगामी मुखात् स्त्रियम् ।
उभयं बस्तिसंजातः शोफो[4] हन्ति न संशयः ॥१९॥"

[योगरत्नाकर : शोथचिकित्सा : पृष्ठ १२४]

---

1. क. परिवर्जयेत् इति षष्ठपुस्तके पाठः ।
   ख. च वर्जयेत् इति प्रथमपुस्तके पाठः ।
2. सदौर्बल्यः इति श्राकरे षष्ठपुस्तके च पाठः ।
3. शोफोपवशंकर: इति षष्ठपुस्तके पाठः ।
4. शोफो इति पंचमपुस्तके पाठः ।

Oedema originating from legs and moving upwards causes death of a male patient. Oedema originating from face and moving downwards causes death of a female patient. If oedema originates in the area of the urinary bladder, then it causes death of both the male and the female patients.

"अनन्योपद्रवकृतः शोथः पादसमुत्थितः[1] ।
पुरुषं हन्ति नारीं च मुखजो गुह्यजो द्वयम् ।
नवोऽनुपद्रवः शोथः साध्योऽसाध्यः[2] पुरेरितः ॥२०॥"

[माधवनिदान : शोथ ३६ : १६]

॥ शोफनिदानम् ॥२१॥

If the oedema originates from the legs and is associated with complications, then the male patient succumbs to death. If the oedema originates from the face then female patient succumbs to death. If oedema originates in the anal region then it leads to the death of both the male and the female patients. Freshly occurring oedema without any complication is curable ; others are incurable.

Thus, ends the diagnosis of oedema.

"शुण्ठीपुनर्नवैरण्डपञ्चमूलशृतं जलम् ।
वातिके श्वयथौ शस्तं पानाहारपरिग्रहे[3] ॥२२॥"

[भैषज्यरत्नावली : शोथरोगाधिकार : ४]

The decoction of *śuṇṭhī*, *punarnavā*, *eraṇḍa* and *pañca mūla* is useful for being used in food and drinks by a patient suffering from *vātika* type of oedema.

---

1. ०समुच्छ्रितः इति पंचमपुस्तकं पाठः ।
2. साध्यं सभिषजेरित इति षष्ठपुस्तके पाठः ।
3. ०परिग्रहं इति प्रथमपंचमपुस्तकयोः पाठः ।

"दशमूलं सर्वथा च शस्तं वाते विशेषतः ॥२३॥"

[भैषज्यरत्नावली : शोथरोगाधिकार : २५]

Decoction of *daśa mūla* is useful in all types of oedema, specially in *vātika* type of oedema.

"क्षीराशनः पित्तकृत्तेऽथ[1] शोथे त्रिवृद्गुडूचीत्रिफलाकषायम् ।

पिबेद् गवां मूत्रविमिश्रितं वा फलत्रिकाच्चूर्णमथाक्षमात्रम् ॥२४॥"

[भैषज्यरत्नावली : शोथरोगाधिकार : ५]

Intake of the decoction of *trivṛt*, *guḍūcī* and *triphalā* and milk preparations as food is useful in *paittika* type of oedema. Such a patient should also use one *akṣa* of *triphalā* powder along with cow's urine.

"अभया दारुमधुकं तिक्ता दन्ती सपिप्पली ।

पटोलं चन्दनं दार्वी त्रायमाणेन्द्रवारुणी ॥२५॥

एषां क्वाथः ससर्पिष्कः श्वयथुज्वरदाहहा ।

विसर्पतृष्णासन्तापसन्निपातविषापहः ॥२६॥"

[भैषज्यरत्नावली : शोथरोगाधिकार : ७-८]

Intake of the decoction of *abhayā*, *deva dāru*, *madhuka*, *tiktā*, *dantī*, *pippalī*, *paṭola*, *candana*, *dārvī*, *trāyamāṇā* and *indra vāruṇī* along with ghee cures oedema, fever, burning sensation, erysipelas, thirst, heating sensation, *sānnipātika* types of diseases and poisoning.

---

1. ०कृत्ते तु इति प्रथमपंचमपुस्तकयोः पाठः ।

"पुराणं[1] माणकं पिष्ट्वा द्विगुणीकृततण्डुलम्[2] ।
साधितं वारितोयाभ्याम[3]भ्यसेत्पायसन्तु तत् ।
हन्ति वातोदरं शोथं ग्रहणीं पाण्डुताम[4]पि ॥२७॥"
[भैषज्यरत्नावली : शोथरोगाधिकार : ३४-३५]

शीतवीर्यैर्हिमजलैरभ्यङ्गादींश्च कल्पयेत् ॥२८॥

Old rhizome of *māṇaka* should be made to a paste, added with double the quantity of rice and required quantity of milk as well as water to prepare a *pāyasa* (a type of milk preparation). Intake of this cures *vātodara*, oedema, *grahaṇī* (sprue syndrome) and anemia.

For a patient of *paittika* oedema, massage, etc. should be done by the ointment prepared of cooling drugs triturated with cold water.

"पुनर्नवाविश्वत्रिवृद्गुडूचीशम्पाकपथ्यामरदारुकल्कम् ।
शोथे कफोत्थे महिषाक्षमूत्रयुक्त[5] पिबेद्वा सलिलं तथैषाम् ॥२९॥"
[भैषज्यरत्नावली : शोथरोगाधिकार : २९]

The paste or decoction of *punarnavā*, *viśva*, *trivṛt*, *guḍūcī*, *śampāka*, *pathyā* and *deva dāru* mixed with *guggulu* and cow's urine is useful in *kaphaja* oedema.

"[6]कफे तु कृष्णासिकतापुराणपिण्याकशिग्रुत्वगुमाप्रलेपः ।
कुलत्थशुण्ठीजलमूत्रसेकश्चण्डागुरुभ्यामनुलेपनश्च ॥३०॥"
[भैषज्यरत्नावली : शोथरोगाधिकार : ६०]

---

1. 'पुराणं—— पाण्डुतामपि' पाठोऽयं प्रथमपुस्तके नोपलभ्यते ।
2. ०कृत्यतंडुलम् इति आदर्शपुस्तकेषु पाठः ।
3. क्षीरतोयाभ्याम० इति आकरे पाठः ।
4. सिद्धो भिषग्भिराख्यातः प्रयोगोऽय निरत्ययः पाठोऽयं आकरे अधिकमुपलभ्यते ।
5. ०मूलयुक्तं इति षष्ठपुस्तके पाठः ।
6. द्रष्टव्यम् योगरत्नाकर : शोथचिकित्सा : पृष्ठ १३३ ।

For *kaphaja* oedema, be paste of *pippalī*, sand, old oil-cake, bask of *sigru* and *umā* should be applied externally. Similarly, water or cow's urine boiled with *kulattha* and *śuṇṭhī* should be used for sprinkl ing, and the paste of *caṇḍā* and *aguru* should be applied externally.

"अजाजिपाठाघनपञ्चकोलव्याघ्रीरजन्यः सुखतोयपीताः ।
शोथं त्रिदोषं चिरजं प्रवृद्धं निघ्नन्ति भूनिम्बमहौषधे च ॥३१॥"

[भैषज्यरत्नावली : शोथरोगाधिकार : १०]

Intake of the luke-warm decoction of *ajāji*, *pāṭhā*, *ghana*, *pañca kola*, *vyāghrī* and *rajanī* cures serious and chronic oedema caused by *sannipāta* (simultaneous vitiation of all the three *doṣas*). The dococtìon of *bhūnimba* and *mahauṣadha* has similar effect.

"[1]पुनर्नवानिम्बपटोलशुण्ठीतिक्तामृतादार्व्यभयाकषायः ।
सर्वाङ्गशोथोदरकास[2]शूलश्वासान्वितं पाण्डुगदं निहन्ति ॥३२॥"

[भैषज्यरत्नावली : शोथरोगाधिकार : २८]

Intake of the decoction of *punarnavā*, *nimba*, *paṭola*, *śuṇṭhī*, *tiktā*, *amṛtā*, *dārvī* and *abhayā* cures general anasarca, *udara roga*, cough, colic pain and anemia associated with asthma.

"आर्द्रकस्य रसः पीतः पुराणगुडमिश्रितः ।
अजाक्षीराशिनां शीघ्रं सर्वशोथहरो भवेत् ॥३३॥

Intake of ginger juice and jaggery along with goat's milk as food quickly cures all types of oedema.

---

1. 'पिप्पल्यादिरजिनी नाम्ना चरके प्रच्यते त्वयम् ।
योगः शुण्ठया पुनः स्थाने ग्राह्या मातंगपिप्पली ॥'
पाठोऽयं पंचमषष्ठपुस्तकयोः अधिकमुपलभ्यते ।
2. ०पार्श्वशूल० इति आकरे पाठः ।

पुनर्नवादारुशुण्ठीक्वाथे[1] मूत्रे च केवले ।
दशमूलरसो[2] वाऽपि गुग्गुलुः[3]' शोथनाशनः ॥३४॥"

[भैषज्यरत्नावली : शोथरोगाधिकार : १४-१५]

Intake of the decoction of *punarnavā*, *deva dāru* and *śuṇṭhī* along with cow's urine or the decoction alone or the decoction of *daśa mūla* along with *guggulu* cures oedema.

"बिल्वपत्ररसं पीतं [illegible] श्वयथौ त्रिजे ।
विड्बधे[5] चैव दुर्नाम्नि विदध्यात् कामलास्वपि[6] ॥३५॥"

[भैषज्यरत्नावली : शोथरोगाधिकार : ३०]

Juice of the leaf of *bilva* has drying effect. It is useful in *sānnipātika* type of oedema, constipation, piles and jaundice.

"गुडपिप्पलिशुण्ठीनां चूर्णं श्वयथुनाशनम् ।
'आमाजीर्णप्रशमनं[7] शूलघ्नं बस्तिशोधनम् ॥३६॥"

[भैषज्यरत्नावली : शोथरोगाधिकार : १७]

The powder of jaggery, *pippalī* and *śuṇṭhī* cures oedema, *āma* (undigested product of food), indigestion and colic pain. It also cleanses the urinary bladder.

---

1. ०क्वाथो इति प्रथमपुस्तके पाठः ।
2. दशमूलरसे इति आकरे पाठः ।
3. 'श्वयथुमूर्द्ध'———गुग्गुलु' पाठोऽयं चतुर्थपुस्तके नोपलभ्यते ।
4. सोषणं इति प्रथमपुस्तके पाठः ।
5. विट्सङ्गे इति आकरे पाठः ।
6. कामलासु च इति आकरे पाठः ।
7. 'आमाजीर्ण०——शोधनम्' पाठोऽयं प्रथमपुस्तके नोपलभ्यते ।

"पथ्यामृताभार्ङ्गिपुनर्नवाग्निदार्वीनिशादारुमहौषधानाम् ।
क्वाथं पिबेच्चोदर[1]पाणिपादवक्त्राश्रितं हन्त्यचिरेण शोथम् ॥३७॥"

[भैषज्यरत्नावली : शोथरोगाधिकार : ६३]

Intake of the decoction of *pathyā*, *amṛtā*, *bhārṅgī*, *punarnavā*, *agni*, *dāru haridrā*, *haridrā*, *deva dāru* and *śuṇṭhī* instantaneously cures oedema affecting abdomen, hands, legs and face.

"बिभीतकानां फलमध्यलेपः शोथेषु[2] दाहार्तिहरः प्रवृष्टः[3] ।
यष्ट्याह्वमुस्तैः सकपित्थपत्रैः[4] सचन्दनैस्तत्पिडकासु[5] लेपः ॥३८॥"

[योगरत्नाकर : शोथचिकित्सा : पृष्ठ १३४]

Application of the ointment prepared of the seed pulp of *bibhītakī* cures burning sensation and pain in a patient suffering from oedema. Application of the ointment of *yaṣṭī*, *mustā*, leaf of *kapittha* and *candana* cures carbuncles.

"पुरं[6] मूत्रेण संसेव्यं[7] पिप्पलीं[8] वा पयोऽन्विताम् ।
गुडेन वाऽभया तुल्या विश्वं वा शोथरोगिणाम्[9] ॥३९॥"

[भैषज्यरत्नावली : शोथरोगाधिकार : १६]

---

1. प्रसह्योदरपाणिपादमुखाश्रितम् इति आकरे पाठः ।
2. सर्वेषु इति आकरे पाठः ।
3. प्रशस्तः इति आकरे पाठः ।
4. सकपित्थमूत्रैः इति आकरे पाठः ।
5. सचन्दनैस्तत्पिटिकासु इति आकरे षष्ठपुस्तके च पाठः ।
6. पुरो इति आकरे पाठः ।
7. सेव्येत इति आकरे पाठः ।
8. पिप्पली इति आकरे पाठः ।
9. शोथनाशनम् इति चतुर्थपुस्तके पाठः ।

The patient suffering from oedema should take *guggulu* along with cow's urine or *pippalī* along with milk or *abhayā* along with jaggery or *śuṇṭhī* along with jaggery.

"गुडार्द्रकं वा गुडनागरं वा गुडाभयां वा गुडपिप्पलीं वा ।
कर्षा[1]भिवृद्ध्या त्रिपलप्रमाणं खादेन्नरः पक्षमथापि मासम् ॥४०॥

शोथप्रतिश्यायगलास्यरोगान्
सश्वासकासारुचिपीनसादीन् ।
जीर्णज्वरार्शोग्रहणीविकारान्
हन्यात्तथाऽन्यान् कफवातरोगान् ॥४१॥"

[भैषज्यरत्नावली : शोथरोगाधिकार : ११-१२]

Intake of jaggery with green ginger, or jaggery with dry ginger, or jaggery with *abhayā* or jaggery with *pippalī* in a dose of three *palas* and increased by one *karṣa* every day for a fortnight or for a month cures oedema, fever, piles, *grahaṇī* (sprue syndrome) and other diseases caused by *kapha* and *vāyu*.

कृष्णाग्निविश्वघनजीरककण्टकारीपाठा-
निशाकरि[2]कणामगधाजयानाम् ।
चूर्णं कटूष्णसलिलैरवलोड्य पीतं
नातः परं श्वयथुरोगहरं नराणाम् ॥४२॥

Intake of the powder of *kṛṣṇā, agni, viśva, ghana, jīraka, kaṇṭakārī, pāṭhā, niśā, gaja pippalī, pippalī* and *jayā* along with hot as well as pungent (by boiling with pungent drugs) water cures oedema. This excells other recipes in its therapeutic efficacy.

---

1. कर्षातिवृद्धया इति प्रथमपंचमपुस्तकयोः पाठः ।
2. ०निशाकरकणा० इति षष्ठपुस्तके पाठः ।

"स्थलपद्ममयं कल्कं पयसालोड्य पाययेत् ।
प्लीहामयहरञ्चैव सर्वाङ्गैकाङ्गशोथजित् ॥४३॥"

[भैषज्यरत्नावली : शोथरोगाधिकार : ३३]

Intake of the paste of *sthala padma* by boiling with milk cures splenic enlargement and oedema in any part of the body or in the whole body.

"दारुगुग्गुलुशुण्ठीनां कल्को मूत्रेण शोथजित् ।
वर्षाभूश्रृङ्गवेराभ्यां कल्को वा सर्वशोथजित् ॥४४॥"

[भैषज्यरत्नावली : शोथरोगाधिकार : १८]

The paste of *deva dāru, guggulu* and *śuṇṭhī* should be taken along with cow's urine which cures oedema. Similarly, the paste of *varṣābhū* and *śṛṅga vera* cures all types of oedema.

"सिंहास्यामृतभण्टाकीक्वाथं कृत्वा समाक्षिकम् ।
पीत्वा शोथं जयेज्जन्तुः कासं श्वासं ज्वरं वमिम् ॥४५॥"

[भैषज्यरत्नावली : शोथरोगाधिकार : २७]

Intake of the decoction of *vāsā, amṛtā* and *bhaṇṭākī* along with honey cures oedema, cough, asthma, fever and vomiting.

"[1]पुनर्नवादेवदारुगुरुचिपाठीसोंठिकूठगोषुरुदारुहरदी। हरदी कटैया भरहटा पीपरि चीता अडूसा सर्वांगशोथपांडुश्वासजा ॥४६॥"

Punarnavā, deva dāru, gudūcī, pāṭhā, śuṇṭhī, kuṣṭha, gokṣura, dāru haridrā, haridrā, kaṇṭakārī, bharahaṭā, pippalī, citraka and *vāsā* cure general anasarca, anemia and dyspnoea.

1. 'पुनर्नवा०———०श्वासजा' पाठोऽयं चतुर्थपंचमषष्ठपुस्तकेषु नोपलभ्यते ।

"पुनर्नवादारुशुण्ठीसिद्धार्थं[1] शिग्रुमेव च ।
पिष्ट्वा[2] चैवारनालेन प्रलेपः सर्वशोथजित्[3] ॥४७॥"

[भैषज्यरत्नावली : शोथरोगाधिकार : ५६]

External application of the paste of *punarnavā*, *deva dāru*, *śuṇṭhī*, *siddhārtha* and *śigru* along with *āranāla* (a type of vinegar) cures all types of oedema.

"भूनिम्बदारुकल्कं जग्ध्वा पेयः पुनर्नवाक्वाथः ।
अपहरति नियतमाशु शोथं सर्वाङ्गिकं[4] नृणाम् ।
शोथनुत्कोकिलाक्षस्य भस्म मूत्रेण वाम्भसा[5] ॥४८॥"

[भैषज्यरत्नावली : शोथरोगाधिकार : ३१-३२]

Intake of the paste of *bhūnimba* and *deva dāru* along with the decoction of *punarnavā* cures general anasarca. Similarly, the ash of *kokilākṣa* along with cow's urine or water cures oedema.

"क्षीरं शोथहरं दारुवर्षाभूनागरैः[6] शृतम् ।
पेयं वा चित्रकव्योषत्रिवृद्दारुप्रसाधितम् ॥४९॥"

[भैषज्यरत्नावली : शोथरोगाधिकार : १९]

1. शिग्रु सिद्धार्थस्तथा इति आकरे पाठः ।
2. अम्लपिष्टैः सुखोष्णोऽयं प्रलेपः सर्वशोथहृत् इति आकरे पाठः ।
3. 'पुनर्नवा —शोथजित्' पाठोऽयं पंचमपुस्तके अधिकमुपलभ्यते ।
4. सर्वाङ्गगं इति प्रथमपंचमपुस्तकयोः पाठः ।
5. चाम्लसा इति प्रथमपुस्तके पाठः ।
6. दाहदारुवर्षा० इति पंचमपुस्तके पाठः ।

Intake of the milk boiled with *deva dāru*, *varṣābhū* and *nāgara* or the milk boiled with *citraka*, *vyoṣa*, *trivṛt* and *deva dāru* cures oedema.

"पुनर्नवादारुकपित्थमूलछिन्नोद्भवाचित्रकमूलसिद्धाः ।
रसा यवाग्वश्च पयांसि यूषाः शोथे प्रदेया दशमूलगर्भाः ॥५०॥"

[भैषज्यरत्नावली : शोथरोगाधिकार : १३]

Meat soup, *yavāgū* (thick gruel), milk or vegetable soup prepared along with the decoction or powder of *punarnavā*, *deva dāru*, root of *kapittha*, *chinnodbhavā* and root of *citraka* or prepared along with the decoction of *daśa mūla* should be administered to the patient suffering from oedema.

"क्षारद्वयं स्याल्लवणानि चत्वार्ययोरजोव्योषफलत्रिके च ।
सपिप्पलीमूलविडङ्गसारं मुस्ताजमोदामरदारुबिल्वम् ॥५१॥
कलिङ्गकश्चित्रकमूलपाठे यष्ट्याह्व चसातिविषं पलांशम् ।
सहिंगुकर्षं त्वयं शुष्कचूर्णं द्रोणं तथा मूलकशुण्ठकानाम् ॥५२॥
स्याद्भस्मनस्तत्सलिलेन साध्य-
मालोड्य यावद्घनमप्रदग्धम्[1] ।
स्त्यानं ततः कोलसमां तु मात्रां
कृत्वा सशुष्कां विधिना प्रयुञ्ज्यात् ॥५३॥
प्लीहोदरश्वित्रहलीमकार्शः पाण्ड्वामयारोचकशोथशोषान् ।
विसूचिकागुल्मगराश्मरींश्च सश्वासकासान् प्रणुदेत् सकुष्ठान् ॥५४॥

1. यावद्घनमप्यदग्धम् इति श्राकरे पाठः ।

सौवर्चलं सैन्धवं च विडमौद्भिदमेव ।
चतुर्लवणमत्र स्याज्जलमष्टगुणं भवेत् ॥५५॥"

॥ क्षारगुटिका[1] ॥

[भैषज्यरत्नावली : शोथरोगाधिकार : २०-२४]

Kṣāra Guṭikā

One *pala* of each of *svarji kṣāra*, *yava kṣāra*, *sauvarcala*, *saindhava*, *viḍa*, *audbhida lavaṇa*, *lauha bhasma*, *vyoṣa*, *triphalā*, *pippalī mūla*, *viḍaṅga* (dehusked), *mustā*, *ajamodā*, *deva dāru*, *bilva*, *kaliṅgaka*, root of *citraka*, *pāṭhā*, *yaṣṭī*, *ativiṣā* and one *karṣa* of *hiṅgu* should be made to a powder. To this, one *droṇa* of the ash of *mūlaka* and *śuṇṭhī* and eight times of water should be added and boiled till it becomes semi-solid but does not get burnt. From out of this paste, pills of one *kola* each should be prepared and dried. Administration of these pills according to prescribed procedure cures *plīhodara*, *śvitra* (leucoderma), *halīmaka* (a serious type of jaundice), piles, anemia, anorexia, oedema, consumption, *visūcikā* (choleric diarrhoea), *gulma* (phantom tumour), poisoning, *aśmarī* (stone in the urinary tract), asthma, cough and *kuṣṭha* (obstinate skin diseases including leprosy).

"पुनर्नवाचित्रकदेवदारुपञ्चोषणक्षारहरीतकीनाम् ।
कल्केन पक्वं दशमूलतोये घृतोत्तमं शोथनिषूदनञ्च ॥५६॥"

॥ पुनर्नवाद्यं घृतम् ॥

[भैषज्यरत्नावली : शोथरोगाधिकार : ६७]

---

1. क्षारादिगुटिका इति आकरे पाठः ।

Punarnavādya Ghṛta

Ghee cooked along with the decoction of *daśa mūla* and the paste of *punarnavā, citraka, deva dāru, pañcoṣaṇa, kṣāra* and *harītakī* cures oedema.

"पुनर्नवाक्वाथकल्कं सिद्धं शोथहरं घृतम् ॥५७॥"

॥ पुनर्नवाघृतम् ॥

[भैषज्यरत्नावली : शोथरोगाधिकार : ६६]

Punarnavā Ghṛta

Ghee cooked with the decoction as well as paste of *punarnavā* cures oedema.

"रसेन[1] पाचयेत्सर्पिः पञ्चकोलकुलत्थयोः ।
पुनर्नवायाः कल्केन घृतं शोथ[2]विनाशनम् ॥५८॥"

॥ पञ्चकोलाद्यं घृतम् ॥

[भैषज्यरत्नावली : शोथरोगाधिकार : १०२]

Pañca Kolādya Ghṛta

Ghee cooked with the decoction of *pañca kola* as well as *kulattha* and the paste of *punarnavā* cures *śotha.*

"विश्वौषधस्य कल्केन दशमूलजले श्रृतम् ।
घृतं निहन्याच्छ्वयथुं ग्रहणीं पाण्डुतामयम् ॥५९॥"

॥ शुण्ठीघृतम् ॥

---

1. रसे विपाचयेत्सर्पिः इति श्राकरे पाठः ।
2. शोथनिषूदनम् इति श्रादर्शपुस्तकेषु पाठः ।

Śuṇṭhī Ghṛta

Ghee cooked with the paste of *śuṇṭhī* and the decoction of *daśa mūla* cures oedema, *grahaṇī* (sprue syndrome) and anemia.

"सचित्रका धान्ययमानिपाठाः सदीप्यकत्र्यूषणवेतसाम्लाः ।
बिल्वात्फलं दाडिमयावशूकं सपिप्पलीमूलमथापि चव्यम् ॥६०॥
पिष्ट्वाऽक्षमात्राणि जलाढकेन
पक्त्वा घृतप्रस्थमथोपयुञ्ज्यात्[1] ।
अर्शांसि गुल्मं श्वयथुं च कृच्छ्रं
निहन्ति वह्निञ्च करोति दीप्तिम् ॥६१॥
॥ चित्रकाद्यघृतम्[2] ॥"

[भैषज्यरत्नावली : शोथरोगाधिकार : ९९-१००]

Citrakādya Ghṛta

One *akṣa* of each of *citraka, dhānya, yamānī, pāṭhā, dīpyaka, tryūṣaṇa, amla vetasa*, fruit of *bilva, dāḍima, yava kṣāra, pippalī mūla* and *cavya* should be boiled in one *āḍhaka* of water. One *prastha* of ghee should be cooked with this decoction. This medicated ghee cures piles, *gulma* (phantom tumour), oedema and dysuria. It stimulates the power of digestion.

"क्षीरं घटे चित्रककल्कलिप्ते दध्यागतं साधु निमथ्य[3] तेन ।
तज्जं घृतं चित्रकमूलकल्कं[4] तक्रेण सिद्धं श्वयथुघ्नमग्र्यम् ।

1. घृतप्रस्थमोपयुक्तम् इति आकरे पाठः ।
2. चित्रकादि घृतम् इति पंचमपुस्तके पाठः ।
3. विमथ्य इति आकरे पाठः ।
4. चित्रकमूलगर्भं इति आदर्शपुस्तकेषु पाठः ।

अर्शोऽतिसारानिलगुल्ममेहांस्तद्धन्ति[1] सवंर्द्धयते च वह्निम् ॥६२॥"

॥ चित्रकघृतम्[2] ॥

[भैषज्यरत्नावली : शोथरोगाधिकार : १०३-१०४]

Citraka Ghṛta

Milk should be kept in a jar smeared with the paste of *citraka* till it becomes curd. Ghee taken out of this curd should be cooked by adding the paste of the root of *citraka* and butter-milk which cures oedema, piles, diarrhoea, *vātika gulma* (phantom tumour) and *prameha* (obstinate urinary disorder including diabetes). It also stimulates the power of digestion.

"माणकक्वाथकल्काभ्यां घृतप्रस्थं विपाचयेत् ।
एकजं द्वन्द्वजं शोथं त्रिदोषञ्च[3] व्यपोहति ॥६३॥"

[भैषज्यरत्नावली : शोथरोगाधिकार : ६५]

Māṇaka Ghṛta

Ghee should be cooked with the decoction as well as paste of *māṇaka*. It cures oedema caused by one *doṣa*, by two *doṣas* and by three *doṣas* vitiated simultaneously.

"स्थलपद्मपलान्यष्टौ त्र्यूषणस्य चतुःपलम् ।
घृतप्रस्थं पचेदेभिः क्षीरं दत्वा चतुर्गुणम् ।
पञ्चकासान् हरेच्छीघ्रं शोथं चैव सुदुस्तरम् ॥६४॥"

॥ स्थलपद्मघृतम्[4] ॥

[भैषज्यरत्नावली : शोथरोगाधिकार : १०१]

---

1. ०मेहानतद्धन्ति इति प्रथमचतुर्थपंचमपुस्तकेषु पाठः ।
2. चित्रकं इति प्रथमचतुर्थपंचमपुस्तकेषु पाठः ।
3. त्रिदोषजमपोहति इति आकरे पाठः ।
4. स्थलपद्मकाद्यं घृतम् इति आदर्शपुस्तकेषु पाठः ।

Sthala Padma Ghṛta

One *prastha* of ghee should be cooked along with eight *palas* of *sthala padma*, four *palas* of *tryūṣaṇa* and four *prasthas* of milk. It instantaneously cures five varieties of cough and serious types of oedema.

"शैलेयकुष्ठागुरुदारुकौन्तीत्वक्पद्मकैलाऽम्बुपलाशमुस्तैः ।
प्रियङ्गुस्थौणेयकहेममांसीतालीशपत्रप्लवपत्रधान्यैः ॥६५॥
श्रीवेष्टकध्यामकपिप्पलीभिः स्पृक्कानखैश्चा[1]ऽपि यथोपलाभम् ।
वातान्वितेऽभ्यङ्गमुशन्ति तैलं सिद्धं सुपिष्टैरपि च प्रदेहम् ॥६६॥"

॥ शैलेयाद्यं तैलम् ॥

[भैषज्यरत्नावली : शोथरोगाधिकार : १०५-१०६]

Śaileyādya Taila

Oil should be cooked along with *śaileya*, *kuṣṭha*, *aguru*, *deva dāru*, *kauntī*, *tvak*, *padmaka*, *elā*, *ambu*, *palāśa*, *mustā*, *priyaṅgu*, *sthauṇeyaka*, *hema* (*nāga kesara*), *māṃsī*, *tālīśa patra*, *plava*, *patra*, *dhānya*, *śrīveṣṭaka*, *dhyāmaka*, *pippalī*, *spṛkkā* and *nakha* depending upon their availability. Massage with this medicated oil is useful in *vātika* type of oedema. Application of the thin paste of the above mentioned drugs also cures oedema.

"शुष्कमूलकवर्षाभूदारुरास्नामहौषधैः ।
पक्वमभ्यञ्जनात्तैलं सशूलं श्वयथुं जयेत् ॥६७॥
॥ मूलकाद्यं[2] तैलम् ॥"

[भैषज्यरत्नावली : शोथरोगाधिकार : ६५]

---

1. ०नखैर्वाऽपि इति श्राकरे पाठः ।
2. क. शुष्कमूलाद्यं इति श्राकरे पाठः ।
   ख. शुष्कमूलकाद्यं तैलम् इति चतुर्थषष्ठपुस्तकयोः पाठः ।
   ग. "शष्कमूलक०——तैलम्" पाठोऽयं प्रथमपुस्तके नोपलभ्यते ।

Mūlakādya Taila

Oil cooked with dry *mūlaka*, *varṣābhū*, *deva dāru*, *rāsnā* and *mahauṣadha* should be used for massage which cures oedema with pain.

"पुनर्नवामृतादारुदशमूलरसाढके ।
आर्द्रकस्वरसप्रस्थे गुडस्य तु तुलां पचेत् ॥६८॥
तत्सिद्धं व्योषपत्रैलात्वक्चव्यैः कार्षिकैः पृथक् ।
चूर्णीकृतैः क्षिपेच्चूर्णं[1] मधुनः कुडवं लिहेत् ॥६९॥
लेहः पौनर्नवो नाम शोथशूलनिषूदनः[2] ।
श्वासकासारुचिहरो बलवर्णाग्निवर्धनः ॥७०॥"

॥ पुनर्नवालेहः[3] ॥

[भैषज्यरत्नावली : शोथरोगाधिकारः : ४३-४४]

Punarnavā Leha

One *āḍhaka* of the decoction of *punarnavā*, *amṛtā*, *deva dāru* and *daśa mūla*, one *prastha* of ginger juice and one *tulā* of jaggery should be cooked. When it is prepared, one *karṣa* of each of the powder of *vyoṣa*, *patra*, *elā*, *tvak* and *cavya* and one *kuḍava* of honey snould be added and mixed well. This is called *punarnavā leha*. It cures oedema, colic pain, dyspnoea, cough and anorexia. This promotes strength, complexion and the power of digestion.

---

1 क्षिपेच्छीते इति आकरे पाठः ।

2. श्लेष्मशोथनिषूदनः इति षष्ठपुस्तके पाठः ।

3. पुनर्नवादिलेहः इति आकरे पाठः ।

"दशमूलकषायस्य कंसे पथ्याशतं पचेत्[1] ।
तुलां गुडात्[2] घने दद्यात्[3] व्योषक्षारचतुः पलम् ॥७१॥
त्रिसुगन्धं[4] तु सुवर्णांशं प्रस्थार्द्धं मधुनो हिमे ।
दशमूलहरीतक्यः शोथान्हन्युः[5] सुदुस्तरान् ॥७२॥"

[योगरत्नाकर : शोथचिकित्सा : पृष्ठ १३०]

'ज्वरारोचकगुल्मार्शोमेहपाण्डूदरामयान्[6] ।
प्रत्येकमेवकर्षांशं त्रिसुगन्धिमितो[7] भवेत् ॥७३॥
कंसहरीतकी चैषा चरके पठ्यतेऽन्यथा ।
एतन्मानेन तुल्यत्वं[8] तेन तत्रापि वर्ण्यते ॥७४॥'

॥ दशमूलीहरीतकी[9] ॥

Daśa Mūla Harītakī

One hundred fruits of *harītakī* should be cooked in one *kaṃsa* of the decoction of *daśa mūla* and one *tulā* of jaggery.

---

1. गुडात् इति आकरे पाठः ।
2. पचेद् इति आकरे पाठः ।
3. तत्र इति आकरे पाठः ।
4. त्रिजातं तु इति आकरे पाठः ।
5. शोफान्घ्नन्ति इति आकरे पाठः ।
6. 'ज्वरारोचक०———वर्ण्यते' पाठोऽयं आकरे नोपलभ्यते ।
7. क. त्रिसुगन्धिसिनो इति पंचमपुस्तके पाठः ।
   ख. त्रिसुगन्धिमितो इति प्रथमपुस्तके पाठः ।
8. तुल्यं त्वतेन इति पंचमपुस्तके पाठः ।
9. दशमूलहरीतकी इति षष्ठपुस्तके पाठः ।

When it becomes semi solid, four *palas* of *vyoṣa kṣāra*, one *suvarṇa* (*karṣa*=unit of weight) of *tri sugandha* and half *prastha* of honey should be added and well mixed. Honey should be added only when the recipe is cooled down. This is called *daśa mūla harītakī*. It cures serious types of oedema, fever, anorexia, *gulma* (phantom tumour), piles, *meha* (obstinate urinary disorder including diabetes anemia and *udara roga* (obstinate abdominal diseases including ascites). Caraka has named this recipe as *kaṃsa harītakī* and used the ingredients in the same weight.

"द्विपञ्चमूलस्य पचेत् कषाये कंसेऽभयानां च शतं गुडाच्च ।
लेहे सुसिद्धे च विनीय चूर्णं व्योषत्रिसौगन्ध्यमुपस्थिते[1] च ॥७५॥
प्रस्थार्द्धमात्रं मधुनः सुशीते किञ्चिच्च चूर्णादपि यावशूकात् ।
एकाभयां प्राश्य ततश्चलेहाच्छु[2]क्तिर्निहन्ति श्वयथुं प्रवृद्धम् ॥७६॥
'कासज्वरारोचकमेहगुल्मप्लीहत्रिदोषोदरपाण्डुरोगान् ।
कार्श्यामवातादसृगम्लपित्तं वैवर्ण्यमूत्रानिलशुक्रदोषान् ॥७७॥'

[चरक : चिकित्सा १२ : ४९-५१]

अत्र व्याख्यान्तरं नोक्तं 'पूर्वे[3] व्याख्यैव यत् श्रुतम्' ॥७८॥"

॥ कंसहरीतकी ॥

[योगरत्नाकर : शोथचिकित्सा : पृष्ठ १३०]

1. ०मुखा स्थिते इति पंचमपुस्तके पाठः ।
2. ०लेहात् शुक्तिं० इति आदर्शपुस्तकेषु पाठः ।
3. 'पूर्वे———श्रुतम्' । पाठोऽयं चतुर्थषष्ठपुस्तकयोः नोपलभ्यते ।

"दशमूलं हरीतक्या तुल्यं कंसहरीतकी ।
मानं तेनात्र तत्रस्थं चरके प्राह जेज्जटः[1] ॥७९॥"

॥ कंसहरीतकी[2] ॥

Kamsa Harītakī

In one *kaṃsa* of the decoction of *daśa mūla*, one hundred fruits of *harītakī* and one hundred *palas* of *guḍa* should be added and cooked. After the linctus is prepared, the powder of *vyoṣa* and *tri sugandhi* should be added. When the linctus is cooled, half a *prastha* of honey should be added along with small quantity of *yava kṣāra*. This should be administered in a dose of one fruit of *abhayā* and one *śukti* (unit of weight) of the linctus. This cures serious type of oedema, cough, fever, anorexia, splenic enlargement, *gulma* (phantom tumour), *ameha* (obstinate urinary disorders including diabetes), *anipātika* type of *udara roga*, anemia, emaciation, *āma vāta* (rheumatism), *rakta pitta* (an ailment characterised by bleeding from various parts of the body), *amla pitta* (acidity in stomach), discoloration of the skin and afflictions of urine, flatus as well as semen. Quantity, etc. of some ingredients are not explained in this recipe and the instructions in the previous recipe should be followed here also which is clarified in the commentary of Jejjaṭa on *Caraka Saṃhitā*.

लेपं त्वरुष्करशोथं निहन्ति तिलदुग्धमधुकनवनीतैः ।
[3]भल्लातकतरोर्मूलमृदालेपश्च शोथजित् ॥८०॥

Treatment of Oedema caused by Poisons

If oedema is caused because of allergic reaction to marking nut (*bhallātaka*), then the body should be anointed with the

1. क. जैज्जटया इति पंचमपुस्तके पाठः ।
   ख. 'दशमूलं——जेज्जट:' पाठोऽयं प्रथमपुस्तके नोपलभ्यते ।
2. पाठोऽयं षष्ठपुस्तके अधिकमुपलभ्यते ।
3. "भल्लातक०———शोथजित्" पाठोऽयं प्रथमपुस्तके नोपलभ्यते ।

paste of *tila*, milk, *madhuka* and butter. The mud collected from the ground on which *bhallātaka* tree grows should also be used externally which cures oedema.

[1]तत्तरुमूर्तिवर्सानलदलैर्व्वार्चिरेण ।
शोथे विषनिमित्ते तु विषोक्ता सम्मता क्रिया ॥८१॥

If oedema is caused by poisoning as a result of contact with poisonous trees, dirty clothes, poisonous smoke or poisonous leaf, then the method prescribed for various types of poisoning should be adopted.

"[2]समूत्रः सवराचूर्णो वल्लो देयः सुधा[3]ग्निधैः [?] ।
[4]शोथोदरं निहन्त्येष सप्तरा[5]त्रानुशीलनात् ॥८२॥

Intake of *triphalā cūrṇa* in a dose of one *valla* along with cow's urine or the solution of *sudhā kṣāra* cures oedema and *udara roga*. This should be administered continuously for one week.

सर्जनीयस्य धूपे तु राठमुस्ताप्रलेपनात् ।
भल्लातकोत्थः श्वयथुर्दुर्वारोऽपि प्रशाम्यति ॥८३॥

Serious type of oedema caused by *bhallātaka* can be cured by fumigation with *sarja rasa* (gum resin of *śāla* tree) or application of the paste of *rāṭha* as well as *mustā*. [There appears to be many errors in verse nos 80-83].

---

1. 'तत्तः———चिरेण' पाठोऽयं चतुर्थषष्ठपुस्तकयोः नोपलभ्यते ।
2. 'समूत्रः———निहन्ति' पाठोऽयं प्रथमपुस्तके नोपलभ्यते ।
3. क. सुधानिधैः इति चतुर्थपुस्तके पाठः ।
   ख. सुधानिधा इति षष्ठपुस्तके पाठः ।
4. शोथं रोगं इति चतुर्थषष्ठपुस्तकयोः पाठः ।
5. सप्तराचातुशीतनात् इति पंचमपुस्तके पाठः ।

यष्टीमधुकलेपोऽरुष्करशोथं निहन्ति ॥८४॥"

Application of the paste of *yaṣṭi madhu* cures oedema caused by *bhallātaka*.

"ग्राम्यानूपं[1] पिशितं लवणं शुष्कशाकं नवान्नम् ।
गौडं पिष्टं दधि सकृशरं[2] विज्जलं[3] मद्यमम्लम् ॥८५॥
धाना वल्लूरमशनमथो[4] गुर्व्यसात्म्यं[5] विदाहि ।
स्वप्नं च रात्रौ श्वयथुगदवान् वर्जयेन्मैथुनं[6] च ॥८६॥"

[चरक : चिकित्सा : १२-२०]

Prohibitions

The patient suffering from oedema should avoid meat of domesticated and marshy animals, salt, freshly harvested cereals, jaggery preparations, pastries, curd, *kṛśarā* (a preparation of rice added with pulses), undiluted alcohol, sour drinks, fried paddy, dried meat, heavy, unwholesome and *vidāhi* (which causes burning sensation) food, sleep at night [?] and sexual intercourse.

इति महाराजाधिराजटोडरमल्लविरचितेटोडरानंदे आयुर्वेदसौख्ये शोथनिदानचिकित्साकथन नाम अष्टचत्वारिंशत्तमो हर्षः ॥८७॥

Thus, ends the 48th Chapter on diagnosis and treatment of oedema in *Āyurveda saukhya* of *Toḍarānanda* composed by the great king Ṭoḍara Malla.

---

1. ग्राम्याब्जानूपं इति प्रथमपुस्तके पाठः ।
2. तिलकृतं इति आकरे पाठः ।
3. मृज्जलं इति चतुर्थषष्ठपुस्तकयोः पाठः ।
4. वल्लूरं समशनमथो इति प्रथमपुस्तके पाठः ।
5. गुर्वसात्म्यं इति आकरे पाठः ।
6. वर्जयेल्लेपनं च इति चतुर्थपंचमषष्ठपुस्तकेषु पाठः ।

CHAPTER XIV

अथ वृद्धिनिदानं चिकित्सा च ।

Diagnosis and Treatment of Vṛddhi (Scrotal Enlargement)

"क्रुद्धो[1]रुद्धगतिर्वायुः शोफशूलकरश्च[2]रन् ।
मुष्कौ वङ्क्षणतः प्राप्य फलकोषाभिवाहिनीः ।
प्रपीड्य धमनीर्वृद्धिं करोति फलकोषयोः ॥१॥

Pathogenesis

The aggravated and obstructed *vāyu*, while causing oedema and pain, moves from groins to the testicular sacs, inflicts

---

1. This is the beginning of the 53rd Chapter of *Āyurveda saukhya* in *Ṭoḍarānanda* and the invocation reads as follows:—
"नवांगनानां नवमण्डले यस्तादृग्वयोमानसमानसंख्यः ।
हैमोद्भवे मारकता इवा धरेजे सदीप्ति विदधातु भूपे ॥
2. ०चरत् इति प्रथमपुस्तके पाठः ।

pressure on channels carrying nourishing material to testicles and increases the vascular size in testicles.

दोषास्त्रमेदोमूत्रान्त्रैः स वृद्धिः सप्तधा गदः ।
मूत्रान्त्रजावप्यनिलाद्धेतुभेदस्तु केवलम् ॥२॥

Varieties

This *vṛddhi* (scrotal enlargement) is of seven types, viz. *vātika, paittika, kaphaja, raktaja, medoja, mūtraja* and *antraja. Mūtra vṛddhi* and *antra vṛddhi* are also caused by *vāyu.* But these are distinguished from *vātika vṛddhi* on account of their etiological factors.

वातपूर्णदृतिस्पर्शो रूक्षो वातादहेतुरुक् ।
पक्वोदुम्बरसंकाशः पित्ताद्[1] दाहोष्मपाकवान् ।
कफाच्छीतो गुरुः स्निग्धः कण्डूमान् कठिनोऽल्परुक् ॥३॥

Vātika, Paittika and Kaphaja Vṛddhi

Vātika vṛddhi is characterised by a touch of the scrotum which feels like a wind inflated blower, roughness and pain without any appreciable reason. In *paittika vṛddhi,* the scrotum appears like a ripe fruit of *udumbara* along with burning as well as heating sensation and suppuration. In *kaphaja vṛddhi,* scrotal growth is cold to touch, heavy, unctuous, associated with itching, hard and less painful.

कृष्णस्फोटावृतः पित्तवृद्धिलिङ्गश्च रक्तजः ।
कफवन्मेदसा[2] वृद्धिर्मृदुस्तालफलोपमः ॥४॥

---

1. पित्ता दाहो॰ इति प्रथमपुस्तके पाठः ।
2. कफवन्मेदसो इति प्रथमपुस्तके पाठः ।

Raktaja and Medoja Vṛddhi

Raktaja vṛddhi shares the signs and symptoms of *pittaja vṛddhi*. In addition, the scrotum is surrounded with black pustules. *Medoja vṛddhi* shares the signs and symptoms of *kaphaja vṛddhi*. In addition, the scrotum is soft to touch like a ripe fruit of *tāla*.

मूत्रधारणशीलस्य मूत्रजः स तु[1] गच्छतः ।
अम्भोभिर्[2]पूर्णदृतिवत् क्षोभं याति सरुङ्मृदुः ।
मूत्रकृच्छ्रमधःस्याच्च चालयन् फलकोषयोः ॥५॥

Mūtra Vṛddhi

The person who habitually suppresses the urge for micturation suffers from *mūtra vṛddhi*. While walking, the enlarged scrotum produces sound as if it is a leather bag containing water. It is associated with pain and is soft to touch. Because of the mobility of the testicles, the patient suffers from dysuria.

वातकोपिभिराहारैः शीततोयावगाहनैः ।
धारणेरणभाराध्वविषमाङ्गप्रवर्त्तनैः[3] ॥६॥
क्षोभणैः क्षोभितोऽन्यैश्च क्षुद्रान्त्रावयवं यदा ।
पवनो विगुणीकृत्य स्वनिवेशादधो नयेत् ।
कुर्याद्वङ्क्षणसन्धिस्थो ग्रन्थ्याभं श्वयथुं तदा ॥७॥

---

1. सतु च गुच्छति इति पंचमपुस्तके पाठः ।
2. अम्भानि इति आदर्शपुस्तकेषु पाठः ।
3. प्रवर्ततैः इति आदर्शपुस्तकेषु पाठः ।

उपेक्ष्यमाणस्य[1] च मुष्कवृद्धिमाध्मानरुक्स्तम्भवती[2] स वायुः ।
प्रपीडितोऽन्तः स्वनवान् प्रयाति प्रध्मापयन्नेति पुनश्च मुक्तः ॥८॥

Antra Vṛddhi (*Inguinal Hernia*)

By the intake of *vāyu* aggravating food, taking bath in cold water, suppression of natural urges, heavy weight, walking a long distance, improper posture of limbs and such other factors which put pressure on the abdomen, the vitiated *vāyu* displaces the small intestine and pushes it downwards as a result of which there appears a small tumour like structure with swelling in the joint of the groin (inguinal canal). If neglected, it causes scrotal enlargement, abdominal distension and pain. If pressed, the growth subsides with gurgling noise of the wind. But when pressure is released, the swelling appears again like a blower.

यस्यांत्रावयवश्लेष[मा]मुष्कयोर्वातसंचयात् ।
अन्त्रवृद्धिरसाध्योऽयं वातवृद्धिसमाकृतिः ।"
[माधवनिदान : वृद्धिनिदान ३७ : १-१०]

रूक्षकृष्णारुणशिरातन्तुजालसमावृता[3] ॥९॥

Prognosis

If because of accumulation of *vāyu* in the testicular region, there is adhesion of the small intestine into the adjoining tissues and if like *vātaja vṛddhi*, it is surrounded by the net work of rough, black and reddish vessels, then it is incurable.

---

1. उपेक्ष० इति आदर्शपुस्तकेषु पाठः ।
2. क. ०ध्मानसाम्रवत्तहि वायु इति षष्ठपुस्तके पाठः ।
   ख. रुकूस्तंभयतीरुवायुः इति प्रथमपुस्तके पाठः ।
3. सुक्ष्मकृष्णा० इति षष्ठपुस्तके पाठः ।

"अत्यभिष्यन्दिगुर्वम्लसेवनान्निचयं[1] गतः ।
करोति वृद्धिवत् शोफं[2] दोषो वंक्षणसंधिषु ।
ज्वरशूलांगसादाद्यं[3] तं ब्रध्नमिति[4] निर्दिशेत् ॥१०॥"

[माधवनिदान : वृद्धिनिदान : ३७ : १० भाषा टीका]

॥ अन्त्रवृद्धिकुरण्डब्रध्ननिदानम्[5] ॥११॥

Bradhna

Because of the intake of *abhiṣyandī* (which obstructs channels of circulation), heavy and sour food as well as drinks, *doṣas* get accumulated in the groin joint to cause swelling like *vṛddhi roga* along with fever, pain and prostration. This is called *bradhna* (tumour in the inguinal region).

Thus, ends the diagnosis of *antra vṛddhi* (inguinal hernia), *kuraṇḍa* (scrotal enlargement) and *bradhna* (tumour in the inguinal region).

गुग्गुलुं रुबुतैलं[6] वा गोमूत्रेण पिबेन्नरः ।
"वातवृद्धिं[7] निहन्त्याशु चिरकालानुबन्धनीम्[8] ॥१२॥

Intake of *guggulu* or castor oil along with cow's urine cures *vātika vṛddhi* even if it is chronic.

---

1. अत्यभिष्यंदिगुर्वम्ल० इति प्रथमपुस्तके पाठः ।
2. ग्रन्थिवच्छोथं इति आकरे पाठः ।
3. ज्वरशूलाङ्गदाहाढ्यं इति आकरे पाठः ।
4. ब्रध्म० इति आदर्शपुस्तकेषु पाठः ।
5. वृद्धिनिदानम इति आकरे पाठः ।
6. गुग्गुलुं रुचुतैलंचा० इति प्रथमपुस्तके पाठः ।
7. वातवृद्धौ पिबेत्स्निग्धं यथाप्राप्तं विरेचनम् इति आकरे पाठः ।
8. ०नुबन्धनीम् इति पंचमपुस्तके पाठः ।

सक्षीरं वा पिबेत्तैलं मासमेरण्डसम्भवम् ।
पुनर्नवायास्तैलं वा तैलं नारायणं तथा ।
पाने बस्तौ रुबोस्तैलं पेयं वा दशकाम्भसा[1] ॥१३॥"

[भैषज्यरत्नावली : वृद्धिरोगाधिकार : २-३]

For the cure of *vāta vṛddhi* following recipes are useful :

1. Intake of castor oil along with milk for one month ;
2. Use of *punarnavādya taila* or *nārāyaṇa taila* as drink and for medicated enema ; and
3. Intake of castor oil along with the decoction of *daśa mūla.*

"चन्दनं मधुकं पद्ममुशीरं नीलमुत्पलम्[2] ।
क्षीरपिष्टैः[3] प्रदेहः स्याद्दाहशोथरुजापहम् ॥१४॥

Candana, *madhuka*, *padma*, *uśira* and *nīlotpala* should be made to a paste by triturating with milk. Application of this paste cures burning sensation, oedema and pain associated with *vṛddhi.*

पञ्चवल्कलकल्केन सघृतेन प्रलेपनम् ।
सर्वं पित्तहरं कार्यं रक्तजे रक्तमोक्षणम् ॥१५॥"

[भैषज्यरत्नावली : वृद्धिरोगाधिकार : ५-६]

The paste of the barks of *nyagrodha*, *udumbara*, *aśvattha*, *pāriṣa* and *plakṣa* should be mixed with ghee and applied

---

1. दशकाम्लसा इति प्रथमपुस्तके पाठः ।
2. पद्ममुत्पलं इति षष्ठपुस्तके पाठः ।
3. क्षीरपृष्टे इति षष्ठपुस्तके पाठः ।

externally and all *pitta* alleviating therapies should be used for the cure of *paittika vṛddhi*. In *raktaja vṛddhi*, blood-letting therapy should be administered.

"श्लेष्मावृद्धिमुष्णवीर्यैर्मूत्रपिष्टैः[1] प्रलेपयेत् ।
पीतदारुकषायञ्च पिबेन्मूत्रेण संयुतम् ॥१६॥"

[भैषज्यरत्नावली : वृद्धिरोगाधिकार : ६]

For the cure of *kaphaja vṛddhi*, drugs having hot potency should be made to a paste by triturating with cow's urine and applied externally. For this, the patient should take the decoction of *pīta dāru* along with cow's urine.

"स्विन्नं मेदःसमुत्थन्तु लेपयेत्सुरसादिना[2] ।
शिरोविरेकद्रव्यैर्वा[3] सुखोष्णैर्मूत्रसंयुतैः[4] ॥१७॥

If the scrotal tumour is caused by *medas* (fat), then first of all, fomentation therapy should be applied over the tumour and thereafter, the luke-warm paste of drugs belonging to *surasādi gaṇa* prepared by triturating with cow's urine should be applied. Similarly, the luke-warm paste of drugs, used for errhine therapy (*śiro-vireka*) prepared by triturating with cow's urine should be applied.

संस्वेद्य मूत्रप्रभवं वस्त्रपट्टेन[5] वेष्टयेत् ।
सेविन्या[6] पार्श्वतोऽधस्ताद्विध्येद् व्रीहिमुखेन वै ॥१८॥"

[भैषज्यरत्नावली : वृद्धिरोगाधिकार : ११-१२]

1. ०मूत्रापिष्टैः इति पंचमपुस्तके पाठः ।
2. ०त्स्वरसादिना इति आदर्शपुस्तकेषु पाठः ।
3. ०दुर्वाच्यैः इति प्रथमपुस्तके पाठः ।
4. ०मूत्र० इति पंचमपुस्तके पाठः ।
5. वस्त्रपदेन इति पंचमपुस्तके पाठः ।
6. सीदत्याः इति प्रथमपुस्तके पाठः ।

Surgical Method

Mūtraja granthi (hydrocele) should first of all be given fomentation therapy and then by wrapping the scrotum with a piece of cloth, it should be punctured at the side and lower part with the help of *brīhi mukha yantra* (trochar and canula).

"शंङ्खोपरि च कर्णान्ते त्यक्त्वा[1] सीवनिमादरात्[2] ।
व्यत्यासाद्वा शिरां[3] विध्येदन्त्रवृद्धिनिवृत्तये[4] ॥१९॥"

[योगरत्नाकर : वृद्धिचिकित्सा : पृष्ठ १३८]

For the cure of *antra vṛddhi* (inguinal hernia), venesection should be performed over the temporal region above the ear. It should be ensured that venesection is not performed over the *sīvani* (suture of the temporal bone) or near about that.

अङ्गुष्ठमध्ये त्वक् छित्वा दहेदङ्ग[5]विपर्यये ॥२०॥

For the cure of *antra vṛddhi* (inguinal hernia) the skin of the thumb of the opposite side should be incised and cauterized.

"रास्नायष्ट्यमृतैरण्डबलागोक्षुरसाधितः ।
क्वाथोऽन्त्रवृद्धिं हन्त्याशु रुबुतैलेन मिश्रितः ॥२१॥

Intake of the decoction of *rāsnā*, *yaṣṭī*, *amṛtā*, *eraṇḍa*, *balā* and *gokṣura* mixed with castor oil instantaneously cures *antra vṛddhi* (inguinal hernia).

---

1. ०भ्यत्का इति पंचमषष्ठपुस्तकयोः पाठः ।
2. ०सादरात् इति पंचमपुस्तके पाठः ।
3. सिरां इति प्रथमपुस्तके पाठः ।
4. ०न्निवृन्तये इति प्रथमपुस्तके पाठः ।
5. दहेप्रागविपर्यये इति षष्ठपुस्तके पाठः ।

तैलमेरण्डजं पीत्वा बलासिद्धं पयोन्वितम् ।
आध्मानशूलोपचितामान्त्रवृद्धिं[1] जयेन्नरः ॥२२॥"

[भैषज्यरत्नावली : वृद्धिरोगाधिकार : १६-१७]

Intake of castor oil cooked with *balā* and milk cures abdominal distension, colic pain and swollen *antra vṛddhi* (inguinal hernia).

"हरीतकीं मूत्रसिद्धां सतैलां[2] लवणान्विताम्[3] ।
प्रातः प्रातश्च सेवेत कफवातमयापहम् ॥२३॥"

[भैषज्यरत्नावली : वृद्धिरोगाधिकार : ६८]

Intake of *harītakī* boiled with cow's urine along with oil and rock-salt every morning cures diseases caused by *kapha* and *vāyu*.

"गोमूत्रसिद्धां रुबुतैलभृष्टां[4] हरीतकीं सैंधवचूर्णयुक्ताम् ।
खादेन्नरः[5] कोष्णजलानुपानं निहन्ति वृद्धिं चिरजां प्रवृद्धाम् ॥२४॥"

[भैषज्यरत्नावली : वृद्धिरोगाधिकार : ७७]

Harītakī, boiled in cow's urine and fried in castor oil should be taken along with rock-salt. Luke-warm water should be taken thereafter. This cures serious type of *vṛddhi roga* of long standing duration.

---

1. ०पचितं अण्डवृद्धिं इति षष्ठपुस्तके पाठः ।
2. सतैलं इति षष्ठपुस्तके पाठः ।
3. लवणान्वितम् इति षष्ठपुस्तके पाठः ।
4. रुबुतैलमिश्रां इति षष्ठपुस्तके पाठः ।
5. क. खादन्नरः इति षष्ठपुस्तके पाठः ।
   ख. पिबेन्नरः इति आकरे पाठः ।

"त्रिफलाक्वाथगोमूत्रं पिबेत्प्रातरतन्द्रितः ।
कफवातोद्भवं हन्ति श्वयथुं[1] वृषणोत्थितम् ॥२५॥"

[भैषज्यरत्नावली : वृद्धिरोगाधिकार : ७२]

Regular intake of the decoction of *triphalā* and cow's urine every morning cures *kaphaja* and *vātaja* types of *vṛddhi roga.*

"सरलागुरुकुष्ठानि देवदारु महौषधम् ।
मूत्रारनालसंयुक्तं[2] शोथघ्नं कफवातनुत् ॥२६॥"

[भैषज्यरत्नावली : वृद्धिरोगाधिकार : ७३]

Intake of *saralā, aguru, kuṣṭha, deva dāru* and *mahauṣadha* along with cow's urine and *āranāla* (a type of sour drink) cures oedema, aggravation of *kapha* as well as *vāyu.*

"भृष्टो रुबुकतैलेन कल्कः पथ्यासमुद्भवः ।
कृष्णासैन्धवसंयुक्तो वृद्धिरोगहरः परः ॥२७॥"

[भैषज्यरत्नावली : वृद्धिरोगाधिकार : २०]

The paste of *harītaki* should be fried with castor oil and mixed with *pippali* as well as rock-salt. Intake of this recipe cures *vṛddhi roga.*

"गव्यं घृतं सैन्धवं च सम्प्रयुक्त शम्बूकभाण्डे निहितं प्रयत्नात्[3] ।
सप्ताहमादित्यकरैर्विपक्वं निहन्ति[4] कुरण्डमतिप्रवृद्धम्[5] ॥२८॥"

[भैषज्यरत्नावली : वृद्धिरोगाधिकार : ७४]

---

1. वृषणं श्वयथूत्स्थिताम् इति षष्ठपुस्तके पाठः ।
2. मूत्रानारलसंपिष्टं इति प्रथमपंचमपुस्तकयोः पाठः ।
3. क. तदेव इति आकरे पाठः ।
   ख. प्रलेपात् इति षष्ठपुस्तके पाठः ।
4. हन्यात् इति आकरे पाठः ।
5. कुरण्डं चिरजं प्रवृद्धम् इति आकरे पाठः ।

Cow's ghee mixed with rock-salt should be kept in a jar prepared of (or containing) sea-shells. This jar should be kept exposed to sun rays for seven days. Intake of this cures serious type of scrotal tumour.

"ऐन्द्रीमूलभवं चूर्णं रुबुतैलेन मर्दितम् ।
त्र्यहाद्[1] गोपयसा पीतं सर्ववृद्धिनिवारणम्[2] ॥२९॥"

[भैषज्यरत्नावली : वृद्धिरोगाधिकार : ७८]

The powder of the root of *aindrī* should be triturated with castor oil and taken for three days with cow's milk which cures all types of *vṛddhi roga.*

रुद्रजटामूललिप्ता[3]करटव्यङ्ग[4]चर्मणा ।
बद्धा वृद्धिः शमं याति चिरजापि न संशयः ॥३०॥

A piece of leather should be smeared with the paste of the root of *rudra jaṭā* and tied over the enlarged scrotum which undoubtedly cures *vṛddhi roga.*

"निष्पिष्टमारनालेन रूपिकामूलवल्कलम् ।
लेपो वृद्ध्यामयं हन्ति बद्धमूलमपि दृढम्[5] ॥३१॥"

[भैषज्यरत्नावली : वृद्धिरोगाधिकार : ७०]

---

1. त्र्यहान् इति आदर्शपुस्तकेषु पाठः ।
2. सर्ववृद्धिहरं परम् इति आकरे पाठः ।
3. ०लिफाकरव्यंग इति षष्ठपुस्तके पाठः ।
4. ०व्यङ्ग० इति चतुर्थपुस्तके पाठः ।
5. ध्रुवम् इति चतुर्थषष्ठपुस्तकयोः पाठः ।

The root bark of *rūpikā* [?] should be made to a paste by triturating with *āranāla* (a sour drink) and applied over the enlarged scrotum for its cure. Application of this paste and then wrapping a piece of cloth with pressure over the scrotum also cure *vṛddhi roga*.

"वचासर्षपकल्केन प्रलेपो[1] वृद्धिनाशनः ।"

[भैषज्यरत्नावली : वृद्धिरोगाधिकार : ७६]

"लज्जागृध्रमलाभ्याञ्च लेपो वृद्धिहरः परः ॥३२॥"

[भैषज्यरत्नावली : वृद्धिरोगाधिकार : २१]

External application of the paste of *vacā* and *sarṣapa* cures *vṛddhi roga*. Similarly, application of the paste of *lajjālu* and stool of vulture cures *vṛddhi roga*.

"मूलं बिल्वकपित्थयोररलुकस्या[2]ग्नेर्बृहत्योर्द्वयोः ।

श्यामापूतिकरञ्जशिग्रुकतरोर्बिभ्यौषधारुष्करम्[3] ॥३३॥

कृष्णाग्रन्थिकचव्यपञ्चलवणक्षाराजमोदान्वितम्[4] ।

पीतं काञ्जिककोष्णतोयमथितैश्चूर्णीकृतं ब्रध्नजित् ॥३४॥

॥ बिल्वादिचूर्णम्[5] ॥

---

1. क. लेपो वृद्धिविनाशनः इति ग्राकरे पाठः ।
   ख. प्रलेपाद्वृद्धिनाशनः इति पंचमपुस्तके पाठः ।
2. बिल्वकापित्थयोरतुलुकस्या० इति प्रथमपुस्तके पाठः ।
3. धातुष्करम् इति द्वितीयपुस्तके पाठः ।
4. ०मोदान्वितः इति पंचमपुस्तके पाठः ।
5. क. पाठोऽयं प्रथमपंचमपुस्तकयोः नोपलभ्यते ।
   ख. बिल्वाद्यं चूर्णम् इति चतुर्थषष्ठपुस्तकयोः पाठः ।

Bilvādi Cūrṇa

Intake of the powder of the roots of *bilva* and *kapittha*, *araluka*, *agni*, *bṛhatī*, *kaṇṭakārī*, *śyāmā*, *pūti karañja*, *śuṇṭhī*, *aruṣkara*, *kṛṣṇā*, *granthika*, *cavya*, *pañca lavaṇa*, *kṣāra* and *ajamodā* along with *kāñjī* (a type of sour drink), luke-warm water or butter-milk cures *bradhna* (growth in the inguinal region).

अविक्षीरेण[1] गोधूमकल्कं कुन्दुरुकस्य[2] वा[3] ।
प्रलेपनं सुखोष्णं स्यात् ब्रध्नशूलहरं[4] परम् ॥३५॥

Wheat and *kunduru* should be made to a paste by triturating with sheep-milk. Application of this luke-warm paste cures pain in *bradhna*.

मृतमात्रे[5] तु वै काके[6] विशस्ते तु प्रवेशयेत् ।
ब्रध्नं[7] मुहूर्त्तं मेधावी तत्क्षणादरुजं[8] भवेत् ॥३६॥

[The meaning of this verse is not clear].

अजाजीहवुषाकुष्ठगोधूमबदराणि च ।
काञ्जिकेन समं पिष्ट्वा कुर्याद् ब्रध्नप्रलेपनम्[9] ॥३७॥"

[भैषज्यरत्नावली : वृद्धिरोगाधिकार : २३-२६]

---

1. क. अजाक्षीरेण इति आकरे पाठः ।
   ख. आविक्षीरेण इति षष्ठपुस्तके पाठः ।
2. कुन्दुककस्य व इति प्रथमचतुर्थपंचमपुस्तकेषु पाठः ।
3. च इति षष्ठपुस्तके पाठः ।
4. ब्रध्म० इति पंचमषष्ठपुस्तकयोः पाठः ।
5. मृत्पात्रे इति पंचमषष्ठपुस्तकयोः पाठः ।
6. पाके इति षष्ठपुस्तके पाठः ।
7. वद्धमूत्रः तु इति षष्ठपुस्तके पाठः ।
8. ०रुजो इति षष्ठपुस्तके पाठः ।
9. ब्रध्ने प्रलेपनम् इति आकरे पाठः ।

Ajājī, havuṣā, kuṣṭha, godhūma and *badara* should be made to a paste by triturating with *kāñji*. Application of this paste cures *bradhna*.

"सैन्धवं मदनं कुष्ठं शताह्वां निचुलं वचाम् ।
ह्रीवेरं मधुकं भार्ङ्गीं देवदारु सनागरम् ॥३८॥
कट्फलं पौष्करं मेदां चविकां चित्रकं शटीम् ।
विडङ्गातिविषां[1] श्यामां वेणुकां[2] नीलिनीं स्थिराम् ॥३९॥
बिल्वाजमोदे[3] कृष्णाञ्च दन्तीं रास्नां[4] प्रपिष्य च ।
साध्यमेरण्डतैलं[5] वा तैलं वा कफवातनुत् ॥४०॥
[6]ब्रध्नोदावर्त्तगुल्मार्शःप्लीहमेहाढ्यमारुतान्[7] ।
आनाहमश्मरीञ्चैव हन्यात्तदनुवासनात् ॥४१॥"

॥ बृहत्सैन्धवाद्यं तैलम् ॥

[भैषज्यरत्नावली : वृद्धिरोगाधिकार : ४३-४६]

Bṛhat Saindhavādya Taila

Castor oil or sesamum oil should be cooked by adding the paste of *saindhava, madana, kuṣṭha, śatāhvā, nicula, vacā, hrīvera, madhuka, bhārṅgī, deva dāru, nāgara, kaṭ phala, puṣkara mūla, medā, cavikā, citraka, śaṭī, viḍaṅga, ativiṣā, śyāmā, veṇukā, nīlinī, sthirā, bilva, ajamodā, kṛṣṇā, dantī* and *rāsnā*. This medicated oil alleviates *kapha* as well as *vāyu* and cures

1. विडङ्गातिविषे इति आदर्शपुस्तकेषु पाठः ।
2. रेणुका नीलिनीं स्थिराम् इति षष्ठपुस्तके आकरे च पाठः ।
3. मोदां इति प्रथमपंचमपुस्तकयोः पाठः ।
4. राष्णां इति आदर्शपुस्तकेषु पाठः ।
5. साध्यमेरण्डजं तैलं इति आदर्शपुस्तकेषु पाठः ।
6. वध्मों० इति षष्ठपुस्तके पाठः ।
7. ०मारुतात् इति प्रथमपंचमपुस्तकयोः पाठः ।

bradhna (inguinal growth), *udāvarta* (upward movement of wind in the abdomen), *gulma* (phantom tumour), piles, splenic enlargement, *prameha* (obstinate urinary disorders including diabetes), *āḍhya vāta*, abdominal distension and *aśmarī* (stone in the urinary tract). This recipe is to be used for *anuvāsana* type of medicated enema.

"[1]शतमेरण्डमूलस्य शुंठ्या पंच यवाढकम् ।
जलद्रोणे [2]चतुर्थांशपयसाष्टगुणानि च ॥४२॥
प्रस्थमेरण्डतैलस्य तन्मूलाश्च चतुःपलम् ।
द्वि[3]पलं शृंगवेरस्य गर्भं दत्त्वा शनैः[4] पचेत् ॥४३॥
[5]तत्पिबेत्प्रयतः शुद्धो नरः क्षीरान्नभुक् सदा ।
अन्त्रवृद्धिं नि[6]हन्त्याशु तैलं गन्धर्वहस्त[7]कम्[8] ॥४४॥"

॥ गन्धर्वहस्ततैलम्[9] ॥

[भैषज्यरत्नावली : वृद्धिरोगाधिकार : ४८-५०]

---

1. शतमेरण्डमूलस्य पलं शुण्ठ्या यवाढकम् इति आकरे पाठः ।
2. विपक्तव्यं यावत्पादावशेषितम् । तेन पादावशेषेण पयसा तत्समेन च इति आकरे पाठः ।
3. त्रिपलं शृंगवेरञ्च इति आकरे पाठः ।
4. विपाचयेत् इति आकरे पाठः ।
5. क. पिबेच्चसतत्रशुद्धातनः इति पंचमपुस्तके पाठः ।
   ख. न पिबेच्च ततः शुद्धो नरः इति षष्ठपुस्तके पाठः ।
6. जयत्याशु इति आकरे पाठः ।
7. क. ०संज्ञिकं इति चतुर्थपुस्तके पाठः ।
   ख. ०संज्ञकं इति षष्ठपुस्तके पाठः ।
8. "शतमेरण्डं......गन्धर्वहस्तकम्" पाठोऽयं प्रथमपुस्तके नोपलभ्यते ।
9. क. गंधर्वतैलम् इति चतुर्थषष्ठपुस्तकयोः पाठः ।
   ख. पाठोऽयं पंचमपुस्तके नोपलभ्यते ।

Gandharva Hasta Taila

One hundred *palas* of the root of *eraṇḍa*, five *palas* of *śuṇṭhī* and one *āḍhaka* of *yava* should be cooked in one *droṇa* of water and reduced to one fourth. To this decoction, eight *prasthas* of milk, one *prastha* of castor oil and four *palas* of the paste of root of *eraṇḍa* and two *palas* of the paste of *śṛṅgavera* should be added and cooked over mild fire. After purification of the body, the patient should take this medicated oil internally. While doing so, he should eat only milk and rice. This is called *gandharva hasta taila* and it cures *antra vṛddhi* (inguinal hernia).

[1]'पातालयन्त्रयोगेन तैलं वृश्चिकसम्भवम् ।
प्रलेपान्नाशयत्येव वृद्धिं मासान्नसंशयः ॥४५॥

॥ वृश्चिकतैलम् ॥[2]

Vṛścika Taila

Oil of *vṛścika* should be extracted with the help of *Pātāla yantra* and applied over the enlarged scrotum which is undoubtedly cured within one month.

विषुरिमांसस्वेदेन कुरण्डो याति ॥४६॥

॥ इति मत्सरहस्यम् ॥

According to Matsya Rahasya

Application of fomentation therapy with the meat of *viṣuri* type of fish cures scrotal tumour.

---

1. 'पातालयन्त्र———लेपः' पाठोऽयं पंचमषष्ठपुस्तकयोः अधिकमुपलभ्यते ।
2. पाठोऽयं षष्ठपुस्तके अधिकमुपलभ्यते ।

गोघृतं सैन्धवोपेतं संबूकस्थं रवेः करैः ।
पक्वं सप्तदिनं हन्यात् शीघ्रं वृद्धि कुरण्डकः ॥४७॥

(A variant reading of the recipe in verse no. 28).

हिंगुलहसुनचित्रकमेलासहिजनात्वचब्रध्मो लेपः ॥४८॥'

The paste of *hiṅgu, laśuna, citraka, bhallātaka, śobhāñjana* (bark) should be applied over *bradhna* (inguinal growth) for its cure.

"घृतं सौरेश्वरं योज्यं ब्रध्नवृद्धिनिवृत्तये ॥४९॥"

[भैषज्यरत्नावली : वृद्धिरोगाधिकार : ४७]

Saureśvara ghṛta should be applied over *bradhna* (inguinal growth) for its cure.

'चित्रकं[1] लशुनं हिंगु भल्लातं शिग्रमूलजम् ।
निम्बुनीरकृतो लेपः स्तीव्रब्रध्मप्रशान्तये ॥५०॥'

Citraka, laśuna, hiṅgu bhallātaka and the bark of the root of *śigru* should be triturated by adding lime juice and made to a paste. Application of this paste cures serious type of *bradhna* (inguinal growth). [This is variant reading in Sanskrit of the recipe at line no 48 above]

"शतपुष्पा[2]देवदारुमरिचं रजनीद्वयम् ।
जीरके द्वे वचा विश्वं[3] त्रिफलां गुग्गुलुं त्वचम् ॥५१॥

1. 'चित्रकं——प्रशान्तये' पाठोऽयं प्रथमपंचमपुस्तकयोः नोपलभ्यते ।
2. शतपुष्पामृतादारु चन्दनं इति आकरे पाठः ।
3. नागत्रिफलागुग्गुलुत्वचम् इति आकरे पाठः ।

मांसी कुष्ठं[1] च पत्रैला रास्ना[2] शृंगी च चित्रकम् ।
कृमिघ्नमश्वगन्धा च शैलेयं कटुरोहिणी ॥५२॥
सैन्धवं तगरं चैव कुटजातिविषैः समैः ।
एतैश्च कार्षिकैः कल्कैर्घृतप्रस्थं विपाचयेत् ॥५३॥
वृषमुण्डितिकैरण्डनिम्बपत्रभवो रसः ।
कण्टकार्यास्तथा क्षीरप्रस्थं प्रस्थं विनिक्षिपेत्[3] ॥५४॥
सिद्धमेतत् घृतं पीतमन्त्रवृद्धिं व्यपोहति ।
वातवृद्धिं तथा[4] घोरां मेदोवृद्धिमथापि वा ॥५५॥
मूत्रवृद्धिं श्लीपदश्च यकृत्प्लीहानमेव च ।
[5]शतपुष्पाघृतञ्चैतद्धन्यादेतन्न संशयः ॥५६॥"

॥ शतपुष्पाद्यं घृतम् ॥

[भैषज्यरत्नावली : वृद्धिरोगाधिकार : ५१-५६]

Śatapuṣpādya Ghṛta

To one *prastha* of ghee, the paste of one *akṣa* of each of *śatapuṣpā*, *deva dāru*, *marica*, *haridrā*, *dāru haridrā*, *śveta jīraka*, *kṛṣṇa jiraka*, *vacā*, *viśva*, *triphalā*, *guggulu*, *tvak*, *māṃsi*, *kuṣṭha*, *patra*, *elā*, *rāsnā*, *śṛṅgī*, *citraka*, *kṛmighna*, *aśva gandhā*, *śaileya*, *kaṭu rohiṇī*, *saindhava*, *tagara*, *kuṭaja* and *ativiṣā*, one *prastha* of each of the juice or decoction of *vṛṣa*, *muṇḍitikā*, *eraṇḍa*, leaves

1. सकुष्ठपत्रैला इति आकरे पाठः ।
2. राष्णा० इति आदर्शपुस्तकेषु पाठः ।
3. पाचयेत् इति चतुर्थषष्ठपुस्तकयोः पाठः ।
4. पित्तवृद्धिं इति आकरे पाठः ।
5. शतपुष्पाद्यमेतद्धि घृतं हन्ति न संशयः इति आकरे पाठः ।

of *nimba* as well as *kaṇṭakārī* and one *prastha* of milk should be added and cooked. Intake of this medicated ghee undoubtedly cures *antra vṛddhī* (inguinal hernia), *vātika vṛddhi*, serious type of *medoja vṛddhi*, *mūtra vṛddhī* (hydrocele), *ślīpada* (filariasis) and liver as well as spleen enlargement. This is called *śata-puṣpādya ghṛta*.

"वेगरोधं[1] पृष्ठयानं व्यायामं मैथुनं तथा ।
अत्याशनं तथा क्रोधं गुरुद्रव्याणि वर्जयेत् ॥५७॥"

Prohibitions

The patient suffering from *vṛddhi roga* should avoid suppression of natural urges, travelling on the back of animals, exercise, sexual intercourse, over-eating, anger and heavy food.

इति श्रीमहाराजाधिराजश्रीटोडरमल्लविरचिते टोडरानन्दे आयुर्वेदसौख्ये अन्त्रवृद्धिकुरण्डनिदानचिकित्साकथनं नाम एकोनपंचासत्तमोहर्षः ॥५८॥

Thus, ends the 49th Chapter dealing with the diagnosis and treatment of *antra vṛddhi* (inguinal hernia) and *kuraṇḍaka* (scrotal tumour) in *Āyurveda saukhya* of *Ṭoḍarānanda* composed by the great king Ṭoḍara Malla.

---

1. द्रष्टव्यम्—भैषज्यरत्नावली: वृद्धिरोगाधिकार : ११७ ।

CHAPTER XV

अथ गलगण्डगण्डमालापचीग्रन्थ्यर्बुदनिदानं चिकित्सा च ।

Diagnosis and Treatment of Galagaṇḍa (Goitre), Gaṇḍa Mālā (Lymphadenitis), Apacī (Suppurated Gland), Granthi (Small Tumour) and Arbuda (Large Tumour)

"निबद्धः[1] श्वयथुर्यस्य[2] मुष्कवल्लम्बते गले ।
महान् वा यदि वा ह्रस्वो गलगण्डं तमादिशेत् ॥१॥

---

1. क. This is the beginning of the 54th Chapter of *Āyurveda saukhya* in *Toḍarānanda* and the invocation reads as follows:—
"कलिंदजासीकरसिच्यमानो ब्रजांगनाभिः कुसुमैः सुरेशैः ।
सुवर्षितः कुंतलषट्यदाभिम्मुं दंगतस्तां विदधातु भूपे ।।"
ख. निबद्धूः इति प्रथमपंचमपुस्तकयोः पाठः ।
2. श्वयथुर्यस्तु इति प्रथमपंचमपुस्तकयोः पाठः ।

Description of Gala Gaṇḍa

A compact growth, small or big, hanging from the neck like scrotum is called *gala gaṇḍa* (goitre).

वातः कफश्चापि गले प्रदुष्टो मन्ये च संसृत्य तथैव मेदः ।
कुर्वन्ति गण्डं क्रमशः स्वलिङ्गैः समन्वितं तं गलगण्डमाहुः ॥२॥

Pathogenesis of Gala Gaṇḍa

Vitiated *vāyu* and *kapha* located in the neck afflict both the sterno-mastoid muscles and the fat as a result of which *gaṇḍa* (tumour like growth) is manifested in association with the signs and symptoms of the concerned *doṣas*. This is called *gala gaṇḍa* (goitre).

तोदान्वितः[1] कृष्णशिरावनद्धः श्यावारुणो[2] वा पवनात्मकस्तु ।
पारुष्ययुक्तश्चिरवृद्धिपाको[3] यदृच्छया पाकमियात्कदाचित् ।
वैरस्यमास्यस्य च तस्य जन्तोर्भवेत्तथा तालुगलप्रशोषः ॥३॥

Vātika Gala Gaṇḍa

Vātika type of goitre is characterised by the following signs and symptoms :

1. Association of pain ;
2. Surrounded by the net work of black vessels ;
3. Gray or reddish colour of the growth ;
4. Rough to touch ;
5. It grows and gets suppurated very slowly ;

---

1. तोदान्वितं इति आदर्शपुस्तकेषु पाठः ।
2. श्यावोऽरुणो इति आकरे पाठः ।
3. वृद्ध्यपाको इति आकरे पाठः ।

6. At times it gets suppurated without any provocating factor ;
7. Distaste in the mouth ; and
8. Dryness of palate as well as throat.

स्थिरः सवर्णो गुरुरुग्रकण्डूः शीतो महांश्चापि कफात्मकस्तु ।
चिराभिवृद्धिं भजते चिराद्वा प्रपच्यते मन्दरुजः कदाचित् ।
माधुर्यमास्यस्य च तस्य जन्तोर्भवेत् तथा तालुगलप्रलेपः ॥४॥

Kaphaja Gala Gaṇḍa

Kaphaja type of goitre is characterised by the following signs and symptoms :

1. It is stable and it's colour is the same as that of the skin ;
2. It is heavy and itching ;
3. It is cold to touch and is big in size ;
4. It grows and get suppurated very slowly ;
5. There is occasional mild pain ; and
6. Sweet taste in the mouth and adhesion of sticky material in the palate and throat.

स्निग्धो गुरुः[1] पाण्डुरनिष्टगन्धो मेदोभवः स्वल्परुजोतिकं[2] च ।
प्रलम्बतेऽलाबुवदल्पमूलो[3] देहानुरूपक्षय"वृद्धियुक्तः[4] ।
स्निग्धास्यता तस्य भवेच्च जन्तोर्गलेन[5] शब्दं कुरुते च नित्यम् ॥५॥

---

1. ०घनः इति चतुर्थषष्ठपुस्तकयोः पाठः ।
2. कण्डुयुतोऽल्परुक् इति आकरे पाठः ।
3. तैलावदल्पमूलो इति पंचमपुस्तके पाठः ।
4. 'वृद्धियुक्तः———संवत्स' पाठोऽयं चतुर्थपुस्तके नोपलभ्यते ।
5. जन्तोर्गलेऽनुशब्दं इति आकरे पाठः ।

Medoja Gala Gaṇḍa

Goitre caused by *medas* (fat) is characterised by the following signs and symptoms :

1. Unctuousness, heaviness, pale colour and foul smell ;
2. Mild pain ;
3. It hangs like the fruit of *alābu* with a thin peduncle ;
4. It gets increased and decreased in size on the basis of the increased and decreased weight of the body ;
5. There will be unctuousness in the mouth ; and
6. His voice resounds from the throat.

कृच्छ्राच्छ्वसन्त मृदुसर्वगात्रं संवत्स''रातीतमरोचकार्तम् ।
क्षीणं च वैद्यो गलगण्डयुक्तं भिन्नस्वरं चापि विवर्जयेच्च ॥६॥

Prognosis

If the patient has difficulty in breathing, if there is softness in his entire body, if the goitre is over one year old, if he has anorexia, emaciation and hoarseness of voice, then he should not be treated by the physician.

कर्कन्धुकोलामलकप्रमाणैः कक्षांसमन्यागलवङ्क्षणेषु ।
मेदःकफाभ्यां चिरमन्दपाकैः स्याद्गण्डमाला[1] बहुभिस्तु गण्डैः ॥७॥

Gaṇḍa Mālā (Lymphadenitis)

Multiple growths of the size as well as shape of *karkandhu*, *kola* and *āmalaki* in axilla, sterno-mastoid region and groin because of vitiated *medas* (fat) and *kapha* are called *gaṇḍa mālā*. These growths get mildly suppurated only after a long time.

---

1. स्याद्गंडुमाला इति प्रथमपुस्तके पाठः ।

ते ग्रन्थयः केचिदवाप्तपाका:[1] स्रवन्ति नश्यन्ति भवन्ति चान्ये ।
कालानुबन्धं चिरमादधाति सैवापचीति प्रवदन्ति केचित्[2] ।।८।।

Apaci (*Suppurated Gland*)

Some of these above mentioned growths get suppurated with secretions and ultimate disappearance. But simultaneously other growths appear. This process takes time and becomes very chronic. This is called *apaci*.

साध्या स्मृताः पीनसपार्श्व"शूल[3]कासज्वरच्छर्दियुतास्[4]त्वसाध्याः ।।९।।

Prognosis of Apacī

Apacī is generally curable. But when the patient gets afflicted with *pīnasa* (chronic rhinitis), pain in the sides of the chest, cough, fever and vomiting, then it is incurable.

वातादयो" मांसमसृक् प्रदुष्टाः संदूष्य[5] मेदश्च "तथा[6] शिराश्च ।
वृत्तोन्नतं विग्रथितं तु[7] शोफं कुर्वन्त्यतो ग्रन्थिरिति प्रदिष्टः ।।१०।।"

***Granthi* (*Small Tumour*)**

Vitiated *vāyu*, *pitta*, *kapha*, *māṃsa* (muscle tissue) and *rakta* (blood) afflict *medas* (fat) as well as vessels to give rise to round,

---

1. केचिदवाप्तकामाः प्रवन्ति इति षष्ठपुस्तके पाठः ।
2. तज्ज्ञाः इति आकरे पाठः ।
3. 'शूलकास०——वातादयो' पाठोऽयं चतुर्थपुस्तके नोपलभ्यते ।
4. ०च्छर्दियुतात्वसाध्य इति प्रथमपंचमपुस्तकयोः पाठः ।
5. पाठोऽयं आदर्शपुस्तकेषु नोपलभ्यते ।
6. 'तथा शिराश्च———प्रदिष्टः' पाठोऽयं षष्ठपुस्तके अधिकमुपलभ्यते ।
7. च शोथं इति आकरे पाठः ।

elevated and knot like compact growth which is called *granthi* (lit. knot) or small tumour.

“आयम्यते[1] वृश्चति तुद्यते च प्रक्षिप्यते[2] मथ्यति भिद्यते च ।

कृष्णो मृदुर्बस्तिरिवाततश्च भिन्नः स्रवेच्चानिलजोऽस्रमच्छम्[3] ॥११॥

Vātika Granthi

Vātika type of *granthi* is characterised by contacting, stinging, puncturing, exploding, twisting and incising types of pain. It is black and soft. In touch, it is like a distended bladder. When it opens up, transparent liquid exudes out of it.

दन्दह्यते धूप्यति चूष्यते च पापच्यते[4] प्रज्वलतीव चापि[5] ।

रक्तः सपीतोऽप्यथवाऽपि पित्ताद्भिन्नः स्रवेदुष्णमतीव चास्रम् ॥१२॥

Paittika Granthi

Paittika type of *granthi* is characterised by different types of pain, viz. burning, fumigating, sucking, suppurating and heating with fire. It is either red or yellow in colour. When it opens up, hot and blood mixed liquid exudes out of it.

शीतोऽविवर्णोऽल्परुजोऽतिकण्डुः पाषाणवत् संहननोपपन्नः ।

चिराभिवृद्धश्च कफप्रकोपाद्भिन्न स्रवेच्छुक्लघनं च पूयम् ॥१३॥

---

1. ‘आयम्यते———संमूर्छिता’ पाठोऽयं प्रथमपंचमपुस्तकयोः नोपलभ्यते ।
2. प्रत्यस्यते इति आकरे पाठः ।
3. ०निलजोऽसमस्त इति षष्ठपुस्तके पाठः ।
4. वापाव्येत इति चतुर्थषष्ठपुस्तकयोः पाठः ।
5. वापि इति आदर्शपुस्तकेषु पाठः ।

Kaphaja Granthi

Kaphaja type of *granthi* is characterised by cold touch, absence of any colour change, mild pain, excessive itching, hardness like stone, compactness and slow growth. When it opens up, pus which is white and dense comes out of it.

शरीरवृद्धिक्षयवृद्धिहानिः स्निग्धो महान् कण्डुयुतोऽरुजश्च ।
मेदःकृतो गच्छति चात्र भिन्ने पिण्याकसर्पिः प्रतिमं तु मेदः ॥१४॥

Medoja Granthi (*Lipoma*)

Granthi caused by *medas* (fat) increases and decreases in size depending upon the increase or decrease of the body weight. It is unctuous, large in size and associated with itching. It is painless. If it opens up, fat like oil cake or ghee comes out of it.

व्यायामजातैरबलस्य तैस्तै-
राक्षिप्य वायुस्तु शिराप्रतानम् ।
संकुच्य संपिड्य विशोष्य चापि
ग्रन्थिं करोत्युन्नतमाशु वृत्तम् ॥१५॥
ग्रन्थिः शिराजः स तु कृच्छ्रसाध्यो
भवेद्यदि स्यात् सरुजश्चलश्च ।
अरुक् स एवाप्यचलो महांश्च
मर्मोत्थितश्चापि विवर्जनीयः ॥१६॥

Śirāja Granthi (*Angioma*)

When a weak person resorts to strenuous exercise, *vāyu* gets vitiated and this vitiated *vāyu* afflicts the net work of vessels by contraction, pressure and dryness as a result of which round and elevated tumours are formed. This is called *śirāja granthi*. If it is mobile and associated with pain, then it is incurable. If it is immobile and without any pain but located in a vital organ, then also it is incurable.

गात्रप्रदेशे क्वचिदेव दोषाः संमूर्च्छिता" मांसमसृक् प्रदूष्य ।
वृत्तं स्थिरं मन्दरुजं महान्तमनल्पमूलं चिरवृद्ध्यपाकम्[1] ।
कुर्वन्ति मांसोच्छ्रयमत्यगाधं तदर्बुदं शास्त्रविदो वदन्ति ॥१७॥

Arbuda (*Large Tumour*)

If in any part of the body, the vitiated *doṣas* afflict *māṃsa* (muscle tissue) and *rakta* (blood) to produce a round, stable, mildly paining, large sized and cessile growth with excessively accumulated muscle tissue, which grows very slowly and which does not get suppurated, then this is called *arbuda* (tumour).

वातेन पित्तेन कफेन चापि रक्तेन मांसेन च मेदसा च[2] ।
तज्जायते तस्य च लक्षणानि ग्रन्थेः समानानि सदा भवन्ति ॥१८॥

Varieties of Arbuda

It is of six types, viz. *vātaja arbuda*, *pittaja arbuda*, *kaphaja arbuda*, *raktaja arbuda māṃsaja arbuda* and *medoja arbuda*. Their signs and symptoms are similar to those of the *granthi*.

दोषः[3] प्रदुष्टो रुधिरं शिरास्तु[4] संकुच्य संपिण्ड्य ततस्त्वपाकम् ।
सास्रावमुन्नह्यति[5] मांसपिण्डं मांसाङ्कुरैरावृतमाशुवृद्धिम्[6] ।
कुर्वन्त्यजस्रं[7] रुधिरप्रवृत्तमसाध्यमेतद् रुधिरात्मकं तु ॥१९॥

1. चिरवृद्धिपाकम् इति आदर्शपुस्तकेषु पाठः ।
2. वा इति आकरे पाठः ।
3. दोषाः प्रदुष्टा इति प्रथमचतुर्थषष्ठपुस्तकेषु पाठः ।
4. शिराश्च इति आकरे पाठः ।
5. सस्रवमुन्नत इति प्रथमपुस्तके पाठः ।
6. मांसाङ्कुरैराचितमाशुवृद्धम् इति आकरे पाठः ।
7. करोत्यजस्रं इति आकरे पाठः ।

रक्तक्षयोपद्रवपीडितत्वात् पांडुर्भवेदर्बुदपीडितस्तु ॥२०॥

Raktaja Arbuda

Following are the characteristic features of *raktaja arbuda* :

1. It is caused by the contracture of and pressure on the vessels because of the vitiated *doṣas* as well as *rakta* (blood) ;
2. It does not get suppurated ;
3. It exudates and gets elevated ;
4. Sharp granular tissues develop over the tumour ;
5. It grows very quickly ;
6. It causes excessive bleeding ; and
7. It is incurable.
8. Because of excessive bleeding, the patient suffers from anemia.

मुष्टिप्रहारादिभिरर्दितेऽङ्गे मांसं प्रदुष्टं जनयेत्तु[1] शोफम् ॥२१॥

अवेदनं स्निग्धमनन्यवर्णमपाकमश्मोपममप्रचाल्यम् ।

प्रदुष्टमांसस्य नरस्य गाढमेतद् भवेन्मांसपरायणस्य ॥२२॥

मांसार्बुदं त्वेतदसाध्यमुक्तं साध्येष्वपीमानि तु वर्जयेच्च ।

संप्रस्रुतं मर्मणि यच्च जातं स्रोतःसु वा यच्च भवेदचाल्यम्[2] ॥२३॥

Māṃsārbuda

Following are the characteristic features of *māṃsārbuda* :

1. It is caused by injury to a particular part of the body because of the blow of fist, etc. which vitiates local muscles and by which that part gets swollen ;

1. जनयेद्धिशोथम् इति आकरे पाठः ।
2. भवेदत्वं इति षष्ठपुस्तके पाठः ।

2. It is painless, unctuous and without any discoloration of the skin ;
3. It does not get suppurated ;
4. It is stony hard and immobile ;
5. The muscle tissue of the local tissue becomes vitiated ;
6. It is deep seated ; and
7. It is generally incurable.

If, there is fluid exudation from such a tumour, if it is located in a vital organ or a channel of circulation and if it is immobile, then also, an otherwise curable patient of *māṃsārbuda* should not be treated.

यज्जायतेऽन्यत्[1] खलु पूर्वजाते ज्ञेयं तदध्यर्बुदमर्बुदज्ञैः ।
यद् द्वन्द्वजातं युगपत् क्रमाद्वा द्विरर्बुदं तच्च भवेदसाध्यम् ॥२४॥

Adhyarbuda and Dvirarbuda

If a tumour appears over another tumour, then it is called *adhyarbuda*. If two tumours appear one after the other or both of them simultaneously, then the condition is called *dvirarbuda*. It is incurable.

न पाकमायान्ति कफाधिकत्वान्मेदोबहुत्वाच्च विशेषतस्तु[2] ।
दोषस्थिरत्वाद् ग्रथनाच्च तेषां सर्वार्बुदान्येव निसर्गतस्तु ॥२५॥

[माधवनिदान : गलगण्डादिनिदानम् ३८ : १-२६]

इति गलगण्डगण्डमालापचीग्रन्थ्यर्बुदनिदानम् ॥२६॥

Cause of Non-Suppuration of Tumour

A tumour does not get suppurated because of the following ;

1. Excess of *kapha* and *medas* in the corpus of the tumour ;

---

1. यज्जायतेन्यः इति प्रथमपंचमपुस्तकयोः पाठः ।
2. विशेषतश्च इति आदर्शपुस्तकेषु पाठः ।

2. Stability and rigid confinement (*grathanāt*) of the *doṣas* in a particular place ; and
3. Natural tendency of all tumours not to get suppurated.

Thus, ends the diagnosis of *gala gaṇḍa*, *gaṇḍa mālā*, *apacī*, *granthi* and *arbuda*.

"यवमुद्गपटोलानि कटुरूक्षञ्च भोजनम् ।
छर्दिं सरक्तमुक्तिञ्च गलगण्डे प्रयोजयेत् ॥२७॥

Line of Treatment

The patient of *gala gaṇḍa* (goitre) should take *yava*, *mudga*, *paṭola* and other pungent as well as ununctuous ingredients as food. He should resort to emetic and blood-letting therapies.

तन्दुलोदकपिष्टेन[1] मूलेन परिलेपितः[2] ।
हस्तिकर्णपलाशस्य गलगण्डः प्रशाम्यति ॥२८॥

The root of *hasti karṇa palāśa* should be added with rice-wash (*taṇḍulodaka*), triturated and made to a paste. Application of this paste cures *gala gaṇḍa* (goitre).

सर्षपान् शिग्रुबीजानि शणबीजातसीयवान् ।
मूलकस्य च बीजानि तक्रेणाम्लेन पेषयेत् ॥२९॥
गलगण्डा[3] ग्रन्थयश्च गण्डमालाः सुदारुणाः ।
प्रलेपात्तेन शाम्यन्ति विलयं यान्ति चाचिरात् ॥३०॥

---

1. तन्दुलोदकम् इति षष्ठपुस्तके पाठः ।
2. परि वा पुनः इति षष्ठपुस्तके पाठः ।
3. क. गन्डानि इति प्रथमपंचमपुस्तकयोः पाठः ।
   ख. गन्डाग्नि इति षष्ठपुस्तके पाठः ।

Seeds of *sarṣapa*, *śigru*, *śaṇa*, *atasī*, *yava* and *mūlaka* should be triturated by adding sour butter-milk. Application of this paste dissolves serious types of *gala gaṇḍa* (goitre), *granthi* (small tumour) and *gaṇḍa mālā* (lymphadenitis).

जीर्णकर्कारुकरसो[1] विडसैन्धवसंयुतः[2] ।
नस्येन हन्ति तरुणं गलगण्डं न संशयः ॥३१॥

Inhalation of the juice of ripe fruit of *karkāruka* mixed with *viḍa* and *saindhava* undoubtedly cures freshly occurred *gala gaṇḍa* (goitre).

जलकुम्भीकजं भस्म पक्वं गोमूत्रगालितम् ।
पिबेत् कोद्रवभक्ताशी[3] गलगण्डप्रशान्तये ॥३२॥

Ash of *jala kumbhī* should be boiled with cow's urine and strained. Intake of this along with food prepared of *kodrava* cures *gala gaṇḍa* (goitre).

सूर्यावर्त्तरसोनाभ्यां गलगण्डोपनाहने ।
स्फोटस्रावे शमं यान्ति गलगण्डः[4] न संशयः ॥३३॥

Upanāha type of fomentation therapy prepared of *sūryāvarta* and *rasona* should be given to the patient of goitre. By this, blisters appear over the goitre and there will be exudation of fluid. This undoubtedly relieves *gala gaṇḍa* (goitre).

---

1. क. जीर्णकर्कातुकरसो इति प्रथमपंचमपुस्तकयोः पाठः।
   ख. 'हस्तिगण्ड पलाशस्य गलगण्डः प्रशाम्यति। सर्षपान् शिग्रुबीजानि बीजातसीय विलयं यान्ति चाचिरात्' पाठोऽयं षष्ठपुस्तके अधिकमुपलभ्यते।
2. विडसैन्धवसंयुतम् इति प्रथमपंचमषष्ठपुस्तकेषु पाठः।
3. क्षौद्रेण तक्राशी इति चतुर्थ षष्ठपुस्तकयोः पाठः।
4. गलगण्डो इति आदर्शपुस्तके पाठः।

तिक्तालाबुफले पक्वे सप्ताहमुषितं[1] जलम् ।
मद्यं वा गलगण्डघ्नं पानात्पथ्यान्नसेविनः[2] ॥३४॥

Ripe fruit of *tiktālābu* should be soaked in water or alcohol for one week. Intake of this along with wholesome food cures *gala gaṇḍa* (goitre).

कट्फलचूर्णान्तर्गलघर्षो गलगण्डामयं[3] हन्ति ।
घृतमिश्रं[4] पीतमपि[5] श्वेतगिरिकर्णिकामूलम् ॥३५॥

Gala gaṇḍa (goitre) is cured if the powder of *kaṭphala* is rubbed over the throat. Intake of the root of the white variety of *giri karṇikā* along with ghee also cures *gala gaṇḍa* (goitre).

महिषीमूत्रविमिश्रं लोहमलं संस्थितं घटे मासम् ।
अन्तर्धूमविदग्धं[6] लिह्यान्मधुनाथ गलगण्डे ॥३६॥

Maṇḍūra (iron rust) should be soaked with buffalo-urine for one month. Then it should be cooked by *antar dhūma* method (without exposure to air, in a sealed jar, it should be burnt and reduced to fine powder form). Intake of this powder along with honey is useful in *gala gaṇḍa* (goitre).

---

1. सप्ताहामुषिते जले इति षष्ठपुस्तके पाठः ।
2. पानात्पक्षानुसेविनाम् इति प्रथमपंचमपुस्तकयोः पाठः ।
3. क. गलगण्डमपहरति इति प्रथमपंचमपुस्तकयोः पाठः ।
   ख. ०र्गलमाधिका विचूर्णिता इति षष्ठपुस्तके पाठः ।
4. घृतं मिश्रं इति प्रथमषष्ठपुस्तकयोः पाठः ।
5. पीतमिव इति आदर्शपुस्तकेषु पाठः ।
6. ०पक्वं इति चतुर्थषष्ठपुस्तकयोः पाठः ।

जिह्वायाः पार्श्वतोऽधस्ताच्छिरा[1] द्वादश कीर्त्तिताः ।
तासां स्थूल[2]शिरे द्वेऽधश्छिन्द्यात्ते च शनैः शनैः ॥३७॥
बडिशेनैव संगृह्य कुशपत्रेण[3] बुद्धिमान् ।
स्रुते रक्ते व्रणे तस्मिन् दद्यात्सगुडमार्द्रकम् ।
भोजनाश्चानभिष्य[4]न्दियूषः कौलत्थ इष्यते ॥३८॥

Surgical Method—Blood-letting

In the sides and below the tongue there are twelve vessels. Two of them are very prominent. These two vessels should be caught with a *baḍiśa* (a type of forceps) and incised with the help of a *kuśa patra* (a thin scalpel). After bleeding is over, jaggery and ginger should be applied over the wound and the patient should be given food which is not *abhiṣyandi* (do not obstruct the channels of circulation) and the soup of *kulattha*. This cures *gala gaṇḍa*.

कर्णयुग्मबहि सन्धिम[5]ध्याभ्यासे स्थितञ्च यत् ।
[6]उपर्य्युपरि तच्छिन्द्याद् गलगण्डे शिरात्रयम् ॥३९॥

Three vessels located one above the other on the outer joints of both the ears should be incised for the cure of *gala gaṇḍa* (goitre).

---

1. ०धूस्तात् शिरा इति आदर्शपुस्तकेषु पाठः ।
2. स्थूले शिरे द्वे च छिन्द्यात्ते च शनैः शनैः इति चतुर्थषष्ठपुस्तकयाः पाठः ।
3. कुशपत्रेण इति आकरे पाठः ।
4. ०भिस्यन्दियूषः इति प्रथमपंचमपुस्तकयोः पाठः ।
5. सन्धिमर्माभ्यासे इति आदर्शपुस्तकेषु पाठः ।
6. उपर्य्ुपरितत्थिद्यात् इति प्रथमपुस्तके पाठः ।

विडङ्गक्षारसिन्धूत्थ[1]राष्णाग्निव्योषदारुभिः ।
कटुतुम्बीफलरसे कटुतैलं विपाचयेत्[2] ।
चिरोत्थमपि नस्येन[3] गलगण्डं विनाशयेत् ॥४०॥

॥ तुम्बीतैलम् ॥

Tumbī Taila

Mustard oil should be cooked with the paste of *viḍaṅga, kṣāra, saindhava, rāsnā, agni, vyoṣa* and *dāru* and the juice of the fruit of *kaṭu tumbī*. Inhalation of this medicated oil cures even chronic *gala gaṇḍa* (goitre).

तैलं पिबेच्चामृतवल्लिनिम्बहिंस्राभया[4]वत्सकपिप्पलीभिः ।
सिद्धं बला[5]भ्याञ्च सदेवदारु हिताय नित्यं गलगण्डरोगी ॥४१॥

॥ अमृताद्यं[6] तैलम् ॥

Amṛtādya Taila

Sesame oil cooked with the paste of *amṛta valli, nimba hiṃsrā, abhayā, vatsaka* and *pippalī*, and the decoction of *balā, nāga balā* as well as *deva dāru* should be taken daily by a patient suffering from *gala gaṇḍa* (goitre).

---

1. ०सिन्धूग्रारास्नाग्निव्योषहिंगुभिः इति आकरे पाठः ।
2. विपाचितम् इति आकरे पाठः ।
3. नश्येन इति आकरे पाठः ।
4. ०हिंस्राह्वयावत्सक० इति आकरे पाठः ।
5. सिद्धमूलाभ्याञ्च इति प्रथमपुस्तकेषु पाठः ।
6. अमृताद्यतैलम् इति प्रथमपंचमपुस्तकयोः पाठः ।

[1]'काञ्चनारत्वचः क्वाथः शुण्ठीचूर्णेन संयुतः ।'
माक्षिकाढ्यः सकृत्पीतः क्वाथो वरुणमूलजः ।
गण्डमालां हरत्याशु चिरकालानुबन्धिनीम् ॥४२॥

Treatment of Gaṇḍa Mālā (Lymphadenitis)

Intake of the decoction of *kāñcanāra* bark mixed with the powder of *śuṇṭhī* and honey cures very chronic *gaṇḍa mālā* (lymphadenitis). Similarly, the decoction of *varuṇa* root (taken only once ?) cures very chronic *gaṇḍa mālā* (lymphadenitis).

पिष्ट्वा ज्येष्ठाम्बुना पीताः काञ्चनारत्वचः शुभाः ।
विश्वभेषजसंयुक्ता गण्डमालापहाः पराः ॥४३॥

Bark of *kañcanāra* should be boiled with cow's urine. Intake of this by adding the powder of *śuṇṭhī* cures *gaṇḍa mālā* (lymphadenitis).

आरग्वधशिफां क्षिप्रं पिष्ट्वा तण्डुलवारिणा ।
सम्यङ्[2] नस्यप्रलेपाभ्यां गण्डमालां समुद्धरेत् ॥४४॥

Root of *āragvadha* should be made to a paste by adding *taṇḍulodaka* (rice-wash). This should be used for inhalation therapy and external application which cures *gaṇḍa mālā* (lymphadenitis).

गण्डमालामयार्त्तानां नस्यकर्मणि योजयेत् ।
निर्गुण्ड्यास्तु शिफां सम्यक् वारिणा परिपेषिताम् ॥४५॥

The root of *nirguṇḍī* should be made to a paste by adding water. It should be used as inhalation therapy for a patient suffering from *gaṇḍa mālā* (lymphadenitis).

---

1. 'काञ्चनार——संयुतः' पाठोऽयं आदर्शपुस्तकेषु नोपलभ्यते ।
2. सम्यक् इति आदर्शपुस्तकेषु पाठः ।

कोषातकीनां स्वरसेन नस्यं तुम्ब्यास्तु वा पिप्पलीसंयुतेन ।
तैलेन वारिष्ठभवेन कुर्याद्वचोपकुल्येनसमाक्षिकेन ॥४६॥[1]

Administration of the inhalation therapy with the juice of *koṣātakī* or the juice of *tumbī* mixed with the powder of *pippalī* or sesame oil cooked with *vacā* as well as *upakulyā* and mixed with honey [cures *gaṇḍa mālā* (lymphadenitis)].

ऐन्द्र्या वा गिरिकर्ण्या वा मूलं गोमूत्रयोगतः ।
गण्डमालां हरेत्पीतं चिरकालोत्थितामपि ॥४७॥

Intake of the root of *aindrī* or *girikarṇī* along with cow's urine cures even chronic *gaṇḍa mālā* (lymphadenitis).

अलम्बुषादलोद्भूतस्वरसं[2] द्वे[3] पले पिबेत् ।
अपच्याः गण्डमालायाः कामलायाश्च नाशनम् ॥४८॥

Intake of the juice of *alambuṣā* leaves in a dose of two *palas* cures *apacī* (suppurated gland), *gaṇḍa mālā* (lymphadenitis) and jaundice.

गलगण्डं गण्डमालां कुरण्डञ्चोपशाम्यति[4] ।
पिष्टं ज्येष्ठाम्बुना लेपान्मूलं ब्राह्मणयष्टिजम् ॥४६॥

Application of the paste of *brāhmaṇa yaṣṭi* root prepared by triturating with cow's urine cures *gala gaṇḍa* (goitre), *gaṇḍa mālā* (lymphadenitis) and *kuraṇḍa* (scrotal tumour).

---

1. कुर्याद् गजोपकुल्येन समाक्षिकेण इति आकरे पाठः ।
2. दलोद्भूतात् सुरसा इति प्रथमपंचमपुस्तकयोः पाठः ।
3. द्विपलं इति आकरे पाठः ।
4. कुरण्डञ्च विनाशयेत् इति आकरे पाठः ।

छुच्छुन्दर्या विपक्वञ्च[1] क्षणात्तैलवरं ध्रुवम् ।
अभ्यङ्गान्नाशयेत् क्षिप्रं[2] गण्डमालां सुदारुणाम् ॥५०॥

Oil cooked with the decoction of *chucchundarī* and *kṣāra* (alkali preparation) should be used for massage which quickly cures serious type of *gaṇḍa mālā.*

गण्डमालापहं तैलं सिद्धं शाखोटकत्वचा ।
बिम्ब्यश्वमारनिर्गुण्डीसाधितं[3] वापि नावनम् ॥५१॥

॥ शाखोटकबिम्बाद्यं तैलम् ॥

Śākhoṭaka Bimbādya Taila

Oil cooked with the bark of *śākhōṭaka, bimbī, aśva māra* and *nirguṇḍī* should be used for inhalation therapy which cures *gaṇḍa mālā* (lymphadenitis).

"निर्गुण्डीस्वरसे चाथ लाङ्गलीमूलकल्कितम् ।
तलं नस्यान्निहन्त्याशु गण्डमालां सुदारुणम् ॥५२॥"

॥ निर्गुण्डीतैलम् ॥

[भैषज्यरत्नावली : गलगण्डादिरोगाधिकार : ५-३०]

Nirguṇḍi Taila

Oil cooked with the juice of *nirguṇḍi* and the paste of *lāṅgalī* should be used for inhalation therapy which quickly cures serious type of *gaṇḍa mālā* (lymphadenitis).

---

1. विपक्वन्तु इति आदर्शपुस्तकेषु पाठः ।
2. अभ्यंगान्नाशयेन्नृणां गण्डमालां सुदारुणम् इति प्रथमपुस्तके पाठः ।
3. चिंव्यश्चमरनिर्गुण्डीसाधितञ्चापि लावणम् इति प्रथमपुस्तके पाठः ।

वनकर्पासिकामूलं तन्दुलैः[1] सह योजितम् ।
पक्त्वा पूपलिकाः[2] खादेदपचीनाशनाय तु ॥५३॥

Treatment of Apacī (Suppurated Gland)

Intake of *pūpalikā* (a type of pastry) prepared of the root of *vana kārpāsa* and rice cures *apacī* (suppurated gland).

शोभाञ्जनं देवदारु काञ्जिकेन तु पेषितम् ।
कोष्णं प्रलेपतो हन्यादपचीमतिदुस्तराम् ॥५४॥

Application of the luke-warm paste of *śobhāñjana* and *deva dāru* prepared by triturating with *kāñjī* (a type of sour drink) cures serious type of *apaci* (suppurated gland).

सर्षपारिष्टपत्राणि दग्ध्वा भल्लातकैः सह ।
छागमूत्रेण सम्पिष्टमपचीघ्नं प्रलेपनम् ॥५५॥

Leaves of *sarṣapa* as well as *ariṣṭa* and *bhallātaka* should be triturated with goat's urine and made to a paste. Its external application cures *apaci* (suppurated glands).

अश्वत्थकाष्ठं निचुलं गतां दन्तञ्च दाहयेत् ।
वराहमज्जसंयुक्तं[3] भस्म हन्त्यपचीव्रणान्[4] ॥५६॥

Wood of *aśvattha*, *nicula* and cow's teeth should be burnt to ashes. This should be made to a paste by adding the bone-marrow of boar. Application of this paste cures ulcers of *apacī* (suppurated gland).

1. तण्डुलैः इति आकरे पाठः ।
2. पक्त्वापि पूलिकां खादेदपची नाशमायतम् इति प्रथमपुस्तके पाठः ।
3. वराहमज्जसम्पृक्तं इति आकरे पाठः ।
4. व्रणात् इति प्रथमपुस्तके पाठः ।

पार्ष्णिं प्रति द्वादश चाङ्गुलानि

भित्वेन्द्रवस्तिं[1] परिवर्ज्य सम्यक् ।

विदार्य मत्स्याण्डनिभानि वैद्यो

निष्पिष्य[2] जालान्यनलं विदध्यात् ॥५७॥

Surgical Treatment

An incision should be made twelve *aṅgulas* (unit of measurement=finger breadth) above the *pārṣṇi* (calcaneum bone) without touching the vital part known as *indra basti.* The wound should be opened, and from inside, the net-work like fish-eggs (*matsyāṇḍa nibha jāla*) should be squeezed out. Then the ulcer should be cauterised. This cures *apacī.*

मणिबन्धोपरिष्टाद्वा कुर्याद्रेखात्रयं[3] भिषक् ।

अङ्गुलान्तरितं सम्यगपचीनां प्रशान्तये ॥५८॥

Over the wrist joint three lines (having one finger space between two lines) should be drawn by cauterisation. This cures *apaci.*

दण्डोत्पलाभवं मूलं बद्धं पुष्येऽपचीं जयेत् ।

अपामार्गस्य वा छिन्द्याज्जिह्वातलगते शिरे ॥५९॥

The root of *daṇḍotpalā* or *apāmārga* should be tied [to the head] in *puṣya* constellation which cures *apaci.* Similarly, incising two [prominent] vessels below the tongue cures *apaci.*

---

1. सिद्धेन्द्रवस्तिं इति प्रथमपंचमपुस्तकयोः पाठः ।
2. क. निष्कृष्ण इति प्रथमपुस्तके पाठः ।
   ख. निष्कृष्य इति पंचमपुस्तके पाठः ।
   ग. वैद्याज्जनिष्य इति षष्ठपुस्तके पाठः ।
3. कुर्याद्रेखाद्वयं इति आकरे पाठः ।

व्योषं विडङ्गमधुकं सैन्धवं देवदारु च ।
तैलमेभिः शृतं नस्यात् कृच्छ्रामप्यपचीं जयेत् ॥६०॥

॥ व्योषाद्यं तैलम् ॥

Vyoṣādya Taila

Inhalation of the oil cooked with *vyoṣa, viḍaṅga, madhuka, saindhava* and *deva dāru* cures even serious type of *apacī*.

चन्दनं साभया लाक्षा वचा कटुकरोहिणी ।
एतैस्तैलं शृतं पीतं समूलामपचीं जयेत् ॥६१॥

Intake of the oil cooked with *candana, abhayā, lākṣā, vacā* and *kaṭu rohiṇī* cures *apacī* right from its root.

गुञ्जाह्वयारिश्यामार्कसर्षपैर्मूत्रसाधितम् ।
तैलन्तु[1] दशधापाकात्कणालवणपञ्चकम्[2] ॥६२॥
मरिचैश्चूर्णितैर्युक्तं[3] सर्वावस्थागतां[4] जयेत् ।
अभ्यङ्गादपचीं नाडीं वल्मीकार्शोगुदव्रणात्[5] ॥६३॥

॥ गुञ्जाद्यं तैलम् ॥

Guñjādya Taila

Oil should be cooked with *guñjā, aśva māra, śyāmā, arka, sarṣapa* and cow's urine for ten times. To this medicated oil,

1. तैलस्तु इति प्रथमपंचमपस्तकयोः पाठः ।
2. दशधा पश्चात्कणालवणपञ्चकैः इति आकरे पाठः ।
3. ०चूर्णितं युक्तं इति प्रथमपंचमपुस्तकयोः पाठः ।
4. ०गताञ्जयेत् इति प्रथमपुस्तके पाठः ।
5. वल्मीकार्शोऽर्बुदव्रणात् इति षष्ठपुस्तके आकरे च पाठः ।

the powder of *kaṇā*, *pañca lavaṇa* and *marica* should be added. Massage with this recipe cures *apacī*, *nāḍi vraṇa* (sinus), *valmīka* (ant-hill like tumour), piles and anal ulcer.

ग्रन्थिष्वपक्वेषु कुर्वीत भिषक् शोथप्रतिक्रियाम् ।
पक्वानापाट्य[1] संशोध्य[2] रोपयेद् व्रणभेषजैः ॥६४॥

Treatment of Granthi (Small Tumour)

Unsuppurated *granthis* should be treated by the physician on the line suggested for the treatment of *śotha* (oedema). If suppurated, then the *granthi* should be incised, purified (disinfected) and healed with the medicines used for ulcers.

हिंस्रा सरोहिण्यमृताथ[3] भार्ङ्गी
श्योनाकबिल्वागुरुकृष्णगन्धाः ।
गोपित्तपिष्टाः सह तालपर्ण्या
ग्रन्थौ विधेयोऽनिलजे[4] प्रलेपः ॥६५॥

Vātika Granthi

Hiṃsrā, *kaṭu rohinī*, *amṛtā*, *bhārṅgī*, *śyonāka*, *bilva*, *aguru*, *kṛṣṇa gandhā* and *tāla parṇī* should be triturated with cow's bile and made to a paste. Application of this paste cures *vātika* type of *granthi*.

---

1. पक्वानुत्पाट्य इति आकरे पाठः ।
2. संयोज्ये रुद्धे प्रमाणभेषजैः इति षष्ठपुस्तके पाठः ।
3. ०मृताथ इति प्रथमपुस्तके पाठः ।
4. ०ऽलजो इति प्रथमपंचमपुस्तकयोः पाठः ।

जलायुका[1] पित्तकृते हितास्तु क्षीरोदकाभ्यां परिषेचयेच्च[2] ।
काकोलिवर्गस्य तु शीतलानि पिबेत्कषायाणि सशर्कराणि ॥६६॥
द्राक्षारसेनेक्षुरसेन वापि चूर्णं पिबेद्वापि हरीतकीनाम् ।
मधूकजम्बवर्जुनवेतसानां त्वग्भिः प्रदेहानवतारयेच्च ॥६७॥

Paittika Granthi

Jalaukā (leech) should be employed over *paittika* type of *granthi*. Thereafter, it should be sprinkled with milk and water. The patient should take cold decoction of drugs belonging to *kākolyādi varga* along with sugar. H… also be given the powder of *harītakī* along with the j… either *drākṣā* or sugar-cane. Over the *granthi* the pas… the bark of *madhūka*, *jambū*, *arjuna* and *vetasa* should be applied.

हृतेषु दोषेषु यथानुपूर्व्या ग्रन्थौ भिषक् श्लेष्मसमुत्थितेषु[3] ।
स्विन्ने तु[4] विम्लापनमेव कुर्यादङ्गुष्ठवेणुदृषदीसुतैश्च[5] ॥६८॥
विकङ्कतारग्वधकाकदन्ती[6]काकादनीतापसवृक्षमूलैः ।
आलेपयेदेनमलाबुभार्गीकरञ्जकालामदनैश्च विद्वान् ॥६९॥

Kaphaja Granthi

In *kaphaja granthi*, first of all the patient should be administered cleansing therapy. Thereafter, fomentation therapy should

---

1. जलायुकाः इति प्रथमपुस्तके पाठः ।
2. परिसेचनञ्च इति प्रथमपंचमपुस्तकयोः पाठः ।
3. श्लेष्मसमुद्भवे तु इति आकरे पाठः ।
4. च इति आकरे पाठः ।
5. ०सुतैस्तु इति आकरे पाठः ।
6. ०काकणन्ती इति आदर्शपुस्तकेषु पाठः ।

be employed over the *granthi*, it should be dissolved (*vimlāpana*) by pressure with finger, bamboo, stone or mercury. The paste of *vikaṅkata*, *āragvadha*, *kāka danti*, *kākādanī*, root of *agastya*, *alābu*, *bhārgī*, *karañja*, *kālā* [?] and *madana* should be applied over it.

दन्तीचित्रकमूलत्वक् सुधार्कपयांसी गुडः[1] ।
भल्लातकास्थिकाशीशं लेपो भिन्द्याच्छिलामपि ॥७०॥

---

1. पलानां दशकं ग्राह्यं कांचनारत्वचः शुभाः ।
षटपलानि पलाग्राह्य व्योषं ग्राह्यं पलं त्रयम् ।
पलैकं वरुणस्यापि त्वगेला पत्रकं तथा ।
कर्षं कषमितं ग्राह्यं सर्वाण्येकत्र चूर्णयेत् ।
सर्वं चूर्णमिदं यावस्तावन्मात्रस्तु गुग्गुलुः ।
संमर्द्य गुटिकाः कार्याः शाणमात्रा स्ततो बुधैः ।
एकैकां भक्षयेद्धीमान्तान् तान् प्रातः सदानरः ।
गंडगालां जयत्युग्रामपचीमर्बुदानि च ।
ग्रन्थीन्व्रणांश्च गुल्मांश्च कुष्ठानि च भगन्दरम् ।
अनुपाने प्रयोक्तव्यः क्वाथो मुंडितिका भवः ।
क्वाथः खदिरसारस्य पथ्याक्वाथोथवोष्मकम् ।
कांचनारो गुग्गुलुः कर्षं शुद्धस्य सूनस्यगन्धकम् वार्द्धकर्षकम् ।
सार्द्धकर्ष ताम्रभस्ममृतकिट्टं त्रिकर्षकम् ।
व्योषं षट्कर्षकं देयं कर्षार्द्धं श्वेतसैंधवम् ।
कांचनारत्वचश्चूर्णं पलत्रयमितं क्षिपेत् ।
गव्याज्यसहितं देयं त्रिपलं शुद्धगुग्गुलोः ।
गंडमालाकंडनोयं रसः परमशोभनः ।
गंधकं टंकणं सिंधुकांचनीनवसादरम् ।
सौवर्चलं यवक्षारं क्षाररक्तं सुवर्चलम् ।
सितं रक्तं च पाषाणं मूषकोत्थं नियोजयेत् ।
जैपालबीजमज्जा च समं जम्बीरपीडितम् ।
शस्त्रैश्छित्वा प्रदातव्यं वेष्ट्ययेरण्डपत्रकैः ।

(*continued on next page*)

Application of the paste of root bark of *dantī* and *citraka*, milky latex of *sudhā* and *arka*, *guḍa*, fruit of *bhallātaka*, *kāśīśa* (iron sulphate) erodes even a stone [what to speak of *granthi*].

ग्रन्थ्यर्बुदादिजिल्लेपो मातृमाहुकीकीट्टजम्[1] ॥७१॥

Application of the paste of the insect called *mātṛ mahuki* cures *granthi* and *arbuda*.

स्वर्जिकामूलकक्षारः शंखचूर्णसमन्वितः ।

प्रलेपो विहितस्तीक्ष्णो हन्ति ग्रन्थ्यर्बुदादिकान् ॥७२॥

The paste prepared of *svarji kṣāra*, *mūlaka kṣāra* and *śaṅkha bhasma* is very sharp. Its application cures *granthi*, *arbuda*, etc.

ग्रन्थीन्[2]मर्मप्रभवान् सुपक्वानुद्धृत्य चाग्निं विदधीत वैद्यः ।

क्षारेण चैतान् प्रतिसारयेत्तु संलिख्य यथोपदेशम् [?] ॥७३॥

(*continued from last page*)

एवं त्र्यहात् स्फुटत्येब दध्यन्नं बंधयेत्ततः ।
गण्डमालोत्थितो ग्रन्थिर्बहिर्निर्याति नान्यथा ।

॥ गण्डमालेयलेपः ॥

गंधकं सूतकं तुल्यमर्कक्षीरेण सैन्धवम् ।
पिष्ट्वा च कांचनीमूलं लेपोयं कण्ठमालिका ।
अदृश्यास्फोटयन्याशुमुंडी द्रावेण पेषिता ।
तन्मलैर्लेपयेत्तत्र सप्ताहं च प्रशाम्यति ।
जलेन लेपयेत्तुल्यं कांचनि चित्रकं विषम् ।
सप्ताहं लेपयस्तु अदृश्यागण्डमालिकाः ।
स्फुटंति नात्र संदेहः स्फोटेलेपमिदं कुरु ।

॥ दीपसारसंग्रहात् ॥

निजद्रावेणसंपिष्टं गण्डीमूलं प्रलेपनात् ।
गण्डमालाक्षयं याति तद्रवं वा पिवेत्पलम् ।"
पाठोऽयं चतुर्थषष्ठपुस्तकयोः अधिकमुपलभ्यते ।

1. मातृवाहककीटजः इति आकरे पाठः ।
2. ग्रन्थिन् मर्मप्रभवान् पक्वानुद्धृत्य इति आकरे पाठः ।

Marmaja Granthi

If *granthi* is located in *marma* (vital part of the body), then it should be removed after it is fully suppurated and thereafter, the ulcer should be cauterised. Alternatively, *kṣāra* (alkali preparation) should be applied over it to scrap it out of its location. [The verse is incomplete.]

ग्रन्थ्यर्बुदानाञ्च यतो विशेषः[1] प्रदेशहेत्वाकृतिदोषदूष्यैः ।
ततश्चिकित्सेद्भिषगर्बुदानि विधानविद्ग्रन्थिचिकित्सितेन ॥७४॥

Treatment of Arbuda

Since *granthi* and *arbuda* have many common features notwithstanding their distinction in location, causative factors, shape, *doṣas* and *dūṣyas*, *arbuda* should be treated on the line suggested for *granthi*.

वातार्बुदे[2] चाप्युपनाहनानि स्निग्धैश्च मांसैरथ वेशवारैः[3] ।
स्वेदं विदध्यात् कुशलस्तु नाड्या शृङ्गेण रक्तं बहुशो हरेच्च ॥७५॥

Treatment of Vātārbuda

In *vātika* type of *arbuda*, hot ointment prepared of meat or *veśavāra* added with unctuous substance, should be applied. It should be fomented according to *nāḍi sveda* method and blood-letting should be performed with deer horn for several times.

1. यतोऽविशेषः इति आकरे पाठः ।
2. वाताब्र्बुदे इति आकरे पाठः ।
3. वेसवारैः इति आदर्शपुस्तकेषु पाठः ।

स्वेदोपनाहा मृदवस्तु[1] पथ्याः पित्तार्बुदे कायविरेचनञ्च ।
विघृष्य[2] चोदुम्बर[3]शाकगोजीपत्रैर्भृशं क्षौद्रयुतं प्रलिम्पेत् ।
श्लक्ष्णीकृतैः सर्जरसप्रियङ्गुपत्तङ्गलोध्रार्जुनयष्टिसंज्ञैः[4] ॥७६॥

Treatment of Pittārbuda

Mild forms of fomentation and *upanāha* (application of hot ointment) therapies are useful in *pittārbuda*. To such patients purgative therapy should be given. The tumour should be rubbed with the leaves of *udumbara*, *śāka* and *goji* repeatedly, and thereafter, the fine paste of *sarja rasa*, *priyaṅgu*, *pattaṅga*, *lodhra*, *arjuna* and *ariṣṭa* mixed with honey should be applied.

लेपनं शंखचूर्णेन सह मूलकभस्मना ।
कफार्बुदापहं कुर्याद्ग्रंथ्यादिषु विशेषतः ॥७७॥
निष्पावपिण्याककुलत्थकल्कैर्मांसप्रगाढैर्दधिमर्दितैश्च ।
लेपं विदध्यात् क्रमयो यथात्र मुञ्चन्त्यपत्यान्यथ[5] मक्षिकाश्च ।
अल्पावशिष्टं क्रिमिभिः प्रजग्धं लिखेत्ततोग्निं विदधीत पश्चात् ।
यदल्पमूलं त्रपुताम्रसीसैः संवेष्ट्य पत्रैरथवायसैर्वा ॥७८॥

Treatment of Kaphajārbuda

In *kaphaja* type of *arbuda*, the paste of *śaṅkha bhasma* and the *kṣāra* (alkali preparation) of *mūlaka* should be applied

---

1. मृदवश्च इति आकरे पाठः ।
2. विकृष्य इति चतुर्थषष्ठपुस्तकयोः पाठः ।
3. चोडुम्बर० इति आकरे पाठः ।
4. ०यष्टिकाह्वैः इति आकरे पाठः ।
5. पतंति मुंचत्यथ इति चतुर्थषष्ठपुस्तकयोः पाठः ।

externally. The paste of *niṣpāva*, *piṇyāka*, *kulattha* and meat triturated with curd should be applied externally till worms (*kṛmis*) and flies (*makṣikā*) lay their eggs in it and eat away a part of the tumour. Then the tumour should be scraped and cauterised. Then the cessile stump of the tumour should be surrounded with tin, copper, lead or iron leaves (thin sheets) and *kṣāra* (alkali preparations), *agni* (cauterisation) as well as *śastra* (surgical operation) therapies should be employed carefully keeping in view the vitality of the patient.

क्षाराग्निशस्त्राण्यवचारयेच्च[1] मुहुर्मुहुः प्राणमवेक्ष्यमाणाः[2] ।
यदृच्छया चोपगतानि पाकं पाकक्रमेणोपचरेद् यथोक्तम् ।।७९।।

If the tumour gets suppurated of its own (without any external aid), then it should be treated on the lines suggested for suppurated ulcers.

उपोदिकारसाभ्यक्तास्तत्[3]पत्रपरिवेष्टिताः ।
प्रणश्यन्त्यचिरान्नृणां पिडकार्बुदजातयः ।।८०।।

Habitual intake of the juice of *upodikā* and surrounding the growth with the leaves of this plant cure *arbuda* (tumour) and *piḍakā* (pimples).

उपोदिका काञ्जिकतक्रपिष्टां तयोपनाहो लवणेन मिश्रः ।
दृष्टो[4]ऽर्बुदानां प्रशमाय कैश्चिद्दिने दिने रात्रिषु मर्मजानाम् ।।८१।।

Application of the hot ointment (*upanāha*) prepared of *upodikā* added with *kāñji* (a type of sour drink) or butter-milk and rock-

---

1. यवतारयेच्च इति आकरे पाठ : ।
2. प्राणमवेक्षमाण: इति आकरे पाठ: ।
3. ०सात्यक्तात्वक् इति प्रथमपुस्तके पाठ: ।
4. कुष्ठार्बुदानाम् इति षष्ठपुस्तके पाठ: ।

salt during day time cures *arbuda*. If the *arbuda* is located in a vital organ, then this ointment should be applied during night.

लेपोर्बुदजिद्रम्भामोचकभस्मतुषशंखचूर्णकृतः[1] ।
सरटरुधिरार्द्रगन्धकयवाग्रजविडङ्गनागरैर्वाथ ॥८२॥

Application of the paste of the *kṣāra* (alkali preparation) of *rambhā, mocaka, tuṣa, śaṅkha bhasma, saraṭa, rudhira, ārdraka*[?], *gandhaka, yava kṣāra, viḍaṅga* and *śuṇṭhī* cures *arbuda*.

स्नुहीनिर्गुण्डीकास्वेदो[2] नाशयेदर्बुदानि च[3] ।
सीसकेनाथ लवणैः पिण्डराकफलेन च ॥८३॥

Fomentation with *snuhī, nirguṇḍī*, lead, salt and the fruit of *piṇḍarāka* cures *arbuda*.

हरिद्रालोध्रपतङ्गगृहधूममनःशिलाः ।
मधुप्रगाढो लेपोऽयं मेदोर्बुदहरः परः ॥८४॥

Haridrā, lodhra, pataṅga, gṛha dhūma and *manaḥ śilā* should be made to a paste by adding adequate quantity of honey. Application of this paste cures *medoja arbuda*.

एतामेव क्रियां कुर्यादशेषां शर्करार्बुदे ॥८५॥

All the above mentioned therapies are also useful in the treatment of *śarkarārbuda* (tumour caused by sugar or sand).

---

1. चूर्णीकृतः इति पंचमपुस्तके पाठः ।
2. स्नुहीगुण्डीका इति प्रथमद्वितीयपुस्तकयोः पाठः ।
3. 'लिप्तं यवक्षारविडङ्गशुण्ठीगंधोत्पलैः सयान्मशली कृतैर्यत् ।
रक्तेन मिश्रैः सुरटस्य घतदर्बुदे शाम्यति नान्यथैनम् ॥'
पाठोऽयं पंचमपुस्तके अधिकमुपलभ्यते ।

इति श्रीमहाराजाधिराजटोडरमल्लविरचिते टोडरानन्दे आयुर्वेदसौख्ये गलगण्डगण्डमालापचीग्रन्थ्यर्बुदनिदान-चिकित्साकथनं नाम पंचाशत्तमो हर्षः ॥८६॥

Thus, ends the 50th Chapter dealing with the diagnosis and treatment of *gala gaṇḍa* (goitre), *gaṇḍa mālā* (lymphadenitis), *apacī* (suppurated gland), *granthi* (small tumour) and *arbuda* (large tumour) in *Āyurveda saukhya* of *Ṭoḍarānanda* composed by the great king Ṭoḍara Malla.

CHAPTER XVI

अथ श्लीपदनिदानं चिकित्सा च ।

Diagnosis and Treatment of Filariasis

यः[1] सज्वरो वङ्क्षणजो[2] भृशार्तिः[3] शोथो नृणां पादगतः क्रमेण ।
तच्छ्लीपदं स्यात् करकर्णनेत्रशिश्नौष्ठनासास्वपि केचिदाहुः ॥१॥

Description

Excessively painful swelling in the groin, spreading gradually to legs and associated with fever is called *ślīpada* (filariasis).

---

1. This is the beginning of the 55th Chapter of *Āyurveda saukhya* in *Toḍarānanda* and the invocation reads as follows :—
   'प्रफुल्लचंपाब्जसुवर्णयूथिके भुजंग भृग्भृंग विहंगनादि ते ।
   अनंगबीजां कुररूपपादपे क्रीडन् हरिः पानुनृपं सदा बने' ॥
2. वक्षंणतो इति प्रथमपुस्तके पाठः ।
3. भृशान्तिं इति प्रथमपुस्तके पाठः ।

According to some physicians, there is swelling also in hands, ears, eyes, pudendum, lips and nose in this disease.

वातजं कृष्णरूक्षं तु स्फुटितं तीव्रवेदनम् ।
अनिमित्तरुजं चापि[1] बहुशो ज्वर एव च ॥२॥

Vātaja Ślīpada

Vātika type of *ślīpada* is characterised by black coloration, roughness, cracking, excessive pain, pain without any perceptible cause and frequent attacks of fever.

पित्तजं पीतसंकाशं दाहज्वरयुतं मृदु ।
श्लैष्मिकं स्निग्धं वर्णं[2] च श्वेतं पाण्डुस्थिरं गुरु ॥३॥

Paittika Ślīpaaa and Kaphaja Ślīpada

In *paittika* type of *ślīpada* there will be fever associated with burning sensation and yellowishness as well as softness of the swelling. In *kaphaja* type of *ślīpada*, the swollen part is unctuous, white as well as pale yellow in colour, stable and heavy.

वल्मीकमिव संजातं कण्टकैरुपचीयते ।
सर्वात्मकं महत्तच्च वर्जनीयं विशेषतः ॥४॥

Sānnipātika Ślīpada

In the *sānnipātika* type of *ślīpada*, the swollen part is surrounded with sharp projections like an ant-hill and the part is excessively enlarged. This type is incurable.

---

1. क. वापि इति षष्ठपुस्तके पाठः ।
   ख. तस्य इति आकरे पाठः ।
2. कृष्णवर्णं इति प्रथमपुस्तकेः पाठः ।

त्रीण्येतानि[1] विजानीयात् श्लीपदानि कफोच्छ्रयात्[2] ।

गुरुत्वं च महत्त्वं च यस्मान्नास्ति विना[3] कफात् ॥५॥

Kapha is predominant even in the remaining three varieties of *ślīpada*, viz. *vātika*, *paittika* and *sānnipātika* because heaviness and enlargement in size, both cannot take place without *kapha.*

पुराणोदकभूयिष्ठाः सर्वर्तुषु च शीतलाः ।

ये देशास्तेषु जायन्ते श्लीपदानि विशेषतः ॥६॥

Predisposing Factor

The disease *ślīpada* occurs specially in those areas which have a lot of accumulated water and which are cool in all seasons.

यच्छ्लेष्मलाहारविहारजातं[4] पुंसः प्रकृत्याऽपि[5] कफात्मकस्य ।

सास्रावमत्युन्नतसर्वलिङ्गं सकण्डुरं श्लेष्मयुतं विवर्ज्यम् ॥७॥

॥ इति श्लीपदनिदानम् ॥८॥

Prognosis

If *ślīpada* (filariasis) is caused by *kapha* aggravating diet and regimens, if the constitution of the patient is dominated by *kapha*, if swelling is associated with exudation, if it is excessively

---

1. त्रीण्यप्येतानि इति आकरे पाठः ।
2. कफोत्थयात् इति प्रथमपुस्तके पाठः ।
3. कफं विना इति आकरे पाठः ।
4. यत् श्लेष्मलाहार० इति आदर्शपुस्तकेषु पाठः ।
5. प्रकृत्या च इति आदर्शपुस्तकेषु पाठः ।

large and is associated with the signs and symptoms of all the three *doṣas* and if there is itching and mucoid exudation, then the patient should not be treated.

Thus, ends the diagnosis of *ślīpada* (filariasis).

लङ्घनालेपनस्वेदरेचनैः रक्तमोक्षणैः[1] ।
प्रायः श्लेष्महरैरुष्णैः श्लीपदं समुपाचरेत् ॥९॥

Line of Treatment

Fasting, external application (*lepana*), fomentation, purgation, blood-letting and such other therapies as are hot and alleviator of *kapha* should be used for the treatment of *ślīpada* (filariasis).

[2]धत्तूरैरण्डनिर्गुण्डीवर्षाभूशिग्रुसर्षपैः ।
प्रलेपः श्लीपदं हन्ति चिरोत्थमपि दारुणम् ॥१०॥

Recipes

External application of the paste of *dhattūra*, *eraṇḍa*, *nirguṇḍī*, *varṣābhū*, *śigru* and *sarṣapa* cures even serious and chronic types of *ślīpada* (filariasis).

निष्पिष्टमारनालेन [3]रूपिकामूलवल्कलम् ।
प्रलेपाच्छ्लीपदं हन्ति बद्धमूलमपि दृढम्[4] ॥११॥

1. रक्तसेचनैः इति आकरे पाठः ।
2. क. धुस्तूरैरण्ड० इति आकरे पाठः ।
   ख. सप्त ताम्बूलपत्राणां कल्कं तप्तेन वारिणा ।
   सम्भृष्ट लवणोपेतं श्लीपदं हन्ति सेवितम् ॥
3. रुपिका० इति आदर्शपुस्तकेषु पाठः ।
4. ध्रुवम् इति षष्ठपुस्तके पाठः ।

Paste should be prepared of the root-bark of *rūpikā* by triturating with *āranāla* (a type of sour drink). Application of this paste cures even deep-seated and compact type of *ślīpada* (filariasis).

पिण्डारकतरुसम्भवबन्दाकशिफा जयति सर्पिषा पीता ।
श्लीपदमुग्रं नियतं बद्धा सूत्रेण जङ्घायाम् ॥१२॥

Intake of the root of *bandāka* growing over *piṇḍāraka* tree along with ghee certainly cures serious type of *ślīpada*. This root should also be tied over the thigh for the cure of *ślīpada* (filariasis).

हितश्चालेपने नियतं चित्रको देवदारु च[1] ।
[2]सिद्धार्थशिग्रुकल्को वा सुखोष्णो मूत्रपेषितः ॥१३॥

Regular application of the luke-warm paste of *citraka*, *deva dāru*, *siddhārtha* and *śigru* prepared by triturating with cow's urine is useful in *ślīpada* (filariasis).

स्नेहस्वेदोपनाहांश्च श्लीपदेऽनिलजे भिषक् ।
कृत्वा गुल्फोपरि शिरां विध्येत्तु चतुरंगुले ॥१४॥

Treatment of Vātika Ślīpada

Oleation therapy, fomentation therapy and *upanāha* (application of hot ointment) should be used for *vātika* type of *ślīpada*. Thereafter, venesection should be performed four *aṅgulas* (finger breadth) above the ankle joint.

---

1. वा इति आकरे पाठः ।
2. सिदार्थ० इति आदर्शपुस्तकेषु पाठः ।

गुल्फस्याधः शिरां विध्येच्छ्लीपदे पित्तसम्भवे[1] ।
पित्तघ्नीश्च[2] क्रियां कुर्यात्पित्तार्बुदे विसर्पवत् ॥१५॥

Treatment of Paittika Ślīpada

In *paittika* type of *ślīpada*, venesection should be performed below the ankle joint and other *pitta* alleviating therapies should be administered as suggested for *paittika* type of *arbuda* (tumour) and *visarpa* (erysipelas).

मञ्जिष्ठां[3] मधुकं[4] रास्नां सहिंस्रां सपुनर्नवाम् ।
पिष्ट्वारनालैर्लेपोऽयं पित्तश्लीपदशान्तये ॥१६॥

Application of the paste of *mañjiṣṭhā*, *madhuka*, *rāsnā*, *hiṃsrā* and *punarnavā* prepared by triturating with *āranāla* (a type of sour drink) cures *ślīpada* (filariasis).

शिरां सुविदितां विध्येदङ्गुष्ठे श्लेष्मश्लीपदे ।
मधुयुक्तानि वा[5] तीक्ष्णकषायाणि[6] पिबेन्नरः ॥१७॥

---

1. क. संभवो इति प्रथमपुस्तके पाठः ।
   ख. निलजे भिषक् इति षष्ठपुस्तके पाठः ।
2. क. पादांगुष्ठसमीपे क्षिप्रमर्मणउर्ध्वं द्वयंगुलात् शिरां व्यध्येत् । पाठोऽयं पंचमपुस्तके अधिकमुपलभ्यते ।
   ख. कृत्वा गुल्फोपरि शिरां विध्येत्तचतुरंगुलं कंठस्याधः शिरां विध्येत् श्लीपदेपित्तसंभवे । पाठोऽयं षष्ठपुस्तके अधिकमुपलभ्यते ।
3. धत्तूरकस्य बीजानि पिप्पलीवर्द्धमानवत् ।
   शीतोदकेन पीतानि श्लीपदं हन्ति दारुणम् ॥
   पाठोऽयं पंचमपुस्तके अधिकमुपलभ्यते ।
4. मधुकां इति प्रथमपुस्तके पाठः ।
5. च इति प्रथमपुस्तके पाठः ।
6. तीक्ष्णकषायादि इति आकरे पाठः ।

Treatment of Kaphaja Ślīpada

In *kaphaja* type of *ślīpada* venesection should be performed over the great toe. The patient should be given the decoctions of drugs having *tīkṣṇa* (sharp) attribute along with honey.

पिबेत्सर्षपतैलेन श्लीपदानां निवृत्तये ।
[1]पूतीकरञ्जच्छदजं रसं वापि यथाबलम् ॥१८॥

The juice of the leaves of *pūtī karañja* should be taken along with mustard-oil in a suitable dose depending upon the strength of the patient which cures *ślīpada.*

अनेनैव विधानेन पुत्रञ्जीवकजं[2] रसम् ।
काञ्जिकेन पिबेच्चूर्णं मूत्रैर्वा वृद्धदारकम्[3] ॥१९॥

Similarly, the juice of *putrañjīvaka* should be given along with *kāñjī* (a type of sour drink) and the powder of *vṛddha dāraka* along with cow's urine.

रजनीं गुडसंयुक्तां गोमूत्रेण पिबेन्नरः ।
वर्षोत्थं श्लीपदं हन्ति दद्रुकुष्ठं[4] विशेषतः ॥२०॥

Intake of turmeric and jaggery along with cow's urine cures *ślīpada* of one year old. This recipe is specially useful for *dadru* (ring worm) type of skin disease.

गन्धर्वतैलभृष्टां हरीतकीं गोजलेन यः पिबति ।
श्लीपदबन्धनमुक्तो भवत्यसौ सप्तरात्रेण ॥२१॥

---

1. गुडूचीं व पिबेदेवं नागरदेवदारुं वा पाठोऽयं चतुर्थषष्ठपुस्तकयोः अधिकमुपलभ्यते ।
2. पुत्रजीवकरंजकम् इति षष्ठपुस्तके पाठः ।
3. वृद्धदारजम् इति आकरे पाठः ।
4. कण्डूकुष्ठं इति षष्ठपुस्तके पाठः ।

Intake of *harītakī* fried in castor oil along with cow's urine for seven days cures *ślīpada* (filariasis).

धान्याम्लं तैलसंयुक्तं कफवातविनाशनम्[1] ।
'जयेच्छ्लीपदकोत्थं[2] च ज्वरं सद्यो न संशयः ।'
श्लीपदघ्नो रसोऽभ्यासा.द्[3] गुडूच्यास्तैलसंयुतः ॥२२॥

Intake of *dhānyāmla* (a type of sour drink) along with oil alleviates *kapha* and *vāyu* and undoubtedly cures fever caused by *ślīpada* (filariasis). Similarly, the juice of *guḍūcī* along with oil should be taken for the cure of *ślīpada*.

"[4]त्रिकटु त्रिफलां चव्यं दार्वीं वरुणगोक्षुरम् ।
अलम्बुषां गुडूचीञ्च समभागानि चूर्णयेत् ॥२३॥
सर्वेषां चूर्णमाहृत्य वृद्धदारस्य[5] तत्समम् ।
काञ्जिकेन ततः[6] पेयमक्षमात्रं प्रमाणतः ॥२४॥
जीर्णे च परिहारं स्याद्भोजनं सर्वकामिकम् ।

---

1. खादेन्मासेण्डरी नरः इति प्रथमपुस्तके पाठः ।
2. क. 'जयेत्——संशयः' पाठोऽयं चतुर्थषष्ठपुस्तकयोः नोपलभ्यते ।
   ख. दीपनं च प्रदोषघ्नमेतत् श्लीपदनाशनम् ।
   गोधापदीमूलयुक्तां खादेन्माखेडरी नरः ।
   कफोत्थं श्लीपदं इतिज्वरं सद्यो न संशयः । पाठोऽयं चतुर्थषष्ठ-पुस्तकयोः अधिकमुपलभ्यते ।
3. रसोभ्वासन् इति आदर्शपुस्तकेषु पाठः ।
4. 'पलाशमूलस्वरसं पिबेद्वा तैलेन तुल्यं सितसर्षपानाम् ।
   मूत्रेण पथ्यामरदारुविश्वं सगुग्गुलुं श्लीपदिभिन्निषेयम् ॥
   पाठोऽयं चतुर्थषष्ठपुस्तकयोः अधिकमुपलभ्यते ।
5. वृद्धदारु च तत्समम् इति आकरे पाठः ।
6. तत्पेयं माषमात्रं इति आकरे पाठः ।

नाशयेच्छ्लीपदस्थौल्यमामवातञ्च दारुणम् ।
गुल्मकुष्ठानिलहरं वातश्लेष्मज्वरापहम् ॥२५॥"

॥ वृद्धदारुकसमचूर्णम्[1] ॥

Vṛddha Dāruka Sama Cūrṇa

One part of each of *trikaṭu*, *triphalā*, *cavya*, *dārvī*, *varuṇa*, *gokṣura*, *alambuṣā* and *guḍūcī*, and twelve parts of *vṛddha dāra* should be made to a powder. This should be taken in a dose of one *akṣa* along with *kāñjī* (a sour drink). After the potion is digested, the patient should take his food. It cures *ślipada* (filariasis), obesity, serious type of *āmavāta* (rheumatism), *gulma* (phantom tumour), *kuṣṭha* (obstinate skin diseases including leprosy), diseases caused by *vāyu* and fever caused by *vāyu* as well as *kapha*.

"पिप्पली त्रिफला दारु नागरं सपुनर्नवम् ।
भागैर्द्विपलिकैरेषां तत्समं वृद्धदारुकम्[2] ॥२६॥
काञ्जिकेन पिबेच्चूर्णं कर्षमात्रं[3] प्रमाणतः ।
जीर्णे च परिहारं स्याद्भोजनं सर्वकामिकम्[4] ॥२७॥
श्लीपदं वातरोगांश्च हन्यात्प्लीहानमेव च ।
अग्निश्च कुरुते घोरं भस्मकञ्च नियच्छति ॥२८॥

॥ पिप्पल्याद्यं चूर्णम् ॥"

[भैषज्यरत्नावली : श्लीपदाधिकार : १-२२]

1. वृद्धदारकसमचूर्णम् इति आदर्शपुस्तकेषु पाठः ।
2. वृद्धदारकम् इति आदर्शपुस्तकेषु पाठः ।
3. माषमात्रं इति आकरे पाठः ।
4. सार्वकामिकम इति आदर्शपुस्तकेषु पाठः ।

Pippalyādya Cūrṇa

Two *palas* of each of *pippalī*, *triphalā*, *deva dāru*, *nāgara* and *punarnavā*, and seven *palas* of *vṛddha dāru* should be made to a powder. This powder should be taken in a dose of one *karṣa* along with *kāñjī* (a sour drink). After the digestion of this potion, the patient should take his food. This cures *ślīpada* (filariasis), diseases caused by *vāyu* and splenic enlargement. It stimulates the power of digestion and cures *bhasmaka* (voracious eating). [This seems to be a variant reading of the previous recipe]

"कृष्णाचित्रकदन्तीनां कर्षमर्द्धपलं पलम् ।
विंशतिश्च हरीतक्या[1] गुडस्य तु पलं द्वयम् ।
मधुना मोदकं खादेत्[2] श्लीपदं हन्ति दुस्तरम् ॥२९॥

॥ कृष्णाद्यो मोदकः ॥

Kṛṣṇādya Modaka

Kṛṣṇā (one *karṣa*), *citraka* (half *pala*) and *dantī* (one *pala*,) *harītakī* (twenty fruits) and *guḍa* (two *palas*) should be added with honey and made to a *modaka* (large size pills). Intake of this cures serious type of *ślīpada* (filariasis).

सुरसा देवकाष्ठञ्च त्रिकटुत्रिफले तथा ।
लवणान्यथ[3] सर्वाणि विडङ्गान्यथ चित्रकम् ॥३०॥
चविका पिप्पलीमूलं गुग्गुलुर्हवुषा वचा ।
यवाग्रजञ्च पाठा च शट्येला वृद्धदारुकम् ॥३१॥

---

1. क. हरीतक्याः इति प्रथमपुस्तके पाठः ।
   ख. हरीतक्यो इति चतुर्थषष्ठपुस्तकयोः पाठः ।
2. खादन् इति आकरे पाठः ।
3. लवणान्यथा इति आदर्शपुस्तकेषु पाठः ।

कल्कैश्च कार्षिकैरेभिर्घृतप्रस्थं[1] विपाचयेत् ।
दशमूलकषायेण[2] धान्ययूषद्रवेण च ॥३२॥
दधिमण्डसमायुक्तं[3] प्रस्थं प्रस्थं पृथक् पृथक् ।
पक्वं स्यादुद्धृतं[4] कल्कात् पिबेत्कर्षद्वयं[5] हविः ॥३३॥
श्लीपदं कफवातोत्थं मांसरक्ताश्रितञ्च यत् ।
मेदःश्रितञ्च[6] वातोत्थं हन्यादेव न संशयः ॥३४॥
अपचीं गण्डमालाञ्च अन्त्रवृद्धिं तथार्बुदम् ।
नाशयेद् ग्रहणीदोषं श्वयथुं गुदजानि च ॥३५॥
परमाग्निकरं[7] हृद्यं कोष्ठक्रिमिविनाशनम् ।
"घृतं[8] सौरेश्वरं नाम श्लीपदं हन्ति सेवितम् ।
जीवकेन कृतं ह्येतत् रोगानीकस्य नाशनम् ॥३६॥
॥ सौरेश्वरी[9] घृतम् ॥

Saureśvara Ghṛta

One *prastha* of ghee should be cooked by adding the paste of one *karṣa* of each of *surasā, deva dāru, trikaṭu, triphalā,*

---

1. ०कार्षितैरेभिः घृतप्रसथं इति प्रथमपुस्तके पाठः ।
2. दशमूली कषायेण इति आदर्शपुस्तकेषु पाठः।
3. दधिमस्तु० इति आकरे पाठः ।
4. सांद्रघृतं कल्कां इति षष्ठपुस्तके पाठः ।
5. पिबेत्तोलार्द्धकम् इति आकरे पाठः ।
6. श्रिताभिद्यातो इति चतुर्थषष्ठपुस्तकयोः पाठः ।
7. परमग्निकरम् इति आदर्शपुस्तकेषु पाठः।
8. 'घृतं——घृतं' पाठोऽयं चतुर्थषष्ठपुस्तकयोः नोपलभ्यते ।
9. सौरेश्वरम् इति चतुर्थषष्ठपुस्तकयोः पाठः ।

pañca lavaṇa, viḍaṅga, citraka, cavya, pippalī mūla, guggulu, havuṣā, vacā, yava kṣāra, pāṭhā, śaṭi, elā and *vṛddha dāruka*, one *prastha* of each of the decoction of *daśa mūla, dhānya yuṣa* and whey. After cooking, the paste should be strained out. This medicated ghee should be administered in a dose of two *karṣas*. It undoubtedly cures *ślīpada* caused by *vāyu* as well as *kapha* and located in *māṃsa* (muscle tissue), *rakta* (blood) and *medas* (fat). It also cures *ślīpada* caused by *vāyu* alone, *apacī* (suppurated glands), *gaṇḍa mālā* (lymphadenitis), *antra vṛddhi* (inguinal hernia), *arbuda* (tumour), *grahaṇī* (sprue syndrome), oedema and piles. It stimulates the power of digestion. It is a cardiac tonic. It cures parasites infesting the intestinal tract. It is called *saureśvara ghṛta* and it is useful for the treatment of *ślīpada*. This recipe is propounded by Jīvaka for the cure of all diseases.

विडङ्गमरिचार्केषु नागरे चित्रके तथा ।
भद्रदार्वेलकाख्ये[1] सर्वेषु लवणेषु च[2] ।
तैलं पक्वं पिबेद्वापि श्लीपदानां निवृत्तये ॥३७॥
॥ विडङ्गादि[3] तैलम् ॥

[भैषज्यरत्नावली : श्लीपदाधिकार : २५-३२]

Viḍaṅgādi Taila

Oil should be cooked with *viḍaṅga, marica, arka, nāgara, citraka, bhadra dāru, elā* and *pañca lavaṇa*. Intake of this medicated oil cures all types of *ślīpada* (filariasis).

---

1. भद्रदार्वेलकाह्वे इति आकरे पाठः ।
2. क. तं इति प्रथमचतुर्थपंचमपुस्तकेषु पाठः ।
   ख. तत् इति षष्ठपुस्तके पाठः ।
3. विडङ्गाद्यं इति प्रथमपुस्तके पाठः ।

"कणावचादारुपुनर्नवानां[1] चूर्णं सविश्वं[2] समवृद्धदारम् ।
अनेन[3] संमर्द्य निहन्ति वल्लः सकाञ्जिकः श्लीपदरोगमुग्रम्[4] ॥३८॥"

[भैषज्यरत्नावली : श्लीपदाधिकार : २३]

Intake of the powder of *kaṇā, vacā, dāru, punarnavā, viśva* and *vṛddha dāra*—all taken in equal quantities, in a dose of one *valla* along with *kāñji* (a sour drink) cures serious type of *ślīpada.*

यवान्नं कटुतैलञ्च कूर्म्ममांसं च योजयेत् ।
श्लीपदानां प्रशान्त्यर्थमशान्तो[5] दाहमग्निनां ॥३९॥

Barley, mustard oil and the meat of tortoise should be taken for the cure of *ślīpada* (filariasis). If the disease is not cured by these, then cauterization therapy should be employed.

इति श्रीमहाराजाधिराजश्रीटोडरमल्लविरचिते टोडरानन्दे आयुर्वेदसौख्ये श्लीपदानां निदानचिकित्साकथनं नाम एकपंचाशत्तमो हर्षः ॥४०॥

Thus, ends the 51st Chapter dealing with the diagnosis and treatment of *ślīpada* (filariasis) in *Āyurveda saukhya* of *Ṭoḍarānanda* composed by the great king Ṭoḍara Malla.

---

1. 'कणा———दाहमग्निनां' पाठोऽयं प्रथमपुस्तके नोपलभ्यते ।
2. सबिल्वं इति आकरे पाठः ।
3. सम्मर्द्य चैतस्य इति आकरे पाठः ।
4. श्लीपदमुग्रवेगम् इति आकरे पाठः ।
5. ०शान्तौ इति षष्ठपुस्तके पाठः ।

CHAPTER XVII

अथ विद्रधिनिदानं चिकित्सा च ।

Diagnosis and Treatment of Vidradhi (Abscess)

"त्वग्[1]रक्तमांसमेदांसि प्रदू[2]ष्यास्थिसमाश्रिताः ।
दोषाः शो[3]थं श[4]नैर्घोरं जयनन्त्युच्छ्रिता भृशम् ॥१॥
महामूलं रुजावन्तं वृत्तं वाऽप्यथवाऽऽयतम् ।
स विद्रधिरिति ख्यातो विज्ञेयः षड्विधश्च सः ॥२॥

---

1. This is the beginning of the 56th Chapter of *Āyurveda saukhya* in *Ṭoḍarānanda* and the invocation reads as follows:—
   ब्रजांगना रासमिता इवैत्यताः प्रतप्त हेमोद्भवजंगमालताः ।
   जिगायकामं जगतां प्रभुत्वकं दद्यात्सदा टोडरमल्लके शुभम् ॥
2. संदूष्यास्थिसमाश्रिताः इति आकरे पाठः ।
3. शोकं इति षष्ठपुस्तके पाठः ।
4. सृतैर्घोरं इति पंचमपुस्तके पाठः ।

Pathogenesis

Doṣas located in the *asthi* (bone tissue), having vitiated skin, blood *māṃsa* (muscle tissue) and *medas* (fat) gradually produce excessively elevated swelling having a wide spread root and pain which is either round or flat. This is called *vidradhi* (abscess). It is of six types.

पृथग्दोषैः समस्तैश्च क्षतेनाप्यसृजा[1] तथा ।
षण्णामपि हि तेषां तु लक्षणं संप्रचक्षते[2] ॥३॥

Varieties

It is of six types, viz. *vātika*, *paittika*, *kaphaja*, *sānnipātika*, *kṣataja* and *raktaja*. Their symptoms are described below.

कृष्णोऽरुणो वा विषमो भृशमत्यर्थवेदनः ।
[3]चित्रोत्थानप्रपाकश्च विद्रधिर्वातसंभवः ॥४॥

Vātika Vidradhi

Vātika type of *vidradhi* is black and reddish in colour, irregular in shape and extremely painful. Its origin and suppuration take place in a irregular manner.

[4]'पक्वोदुम्बरसंकाशः श्यावो वा ज्वरदाहवान् ।
क्षिप्रोत्थानप्रपाकश्च विद्रधिः पित्तसंभवः ॥५॥

---

1. क्षतेनाहृयसृजा इति षष्ठपुस्तके पाठः ।
2. संप्रचक्ष्यते इति आकरे पाठः ।
3. चिरोत्थानप्रपाकश्च इति षष्ठपुस्तके पाठः ।
4. 'पक्वोदुंवर— —पित्तसम्भव;' पाठोऽयं पंचमपुस्तके अधिकमुपलभ्यते ।

Paittika Vidradhi

Paittika type of *vidradhi* is like a ripe fruit of *udumbara* and grayish in colour. It is associated with fever and burning sensation. It originates and suppurates very quickly.

शरावसदृशः पाण्डु शीतः स्निग्धोऽल्पवेदनः ।

चिरोत्थानप्रपाकश्च विद्रधिः कफसंभवः ॥६॥

Kaphaja Vidradhi

Kaphaja type of *vidradhi* is flat and elevated like a plate, pale-yellow in colour, cold to touch, unctuous and less painful. It takes a long time to manifest and then to get suppurated.

तनुपीतसिताश्चैषामास्रावाः[1] [2] क्रमशः स्मृताः ॥७॥

The pus of *vātika vidradhi* is thin, of *paittika vidradhi* is yellow in colour and of *kaphaja vidradhi* is white in colour.

नानावर्णरुजास्रावो घाटालो[3] विषमो महान् ।

विषमं पच्यते चापि विद्रधिः सान्निपातिकः ॥८॥

Sānnipātika Vidradhi

Sānnipātika type of *vidradhi* is characterised by different types of colour, pain and exudation, unevenness and is irregularly large. It gets suppurated in an irregular manner.

---

1. ०शितश्चै० इति प्रथमपंचमपुस्तकयोः पाठः ।
2. श्रावा इति प्रथमपुस्तके पाठः ।
3. क. घंटाभो इति चतुर्थपुस्तके पाठः ।
   ख. पाठाभो इति षष्ठपुस्तके पाठः ।

तैस्तैर्भावैरभिहते[1] क्षते चापथ्यकारिणः ।
क्षतोष्मा वायुमाश्रित्य[2] सरक्तं पित्तमीरयेत् ॥९॥
ज्वरस्तृष्णा च दाहश्च जायते तस्य देहिनः ।
आगंतुर्विद्रधिह्येष[3][4] पित्तविद्रधिलक्षणः ॥१०॥

Kṣataja or Āgantuja Vidradhi

If a person, having been afflicted with various causative factors, resorts to unwholesome food, then the heat of the injured part, being carried by *vāyu*, vitiates blood and *pitta* as a result of which the patient suffers from fever, thirst and burning sensation. This exogenous type of *vidradhi* has the signs and symptoms of *paittika vidradhi.*

कृष्णस्फोटावृतः श्यावस्तीव्रदाहरुजाकरः[5] ।
पित्तविद्रधिलिङ्गस्तु रक्तविद्रधिरुच्यते[6] ॥११॥"

[माधवनिदान : विद्रधिनिदान ४० : १-११]

Raktaja Vidradhi

In *raktaja* type of *vidradhi*, the growth is surrounded by black pustules which are grayish in colour. These are associated with acute burning sensation and pain. Other signs and symptoms of *paittika vidradhi* are also manifested in *raktaja vidradhi*.

---

1. स्तौ० इति षष्ठपुस्तके पाठः ।
2. वायुविसृत: इति आकरे पाठ: ।
3. एष विद्रधिरागन्तुः इति आकरे पाठः ।
4. ०विद्रधिस्त्वेष इति माधवनिदाने पाठ: ।
5. ०रुजाज्वर: इति आकरे पाठः ।
6. ०विद्रधि उच्यते इति आदर्शपुस्तकेषु पाठः ।

"स्त्रीणामपप्रजातानां प्रजातानां तथाऽहितैः[1] ।
दाहज्वरकरो घोरो जायते रक्तविद्रधिः ॥१२॥"

[सुश्रुत : निदान ९ : २६]

Rakta Vidradhi in Ladies

If there is improper delivery and if after proper delivery, ladies use unwholesome food and regimens, then *rakta vidradhi* is formed causing serious type of burning sensation and fever.

"उक्ता विद्रधयो ह्येते तेष्वसाध्यस्तु सर्वजः ।
आभ्यन्तरगतांश्[2]चैव विद्रधीन् परिचक्ष्महे[3] ॥१३॥"

[सुश्रुत : निदान ९ : ४-१५]

Prognosis

Out of the above mentioned varieties of *vidradhi*, the *sānnipātika* variety is incurable. Internal type of abscess is being described below.

"गुर्वसात्म्यविरुद्धान्नशुष्क[4]शाकान्नभोजनात् ।
अतिव्यवायव्यायामा[5]वगाहातपसेविनः ॥१४॥"

---

1. तथा हितैः इति आदर्शपुस्तकेषु पाठः ।
2. क. अल्पत्तरगतां० इति प्रथमपुस्तके पाठः ।
   ख. आभ्यन्तरानतस्तूर्ध्वं इति आकरे पाठः ।
3. परिचक्षते इति आकरे पाठः ।
4. ०शुष्कसंसृष्टभोजनात् इति आकरे पाठः ।
5. ०व्यायामवेगाघातविदाहिभिः इति आकरे पाठः ।

"पृथक् संभूय वा दोषाः कुपिता गुल्मरूपिणम् ।
बल्मीकवत्समुन्नद्धमन्तः[1] कुर्वन्ति विद्रधिम् ॥१५॥
गुदे बस्तिमुखे नाभ्यां कुक्षौ वङ्क्षणयोस्तथा ।
वृक्कयोप्लीह्नि यकृति हृदि[2] वा क्लोम्नि वाप्यथ ॥१६॥
एषामुक्तानि लिङ्गानि बाह्यविद्रधिलक्षणैः ।
आमपक्वैषणीयाच्च[3] पक्वापक्वं विनिर्दिशेत् ॥१७॥

Internal Abscess

By the intake of heavy, unwholesome and mutually contradictory ingredients of food, dry vegetables and dry food and by indulging in excessive sexual intercourse, physical exercise, bath [?] and exposure to sun, *doṣas*, individually or all together, get vitiated to cause an internal abscess like a *gulma* (phantom tumour) or an ant-hill in anus, opening of the urinary bladder, umbilicus, pelvis, groin, kidneys, spleen, liver, heart or lungs. Their signs and symptoms are like those of external abscesses. Its unsuppurated (*āma*) and suppurated (*pakva*) states are described in the *Āma-pakveṣaṇīya* chapter [of *Suśruta Saṃhitā*]

अधिष्ठानविशेषेण लिङ्गं शृणु विशेषतः ।
गुदे वातनिरोधस्तु बस्तौ कृच्छ्राल्पमूत्रता ॥१८॥
नाभ्यां हिक्का तथाऽऽटोपः कुक्षौ मारुतकोपनः[4] ।
कटीपृष्ठग्रहस्तीव्रो वङ्क्षणोत्थे तु विद्रधौ ॥१९॥

1. मन्तकुर्वन्ति इति आदर्शपुस्तकेषु पाठः ।
2. हृदये इति आकरे पाठः ।
3. आमपक्वेषणीये च इति आदर्शपुस्तकेषु पाठः ।
4. ०कोपनम् इति आकरे पाठः ।

वृक्कयोः[1] पार्श्वसङ्कोचः प्लीह्नि[2] श्वासावरोधनम् ।
सर्वाङ्गप्रग्रहस्तीव्रो हृदि कासश्च जायते ।
श्वासो यकृति तृष्णा[3] च पिपासा क्लोमजेऽधिका ॥२०॥

Depending upon their locations, these internal abscesses produce different additional signs and symptoms as given below:

Location of Abscess		*Signs and Symptoms*
1. Anus	—	obstruction to the passage of flatus.
2. Opening of urinary bladder	—	dysuria and oliguria.
3. Umbilicus	—	hiccup and gurgling noise in abdomen.
4. Pelvis	—	aggravation of wind.
5. Groin	—	extreme stiffness in lumber region and back.
6. Kidneys	—	contraction of the sides of the abdomen.
7. Spleen	--	obstruction to breathing.
8. Heart	—	extreme stiffness all over the body.
9. Liver	—	dyspnoea and thirst.
10. Kloman (Lungs or Pancreas ?)	—	thirst.

आमो वा[4] यदि वा पक्वो महान् वा यदि वेतरः ।
सर्वो मर्मोत्थितश्चापि विद्रधि कष्ट उच्यते ॥२१॥

---

1. वृक्कायोः इति आदर्शपुस्तकेषु पाठः ।
2. प्लीह्नयुच्छ्वासावरोधनम् इति आकरे पाठः ।
3. हिक्का इति आदर्शपुस्तकेषु पाठः ।
4. वाप्यपक्व वा इति आदर्शपुस्तकेषु पाठः ।

Prognosis

All internal abscesses located in vital organs are difficult of cure irrespective of their *āma* (unsuppurated) or *pakva* (suppurated) stages and large or small size.

नाभेरुपरिजाः पक्वा[1] यान्त्यूर्ध्व[2]मितरे त्वधः[3] ।
अधः स्रुतेषु जीवेत्तु स्रुतेषूर्ध्वं न जीवति ॥२२॥

Internal abscesses located above the umbilicus, when suppurated, get eliminated through the upward tracts and those located below the umbilicus get eliminated through the downward tracts. When it gets eliminated through the downward tracts, it is curable and if it gets eliminated through the upward tracts, then it is incurable.

हृन्नाभि[4]बस्तिवर्ज्या ये तेषु भिन्नेषु बाह्यतः ।
जीवेत् कदाचित् पुरुषो नेतरेषु कदाचन ॥२३॥"

[सुश्रुत : निदान ६ : १५-२५]

If the internal abscesses, located in places other than heart, umbilicus and urinary bladder, get eliminated through the exterior, then occasionally, the patient survives. Otherwise, the patient succumbs to death.

---

1. पाक्वाः इति प्रथमपुस्तके पाठः ।
2. जात्यूर्द्धमि० इति प्रथमपुस्तके पाठः ।
3. यः पक्वः सोऽप्यसाध्यः स्याद्यश्चोर्ध्वमुरे तथा पाठोऽयं आकरे अधिकमुपलभ्यते ।
4. वस्ति इति आदर्शपुस्तकेषु पाठः ।

साध्या विद्रधयः पंच विवर्ज्यः सान्निपातिकः[1] ।
आमपक्वविदग्धत्वं तेषां शोफवदादिशेत् ॥२४॥

Five varieties of external abscesses excluding *sānnipātika* variety are curable. The patient with *sānnipātika* variety of abscess should not be treated. Their three stages, viz. *āma* (immature or unsuppurated), *pakva* (mature or suppurated) and *vidagdhatva* (over matured or over suppurated) should be determined on the lines suggested for *śopha* (oedema).

आध्मातं[2] बद्धनिष्यन्दं छर्दिहिक्कातृषान्वितम् ।
रुजाश्वाससमायुक्तं विद्रधिर्नाशयेन्नरम् ॥२५॥

[माधवनिदान : विद्रधि ४० : ११-२०]

If the patient of *vidradhi* suffers from abdominal distension, if the exudation is arrested, if he gets vomiting, hiccup, thirst, pain and dyspnoea, then he succumbs to death.

हृन्नाभिबस्तिजः[3] पक्वो वर्ज्यो यश्च त्रिदोषजः ॥२६॥

[सुश्रुत : निदान ६ : ३४]

Suppurated abscess located in heart, umbilicus and urinary bladder and the abscess caused by *sannipāta* (simultaneous vitiation of all the three *doṣas*) should not be treated.

---

1. सानिपातिकः इति आदर्शपुस्तकेषु पाठः ।
2. आध्मानवचनिस्पंदं इति प्रथमपुस्तके पाठः ।
3. ०वस्तिजः इति आदर्शपुस्तकेषु पाठः ।

तथा च भोजः

"असाध्यो मर्मजो ज्ञेयः पक्वोऽपेक्षश्च विद्रधिः ।
सन्निपातोत्थितेप्येवं पक्व एव तु बस्तिजः ॥२७॥"

[माधवनिदान : विद्रधिनिदान ४० : २० टीका]

If the abscess is located in a vital organ and gets suppurated, then, it should not be treated. Similarly, *sānnipātika* variety of abscess and the abscess located in the urinary bladder should not be treated.

मुष्टिप्रमाणो गुल्मस्तु विद्रधिस्तु ततः परम् ।
गुल्मस्तिष्ठति दोषेषु विद्रधिर्मांसशोणिते ।
विद्रधिः पच्यते तस्माद् गुल्मश्चापि न पच्यते ॥२८॥

॥ विद्रधिनिदानम् ॥२९॥

Differential Diagnosis between Gulma and Vidradhi

Gulma (phantom tumour) is of the size of a fist (*muṣṭi*) and the size of the *vidradhi* (abscess) is larger than this. *Gulma* is located in the *doṣas* where as *vidradhi* is located in muscle tissue and blood. Therefore, *vidradhi* (abscess) gets suppurated where as *gulma* (phantom tumour) does not.

Thus, ends the description of the diagnosis of *vidradhi* (abscess).

एवमेव स्तनसिराः[1] विकृताः प्राप्य योषिताम् ।
सूतानां गर्भिणीनां[2] च संभवेत् श्वयथुर्घनः ॥३०॥

---

1. ०सिराविकृताः इति द्वितीयपुस्तके पाठः ।
2. श्वयथुनां इति षष्ठपुस्तके पाठः ।

स्तने सदुग्धेऽदुग्धे वा बाह्यविद्रधिलक्षणाः ।
नाडीनां सूक्ष्मछिद्राणां[1] कन्यानां तु न[2] जायते ॥३१॥

॥ स्तनविद्रधिनिदानम् ॥३२॥

Breast Abscess

Similarly, in women, after delivery or during pregnancy, the vitiated *doṣas* affecting the vessels in their breasts cause hard swelling. It might occur during lactation or in its absence. Signs and symptoms of external type of abscess are manifested in this condition. These breast abscesses do not occur in young girls bccause of the subtleness of the channels of circulation in their breasts.

Thus, ends the description of the diagnosis of breast abscess.

"जलौकः पातं शस्ततं सर्वाभिन्ने व विद्रधौ ।
मृदुर्विरेको लघ्वन्नं स्वेदः पित्तोद्भवं विना ॥३३॥

Line of Treatment

In all types of unsuppurated abscesses, application of leeches (*jalaukā*) for blood-letting, mild purgation, light food and fomentation therapies are useful. However, fomentation therapy should not be applied over *paittika* type of *vidradhi* (abscess).

वातघ्नमूलकल्कैस्तु[3] वसातैलघृताप्लुतैः[4] ।
सुखोष्णो बहलो लेपः प्रयोज्यो वातविद्रधौ ॥३४॥

1. सूक्ष्मवक्रत्वात् इति चतुर्थषष्ठपुस्तकयोः पाठः ।
2. तनजायते इति षष्ठपुस्तके पाठः ।
3. वातघ्नौषधकल्कैर्वा इति चतुर्थषष्ठपुस्तकयोः पाठः ।
4. वसातैलघृतान्वितैः इति ग्राकरे पाठः ।

Treatment of Vātika Vidradhi

In *vātika* type of *vidradhi*, a thick layer of the luke-warm paste of *vāyu* alleviating drugs mixed with *vasā* (muscle fat), oil or ghee should be applied.

स्वेदोपनाहाः कर्त्तव्याः शिग्रुमूलसमन्विताः ।
यवगोधूममुद्‌गैश्च सिद्धपिष्टैः[1] प्रलेपयेत्[2] ।
विलीयन्ते क्षणेनैवमपक्वश्चैव विद्रधिः ॥३५॥

Fomentation therapy and *upanāha* (application of hot ointment) should be done with the root of *śigru*. Over the abscess, the paste of barley, wheat or *mudga* should be applied.

पुनर्नवादारुविश्वदशमूलाभयाम्भसा[3] ।
गुग्गुलुं रुबुतैलं वा पिबेन्मारुतविद्रधौ ॥३६॥

The patient should take *guggulu* or castor oil along with the decoction of *punarnavā*, *deva dāru*, *śuṇṭhī*, *daśa mūla* and *abhayā* for the cure of *vātika vidradhi*.

पैत्तिकं शर्करालाजमधुकैः सारिवायुतैः ।
प्रदिह्यात्[4] क्षीरपिष्टैर्वा पयस्योशीरचन्दनैः[5] ॥३७॥"

[भैषज्यरत्नावली : विद्रधिरोगाधिकार : १-६]

---

1. सिद्धपिष्टैश्च लेपयेत् इति आकरे पाठः ।
2. प्रलेपनात् इति चतुर्थषष्ठपुस्तकयोः पाठः ।
3. ०दशमूलाभयाम्लसा इति प्रथमद्वितीयपुस्तकयोः पाठः ।
4. प्रतिह्यत् इति प्रथमपुस्तके पाठः ।
5. ०यस्यौशीरचन्दनैः इति आकरे पाठः ।

Treatment of Paittika Vidradhi

Over *paittika vidradhi*, the paste of *śarkarā*, *lājā*, *madhuka*, *sārivā*, *uśīra* and *candana* prepared by adding milk or water should be applied.

पिबेद्वा[1] त्रिफलाक्वाथं त्रिवृत्कल्काक्षसंयुतम् ॥३८॥

Decoction of *triphalā* added with one *akṣa* of the paste of *trivṛt* should be taken by the patient suffering from *paittika* type of abscess.

"पञ्चवल्कलकल्केन घृतमिश्रेण लेपनम् ।
यष्ट्याह्वशारिवादूर्वानलमूलैः सचन्दनैः ।
क्षीरपिष्टैः प्रलेपस्तु पित्तविद्रधिशान्तये ॥३९॥

Application of the paste of *pañca valkala* mixed with ghee or the paste of *yaṣṭi*, *śārivā*, *dūrvā*, root of *nala* and *candana* prepared by triturating with milk relieves *paittika* type of abscess.

'इष्टका[2]सिकतालोहगोशकृत्तु[3]षपांशुभिः ।
मूत्र[4]पिष्टैश्च सततं स्वेदयेच्छ्लेष्मविद्रधिम् ॥४०॥'

Treatment of Kaphaja Vidradhi

Kaphaja type of abscess should be given fomentation therapy with the paste of brick, sand, iron, cow-dung, husk of paddy and ash prepared by triturating with cow's urine.

---

1. पिबेच्चत्रिफलाक्वाथं इति षष्ठपुस्तके पाठः ।
2. 'इष्टका०—— ०विद्रधिम्, पाठोऽयं षष्ठपुस्तके नोपलभ्यते ।
3. शकृद्रसपांशुभिः इति प्रथमपुस्तके पाठः ।
4. मूत्रैरुष्णैश्च इति प्रथमपंचमपुस्तकयोः पाठः ।

दशमूलीकषायेण सस्नेहेन रसेन वा ।
शोथं व्रणं[1] वा कोष्णेन सशूलं परिषेचयेत् ॥४१॥

Oedema or ulcer associated with pain should be sprinkled with the luke-warm decoction or juice of *daśa mūla* added with *sneha* (fat).

त्रिफलाशिग्रुवरुण[2]दशमूलाम्भसा पिबेत् ।
गुग्गुलुं मूत्रयुक्तं वा विद्रधौ कफसम्भवे ॥४२॥"

[भैषज्यरत्नावली : विद्रधिरोगाधिकार : ७-११]

The patient suffering from *kaphaja* type of abscess should take *guggulu* along with cow's urine or the decoction of *triphalā, śigru, varuṇa* and *daśa mūla.*

"पित्तविद्रधिवत्सर्वां क्रियां निरवशेषतः ।
विद्रध्योः कुशलः कुर्याद्रक्तागन्तु[3]निमित्तयोः ॥४३॥

Treatment of Kṣataja and Raktaja Vidradhis

For the treatment of *kṣataja* (caused by external injury) and *raktaja* (caused by vitiation of blood) types of abscess, all the therapies prescribed for *paittika vidradhi* should be adopted.

[4]सौभाञ्जनकनिर्यूहो हिंगुसैन्धवसंयुतः ।
अचिरात् विद्रधिं[5] हन्ति प्रातः प्रात[6]र्निषेवितः ॥४४॥

---

1. व्रणञ्च इति प्रथमपंचमपुस्तकयोः पाठः ।
2. ०लवण० इति प्रथमपंचमपुस्तकयोः पाठः ।
3. क. निवृन्तयोः इति प्रथमपुस्तके पाठः ।
   ख. निवृत्तयो इति पंचमपुस्तके पाठः ।
4. शोभाञ्जन० इति आकरे पाठः ।
5. विद्रधीन् इति आदर्शपुस्तकेषु पाठः ।
6. ०र्न्नि० इति आदर्शपुस्तकेषुः पाठः ।

Intake of the decoction of *śobhāñjana* mixed with *hiṅgu* and *saindhava* every morning instantaneously cures abscess.

शिग्रुमूलं[1] जले धौतं दरपिष्टं प्रगालयेत् ।
तद्रसं मधुना पीत्वा हन्त्यन्तर्विद्रधिं नरः ॥४५॥

Treatment of Internal Abscess

Roots of *śigru* should be washed with water, coarsely pounded and strained through a cloth. Intake of this juice with honey cures internal abscess.

श्वेतवर्षाभुवो मूलं मूलं वरुणकस्य च ।
जलेन क्वथितं पीतमपक्वं विद्रधिं जयेत् ॥४६॥"

[भैषज्यरत्नावली : विद्रधिरोगाधिकार : १३-१६]

Intake of the decoction of the root of *punarnavā* or the root of *varuṇa* prepared by boiling with water, cures unsuppurated abscess.

"वरुणादिगणक्वाथमपक्वेऽभ्यन्तरोत्थिते[2] ।
ऊषकादिप्रतीवापं[3] पिबेत्संशमनाय वै ॥४७॥"

[भैषज्यरत्नावली : विद्रधिरोगाधिकार : १२]

Decoction of the drugs belonging to *varuṇādi gaṇa* should be sprinkled with the powder of drugs belonging to *ūṣakādi gaṇa*. Intake of this potion cures unsuppurated internal abscess.

---

1. "त्रीणि पलानि फलत्रितयश्च द्वेपले तुलिते मगधायाः । पञ्चपलानि भवन्ति पुरस्यात्सफलत्रिक गुग्गुलु योगः ।' पाठोऽयं प्रथमपुस्तके नोपलभ्यते ।
2. ०पक्वोभ्यन्तरोत्थिते इति प्रथमपुस्तके पाठः ।
3. प्रतिवापं इति पंचमपुस्तके पाठः ।

"शमयति पाठामूलं[1] क्षौद्रयुक्तं तण्डुलाम्भसा पीतम् ।
अन्तर्भूतं विद्रधिमुद्धतमाश्वेव मनुजस्य ॥४८॥
अपक्वे[2] त्वेतन्निर्दिष्टं[3] पक्वे तु व्रणवत् क्रिया ॥४९॥

Intake of the paste of *pāṭhā* along with honey and *taṇḍulodaka* (rice wash) instantaeously cures serious type of internal abscess when it is in an unsuppurated state. When the internal abscess gets suppurated, then it should be treated on the lines suggested for the treatment of ulcers.

स्रुतेऽप्यूद्ध्र्वमधश्चैव मैरेयाम्लसुरासवैः[4] ।
पेयो वरुणकादिश्च[5] मधुशिग्रुरसोऽथवा ॥५०॥"

[भैषज्यरत्नावली : विद्रधिरोगाधिकार : १७-१९]

If the pus, etc. of the internal abscess comes out through either the upward tracts or downward tracts, then the patient should be given the decoction of drugs belonging to *varuṇādi*

---

1. मानकमूलं इति चतुर्थषष्ठपुस्तकयोः पाठः ।
2. मन: शिलाभल्लातसूक्ष्मैलागुरुचन्दनैः ।
जातिपल्लव तर्कैश्च निम्बतैलं विपाचयेत् ।
बल्मीकं नाशयेत् तद्धि बहुछिद्रं बहुव्रणम् ।
॥ इति निम्बतिलम् ॥
पाठोऽयं चतुर्थषष्ठपुस्तकयोः अधिकमुपलभ्यते ।
3. तुनन्निर्दिष्टं इति षष्ठपुस्तके पाठः ।
4. क. शैलयोम्लसुरासुरैः इति षष्ठपुस्तके पाठः ।
ख. मैरेयाम्लसुरासुरैः इति प्रथमपुस्तके पाठः ।
5. ०वरुणकारिमर्कशिग्रुरसोथवा इति षष्ठपुस्तके पाठः ।

gaṇa or the juice of *madhu śigru* along with *maireya* (a type of vinegar), sour juice, *surā* or *āsava* (different types of alcoholic preparations).

“प्रियङ्गु[1]धातकीलोध्रकट्फलं तिनि[2]शत्वचम् ।
एतैस्तैलं विपक्तव्यं विद्रधौ रो[3]पणं परम् ॥५१॥”
॥ प्रियङ्ग्[4]वाद्यं तैलम्[5] ॥

[भैषज्यरत्नावली : विद्रधिरोगाधिकार : २३]

Priyaṅgvādya Taila

The oil cooked with *priyaṅgu*, *dhātakī*, *lodhra*, *kaṭ phala* and bark of *tiniśa* is an excellent recipe for the healing of ulcers.

---

1. प्रियङ्गुत्वक्फलं लोध्रं इति षष्ठपुस्तके पाठः ।
2. तिनिशन्वचं इति षष्ठपुस्तके पाठः ।
3. व्रणरोपणम् इति आकरे पाठः ।
4. पाठोऽयं प्रथमपंचमपुस्तकयोः नोपलभ्यते ।
5. त्रायन्ती त्रिफलानिम्बकटुकामधुकं समम् ।
तृवृत्पटोलमूलाभ्यां चत्वारांशा पृथक् पृथक् ।
मसूरानिस्तुषं यष्टी तत्क्काथो साघृतो जयेत् ।
मनःशिलालभल्लातसूक्ष्मैलागुरुचन्दनैः ।
जातिपल्लवतक्रं च निम्बतैलं विपाचयेत् ।
बल्मीकनाशयेत्तद्धि बहुछिद्रं बहुव्रणम् ।
॥ निम्बतैलम् ॥
द्विवल्लः समधु हन्ति लोकनाथस्तु विद्रधिम् ।
अथवा बोलसहितोद्विवल्लः पर्पटी रसः ।
हिंगुकासीससिन्धूत्थसिलाजतुविमिश्रितः ।
वरुणत्वग्भवः क्वाथो हन्याद्विद्रधिमुत्कटम् ।
पाठोऽयं चतुर्थपंचमषष्ठपुस्तकेषु अधिकमुपलभ्यते ।

इति श्रीमहाराजाधिराजश्रीटोडरमल्लविरचिते टोडरानन्दे आयुर्वेदसौख्ये विद्रधिनिदानचिकित्साकथनं नाम द्विपंचाशत्तमो हर्षः ॥५२॥

Thus, ends the 52nd Chapter dealing with the diagnosis and treatment of *vidradhi* (abscess) in *Āyurveda saukhya* of *Todarānanda* composed by the great king Todara Malla.

CHAPTER XVIII

अथ व्रणनिदानं चिकित्सा च ।

Diagnosis and Treatment of Ulcers

"एकदेशोत्थितः[1] शोथो व्रणानां[2] पूर्वलक्षणम् ।

षड्विधः[3] स्यात् पृथक् सर्वदोषैश्चागन्तुरक्तजः[4] ॥१॥

शोफा[5] एते तु विज्ञेयाः प्रागुक्तैः शोथलक्षणैः ।

विशेषः कथ्यते चैषां पक्वापक्वादिनिश्चये[6] ॥२॥

---

1. This is the beginning of the 57th Chapter of *Āyurveda saukhya* in *Ṭoḍarānanda* and the invocation reads as follows :
   ग्रस्तं भुजं गाधि पकेन तातं त्राहितियो वा विपिने वदं तम् ।
   अमोचयट्टोडरमल रुपं पायद्धरिः कल्पतरु स्वरुपम् ।।
2. व्रणानामुपलक्षणं इति षष्ठपुस्तके पाठः ।
3. द्विविधः इति षष्ठपुस्तके पाठः ।
4. सर्वरक्तागन्तुनिमित्तजः इति आकरे पाठः ।
5. शोथाः षडेते विज्ञेयाः इति आकरे पाठः ।
6. ०निश्चयः इति षष्ठपुस्तके पाठः ।

Premonitory Signs and Varieties

The premonitory signs of all types of ulcers is a localised swelling. It is of six types, viz. *vātika*, *paittika*, *kaphaja*, *sānnipātika*, exogenous and *raktaja* (caused by vitiation of blood). Their signs and symptoms are similar to those described for the respective varieties of *śotha* (oedema). For determining different stages of these ulcers, viz. *pakva* (suppurated), *apakva* (unsuppurated), etc., their special characteristics are being described below.

विषमं पच्यते वातात् पित्तोत्थश्चाचिरं[1] चिरम् ।
कफजः पित्तवच्छोफो[2] रक्तागन्तुसमुद्भवः ॥३॥

In *vātika* type of ulcer, suppuration takes place in an irregular manner, *paittika* type of ulcer suppurates quickly and *kaphaja* type of ulcer suppurates very slowly. *Raktaja* and exogenous types of ulcer suppurates quickly like *paittika* type of ulcer.

मन्दोष्मताऽल्पशोफत्वं[3] काठिन्यं त्वक्सवर्णता ।
मन्दवेदनता चैवं[4] शोफानामामलक्षणम् ॥४॥

Āma (*unsuppurated*) *Ulcer*

In the unsuppurated stage of the ulcer, there will be less of heat, less of oedema, hardness, colour is similar to that of the skin and less of pain.

1. ०चिराच्चिरम् इति आक. पाठः ।
2. ०छोथो इति आकरे पाठः ।
3. ०ताऽल्पशोथत्वं इति आकरे पाठः ।
4. चैतच्छोथाना० इति आकरे पाठः ।

दह्यते दहनेनेव क्षारेणेव च पच्यते ।
पिपीलिकागणेनेव दश्यते छिद्यते तथा ॥५॥
भिद्यते चैव शस्त्रेण दण्डेनेव च ताड्यते ।
पीड्यते पाणिनेवान्तः सूचीभिरिव[1] तुद्यते[2] ॥६॥
सोषाचोषो विवर्णः स्यादङ्गुल्येवावपीड्यते[3] ।
आसने शयने स्थानेऽशान्तिः वृश्चिकविद्धवत् ॥७॥
न गच्छेदाततः[4] शोफो[5] भवेदाध्मानबस्तिवत्[6] ।
ज्वरस्तृष्णाऽरुचिश्चैव[7] पच्यमानस्य लक्षणम् ॥८॥

Pacyamāna (beginning of suppuration) Ulcer

In *pacyamāna* stage when the ulcer begins to get suppurated (not yet fully suppurated), following signs and symptoms are manifested :

1. It burns as if touched by fire, it gets cooked as if touched by *kṣāra* (alkali preparation) and it pains as if bitten by a group of ants or incised by a weapon or injured by a staff or strongly pressed by hand or pricked by a needle;
2. If pressed by finger, the patient feels as if a current of heat is passed or as if the part is being strongly sucked and the area becomes discoloured;

---

1. शुचिभिरव इति द्वितीयपुस्तके पाठः ।
2. नुद्यते इति प्रथमपुस्तके पाठः ।
3. ०वावघट्यते इति आकरे पाठः ।
4. ०दातुरः इति प्रथमपंचमपुस्तकयोः पाठः ।
5. शोथो इति आकरे पाठः ।
6. ०ध्मातबस्तिवत् इति आकरे पाठः ।
7. ०रुचिस्तृकिः इति षष्ठपुस्तके पाठः ।

3. The patient does not get peace in sitting, sleeping or standing as if stung by a scorpion;
4. There is no pitting on pressure and the swelling appears like an inflated leather bag; and
5. The patient suffers from fever, thirst and anorexia.

वेदनोपशमः[1] शोथोऽलोहितोऽल्पो न चोन्नतः ।
प्रादुर्भावो वलीनां च तोदः कण्डूर्मुहुर्मुहुः ॥९॥
उपद्रवाणां प्रशमो निम्नता स्फुटनं त्वचः[2] ।
बस्ताविवाम्बुसंचारः स्याच्छोफेऽङ्गुलिपीडिते ॥१०॥
पूयश्च[3] पीडयत्येकमन्ते अन्ते च पीडिते ।
भक्ताकांक्षा[4] भवेच्चैव शोफानां पक्वलक्षणम् ॥११॥

Pakva (*fully suppurated*) *Ulcer*

When the ulcer is fully suppurated, following signs and symptoms are manifested:

1. Reduction in pain, oedema, redness and elevation;
2. Wrinkles appear over the skin;
3. Frequent pain and itching;
4. Alleviation of complications;
5. Depression in the swollen part;
6. Cracking of the skin;
7. If pressed through the finger, it feels like a leather bag filled with water and the pus gets reduced from the side of the pressure and accumulates in the other side; and
8. The patient feels hungry.

---

1. कफजेषु च शोथेषु गम्भीरं पाकमेत्यसृक् पाठोऽयं पंचमपुस्तके अधिकमुपलभ्यते ।
2. त्वचाम् इति आकरे पाठः ।
3. पूयस्य इति आकरे पाठः ।
4. भुक्ताकांक्षा इति पंचमपुस्तके पाठः ।

कफजेषु च शोथेषु गम्भीरं पाकमेत्यसृक्[1] ।
पक्वलिङ्गं ततः स्पष्टं यत्र स्याच्छीतशोफताम्[2] ॥१२॥
त्वक्सवर्णं रुजाऽल्पत्वं[3] घनस्पर्शत्वमश्मवत् ।
रक्तपाकमिति ब्रूयात्तं प्राज्ञो मुक्तसंशयः ॥१३॥

Rakta Pāka

In *kaphaja* type of oedema, the blood located very deep in the body gets suppurated. Then the signs and symptoms of suppuration are clearly manifested even though the oedematous part is cold to touch. There is no change in the colour of the skin, there will be less of pain and on touch, the oedematous portion will feel like a compact and stony hard mass. The physician should describe this condition as *rakta pāka* (suppuration of blood) without any doubt.

'तत्रा[4]निलाद्रुक् न विना च पित्तं
पाकःकफाच्चापि विना न पूयः ।
तस्मात्[5] समस्ताः परिपाककाले
पचन्ति शोफास्त्रिभिरेव[6] दोषैः ॥१४॥

1. पाकमन्त्रसृक् इति षष्ठपुस्तके पाठः ।
2. ०शोफना इति षष्ठपुस्तके पाठः ।
3. रुजो० इति प्रथमपुस्तके पाठः ।
4. नर्ते रुजा वातमृते च पित्तं इति आकरे पाठः ।
5. तस्माद्विपाकं इति आकरे पाठः ।
6. ०चैव इति षष्ठपुस्तके पाठः ।

कालान्तरेणाभ्युदितं तु पित्तं
कृत्वा वशे वातकफौ प्रसह्य ।
पचत्यतः शोणितमेव पाको
मतोऽपरेषां विदुषां द्वितीयः[1] ॥१५॥'

[सुश्रुत : सूत्र १७ : ७-८]

Role of Doṣas

There is no pain without *vāyu*, no suppuration without *pitta* and no pus formation without *kapha*. Therefore, during the process of suppuration, all the three *doṣas* play their roles. Some other physicians however hold the view that *rakta* (blood), in due course of time, aggravates *pitta* and suppresses the activities of *vāyu* as well as *kapha* to cause suppuration.

'कक्षं समासाद्य यथैव वह्नि-
र्वाय्वीरितः संदहति प्रसह्य ।
तथैव पूयोऽप्यविनिःसृतो[2] हि
मांसंसिराः स्नायु च खादतीह ॥१६॥'

[सुश्रुत : सूत्र १७ : १६]

As fire having entered into a fuel chamber and supported by wind bur ns evrything vigorously, similarly pus which is no taken out of the abscess causes devastation to the adjoining muscle tissues, vessels and ligaments.

---

1. द्वितीयं इति आदर्शपुस्तकेषु पाठः ।
2. सृतोयं इति प्रथमपुस्तके पाठः ।

आमं विदह्यमाणं च सम्यक् पक्वं च यो भिषक् ।
जानीयात् स भवेद्वैद्यः शेषास्तस्करवृत्तयः[1] ॥१७॥

The person who is able to correctly recognise the *āma* (unsuppurated), *pacyamāna* (beginning of suppuration) and *pakva* (fully suppurated) stages of an ulcer is entitled to be called a *vaidya* (physician or surgeons). All the rest are cheats.

यच्छिनत्त्याममज्ञानाद्यश्च[2] पक्वमुपेक्षते ।
श्वपचाविव विज्ञेयौ तावनिश्चितकारिणौ ॥१८॥"

॥ व्रणशोफनिदानम्[3] ॥१९॥

[माधवनिदान : व्रणशोफनिदान : १-१५]

If a physician incises an ulcer in *āma* (unsuppurated) stage and neglects the incision in *pakva* (fully suppurated) stage of an ulcer, then such are like lowcaste people not worth their profession.

Thus, ends the diagnosis of ulcerative oedema (*vraṇa śopha*).

"द्विधा व्रणः परिज्ञेयः[4] शारीरागन्तुभेदतः ।
दोषैराद्यस्तयोरन्य शस्त्रादिक्षतसंभवः ॥२०॥

---

1. शोषाः इति प्रथमपुस्तके पाठः ।
2. क. यश्छिनत्त्याममज्ञानाद्यो वा इति आकरे पाठः ।
   ख. ०ममज्ञानात् यत योरन्यशस्त्रादिक्षमेतच्च । इति षष्ठपुस्तके पाठः ।
3. व्रणशोथनिदानम् इति आकरे पाठः ।
4. स विज्ञेयः इति आकरे पाठः ।

Two Types of Ulcers

Ulcers are of two types, viz. *śārīra* (endogenous) and *āgantu* (exogenous). The former is caused by the vitiated *doṣas* and the latter by external injury by weapons, etc.

स्तब्धः[1] कठिनसंस्पर्शो मन्दस्रावो महारुजः ।
तुद्यते स्फुरति श्यावो व्रणो मारुतसंभवः ॥२१॥

Vātika Ulcer

Stiffness, hardness in touch, less of excretion, excessive pain including pinching and fluttering pain and grayish colour—these are the characteristic features of *vātika* type of ulcer.

तृष्णामोहज्वरक्लेददाहदुष्ट्यवदारणैः[2] ।
व्रणं पित्तकृतं[3] विद्यादगन्धैः स्रावैश्च[4] पूतिकैः ॥२२॥

Paittika Ulcer

Paittika type of ulcer is characterised by thirst, unconsciousness, fever, stickiness, burning sensation, vitiation, cracking and putried smell of the excretion.

बहुपिच्छो गुरुः स्निग्धः स्तिमितो मन्दवेदनः ।
पाण्डुवर्णोऽल्पसंक्लेदश्चिरपाकी कफव्रणः ॥२३॥

---

1. क. स्तद्धः इति प्रथमपुस्तके पाठः ।
   ख. तच्च इति षष्ठपुस्तके पाठः ।
2. ०पाकावदारुणौः इति चतुर्थषष्ठपुस्तकयोः पाठः ।
3. पित्तकर इति षष्ठपुस्तके पाठः ।
4. श्रावैश्च इति प्रथमपुस्तके पाठः ।

Kaphaja Ulcer

Kaphaja type of ulcer is characterised by excessive slimness, heaviness, unctuousness, numbness, less of pain, yellowish white coloration, less of stickiness and delayed suppuration.

रक्तो रक्तस्रुती रक्तात्[1] द्वित्रिजः स्यात्तदन्वयैः ॥२४॥

Raktaja, Dvandvaja and Sānnipātika Ulcers

In *raktaja* type of ulcer there will be more of bleeding. In *dvandvaja* type of ulcers signs and symptoms of the respective two *doṣas* are manifested. In *sānnipātika* type of ulcer signs and symptoms of all the three *doṣas* are manifested.

त्वङ्मांसजः सुखे देशे तरुणस्यानुपद्रवः ।
धीमतोऽभिनवः काले सुखे साध्यः सुखं व्रणः[2] ॥२५॥
गुणैरन्यतमैर्हीनस्ततः कृच्छ्रो व्रणः स्मृतः ।
सर्वैर्विहीनो विज्ञेयस्त्वसाध्यो निरुपक्रमः[3] ॥२६॥

Prognosis

If the ulcer is located in skin and muscle tissue, if it is not located in any vital organ, if the patient is young, if the ailment is not associated with any complication, if the physician is wise, if the ulcer is of short origin, if the time is suitable for treatment and if the ulcer is not of serious nature, then it is curable. If some of these features are absent then the patient is difficult of cure. If, however, all these characteristics are absent then the patient is not curable.

---

1. रक्तोरक्तजः इति षष्ठपुस्तके पाठः ।
2. पुनः इति षष्ठपुस्तके पाठः ।
3. निरुपद्रवः इति चतुर्थषष्ठपुस्तकयोः पाठः ।

पूतिः[1] पूयातिदुष्टासृक्स्राव्युत्सङ्गी चिरस्थितिः ।
दुष्टव्रणोऽतिगन्धादिः शुद्धलिंगविपर्ययः ॥२७॥

Duṣṭa Vraṇa and Śuddha Vraṇa

Presence of putried pus and vitiated blood, excessive excretion of pus, excessive swelling, long duration, excessively foul smell, etc., characterise *duṣṭa vraṇa* (vitiated ulcer). Otherwise, the ulcer is called *śuddha vraṇa* (clean ulcer).

जिह्वातलाभोऽतिमृदुः[2] स्निग्धो[3] विगतवेदनः[4] ।
सुव्यवस्थो निरास्रावः[5] शुद्धो व्रण इति स्मृतः ॥२८॥"

[माधवनिदान : शरीरव्रणनिदान १-८]

If the ulcer is very soft like the bottom of the tongue, unctuous, painless, well shaped and free from excretion then it is called clean (*śuddha vraṇa*).

व्रण शुद्ध्यति बन्धेन मृदुत्वं चोपगच्छति ।
रोहित्यपि च निःशंकं तस्माद्बंधः प्रशस्यते ॥२९॥

Bandage

Bandage makes the ulcer clean as well as soft and it helps in healing. Therefore, without any fear, bandage should be applied over the ulcer.

---

1. क. पूतिपूयोति इति प्रथमपुस्तके पाठः ।
   ख. पूतिपूयाति इति षष्ठपुस्तके पाठः ।
2. ०तलात्तोतिमृदुः इति प्रथमपुस्तके पाठः ।
3. स्निग्धोऽल्पवेदनः इति आकरे पाठः ।
4. वदनः इति षष्ठपुस्तके पाठः ।
5. स्रावोः इति चतुर्थपुस्तके पाठः ।

दोषप्रकोपाद् व्यायामादभिघातादजीर्णतः ।
हर्षात् क्रोधाद्भयात् चापि व्रणो रूढो विदीर्यते[1] ॥३०॥

Even a healed ulcer bursts because of aggravation of *doṣas*, exercise, injury, indigestion, exhileration, anger and fear.

"कपोतवर्णप्रतिमाः[2] यस्यान्ताः क्लेदवर्जिताः ।
स्थिराश्च पिडकावन्तो[3] रोहतीति[4] तमादिशेत्[5] ॥३१॥

Healing Ulcer

If the margin of the ulcer has the colour of a pigeon, if the border is free from sticky material, if it is stable (non-spreading) and if it is with granules, then it is called healing ulcer.

रूढवर्त्मानमग्रन्थिमशूनमरुजं[6] व्रणम् ।
त्वक्सवर्णं समतलं सम्यक्[7] रूढं तमादिशेत् ॥३२॥

Healed Ulcer

If the opening of the ulcer is closed without any nodules, if there is no swelling and no pain, if it has the colour of the skin and if it's surface is even, then the ulcer to be considered as healed.

---

1. विवर्द्धते इति षष्ठपुस्तके पाठः ।
2. क. ०प्रतिमा इति प्रथमपुस्तके पाठः ।
   ख. प्रतिमो इति षष्ठपुस्तके पाठः ।
3. ०वत्तो इति पंचमपुस्तके पाठः ।
4. राहतीति इति षष्ठपुस्तके पाठः ।
5. समादिशेत् इति प्रथमपुस्तके पाठः ।
6. क. ०मनुजं इति प्रथमपुस्तके पाठः ।
   ख. ०ग्रन्थिमस्तनं सरुजं इति षष्ठपुस्तके पाठः ।
7. सम्यग्रढं विनिर्दिशेत् इति आकरे पाठः ।

कुष्ठिनां विषदुष्टानां शोषिणां मधुमेहिनाम् ।

व्रणाः कृच्छ्रेण सिद्ध्यन्ति येषां चापि[1] व्रणे व्रणाः ॥३३॥

Delayed Healing

Ulcers in patients suffering from *kuṣṭha* (obstinate skin diseases including leprosy), poisoning and *madhu meha* (diabetes mellitus) heal with difficulty. If ulcer takes place over another ulcer, then also it heals with difficulty.

वसां मेदोऽथ मज्जानं मस्तुलुङ्गं च यः स्रवेत् ।

आगन्तुजो व्रणः सिध्येन्न सिद्ध्येद्दोषसंभवः ॥३४॥

Prognosis

If, in an exogenous ulcer, there is excretion of *vasā* (muscle fat), *medas* (fat), *majjā* (bone marrow) and *mastuluṅga* (brain matter), then it can be cured. But if these types of excretions take place in an endogenous type of ulcer, then it does not get cured.

मद्यागुर्वाज्यसुमनः पद्मचन्दनचम्पकैः ।

[2]सुगन्धा दिव्यगंधाश्च मुमूर्षणां व्रणाः स्मृताः ॥३५॥

Smell of alcohol, *aguru*, ghee, jasmin flower, lotus, sandal wood and *campaka* and other heavenly smell in the ulcer indicate that the patient is moribund.

ये च मर्मसु [3]संभूता भवन्त्यत्यर्थवेदनाः ।

दह्यन्ते चान्तरत्यर्थं बहिःशीताश्च ये व्रणाः ॥३६॥

---

1. पिच इति आदर्शपुस्तकेषु पाठः ।
2. सगन्धा इति आकरे पाठः ।
3. मर्मस्वसंभूता इति आकरे पाठः ।

दह्यन्ते बहिरत्यर्थं भवन्त्यन्तश्च शीतलाः ।
प्राणमांसक्षयश्वासकासारोचकपीडिताः[1] ॥३७॥
प्रवृद्धपूयरुधिरा व्रणा येषां[2] च मर्मसु ।
क्रियाभिः सम्यगारब्धा न सिध्यन्ति च ये व्रणाः ।
वर्जयेदपि तान्वैद्यः संरक्षन्नात्मनो यशः ॥३८॥"

[माधवनिदान : शारीरव्रण निदान ४२ : ६-१७]

॥ इति व्रणनिदानम्[3] ॥३९॥

The physician desirous of protecting his own fame should not treat the following types of ulcers:

1. When the ulcer is located in a vital organ;
2. Extremely painful ulcers;
3. Burning sensation in the interior but cool to touch in the exterior;
4. Burning sensation in the exterior but feeling of coolness in the interior;
5. If the patient is reduced of its vitality and muscle tissue;
6. If the patient, in addition, is suffering from dyspnoea, cough and anorexia;
7. If the ulcer located in the vital organs excretes excess of pus and blood; and
8. If the administration of appropriate therapy do not cause healing of the ulcer.

Thus, ends the diagnosis of endogenous types of ulcer.

---

1. ०कासाद्रोचक० इति प्रथमपुस्तके पाठः ।
2. यषाम् इति षष्ठपुस्तके पाठः ।
3. शारीरव्रणनिदानम् इति आकरे पाठः ।

"नानाधारमुखैः[1] शस्त्रैर्नानास्थाननिपातितः ।
भवन्ति नानाकृतयो व्रणास्तांस्तान्निबोध मे ॥४०॥

Different types of weapons having different types of edges and tips cause different types of ulcers (wounds) when they injure various places of the body. These different types of ulcers are being described below:

छिन्नं भिन्नं तथा विद्धं क्षतं पिच्चितमेव च ।
घृष्टमाहुस्तथा षष्ठं[2] तेषां वक्ष्यामि लक्षणम् ॥४१॥

Varieties

Wounds are of six varieties, viz. *chinna* (cut), *bhinna* (perforation), *viddha* (punctured wound), *kṣata* (lacerated wound), *piccita* (contusion) and *ghṛṣṭa* (abraison). Their characteristics are being described below.

तिर्यक् छिन्नं ऋजुर्वाऽपि यो व्रणस्त्वायतो भवेत् ।
गात्रस्य पातनं[3] तद्धि[4] छिन्नमित्यभिधीयते ॥४२॥

Chinna (cut) Type of Wound

If a portion gets separated from the body by an oblique or straight cut with wide spread wound, then it is called *chinna vraṇa*

शक्तिकुन्तेषुखड्गाग्रविषाणैराशयो हतः ।
यत्किंचित् प्रस्रवेत्तद्धि भिन्नलक्षणमुच्यते ॥४३॥

1. ०धारैर्मुखेशस्त्रैनाना इति पंचमपुस्तके पाठः ।
2. घष्ठं इति प्रथमपुस्तके पाठः ।
3. गात्रस्यावंतरं इति प्रथमपुस्तके पाठः ।
4. तच्च इति आकरे पाठः ।

Bhinna (*perforated*) *Type of Wound*

If a viscera get perforated by any sharp edged weapon like *śakti*, *kunta*, tip of a sword or horn resulting in the excretion of the contents of that viscera, then it is called *bhinna vraṇa.*

स्थानान्यामाग्निपक्वानां मूत्रस्य रुधिरस्य च ।
हृदुण्डुकः फुप्फुसश्च कोष्ठ इत्यभिधीयते ॥४४॥

Āmāśaya (stomach), *agnyāśaya* (small intestine including duodenum), *pakvāśaya* (colon), *mūtrāśaya* (urinary bladder), *rudhirāśaya* (liver and spleen), *hṛt* (heart), *uṇḍuka* (caecum) and *phuphusa* (lungs)—these taken together are called *koṣṭha.*

तस्मिन् भिन्ने रक्तपूर्णे ज्वरो दाहश्च जायते ।
मूत्रमार्गगुदास्येभ्यो[1] रक्तं घ्राणाच्च गच्छति ॥४५॥
मूर्च्छा श्वासस्तृषाऽऽध्मानमभक्तच्छन्द एव च ।
विण्मूत्रवातसङ्गश्च स्वेदास्रावोऽक्षिरक्तता ॥४६॥
लोहगन्धत्वमास्यस्य[2] गात्रदौर्गन्ध्यमेव च ।
हृच्छूलं पार्श्वयोश्चापि[3] विशेषं चात्र मे शृणु ॥४७॥

If there is perforation to any of the above mentioned visceras, then it will be filled with blood and there will be fever and burning sensation. There will be bleeding from urethra, anus, mouth and nose. The patient will suffer from fainting, dyspnoea, thirst, abdominal distension, loss of appetite, obstruc-

1. क. ०गुदस्य० इति षष्ठपुस्तके पाठः ।
   ख. गुदस्येभ्यो इति आकरे पाठः ।
2. लोहगन्धित्व० इति आकरे पाठः ।
3. पार्श्वयेश्चापि इति प्रथमपुस्तके पाठः ।

tion to the passage of stool, urine and flatus, perspiration, redness of eyes, iron-smell from the mouth, foul smell from the mouth, foul smell from the body, cardiac pain and pain in the sides of the chest. Other characteristics of these wounds will be described below.

आमाशयस्थे रुधिरे रुधिरं छर्दयत्यपि ।
आध्मानमतिमात्रं च शूलं च भृशदारुणम् ॥४८॥

If blood accumulates in the stomach, then there will be blood vomiting, abdominal distension in excess and serious type of colic pain.

पक्वाशयगते चापि रुजा गौरवमेव च ।
अधःकाये विशेषेण शीतता चोपजायते[1] ॥४९॥

[माधवनिदान : सद्योव्रण ४३ : १-१०]

If blood accumulates in the colon, then there will be pain, heaviness and coldness specially in the lower abdomen.

"अभिन्नेऽप्याशयेऽन्त्राणां खैः[2] सूक्ष्मैरन्त्रपूरणम् ।
पिहितास्यो[3] घटे यद्वल्लक्ष्यते[4] तस्य गौरवम् ॥५०॥

Even if the viscera is not perforated, the intestines get filled up through the subtle channels like a sealed jar kept in water gets filled up with water through it's pores. Therefore, there is heaviness in the intestines.

---

1. क. चापजायते इति षष्ठपुस्तके पाठः ।
   ख. च भवेदिह इति आकरे पाठः ।
2. वैः इति आदर्शपुस्तकेषु पाठः ।
3. पिहितास्ये इति आकरे पाठः ।
4. क. यद्वल्लभ्यते इति प्रथमपुस्तके पाठः ।
   ख. यद्वल्लजते इति षष्ठपुस्तके पाठः ।

सूक्ष्मास्यशल्याभिहतंयदङ्गं[1] त्वाशयं विना ।
उत्तुण्डितं निर्गतं वा तद्विद्धमिति निर्दिशेत् ॥५१॥

Viddha (*Punctured*) *Wound*

If any part of the body, other than visceras, gets injured by a sharp and pointed weapon where the tissues either remain projected outside (*uttuṇḍita*) or come out of the body (*nirgata*), then it is called *viddha vraṇa* (punctured wound).

नातिच्छिन्नं नातिभिन्नमुभयोर्लक्षणान्वितम् ।
विषमं व्रणमङ्गे यत्तत्[2] क्षतं[3] वापि[4] निर्दिशेत् ॥५२॥

Kṣata (*Lacerated*) *Wound*

If the wound is neither cut excessively nor perforated in excess, and is irregular in shape, then it is called *kṣata vraṇa* (lacerated wound).

प्रहारपीडनाभ्यां तु यदङ्गं पृथुतां गतम् ।
सास्थि तत् पिच्चितं विद्यान्मज्जारक्तपरिप्लुतम् ॥५३॥

Piccita (*Contusion*) *Wound*

If by the impact of beating, a part of the body including the bone gets swollen and the wound is filled with blood as well as bone-marrow, then it is called *piccita vraṇa* (contusion).

---

1. क. यदंगाशयम् इति षष्ठपुस्तके पाठः ।
   ख. त्वाशयाद् विना इति आकरे पाठः ।
2. यन्त इति प्रथमपुस्तके पाठः ।
3. कृतं इति षष्ठपुस्तके पाठः ।
4. क. चापि इति चतुर्थपुस्तके पाठः ।
   ख. त्वाभिनिर्दिशेत् इति आकरे पाठः ।

घर्षणादभिघाताद्वा यदङ्गं विगतत्वचम् ।
उष्मास्रावान्वितं[1] तद्धि[2] घृष्टमित्यभिधीयते ॥५४॥"

[सुश्रुत : चिकित्सा २ : १८-२३]

Ghṛṣṭa Vraṇa (Abraison)

If because of rubbing (*gharṣaṇa*) or injury (*abhighāta*), the skin of the body gets peeled off and there is exudation of warm liquid, then it is called *ghṛṣṭa vraṇa* (abraison).

"श्यावं सशोथं पिडकाचितं च मुहुर्मुहुः शोणितवाहिनं[3] च ।
मृदूद्गतं बुद्बुदतुल्यमांसं व्रणं सशल्यं सरुजं वदन्ति ॥५५॥
त्वचोऽतीत्य शिरादीनि भित्त्वा च परिहृत्य वा[4] ।
कोष्ठे प्रतिष्ठितं शल्यं कुर्यादुक्तानुपद्रवान्[5] ॥५६॥

Wound Containing Foreign-Body

Grayish colour, oedema, appearance of pimples, frequent bleeding, soft elevation, bubble like appearance over the wounded muscle tissue and pain indicate the presence of foreign body in the wound. These complications arise when the foreign body while penetrating the skin and cutting or bringing out vessels, gets lodged in any of the visceras.

---

1. उषास्रावान्वितं इति आकरे पाठः ।
2. तत्तु इति आकरे पाठः ।
3. वाहनम् इति षष्ठपुस्तके पाठः ।
4. च इति षष्ठपुस्तके पाठः ।
5. कुर्यान्नेतानुपद्रवान् इति षष्ठपुस्तके पाठः ।

तत्रान्तर्लोहितं[1] पाण्डुशीतपादकराननम्[2] ।
शीतोच्छ्वासं रक्तनेत्रमानद्धं च विवर्जयेत् ॥५७॥

Prognosis

If the ulcer is red in colour inside, if the patient is pale-yellow in colour, if his legs, hands and face are cold to touch, if his breathing is heavy and cold and if his eyes are fixed and red in colour, then such a patient should not be treated.

भ्रमः प्रलापः पतनं[3] प्रमोहो विचेष्टनं[4] ग्लानिरथोष्णता च ।
स्रस्ताङ्गता मूर्च्छनमूर्द्धवातस्तीव्रा[5] रुजो[6] वातकृताश्च तास्ताः[7] ॥५८॥
मांसोदकाभं[8] रुधिरं च गच्छेत् सर्वेन्द्रियार्थोपरमस्तथैव ।
दशार्द्धसंख्येष्वथ[9] विक्षतेषु सामान्यतो मर्मसु लिङ्गमुक्तम् ॥५९॥

Signs and Symptoms of Wound in Vital Organ

Giddiness, delirium, fall, unconsciousness, irregular movement of the body, drowsiness (*glāni*), rise in temperature, prostration, fainting, *ūrdhva vāta* (upward movement of the wind), excruciating pain, appearance of signs of aggravated *vāyu*, excretion of blood appearing like the water washed with flesh and withdrawal from the objects of senses—these are the signs and symptoms of injury to the five vital organs.

---

1. सव्वातिलर्लोहितं इति षष्ठपुस्तके पाठः ।
2. ०णीत० इति षष्ठपुस्तके पाठः ।
3. पततं इति प्रथमपुस्तके पाठः ।
4. विवेष्टनम् इति प्रथमपुस्तके पाठः ।
5. ०मूर्द्धवात० इति आदर्शपुस्तकेषु पाठः ।
6. ०रुजा इति षष्ठपुस्तके पाठः ।
7. तास्ता इति आदर्शपुस्तकेषु पाठः ।
8. मांसादकाभं इति षष्ठपुस्तके पाठः ।
9. ०संख्यष्त्वथ इति चतुर्थषष्ठपुस्तकयोः पाठः ।

सुरेन्द्रगोपप्रतिमं प्रभूतं
रक्तं स्रवेत्तत्क्षतजश्च[1] वायुः ।
करोति रोगान् विविधान् यथोक्तान्
शिरासु[2] छिन्नास्वथ[3] वा क्षतासु ॥६०॥

Injury to Vessels

If the vessel is cut or injured, then there will be excessive bleeding of the colour of *indra gopa* and the *vāyu*, aggravated as a result of this, produces several diseases.

कौब्ज्यं[4] शरीरावयवावसादः
क्रियास्वशक्तिस्तुमुला रुजश्च ।
चिराद् व्रणो रोहति यस्य चापि
तं स्नायुबिद्धं पुरुषं व्यवस्येत् ॥६१॥

Injury to Ligaments and Nerves (Snāyu)

If the ligaments or nerves are cut, then there will be *kaubjya* (hunch back), immobility of limbs, inability to perform any activity and excruciating pain. The ulcer in such cases takes a long time to heal.

---

1. क. क्षवजश्च इति प्रथमपुस्तके पाठः ।
   ख. क्षपयश्च इति षष्ठपुस्तके पाठः ।
2. सिरासु० इति प्रथमपुस्तके पाठः ।
3. विद्धास्वथ इति आकरे पाठः ।
4. कोष्ठशरीरा० इति षष्ठपुस्तके पाठः ।

[1]शोथाभिवृद्धिस्तुमुला रुजश्च बलक्षयः सर्वत एव शोथः ।
क्षतेषु सन्धिष्वचलाचलेषु स्यात् सर्व[2]कर्मोपरमश्च लिङ्गम् ॥६२॥

Injury to Joints

If there is injury to the joints, whether mobile of immobile, then there will be excess of oedema, excruciating pain, loss of strength, general anasarca and inability to perform any activity.

घोरा रुजो य.य निशादिनेषु
सर्वास्ववस्थासु च नैति शान्तिम् ।
भिषग्विपश्चिद्विदितार्थसूत्र-
स्तमस्थिविद्धं पुरुषं व्यवस्येत् ॥६३॥

Injury to Bone

If there is excruciating pain during the day and the night and absence of peace in any situation then the wise physician who is well versed with the science of surgery should diagnose this as injury to the bones.

यथास्वमेतानि विभावयेच्च[3]
लिङ्गानि मर्मस्वभिताडितेषु ।
पाण्डुर्विवर्णः स्पृशितं[4] न वेत्ति
यो मांसमर्म[5]ण्यभिपीडितः स्यात् ॥६४॥

1. क. शोथाति इति पंचमपुस्तके पाठः ।
   ख. शोषाभिवृद्धि० इति आकरे पाठः ।
2. कर्म्मो० इति प्रथमपुस्तके पाठः ।
3. ०येश्च इति प्रथमपुस्तके पाठः ।
4. स्परशं भवन्ति इति प्रथमपुस्तके पाठः ।
5. ०मर्म्मस्वभिताडितः इति प्रथमपुस्तके पाठः ।

Injury to a Vital Muscle

If any vital organ is injured, then the signs and symptoms of injury in respect of that particular organ will be manifested. If a *māṃsa marma* is injured, then there will be pale-yellow and other forms of discoloration and the patient will be insensitive to any touch sensation.

विसर्प-पक्षाघातश्च शिरास्तम्भोऽपतानकः ।
मोहोन्मादौ[1] व्रणरुजो ज्वरस्तृष्णा हनुग्रहः ॥६५॥
कासश्छर्दिरतीसारो हिक्का श्वासः सवेपथुः ।
षोडशोपद्रवाः प्रोक्ता व्रणानां व्रणचिन्तकैः ॥६६॥

॥ सद्योव्रणनिदानम् ॥६७॥

[माधवनिदान : सद्योव्रणाधिकार : १५-२६]

Complications

Erysipelas, hemiplegia, stiffness of vessels, *apatānaka*, unconsciousness, insanity, pain in ulcer, fever, thirst, *hanu graha* (lock-jaw), cough, vomiting, diarrhoea, hiccup, dyspnoea and trembling—these are the sixteen complications of injury.

Thus, ends the diagnosis of *sadyo-vraṇa* (fresh-wounds).

"आदौ विम्लापनं कुर्याद् द्वितीयमवसेचनम् ।
तृतीयमुपनाहञ्च चतुर्थीं पाटनक्रियाम् ॥६८॥
पञ्चमं शोधनं चैव[2] षष्ठं रोपणमिष्यते ।
एते क्रमा व्रणस्योक्ताः सप्तमो वैकृतापहः ॥६९॥

[भैषज्यरत्नावली : व्रणशोथाधिकार : १-२]

---

1. मोहोन्मादव्रणरुजो इति आकरे पाठः ।
2. कुर्यात् इति आकरे पाठः ।

Line of Treatment

Ulcers should be treated according to the following seven stages:

Stage		*Nature of the Therapy*
First stage	—	*Vimlāpana* (dissolution of oedema or the accumulated material)
Second stage	—	*avasecana* (sprinkling of medicated liquids)
Third stage	—	*upanāha* (application of hot ointment)
Fourth stage	—	*pāṭana* (opening the wound by incission)
Fifth stage	—	*śodhana* (cleansing the wound by medicated decoctions, etc.)
Sixth stage	—	*ropaṇa* (application of healing ointments, etc.)
Seventh stage	—	*vāikṛtāpaha* (correction of deformities).

"मातुलुंगा[1]ग्निमन्थौ च सुरदारु[2]महौषधम् ।
अहिंस्रा चैव रास्ना[3] च प्रलेपो वातशोथहा ॥७०॥"

[भैषज्यरत्नावली : व्रणशोथाधिकार : ६]

Treatment of Vātika Oedema

Application of the paste of *mātuluṅga, agni mantha, sura dāru, mahauṣadha, ahiṃsrā* and *rāsnā* cures *vātika* type of oedema in an ulcer.

1. मातुलुङ्गा इति आकरे पाठ: ।
2. भद्रदारु इति आकरे पाठ: ।
3. राष्णा इति आदर्शपुस्तकेषु पाठ: ।

"कल्कः काञ्जिकसम्पिष्टः स्निग्धः शाखोटकत्वचः ।
सुपर्ण इव नागानां वातशोथविनाशनः ॥७१॥

[भैषज्यरत्नावली : व्रणशोथाधिकार : ५]

The bark of *śākhoṭaka* should be made to a paste by triturating with *kāñji* (a sour drink) and oil. Application of this paste cures *vātika* type of oedema in an ulcer as snakes are overpowered by the bird *garuḍa*

दूर्वा च नलमूलञ्च मधुकं चन्दनं तथा ।
शीतलैश्च[1] गणैः[2] सर्वैः प्रलेपः पित्तशोफजित्[3] ॥७२॥"

[योगरत्नाकर : व्रणशोथचिकित्सा : (उत्तरार्द्धम) पृष्ठ १७३]

Treatment of Paittika Oedema

Application of the paste of *dūrvā*, root of *nala*, *madhuka*, *candana* and other cooling drugs cures *paittika* type of oedema.

"न्यग्रोधोदुम्बराश्वत्थप्लक्षवेतसवल्कलैः ।
ससर्पिष्कैः प्रलेपः स्याच्छोथ[4]निर्वापणः परः ॥७३॥

Barks of *nyagrodha*, *udumbara*, *aśvattha*, *plakṣa* and *vetasa* should be made to a paste. Application of this paste along with ghee dissolves oedema in an ulcer.

---

1. शीतलाश्च इति प्रथमपंचमपुस्तकयोः पाठः ।
2. गणाः इति प्रथमपंचमपुस्तकयोः पाठः ।
3. पित्तशोथहा इति आदर्शपुस्तकेषु पाठः ।
4. स्यात् शोथ इति प्रथमपंचमपुस्तकयोः पाठः ।

आगन्तौ शोणितोत्थे वा एष एव क्रियाक्रमः ॥७४॥

Treatment of Exogenous and Raktaja Oedema

For the treatment of exogenous and *raktaja* types of oedema, the above mentioned therapies [prescribed for *paittika* type of oedema] should be employed.

अजगन्धाऽश्वगन्धा च काला सरलया[1] सह ।
एकैषिका[2] च शृङ्गी च प्रलेपः श्लेष्मशोथहा ॥७५॥

Treatment of Kaphaja Oedema

Application of the paste of *aja gandhā, aśva gandhā, kālā, saralā, ekeṣikā* and *śṛṅgī* cures *kaphaja* type of oedema in an ulcer.

पुनर्नवाशिग्रुदारुदशमूलमहौषधैः[3] ।
कफवातकृते शोथे लेपः कोष्णो विधीयते ॥७६॥

In oedema of *kapha-vātaja* type, the luke-warm paste of *punarnavā, śigru, deva dāru, daśa mūla* and *śuṇṭhi* should be applied.

न रात्रौ लेपनं दद्याद्दत्तञ्च पतितं तथा ।
न च पर्युषितं शुष्यमाणं नैवावधारयेत् ॥७७॥

Paste should not be applied at night. The paste which has come out after application should not be used again. The paste which is stale (kept over night) and which has dried up should not be applied.

---

1. सरणया इति षष्ठपुस्तके पाठः ।
2. एकैधिकाजश्शृङ्गी इति प्रथमपंचमपुस्तकयोः पाठः ।
3. ०महौषधौ इति प्रथमपुस्तके पाठः ।

शुष्यमाणमुपेक्षेत प्रदेहं पीडनं प्रति ।

न चापि मुखमालिम्पेत्तेन दोषः प्रसिच्यते ॥७८॥

If the intention is to squeeze out pus, etc., from the wound, then *pradeha* (thick ointment) should be left over the wound even if it has dried up after application. However, the opening of the wound should not be covered with the paste to facilitate pus, etc. to come out of the wound.

स्थिरान् मन्दरुजान्[1] शोथान्[2]स्नेहैर्वातकफापहैः ।

अभ्यज्य स्वेदयित्वा[3] च वेणुनाड्या ततः शनैः ॥७९॥

विम्लापनार्थं मृद्नीयात्[4] तलेनांगुष्ठकेन वा[5] ।

रक्तावसेचनं कुर्यादादावेव विचक्षणः ॥८०॥

If the oedema in the ulcer is stable (not spreading) and is having mild pain, then it should be massaged with medicated oil prepared of drugs alleviating *vāyu* as well as *kapha*, and fomentation therapy should be given over it with the help of a bamboo tube. Thereafter, with the palm or thumb, the oedema should be gently rubbed with a view to dissolving the internal material (*vimlāpana*). Thereafter, blood-letting therapy should be applied by an experienced physician.

---

1. मन्दरुजः इति आदर्शपुस्तकेषु पाठः ।
2. शोथो इति षष्ठपुस्तके पाठः ।
3. स्नेहयित्वा इति प्रथमपुस्तके पाठः ।
4. क. मृद्नीयान्तलेनांगुष्ठकेन इति पंचमपुस्तके पाठः ।
   ख. गृह्णीयात्तलेनांगुष्ठकेन इति षष्ठपुस्तके पाठः ।
5. च इति पंचमपुस्तके पाठः ।

शोथे महति संवृद्धे[1] वेदनावति वा[2] व्रणे[3] ।
यो न याति शमं[4] लेपस्वेदसेकापतर्पणैः ।
सोऽपि नाशं व्रजत्याशु[5] शोथ शोणितमोक्षणात् ॥८१॥

If there is excessive aggravation of oedema, if there is excessive pain in the ulcer and if there is no alleviation of these symptoms by the application of ointments, fomentation therapy, sprinkling of medicated liquids and *apatarpaṇa* (cooling applications), then blood-letting therapy should be employed by which the oedema will subside quickly.

एकतश्च क्रिया सर्वा रक्तमोक्षणमेकतः[6] ।
रक्तं ह्यत्यम्लतां[7] याति तच्चेन्नास्ति[8] न चास्ति रुक् ॥८२॥

Importance of Blood-Letting Therapy

In an ulcer, sourness appears in the blood and pain is caused by this vitiated blood. If there is no vitiated blood then there will be no pain. This vitiated blood can be removed by blood-letting. Therefore, blood-letting therapy is equal to the administration of all the remaining therapies in therapeutic efficacy.

---

1. संरब्धे इति आदर्शपुस्तकेषु पाठः ।
2. चाव्रणे इति प्रथमपुस्तके पाठः ।
3. निवारणाय पाकस्य वेदनोपशमाय च पाठोऽयं आकरे अधिकमुपलभ्यते ।
4. समं लेपान् स्वेद० इति प्रथमपंचमपुस्तकयोः पाठः ।
5. व्रजन्त्याशु इति प्रथमपुस्तके पाठः ।
6. रक्तमोक्षणमथै इति षष्ठपुस्तके पाठः ।
7. रक्तं हि व्यम्लतां इति आकरे पाठः ।
8. तच्च नास्ति इति आकरे पाठः ।

स चेदेवमुपक्रान्तः[1] शोथो न प्रशमं व्रजेत् ।
तस्योपनाहैः पक्वस्य पाटनं हितमुच्यते ॥८३॥"

[भैषज्यरत्नावली : व्रणशोथाधिकार : ७-१७]

If the oedema does not get subsided by blood-letting therapy, the *upanāha* (hot ointment) should be applied over the wound for suppuration, and thereafter, it should be incised.

"तैलेन सर्पिषा वापि ताभ्यां वा शक्तुपिण्डका ।
सुखोष्णः शोथपाकार्थमुपनाहः[2] प्रशस्यते ॥८४॥

Upanāha

Application of the luke-warm paste of *śaktu* (roasted barley flour) in a bolus form (*piṇḍikā*) along with oil or ghee or both oil and ghee helps in the suppuration of the oedema. This is called *upanāha*.

सतिला सातसीबीजा दध्यम्ला शक्तुपिण्डिका ।
सकिण्व[3]कुष्ठलवणा शस्ता[4] स्यादुपनाहने ॥८५॥"

[भैषज्यरत्नावली : व्रणशोथाधिकार : २४-२५]

A paste should be prepared of *śaktu* (roasted barley flour), *tila*, seeds of *atasī*, *kiṇva*, *kuṣṭha* and salt. In a bolus form, this paste should be applied over the oedema as *upanāha* (to cause suppuration of the wound).

---

1. स वेदेवमुपक्रान्तः इति प्रथमपुस्तके पाठः ।
2. क. सुखपाकार्थमुपनाह इति आकरे पाठः ।
   ख. सुखोष्णसस्तपाकार्थमुपनाहः इति षष्ठपुस्तके पाठः ।
3. सकिण्डु० इति प्रथमपुस्तके पाठः ।
4. लवणा इति आदर्शपुस्तकेषु पाठः ।

"बालवृद्धासहक्षीणभीरुणां योषितामपि ।
मर्मोपरि च जाते च पक्वे शोथे च [1]दारुणे ॥८६॥
[2]गवां दन्तं जले घृष्टं विन्दुमात्रं [3]प्रलेपयेत् ।
[4]अत्यर्थकठिने चापि शोथे पाचनभेदनम् ॥८७॥"

[भैषज्यरत्नावली : व्रणशोथाधिकार : १८-१९]

If the patient is a child, old man, intolerant to therapies (*asaha*), emaciated, fearful or a woman; if the wound is over a vital organ and if the suppurated oedema is of serious nature, then one drop of the paste of cow's tooth prepared by rubbing over a stone along with water should be applied over the wound. This helps in the suppuration and opening up of the wound. This is also useful if the oedema is exceedingly hard.

"कटुतैलान्वितैर्लेपात् सर्पनिर्मोकभस्मभिः ।
चयः शाम्यति गण्डस्य [5]प्रकोपः स्फुटति द्रुतम् ॥८८॥

The ash of the dead skin of the snake should be mixed with mustard oil and made to a paste. Application of this suppresses the unmatured wound and opens up of the suppurated wound quickly.

---

1. दारणम् इति आकरे पाठः ।
2. गजम् इति चतुर्थपुस्तके पाठः ।
3. प्रलेपनात् इति आकरे पाठः ।
4. क. अत्यन्तकठिने इति आकरे पाठः ।
   ख. अव्यथाकठिने इति षष्ठपुस्तके पाठः ।
   ग. हस्तिदंतं जले घृष्ट्वा विन्दुमात्रं प्रलेपयेत् पाठोऽयं षष्ठपुस्तके अधिकमुपलभ्यते ।
5. पक्वस्तु इति आकरे पाठः ।

चिरबिल्वाग्निको दन्ती चित्रको हयमारकः ।
कपोतकङ्कगृध्राणां[1] पुरीषाणि च दारणम्[2] ।"
[भैषज्यरत्नावली : व्रणशोथाधिकार : २१-२२]
क्षारद्रव्याणि यावन्ति क्षारो वा दारणं परम् ॥८९॥

Application of the paste of *cira bilva, agnika, dantī, citraka, haya māraka*, stool of *kapota*, stool of *kaṅka* or the stool of *gṛdhra* opens up the wound. Similarly, application of the paste of drugs which are used for alkali preparations (*kṣāra dravyas*) and the alkali preparations (*kṣāras*) also help in the opening up of the wound.

"द्रव्याणां पिच्छिलानां तु त्वङ्मूलानि प्रपीडनम्[3] ।
यवगोधूममाषाणां चूर्णानि च समासतः[4] ॥९०॥"
[भैषज्यरत्नावली : व्रणशोथाधिकार : २६]

Barks and roots of all slimy drugs in general and the powders of *yava, godhūma* and *māṣa* in special squeeze out pus from a wound when applied in the form of a paste.

ततः प्रक्षालने क्वाथः पटोलीनिम्बपत्रजः ।
अविशुद्धे[5] विशुद्धे तु न्यग्रोधादित्वगुद्भवः ॥९१॥

---

1. ०कङ्ग० इति प्रथमपुस्तके पाठः ।
2. दारुणम् इति आदर्शपुस्तकेषु पाठः ।
3. क. प्रपीडितम् इति षष्ठपुस्तके पाठः ।
   ख. निपीडनम् इति आकरे पाठः ।
4. क. समासनः इति चतुर्थपुस्तके पाठः ।
   ख. चूर्णानि ससमासतः इति पंचमपुस्तके पाठः ।
5. अविशुद्धं विशुद्धे तु न्यग्रोध० इति षष्ठपुस्तके पाठः ।

Thereafter, the wound should be washed with the decoction of *paṭoli* and leaves of *nimba* if it is not clean. If it is clean, then the wound should be washed with decoction of the bark of *nyagrodha*, etc.

पञ्चमूलद्वयं वाते न्यग्रोधादिश्च पैत्तिके ।
आरग्वधादिको योज्यः कफजे[1] सर्वकर्म्मसु ॥६२॥

The decoction of *daśa mūla* should be used in all therapies for the treatment of *vātika* ulcer, the decoction of drugs belonging to *nyagrodhādi gaṇa* should be used in all recipes for the treatment of *paittika* ulcer and the decoction of drugs belonging to *āragvadhādi gaṇa* should be used in all recipes for the treatment of *kaphaja* type of ulcer.

"तिलकल्कः सलवणो[2] द्वे हरिद्रे त्रिवृद् घृतम् ।
मधूकं निम्बपत्रञ्च[3] लेपः स्याद् व्रणशोधनः ॥६३"।
॥ तिलाष्टकः[4] ॥

Tilāṣṭaka

Application of the paste of *tila*, *lavaṇa* (rock-salt), *haridrā*, *dāru haridrā*, *trivṛt*, ghee, *madhūka* and leaves of *nimba* helps in cleansing the ulcer.

---

1. कफजः इति षष्ठपुस्तके पाठः ।
2. लवणे इति प्रथमपुस्तके पाठः ।
3. निम्बपत्राणि इति आदर्शपुस्तकेषु पाठः ।
4. क. तिलावष्टकः पंचमपुस्तके पाठः ।
   ख. तिलाष्टकम् इति आकरे पाठः ।

निम्बपत्रं तिला दन्ती त्रिवृत्[1] सैन्धवमाक्षिकम्[2] ।
दुष्टव्रणप्रशमनो लेपः शोधनकेशरी ।
एकं[3] वा सारिवामूलं[4] सर्वव्रणविशोधनम् ॥९४॥"

[भैषज्यरत्नावली : व्रणशोथाधिकार : २८-३०]

Application of the paste of leaves of *nimba*, *tila*, *dantī*, *trivṛt*, rock-salt and honey relieves vitiated wounds and cleanses them effectively. The paste of the root of *śārivā* alone cleanses all types of ulcers.

"पटोलीतिलयष्ट्याह्व[5]त्रिवृद्दन्तीनिशाद्वयम् ।
निम्बपत्राणि चालेपः[6] सपटुर्व्रणशोधनः[7] ॥९५॥"[8]

[भैषज्यरत्नावली : व्रणशोथाधिकार : २७]

Application of the paste of *paṭolī*, *tila*, *madhu yaṣṭī*, *trivṛt*, *dantī*, *niśā*, *dāru niśā*, leaves of *nimba* and rock-salt cleanses all types of ulcer.

"निम्बकोलकपत्राणां कषायः शोधने हितः ॥९६॥"

[भैषज्यरत्नावली : व्रणशोथाधिकार : ३१]

---

1. तृवृत् इति आदर्शपुस्तकेषु पाठः ।
2. ०सैंधवमक्षिकै इति प्रथमपुस्तके पाठः ।
3. एकवामानिवा इति षष्ठपुस्तके पाठः ।
4. शारिवामूलं इति आकरे पाठः ।
5. ०तिलयष्ट्याट्कतृवृत्० इति प्रथमपुस्तके पाठः ।
6. च लेपः इति प्रथमपुस्तके पाठः ।
7. सपठ्व्रंणः इति प्रथमपुस्तके पाठः ।
8. त्रिफला खादिरो दार्वी न्यग्रोधादिबलाकुशाः । पाठोऽयं चतुर्थषष्ठ-पुस्तकयोः अधिकमुपलभ्यते ।

Washing the wound with the decoction of the leaves of *nimba* as well as *kola* also helps in cleaning the ulcer.

"अपेतपूतिमांसानां मांसस्थानामरोहताम् ।
कल्कः संरोपणः कार्यस्तिलानां[1] मधुकान्वितः ॥९७॥"

[भैषज्यरत्नावली : व्रणशोथाधिकार : ३४]

If the ulcer located in the muscle tissue does not get healed up, then from this ulcer the putrified muscle tissues should be removed and the paste of *tila* and *madhuka* should be applied over it which helps in healing.

निम्बपत्रमधुभ्यान्तु युक्तः संशोधनः स्मृतः ।
पूर्वाभ्यां सर्पिषा वापि[2] युक्तश्चाप्युपरोपणः[3] ॥९८॥

Application of the leaves of *nimba* and honey helps in the cleansing of the ulcer. Thereafter, the paste of the earlier mentioned two drugs, [*tila* and *madhuka*] along with ghee should be applied over the ulcer for its healing.

निम्बपत्रतिलैः कल्को मधुना[4] क्षतशोधनम्[5] ।
रोपणं सर्पिषा युक्तो यवकल्कोप्ययं विधिः ॥९९॥

The paste of the leaves of *nimba* and *tila* along with honey cleanses the ulcer. Application of the paste of *yava* along with ghee helps in the healing of ulcers.

---

1. कार्यस्तिलजो मधुसंयुतः इति आकरे पाठः ।
2. चापि इति षष्ठपुस्तके पाठः ।
3. युक्तः संशोधनः स्मृतः इति षष्ठपुस्तके पाठः ।
4. मधुनः इति षष्ठपुस्तके पाठः ।
5. क्षतशोधनः इति चतुर्थषष्ठपुस्तकयोः पाठः ।

"निम्बपत्रघृतक्षौद्रदार्वीमधुकसंयुता ।

वर्तिस्तिलानां कल्को वा शोषयेद्रोपयेत्[1] व्रणान् ॥१००॥"

[भैषज्यरत्नावली : व्रणशोथाधिकार : ४५]

Application of the *varti* (elongated pill) prepared of leaves of *nimba*, ghee, honey, *dāru haridrā* and *madhuka* or the paste of *tila* absorbs the pus and heals the ulcer.

"सप्तदलदुग्धकल्कः शमयति दुष्टव्रणं प्रलेपेन[2] ।

मधुयुक्ता शरपुंखा सर्वव्रणरोपणी[3] कथिता ॥१०१॥

Application of the paste of *sapta dala* prepared by triturating with milk is useful in the treatment of vitiated ulcers (*dusṭa vraṇa*). The paste of *śarapuṅkhā* mixed with honey should be applied for the healing of all types of ulcer.

मानुषशिरःकपालं तदस्थिलेपनञ्च मूत्रेण ।

रोहणमिदं क्षतानां योगशतैरप्यसाध्यानाम् ॥१०२॥"

[भैषज्यरत्नावली : व्रणशोथाधिकार : ३५-३६]

The skull bone of human beings should be made to a paste by triturating with cow's urine. Application of this helps in the healing of ulcers which were not amenable to hundreds of other recipes.

व्रणान्विशोधयेद्वर्त्या सूक्ष्मास्यान् सन्धिमर्मगान्[4] ॥१०३॥

---

1. शोधयेद्रोपयेत् व्रणाम् इति षष्ठपुस्तके पाठः ।
2. क. लेपात् इति आकरे पाठः ।
   ख. प्रलेपेणा इति षष्ठपुस्तके पाठः ।
3. क. सर्वव्रणरोपणाकथिता इति प्रथमपुस्तके पाठः ।
   ख. दुष्टव्रणरोपणी इति आकरे पाठः ।
4. सन्धिमार्गमान् इति षष्ठपुस्तके पाठः ।

Vartis (elongated pills) should be used for cleansing such ulcers which have small opening and which are located in the joints and vital organs.

[1]अभयात्रिवृतादन्तीलांगलीमधुसैंधवाः ।
[2]सुषवीपत्रधत्तूरकर्णमोटकुठेरकाः ।
पृथगेते प्रलेपेन गंभीरव्रणरोपणाः ॥१०४॥

Abhayā, trivṛt, dantī, lāṅgalī, madhu, saindhava, leaves of *suṣavī, dhattūra, karṇa moṭa* and *kuṭheraka*—all these drugs applied individually help in the healing of deep seated ulcers.

"पञ्चवल्कलचूर्णैर्वा शुक्तिचूर्णसमायुतैः ।
धातकीचूर्णलोध्रैर्वा तथा रोहन्ति ते व्रणाः[3] ॥१०५॥"

[भैषज्यरत्नावली : व्रणशोथाधिकार : ३७]

Ulcers get healed up by the powder of either *pañca valkala* and *śukti*, or *dhātakī* and *lodhra*.

[4]सदाहा वेदनावन्तो ये व्रणाः मारुतोद्भवाः ।
[5]तेषां तिलानुमांश्चैव भृष्टान् पयसि निर्वृतान् ।
तेनैव पयसा पिष्ट्वा दद्यादालेपनं भिषक् ॥१०६॥

If the ulcer is caused by aggravated *vāyu* and is associated with burning sensation as well as pain, then the paste prepared of roasted *tila* and *atasī* boiled in milk and then triturated with the same milk should be applied which is useful.

---

1. कृतया० इति प्रथमद्वितीयपुस्तकयोः पाठः ।
2. सुखाविपत्र० इति चतुर्थषष्ठपुस्तकयोः पाठः ।
3. तैर्व्रणः इति षष्ठपुस्तके पाठः ।
4. सदाहवेदना० इति षष्ठपुस्तके पाठः ।
5. माषान् इति षष्ठपुस्तके पाठः ।

वाताभिभूतान्[1] संस्रवान् धूपयेदुग्रवेदनान् ।
यवाज्यभूर्ज[2]मदनश्रीवेष्टकसुराह्वयैः ॥१०७॥

Fumigation

If the ulcer is afflicted by *vāyu* and is associated with secretions and excruciating pain, then it should be fumigated with *yava*, ghee, *bhūrja*, *madana*, *śriveṣṭaka* and *deva dāru*.

श्रीवासगुग्गुल्वगुरुशालनिर्यासधूपिताः ।
कठिनत्वं व्रणाः[3] यान्ति नश्यन्त्या[4]स्राववेदनाः[5] ॥१०८॥

By the fumigation with *śrīvāsa*, *guggulu*, *aguru* and resin from *śāla*, the ulcerated tissues become hard thereby reducing secretions and pain in the wound.

तिलः[6] पयः सिताः[7] क्षौद्रं तैलं मधुकचन्दनम् ।
लेपेनं[8] शोथरुग्दाहरक्तं निर्वापयेद् व्रणात्[9] ।[10]
पित्तविद्रधिवीसर्पशमनं लेपनादिकम् ॥१०९॥

---

1. भूतां इति पंचमपुस्तके पाठः ।
2. ०ज्यमूर्व्यमदनश्री० इति षष्ठपुस्तके पाठः ।
3. व्रणा यान्ति इति प्रथमपुस्तके पाठः ।
4. नश्यन्ताश्राववेदना इति पंचमपुस्तके पाठः ।
5. वेदनाः इति षष्ठपुस्तके पाठः ।
6. तिलाः इति षष्ठपुस्तके पाठः ।
7. सिता इति चतुर्थपंचमषष्ठपुस्तकेषु पाठः ।
8. क. लोपनं इति चतुर्थपुस्तके पाठः ।
   ख. लेपनं इति षष्ठपुस्तके पाठः ।
9. क. व्रणान् इति चतुर्थपुस्तके पाठः ।
   ख. ०व्रणाम् इति पंचमपुस्तके पाठः ।
10. 'करञ्जारिष्ट निर्गुण्डीरसो हन्याद्व्रणः कृमीन् ।
    कलायविदलापत्राकौशास्त्रास्थि च पूरणम् ।
    सुरसादि रसैः सेकालेपनं लशने नवा ।'
    पाठोऽयं षष्ठपुस्तके अधिकमुपलभ्यते ।

Application of the paste of *tila*, milk, sugar, honey, oil, *madhuka* and *candana* cures oedema, pain, burning sensation and bleeding. The paste, etc., described in the treatment of *paittika vidradhi* (abscess) and *visarpa* (erysipelas) should also be used in this condition.

अथाग्निदग्धलक्षण[1]चिकित्सा वक्ष्यते ॥११०॥

Burns and Scalds

Now the diagnosis and treatment of *agni dagdha* (burns and scalds) will be described.

"तत्र, स्निग्धं रूक्षं वाऽऽ(चा) श्रित्य द्रव्यमग्निर्दहति; अग्निसंतप्तो हि स्नेहः सूक्ष्मसि[2]रानुसारित्वात्त्वगादीननुप्रविश्याशु दहति; तस्मात् स्नेहदग्धेऽ[3]धिका रुजो भवन्ति ॥१११॥

The fire burns with the help of unctuous (*sneha*) or ununctuous (*rūkṣa*) media. The *sneha dravya* (oil, ghee or fat) has the natural attribute of quickly entering into the subte channels. When hot, it enters into the skin, etc., and instantaneously causes burn. Therefore, in a burn (scald) caused by oil, ghee or fat, there is excessive pain.

तत्र प्लुष्टं दुर्दग्धं सम्यग्दग्धमतिदग्धं चेति चतुर्विधमग्निदग्धम् । तत्र यद्विवर्णं [4]प्लुष्यतेऽतिमात्रं तत् प्लुष्टं; यत्रो[5]त्तिष्ठन्ति स्फोटास्तीव्रा[6]श्चोषदाहरागपाकवेदनाश्चि[7]राच्चोपशा-

1. ०दग्धनिदान चिकित्सा० इति चतुर्थषष्ठपुस्तकयोः पाठः ।
2. शिरा० इति आदर्शपुस्तकेषु पाठः ।
3. ०दग्धोधिका इति षष्ठपुस्तके पाठः ।
4. चूष्यतेतिमात्रं इति प्रथमपुस्तके पाठः ।
5. यत्रोस्तिष्ठन्ति इति षष्ठपुस्तके पाठः ।
6. ०श्चादोषदाहवेदाहवेदना० इति चतुर्थषष्ठपुस्तकयोः पाठः ।
7. ०श्चिराश्चोप इति प्रथमपुस्तके पाठः ।

स्यन्ति तद्दुर्दग्धं; सम्यग्दग्धमनवगाढं तालवर्णं सुसंस्थितं पूर्वलक्षणयुक्तं च; अतिदग्धे मांसावलम्बनं[1] गात्रविश्लेषः सिरा-[2] स्नायुसन्ध्यस्थिव्यापादमतिमात्रं ज्वरदाहपिपासामूर्च्छाश्चोपद्रवा भवन्ति, व्रणश्चास्य चिरेण रोहति, रूढश्च विवर्णो भवति। तदेतच्चतुर्विधमग्निदग्धलक्षणमात्मकर्मप्रसाधकं भवति ॥११२॥

Varieties and Characteristics

Agni dagdha (burn) is of four types, viz. *pluṣṭa* (mild burn), *durdagdha* (severe burn), *samyak dagdha* (moderate burn) and *ati dagdha* (excessive burn). Excessive discoloration of the skin and burning sensation are the characteristic features of *pluṣṭa* (mild burn). If the place of burn is elevated with pustules and if there is acute form of heating sensation, burning sensation, redness, suppuration as well as pain, and if healing takes place after a long time, then it is called *durdagdha* (severe burn). *Samyak dagdha* (moderate burn) is not very deep. It is like a ipe fruit of *tāla* and is associated with the signs and symptoms described before for *durdagdha.* In *ati dagdha* (excessive burn), muscles hang out, the body loses its compactness, there is cxessive damage to *śirā* (vessels), *snāyu* (ligaments includinge nerves), *sandhi* (joints) as well as *asthi* (bones), and the patient suffers from complications like fever, burning sensation, thirst and fainting. The ulcer takes a long time to heal and even after healing there will be discoloration. Determination of these four varieties of burn helps in the administration of therapies.

भवन्ति चात्र—

अग्निना कुपितं रक्तं भृशं जन्तोः प्रकुप्यति ।
ततस्तेनैव वेगेन पित्तमस्याप्युदीर्यते[3] ॥११३॥

1. त्वङ्मांसा० इति चतुर्थषष्ठपुस्तकयोः पाठः ।
2. शिरा० इति आदर्शपुस्तकेषु पाठः ।
3. पित्तमस्याह्युदीर्यते इति षष्ठपुस्तके पाठः ।

तुल्यवीर्ये उभे ह्येते रसतो वीर्यतस्तथा[1] ।
तेनास्य वेदनास्तीव्राः प्रकृत्या च विदह्यते ।
स्फोटाः शीघ्रं विजायन्ते[2] ज्वरस्तृष्णा च वर्द्धते[3] ॥११४॥[4]

Thus it is said:

Blood gets extremely vitiated by the heat of fire, ana similarly, the *pitta* of the patient gets extremely aggravated. Both the *rakta* (blood) and *pitta* are similar in taste (*rasa*) and dotency (*vīrya*). Therefore, there will be acuie form of pain and burning sensation, quick appearance of pustules and aggravated form of fever as well as thirst.

दग्धस्योपशमार्थाय चिकित्सा संप्रवक्ष्यते ।
प्लुष्टस्याग्निप्रतपनं कार्यमुष्णं तथौषधम्[5] ॥११५॥
शरीरे स्विन्नभूयिष्ठे स्विन्नं भवति शोणितम् ।
प्रकृत्या ह्युदकं[6] शीतं स्कन्दयत्यति शोणितम् ।
तस्मात्[7] सुखयति ह्युष्णं[8] न तु[9] शीतं कथंचन ॥११६॥

Treatment of Pluṣṭa (Mild Burn)

Now the treatment of burn will be described. For the treatment of *pluṣṭa* (mild burn) heat should be applied and other

---

1. द्रव्यतस्तथा इति आकरे पाठः ।
2. प्रजायन्ते इति आकरे पाठः ।
3. बाधते इति आकरे पाठः ।
4. 'तिलतैलं यवादग्धा एतल्लेपननिश्चितम्
   अग्निदग्ध लक्षणमात्मकर्म्मसाधकं भवति ।
   व्रणोरोहन्यति दुःखं प्रशाम्यति ।
   ॥ इति अग्निदग्धनिदानम्' ॥
   पाठोऽयं चतुर्थषष्ठपुस्तकयोः अधिकमुपलभ्यते ।
5. तथौखधम् इति प्रथमपुस्तके पाठः ।
6. ह्क्रुदकं इति प्रथमपुस्तके पाठः ।
7. तस्यात् इति षष्ठपुस्तके पाठः ।
8. ह्क्रुष्णं इति प्रथमपुस्तके पाठः ।
9. नु इति प्रथमपुस्तके पाठः ।

heating drugs should be employed. Because of excessive heat in the body, the blood becomes *svinna* (liquefied). Water is by nature cold and it exceedingly condenses or coagulates (*skandana*) the blood. Therefore, heating therapies give relief and cooling therapies are not useful at all.

शीतामुष्णां[1] च दुर्दग्धे क्रियां कुर्याद्भिषक् पुनः ।
घृतालेपनसेकांस्तु[2] शीतानेवास्य[3] कारयेत् ॥११७॥

Treatment of Durdagdha (Severe Burn)

In *durdagdha* (severe burn), the physician should employ both the heating and cooling therapies. Ghee should be applied and water should be sprinkled over it.

सम्यग्दग्धे तुगाक्षीरीप्लक्ष[4]चन्दनगैरिकैः ।
सामृतैः सर्पिषा स्निग्धैरालेपं कारयेद्भिषक् ॥११८॥
ग्राम्यानूपौदकैश्चैनं[5] पिष्ट्वा[6] मांसैः प्रलेपयेत् ।
पित्तविद्रधिवच्चैनं संततोष्माणमाचरेत् ॥११९॥

Treatment of Samyak Dagdha (Moderate Burn)

In *samyak dagdha* (moderate burn), the paste of *tugā kṣīrī*, *plakṣa*, *candana*, *gairika* and *amṛtā* along with ghee should be

---

1. शीतामुष्णम् इति षष्ठपुस्तके पाठः ।
   घृतालेपां सेकस्तु इति पंचमपुस्तके पाठः ।
3. शीतानैवास्य इति पचमपुस्तके पाठः ।
4. तुगाक्षीरीरक्तचन्दनगैरिकैः षष्ठपुस्तके पाठः ।
5. ग्राम्यनूपोदकैश्चेनं इति आदर्शपुस्तकेषु पाठः ।
6. पिष्टैर्मांसैः इति आकरे पाठः ।

applied. The paste of the meat of domesticated, marshy and aquatic animals should be applied over it. This condition of constant heat should be treated on the lines suggested for *paittika v idradhi* (abscess).

अतिदग्धे विशीर्णानि मांसानुत्कृत्य[1] शीतलाम्[2] ।
क्रियां[3] कुर्याद्भिषक् पश्चात्[4] शालितण्डुलकण्डनैः[5] ॥१२०॥
तिन्दुकीत्वक्कपालैर्वा घृतमिश्रैः प्रलेपयेत् ।
व्रणं गुडूचीपत्रैर्वा छादयेदथवोदकैः[6] ॥१२१॥
क्रियां[7] च निखिलां[8] कुर्याद्भिषक् पित्तविसर्पवत् ॥१२२॥

Treatment of Ati Dagdha (Excessive Burn)

In *ati dagdha* (excessive burn), first of all, the loosely hanging muscles should be separated. Thereafter, cooling therapies should be employed. The husk of *śāli* type of rice mixed with the bark or epicarp of the fruit of *tinduka* should be made to a paste, and applied over it. The ulcer should be covered with the leaves of *guḍūcī* or aquatic plants. All therapies described

1. मांसान्युद्धृत्य इति आकरे पाठः ।
2. शीतलम् इति षष्ठपुस्तके पाठः ।
3. कृयां इति प्रथतपुस्तके पाठः ।
4. यत्नात् इति षष्ठपुस्तके पाठः ।
5. क. शशितंडुलखंडनैः इति प्रथमपुस्तके पाठः ।
   ख. पश्चाच्छालितण्डुलकण्डनैः इति आकरे पाठः ।
6. क्षादयेतथ ओदकैः इति पंचमपुस्तके पाठः ।
7. क. कृया इति प्रथमपुस्तके पाठः ।
   ख. 'क्रियां——विसर्पवत्' पाठोऽयं पंचमपुस्तके नोपलभ्यते ।
8. कुर्यानिखिलां भिखक् पित्र विसर्पवत् इति प्रथमपुस्तके पाठः ।

for the treatment of *paittika visarpa* (erysipelas) should be used for *ati dagdha* (excessive burn).

मधूच्छिष्टं समधुकं[1] रोध्रं सर्जरसं तथा ।
मञ्जिष्ठां चन्दनं मूर्वां पिष्ट्वा सर्पिर्विपाचयेत् ।
सर्वेषामग्निदग्धानामेतद्रोपणमिष्यते[2] ॥१२३॥[3]
स्नेहदग्धे क्रियां रूक्षां[4] विशेषेणावचारयेत् ॥१२४॥"

[सुश्रुत : सूत्रस्थान १२ : १५-२६]

Ghee should be cooked with the paste of *madhūcchiṣṭa*, *madhuka*, *rodhra*, *sarja rasa*, *mañjiṣṭhā*, *candana* and *mūrvā*. It helps in the healing of ulcers of all types of burn. If the burn is caused by *sneha* (boiling ghee, oil, etc.), then ununctuous therapies should be employed.

"उष्णवातातपैर्दग्धे शीतः कार्यो विधिः सदा[5] ।
शीतवर्षानिलैर्दग्धे[6] स्निग्धमुष्णश्च शस्यते ।
तथाऽतितेजसा[7] दग्धे सिद्धिर्नास्ति[8] कदाचन[9] ॥१२५॥

1. समधुलो इति षष्ठपुस्तके पाठः ।
2. ०द्रोपणमुत्तमम् इति आकरे पाठः ।
3. 'तिलतैलं जवादग्ध्वा एतल्लेपेननिश्चितम् ।
अग्निदग्धाव्रणा रोहंयाति दुःखं प्रशाम्यति ।
॥मधुच्छिष्टाद्यं घृतम् ॥'
पाठोऽयं पंचमपुस्तके अधिकमुपलभ्यते ।
4. रुग्धे क्रियां रुक्षां इति चतुर्थपुस्तके पाठः ।
5. स्तथा इति षष्ठपुस्तके पाठः ।
6. हिमशीतानिलैर्दग्धै इति षष्टपुस्तके पाठः ।
7. अथाग्नितेजसा दग्धे इति षष्ठपुस्तके पाठः ।
8. क. सिधिन्नास्ति इति पंचमपुस्तके पाठः ।
ख. सिद्धिर्नास्ति इति चतुर्थषष्ठपुस्तकयोः आकरे च पाठः ।
9. कथंचन इति आकरे पाठः ।

इन्द्रवज्राग्निदग्धेऽपि जीवति प्रतिकारयेत् ।
स्नेहाभ्यङ्गपरीषेकैः प्रदेहैश्च तथा भिषक् ॥१२६॥

[सुश्रुत : सूत्र १२ : ३८-३९]

Heat and Cold Strokes

Burns caused by exposure to hot wind and hot sun should be treated with cooling therapies. For the treatment of burns caused by exposure to cold rain (snow fall) or cold wind, unctuous and hot therapies should be employed. If the patient is burnt by exposure to extremely dazzling light, then he cannot be cured. If there is burn by thunder-bolt, then even the patient may survive and he should be treated with oleation, massage as well as sprinkling therapies and by the application of ointments.

अग्निदग्धे व्रणे[1] सम्यक् प्रयुञ्जीत चिकित्सकः[2] ।
"महाराष्ट्रीजटालेपो दग्धे पिष्टावचूर्णनम्[3] ।
जीर्ण[4]गृहतृणाच्चूर्णं दग्धव्रणहरं परम् ॥१२७॥"

[भैषज्यरत्नावली : सद्योव्रणाधिकार : १२]

In *ati dagdha* (excessive burn), the physician should apply the paste of the root of *mahārāṣṭrī* and the powder of this root should be sprinkled over the affected parts. Sprinkling of the powder of the old straw used for roofing is also useful in curing ulcer caused by burn.

---

1. व्रणै इति षष्ठपुस्तके पाठः ।
2. चिकित्सितम् इति षष्ठपुस्तके पाठः ।
3. ०चूर्णणाम् इति षष्ठपुस्तके पाठः ।
4. जीर्णगेहतृणात् इति प्रथमपुस्तके पाठः ।

"जीरकपक्वं पश्चात् सिक्थक[1]सर्जरसमिश्रितं हरति ।
घृतमभ्यङ्गात् पावकदग्ध[ज]दुःखं क्षणार्द्धेन ॥१२८॥"

[भैषज्यरत्नावली : सद्योव्रणाधिकार : १५]

Ghee cooked with *jīraka* and mixed later with *sikthaka* and *sarja rasa* should be applied over the affected part. It quickly relieves pain caused by burn.

"अन्तर्दग्धकुठारको[2] दहनजं लेपान्निहन्ति व्रणम् ।
अश्वत्थस्य विशुष्कवल्कलकृतं चूर्णं तथा गुण्डनात्[3] ॥१२९॥

Application of the paste of *kuṭhāraka* burnt in a sealed jar without exposure to air cures ulcers caused by burn. Spraying the powder of dried barks of *aśvattha* also cures ulcers caused by burn.

अभ्यङ्गाद्विनिहन्ति तैलमखिलं गण्डूपदैः[4] साधितम् ।
पिष्ट्वा शाल्मलितूलकैर्जलगता लेपात्तथा वालुका[5] ॥१३०॥

[भैषज्यरत्नावली : सद्योव्रणाधिकार : १३-१४]

---

1. सित्द्कं इति षष्ठपुस्तके पाठः ।
2. ०कुठारका इति प्रथमपुस्तके पाठः ।
3. गुण्ठनात् इति षष्ठपुस्तके पाठः ।
4. गण्डूपलै इति षष्ठपुस्तके पाठः ।
5. 'शस्त्रक्षते च दशनच वितुवाण पुंखामूलोद्भव विनिदधीतरसं प्रयत्नात् । तस्मिन्पुरीषमथवा माहिषीसुतस्य प्राङ्गि सृतं मशृत् चूर्णितमाशु दद्यात् । लज्जालुका सरपुंखाभागीनां मध्यतः प्रलेपानां एकैकस्य जलैः पिष्टं मूलं शस्त्रक्षते ॥
   घृतेनलीर्गुल्याकं देनवीलेपते व्रणमुखे सद्योनियाति जवात्स्वल्पं चिरकालमपि तृणतालराजकस्य मूलं व मूलमूत्ररणी भवं जल-पिष्टप्रलेपेन नष्टशल्यं समुद्धरेत ॥' पाठोऽयं पंचमपुस्तके अधिकमुपलभ्यते ।

External application of the oil cooked by adding *gaṇḍū pada* (earth worm) cures burns. Similarly, sand collected from inside water should be made to a paste by adding the cotton of *śālmalī* and applied over the burn which is useful.

"सद्यः क्षतं व्रणं वैद्यः सशूलं परिषेचयेत्[1] ।
यष्टीमधुकयुक्तेन[2] किञ्चिदुष्णेन सर्पिषा ॥१३१॥"

[भैषज्यरत्नावली : सद्योव्रणाधिकार : १]

Luke-warm ghee cooked with the paste of *yaṣṭi madhu* should be sprinkled over a fresh wound associated with pain.

बुद्ध्वागन्तुव्रणं वैद्यो घृतक्षौद्रसमन्वितम् ।
शीतां क्रियां प्रयुञ्जीत रक्तपित्तोष्मनाशिनी[3] ॥१३२॥

In exogenous type of ulcer, the physician should employ ghee, honey and other cooling therapies for the alleviation of vitiated blood, *pitta* and heat.

[4]क्रान्तक्रामकमेकं सुश्लक्ष्णं गव्यसर्पिषा पिष्टम् ।
शमयति लेपान्नियतं व्रणमागन्तुजं न संदेहः ॥१३३॥

One *krānta krāmaka* [?] should be made to a fine paste by adding cow's ghee. Application of this undoubtedly cures exogenous types of ulcers.

---

1. परिसेचयेत् इति प्रथमपुस्तके पाठः ।
2. यष्टीमुधककल्केन इति आदर्शपुस्तकेषु पाठः ।
3. ०नाशनी इति प्रथमपुस्तके पाठः ।
4. क. कान्तक्रामकमेकं इति प्रथमपुस्तके पाठः ।
   ख. क्रान्तक्रामकमुक्तं इति षष्ठपुस्तके पाठ ।

"अपामार्गस्य संसिक्तं पत्रोत्थेन रसेन च[1] ।
सद्योव्रणेषु रक्तं तु प्रवृत्तं परितिष्ठति ॥१३४॥

If the juice of the leaf of *apāmārga* is applied over a fresh wound, then bleeding stops.

कर्पूरपूरितं बद्धं सघृतं सम्प्ररोहति[2] ।
सद्यः शस्त्रक्षतं पुंसां व्यथापाकविवर्जितम् ॥१३५॥

Ghee mixed with camphor should be applied over the ulcer and bandaged tightly. It removes pain, prevents suppuration and helps in healing of the freshly occurring ulcer caused by weapon.

शरपुङ्खा काकजङ्घा प्रथमं महिषीसुतमलम्[3] ।
लज्जालुका[4] च सद्यः[5] क्षतव्रणघ्नं पृथगेव तु ॥१३६॥

Śarapuṅkhā, *kāka jaṅghā*, first stool (meconium) of the male calf of buffalo and *lajjālu*—these drugs used separately cure freshly occurring ulcers caused by weapons.

शुनो जिह्वाकृतश्चूर्णः सद्यः क्षतविरोहणः[6] ।

[भैषज्यरत्नावली : सद्योव्रणाधिकार : २-५]

चक्रतैलं क्षते बिद्धे रोपणं परमं मतम्[7] ॥१३७॥

1. वा इति षष्ठपुस्तके पाठः ।
2. सम्प्ररोहयेत् इति षष्ठपुस्तके पाठः ।
3. महिषीसुतात् इति आकरे पाठः ।
4. मलं लज्जा च इति आकरे पाठः ।
5. सद्यस्कव्रणघ्नं इति आकरे पाठः ।
6. क्षतविरोहति इति चतुर्थषष्ठपुस्तकयोः पाठः ।
7. 'शस्त्रक्षते दशनचर्वितवाणपुंखामूलोद्भवं विनिदधतिर संप्रयत्नात् ।
तस्मिन् पुरीषमथवामहिषी सुतस्य प्राग्नि सृतं मसृणचूर्णितमाशु

(*Continued on next page*)

The powder of the tongue of the dog also helps in the healing of the fresh wound. *Cakra taila* is exceedingly helpful for healing a lacerated or punctured wound.

यवक्षारं भक्षयित्वा पिण्डं दद्याद् व्रणोपरि ।
शृगालकोल[1]मूलेन नष्टशल्यं विनिःसरेत् ।
लाङ्गलीमूललेपाद्वा गवाक्षीमूलकस्तथा ॥१३८॥

Extraction of Foreign Body

If a portion of the weapon remains inside the wound, then the patient should take *yava kṣāra* and a bolus of the paste of the root of either *śṛgāla kola*, *lāṅgalī* or *gavākṣī* should be applied over the wound. By this, the part of the weapon which has remained inside the wound comes out.

क्षतोष्मणो निग्रहार्थं तत्कालं विसृ[2]तस्य च ।
कषाय[3]शीतमधुराः स्निग्धलेपादयो हिताः ॥१३९॥

Immediately after the extraction of the foreign body, for the alleviation of heat of the wound, application of the unctuous paste, etc. of astringent, cooling and sweet drugs is useful.

"आमाशयस्थे रुधिरे वमनं पथ्यमुच्यते ।
पक्वाशयस्थे देयं च विरेचनमसंशयम् ॥१४०॥"

[सुश्रुत : चिकित्सा २ : ५२]

(*Continued from last page*)

दद्यात् । लज्जालुका शरपुखाभाङ्गीनां मध्यतः प्रलेपेन । एकैकस्य जलैः पिष्टं मूलं शस्त्र क्षते हितम् । घृतैन लांगलक्याः कंदेन विलेपिते व्रणस्य मुखे । सदया निर्गातिजवात् शल्यं चिरकालमपि । तृणराजस्य मूलं व मूलमूत्र रणीभवम् । जलपिष्टं प्रलेपेन नष्टशल्यं समुद्धरेत् ।' पाठोऽयं चतुर्थषष्ठपुस्तकयोः अधिकमुपलभ्यते ।

1. ०कोलिमूलेन इति षष्ठपुस्तके पाठः ।
2. निःसृतस्य इति चतुर्थषष्ठपुस्तकयोः पाठः ।
3. कषायाः इति चतुर्थपुस्तके पाठः ।

If blood is accumulated in the stomach then emetic therapy is useful and if the blood is accumulated in the colon, then purgation therapy should undoubtedly be administered.

"क्वाथो वशांत्वगेरण्डश्वद्रंष्ट्राश्मभिदा कृतः ।
सहिंगुसैन्धवः[1] पीतः कोष्ठस्थं स्रावयेदसृक् ॥१४१॥

Intake of the decoction of the bark of *vamśa*, *eraṇḍa*, *śvadaṃṣṭrā* and *pāṣāṇa bheda* along with asafoetida and rock-salt eliminates accumulated blood from the *koṣṭha* (alimentary tract).

यवकोलकुलत्थानां निस्नेहेन रसेन वा[2] ।
भुञ्जीतान्नं यवागूं वा पिबेत्सैन्धवसंयुताम् ॥१४२॥"
[योगरत्नाकर : सद्योव्रणचिकित्सा : पृष्ठ १८३]

Diet

After the blood is eliminated from the alimentary canal, the patient should be given food along with the soup of *yava*, *kola* and *kulattha* without adding any fat or he should be given *yavāgū* (thick gruel) along with rock-salt to eat.

अत्यर्थमस्रं स्रवति प्रायशोऽथात्रविक्षते[3] ।
ततो रक्तक्षयाद्वायौ[4] कुपितेऽतिरुजाकरे ॥१४३॥
"स्नेहपानपरिषेकस्नेहलेपोपनाहनम्[5] ।

---

1. हिङ्गुसैन्धवसंयुक्तः इति आकरे पाठः ।
2. च इति आकरे पाठः ।
3. क. प्रायशोथत्रविक्षिते इति पंचमपुस्तके पाठः ।
   ख. प्रायशोथत्रवीक्षते इति षष्ठपुस्तके पाठः ।
4. रक्तं तु या द्वायौ कुपिते तु रुजा करे इति पंचमपुस्तके पाठः ।
5. ०परिषेकलेपस्वेदोपदाहनम् इति आकरे पाठः ।

स्नेहबस्तिश्च[1] कुर्वीत वातघ्नौषधसाधितम् ॥१४४॥"

[योगरत्नाकर : सद्योव्रणचिकित्सा : १८२]

When blood comes out in a large quantity, then generally *vāyu* gets aggravated to cause excruciating pain. In this condition, *sneha* (fat) should be used for drinking, sprinkling, external application and *upanāha* (application of hot paste). The patient should be given medicated enema with unctuous substance cooked by adding *vāyu*-alleviating drugs.

"इति सप्ताहिकः[2] प्रोक्तः[3] सद्योव्रणहितो विधिः ।
सप्ताहात्परतः कुर्यात्[4] शरीरव्रणवत्क्रियाम् ॥१४५॥"

[भैषज्यरत्नावली : सद्योव्रणाधिकार : ६]

In the above mentioned manner, therapies should be administered for one week to a patient having fresh wounds. After seven days, such patients should be treated on the lines suggested for endogenous ulcers.

"करञ्जारिष्टनिर्गुण्डीरसो[5] हन्याद्व्रणक्रमीन् ॥१४६॥"

[भैषज्यरत्नावली : व्रणशोथाधिकार : ४७]

Treatment of Magots and Germs

If magots are formed in the ulcer, then the juice of *karañja*, *ariṣṭa* and *nirguṇḍī* should be applied over it.

---

1. कुर्वीत स्नेह बस्तिं च मारुतघ्नौषधैः श्रृतैः इति आकरे पाठः ।
2. साप्ताहिकः इति आकरे पाठः ।
3. कार्यः इति आकरे पाठः ।
4. कुर्याच्छरीर० इति आकरे पाठः ।
5. ०लेपो इति आकरे पाठः ।

कलापविदलीपत्रं कोषाम्रास्थि[1] च पूरणात् ।
सुरसादिरसैः सेको[2] लेपनं लशुनेन वा ॥१४७॥

To remove magots, the ulcer should be filled with the leaf of *kalāpa vidalī* or the seed pulp of *koṣāmra* or sprinkled with the juice of drugs belonging to the *surasādi gaṇa* or anointed with the paste of *laśuna*.

"निम्बशम्याकजात्यर्क[3]सप्तपर्णा[4]श्वमारका[5]: ।
क्रिमिघ्ना मूत्रसंयुक्ताः सेकालेपनधावनैः[6] ॥१४८॥"

[योगरत्नाकर : व्रणशोधनरोपणविधि : पृष्ठ १७६]

Nimba, śamyāka, jātī, arka, sapta parṇa and *aśva māraka*—these drugs destroy *kṛmis* (parasites). Along with cow's urine, these drugs should be used for sprinkling, anointment and washing.

प्रच्छाद्य[7] मांसपेष्यो वा कृमीनपहरेत्[8] व्रणात्[9] ।
"लशुनेनाथवा[10] दद्यात् लेपनं कृमिनाशनम् ॥१४९॥"

[योगरत्नाकर : व्रणशोधनरोपणविधि : पृष्ठ १०८]

---

1. कोलास्रास्थि इति चतुर्थषष्ठपुस्तकयो: पाठः ।
2. सको इति षष्ठपुस्तके पाठ: ।
3. ०संपाकजात्यर्क इति पंचमपुस्तके पाठः ।
4. सप्तकर्णाश्च इति षष्ठपुस्तके पाठ: ।
5. सप्तपर्णाश्व इति पंचमपुस्तके पाठ: ।
6 सकलेपनधावनै: इति चतुर्थषष्ठपुस्तकयोः पाठः ।
7. क. प्रसार्यमांसपेष्यो इति चतुर्थपुस्तके पाठः ।
   ख. प्रक्षाद्यमांसपेष्यो इति पंचमपुस्तके पाठः ।
8. कृमीनुपहरेत् इति षष्ठपुस्तके पाठः ।
9. व्रणात् इति चतुर्थषष्ठपुस्तकयोः पाठः ।
10. लशुनेनाद्यवादद्यात् इति प्रथमद्वितीयपुस्तकयोः पाठ; ।

By scraping the muscle tissue over the ulcer, parasites (magots) should be removed or the paste of *laśuna* should be applied over the ulcer for destroying the parasites.

"धूपनं[1] कृमीनुत्सा[ज्यं] निम्बाग्निर्हिंगुसैंधवैः ॥१५०॥"

Fumigation with *nimba*, *agni*, *hiṅgu*, *saindhava* and ghee destroys parasites or germs in the ulcers.

"ये[2] क्लेदपाकस्रुतिगन्धवन्तो व्रणा महान्तः सरुजः सशोथाः ।
प्रयान्ति ते गुग्गुलुमिश्रितेन पीतेन[3] शान्तिं त्रिफलारसेन ॥१५१॥"

॥ त्रिफलागुग्गुलुः ॥"

[भैषज्यरत्नावली : व्रणशोथाधिकार : ४६]

[योगरत्नाकर : व्रणशोधनरोपणविधि : पृष्ठ १७७]

Triphalā Guggulu

Ulcers with stickiness, suppuration, exudation and foul smell and ulcers which are big in size with pain and oedema get relieved by the intake of the decoction of *triphalā* added with *guggulu*.

"त्रिफलाचूर्णसंयुक्तो[4] गुग्गुलुर्वटकीकृतः[5] ।

---

1. 'धूपनं———सैंधवैः' पाठोऽयं प्रथमपंचमपुस्तकयोः नोपलभ्यते ।
2. तत् इति षष्ठपुस्तके पाठः ।
3. पानेन नाशं इति चतुर्थषष्ठपुस्तकयोः पाठः ।
4. नरकपालकच्छपास्थि अतसीनृकेश जीर्णवस्त्र समजारि चूर्ण कर व खैर मिलाई व्रण पर तीसिभिका तैल मिलै उपर पूर्वो चूर्णमल व सर्वथा शीघ्रव्रण नाश होय । पाठोऽयं पंचमपुस्तके अधिकमुपलभ्यते ।
5. गुग्गुलर्वटकीकृतः इति आदर्शपुस्तकेषु पाठः ।

निर्यन्त्रणो विबन्धघ्नो व्रणशोधनरोपणः ॥१५२॥

॥ अमृतागुग्गुलुः[1] ॥"

[योगरत्नाकर : व्रणशोधनरोपणविधि : पृष्ठ १७७]

Amṛtā Guggulu

Guggulu added with the powder of *triphalā* should be made to pills. Intake of this relieves pain and constipation. It also cleanses and heals ulcer. [*Amṛtā* is also a synonym of *harītakī*, one of the ingredients of *triphalā*; hence the name of the recipe]

शस्त्रोद्धृतं तैलं च बज्रकम् ॥१५३॥

[This seems to be a part of a verse which is missing perhaps because of calligraphic errors].

"विडङ्गत्रिफलाव्योषचूर्णं गुग्गुलुना समम्[2] ।
सर्पिषा वटिकां[3] कृत्वा खादेद्वा हितभोजनः ।
दुष्टव्रणापचीमेहकुष्ठ[4]नाडीविशोधनः[5] ॥१५४॥"

॥ गुग्गुलुवटिका[6] ॥

[भैषज्यरत्नावली : व्रणशोथाधिकार : ५०]

---

1. क. गुग्गुलुवटकः इति आकरे पाठः ।
   ख. त्रिफलागुग्गुलुः इति चतुर्थषष्ठपुस्तकयोः पाठः ।
2. गुग्गुलुनाशनम् इति प्रथमपुस्तके पाठः ।
3. वटकान् कुर्यात् खादेद्वा हितभोजनः इति आकरे पाठः ।
4. ०कुष्ठव्रणनाडी० इति प्रथमषष्ठपुस्तकयोः पाठः ।
5. ०विशोधनान् इति आकरे पाठः ।
6. विडङ्गादिगुग्गुलुः इति आकरे पाठः ।

Vaṭikā Guggulu

One part of each of *viḍaṅga*, *triphalā* and *trikaṭu* should be added with seven parts of *guggulu*. From out of this paste, pills should be prepared by adding ghee. Intake of these pills along with wholesome food cures *duṣṭa vraṇa* (vitiated ulcer), *apacī* (suppurated gland), *meha* (obstinate urinary disorders including diabetes), *kuṣṭha* (obstinate skin diseases including leprosy) and *nāḍī vraṇa* (sinus).

अमृतापटोलमूलत्रिफलात्रिकटुकृमिघ्नानाम् ।
समभागानां[1] चूर्णं सर्वसमो गुग्गुलोर्भागः ॥१५५॥
प्रतिवासरमेकैकां खादेदक्षपरिमाणम्[2][3] ।
जेतुं व्रणवातासृक्गुल्मोदरश्वयथुपाण्डुरोगांश्च[4][5] ॥१५६॥
॥ अमृतावटिका गुग्गुलुः[6] ॥

[योगरत्नाकर : व्रणशोधनरोपणविधि : उत्तरार्द्ध : पृष्ठ १७७]

Amṛtā Vaṭikā Guggulu

One part of the powder of each of *amṛtā*, *paṭola* (root), *triphalā*, *trikaṭu* and *kṛmighna* and nine parts of *guggulu* should be mixed and made to pills of one *akṣa* each. Intake of one pill every day cures ulcer, *vāta rakta* (gout), *gulma* (phantom tumour), *udara* (obstinate abdominal diseases including ascites), oedema and anemia.

---

1. क. सर्वसमभागचूर्णं इति षष्ठपुस्तके पाठः ।
   ख. कृत्वा समभागचूर्णं तत्तुल्यो गुग्गुलुर्योज्यः इति आकरे पाठः ।
2. गुटिकां खादेदक्षपरिमाणम् इति षष्ठपुस्तके पाठः ।
3. ०अपरिमाणाम् इति चतुर्थपुस्तके आकरे च पाठः
4. व्रणवातास्रं गुल्मोदरपाण्डुशोथादीन् इति आकरे पाठः ।
5. क. पाण्डुरोगात् इति चतुर्थपुस्तके पाठः ।
   ख. रोगान् इति षष्ठपुस्तके पाठः ।
6. अमृताद्यो गुग्गुलुः इति आकरे पाठः ।

स्वर्जिका[1] च यवक्षारं[2] कम्पिल्लं च मेहेन्दिका:[3] ।
टङ्कणः[4] श्वेतखदिरं तुत्थं चूर्णं च गोघृतैः ।
सर्वं समांशं संचूर्ण्य मर्दयेत्प्रहरं द्वयम्[5] ॥१५७॥
एवं सर्वव्रणविशोधनम् ।
पूरणं कृमिकण्डुघ्नं शीघ्रपाटवकारकम् ॥१५८॥"
॥ स्वर्जिकादिघृतम्[6] ॥

[योगरत्नाकर : व्रणशोधनरोपणविधि : पृष्ठ १७८]

Svarjikādi Ghṛta

Svarji kṣāra, *yava kṣāra*, *kampilla*, *mehendikā*, *ṭaṅkaṇa*, *śveta khadira* and *tuttha*—powder of all these drugs taken in equal quantities should be triturated by adding cow's ghee for two *praharas*. This cleanses and heals all types of ulcers and cures *kṛmi* (parasitic infestation) as well as itches. It is effective very quickly. [The last but one line is incomplete because of calligraphic error, perhaps in the original manuscript].

"जातीनिम्बपटोलपत्रकटुकादार्वीनिशासारिवा-[7]
मञ्जिष्ठामयसिक्थतुत्थमधुकैर्नक्ताह्वबीजैः[8] समैः ॥१५९॥

---

1. 'स्वर्जिका———स्वर्जिकाद्यं घृतम्' पाठोऽयं षष्ठपुस्तके अधिकमुपलभ्यते ।
2. यवक्षारः इति आकरे पाठः ।
3. हरेणुका इति आकरे पाठः ।
4. टङ्कणं श्वेतखदिरं इति आकरे पाठः ।
5. दृढम् इति आकरे पाठः ।
6. स्वर्जिकाद्यं इति आकरे पाठः ।
7. जातीपत्रपटोलनिम्ब० इति योगरत्नाकरे पाठः ।
8. ०र्नक्ताह्वबीजान्विताः इति योगरत्नाकरे पाठः ।

सर्पिः सिद्धमनेन सूक्ष्मवदना मर्माश्रिताः स्राविणो
गम्भीराः सरुजो व्रणाः[1] सगतिकाः शुद्धयन्ति रोहन्ति च ॥१६०॥

॥ जात्याद्यं[2] घृतम् ॥

[भैषज्यरत्नावली : व्रणशोथाधिकार : ५१]

[योगरत्नाकर : व्रणशोधनरोपणविधि : पृष्ठ १७७-१७८]

Jātyādya Ghṛta

Ghee should be cooked with *jāti*, *nimba*, *paṭola* (leaf), *kaṭukā*, *dāru haridrā*, *haridrā*, *sāriva*. *mañjiṣṭhā*, *kuṣṭha*, *siktha*, *tuttha*, *madhuka* and *naktāhva* (seed)—all these drugs should be taken in equal quantities. Application of this medicated ghee cleanses and heals ulcers having small openings, located in vital organs, with exudations, and ulcers which are deep seated, painful as well as spreading.

"गौरा हरिद्रा मञ्जिष्ठा मांसी मधुकमेव च ।
प्रपौण्डरीकं ह्रीबेरं भद्रमुस्तं सचन्दनम् ॥१६१॥
जातीनिम्बपटोलञ्च[3] करञ्जं[4] कटुरोहिणी[5] ।
मधूच्छिष्टं[6] समधूकं महामेदा तथैव च ॥१६२॥
पञ्चवल्कलतोयेन घृतप्रस्थं विपाचयेत् ।
एष गौरो महावीर्यः[7] सर्वव्रणविशोधनः ॥१६३॥

---

1. व्रणोः इति प्रथमपुस्तके पाठः ।
2. जात्यादिघृतम् इति योगरत्नाकरे पाठः ।
3. जाति इति आदर्शपुस्तकेषु पाठः ।
4. करञ्जे इति षष्ठपुस्तके पाठः ।
5. कटुरोहिणीम् इति प्रथमषष्ठपुस्तकयोः पाठः ।
6. मधुच्छिष्टं इति पंचमपुस्तकेषु पाठः ।
7. महायोगः इति आकरे पाठः ।

आगन्तुसहजाश्चैव[1] सुचिरोत्थाश्च ये व्रणाः ।
विषमामपि नाडीन्तु शोधयेच्छीघ्रमेव[2] तु ॥१६४॥

॥ गौराद्यं घृतम् ॥

Gaurādya Ghṛta

One *prastha* of ghee should be cooked with the decoction of *pañca valkala* and the paste of *gaurā, haridrā, mañjiṣṭhā, māṃsī, madhuka, prapauṇḍarīka, hrībera, bhadra mustā, candana, jātī, nimba, paṭola, karañja, kaṭu rohiṇī, madhūcchiṣṭa, madhūka* and *mahā medā*. It is a very potent recipe for the cleansing of all types of ulcer, viz. exogenous, endogenous and chronic ulcers. It quickly cleanses irregularly formed si uses also.

गौराद्यं जातिकाद्यं[3] च तैलमेवं प्रसाध्यते ।
तैलं सूक्ष्मानने दुष्टे व्रणे गम्भीर एव च ॥१६५॥

[भैषज्यरत्नावली : व्रणशोथाधिकार : ५२-५६]

Gaurādya and Jātikādya Tailas

In the above mentioned two recipes, oil can be used for cooking in the place of ghee. Then these recipes are called *gaurādya taila* and *jātikādya taila*. These medicated oils are useful in the treatment of ulcers having small openings, putrified ulcers and deep-seated ulcers.

---

1. ०सहजोत्थश्च इति षष्ठपुस्तके पाठः ।
2. क. शोध्येत्शीघ्रमेव इति पंचमपुस्तके पाठः ।
   ख. शोध्येच्छीघ्रमेव तु इति चतुर्थषष्ठपुस्तकयोः पाठः ।
3. जातीकाद्यं इति आदर्शपुस्तकेषु पाठः ।

"नक्तमालस्य पत्राणि[1] तरुणानि फलानि च ।
सुमनायाश्च पत्राणि पटोलारिष्टयोस्तथा[2] ॥१६६॥
द्वे हरिद्रे मधूच्छिष्टं[3] मधुकं तिक्तरोहिणी ।
मञ्जिष्ठा[4] चन्दनोशीरमुत्पलं[5] सारिवे[6] त्रिवृत्[7] ॥१६७॥
एतेषां कार्षिकैर्भागैर्घृत[8]प्रस्थं विपाचयेत् ।
दुष्टव्रणप्रशमनं तथा नाडीविशोधनम् ।
सद्यश्छिन्नव्रणानाञ्च करञ्जाद्यमिदं शुभम्[9] ॥१६८॥
॥ करञ्जाद्यं घृतम् ॥"

[भैषज्यरत्नावली : व्रणशोथाधिकार : ७४-७६]

Karañjādya Ghṛta

One *prastha* of ghee should be cooked by adding one *karṣa* of each of *nakta māla* (leaves and tender fruits), *sumanā* (leaves), *paṭola* (leaves), *ariṣṭa* (leaves), *haridrā*, *dāru haridrā*, *madhūcchiṣṭa*, *madhuka*, *tikta rohiṇī*, *mañjiṣṭhā*, *candana*, *uśīra*, *utpala*, *kṛṣṇa sārivā*, *śveta sārivā* and *trivṛt*. This medicated

1. पणसिराणि इति षष्ठपुस्तके पाठः ।
2. पटोलारिष्टके तथ इति ग्राकरे पाठः ।
3. मधुछिष्टं इति षष्ठपुस्तके पाठः ।
4. मंजिष्णा इति षष्ठपुस्तके पाठः ।
5. ०शीरमूम्पल इति षष्ठपुस्तके पाठः ।
6. सारिंचे इति षष्ठपुस्तके पाठः ।
7. भृष्टता इति षष्ठपुस्तके पाठः ।
8. ०र्भागोघृत० इति षष्ठपुस्तके पाठः ।
9. स्मृतम इति षष्ठपुस्तके पाठः ।

ghee called *karañjādya ghṛta* relieves putrified ulcer, cleanses sinus and is useful for fresh cut-wounds.

"प्रपौण्डरीक[1]मञ्जिष्ठामधुकोशीरपद्मकैः ।
सहरिद्रैः कृतं[2] सर्पिः सक्षीरं व्रणरोपणम् ॥१६९॥
॥ प्रपौण्डरीकाद्यं घृतम् ॥"
[भैषज्यरत्नावली : व्रणशोथाधिकार : ७८]

Prapauṇḍarīkādya Ghṛta

Ghee cooked with *prapauṇḍarīka*, *mañjiṣṭhā*, *madhuka*, *uśīra*, *padmaka*, *haridrā* and milk helps in the healing of ulcers.

"तिक्तासिक्थनिशायष्टी[3]नक्ताह्वफलपल्लवैः ।
पटोलमालतीनिम्बपत्रैर्व्रण्यं[4] घृतं स्मृतम्[5] ॥१७०॥"
॥ तिक्ताद्यं घृतम् ॥
[भैषज्यरत्नावली : व्रणशोथाधिकार : ७७]

Tiktādya Ghṛta

Ghee cooked with *tiktā*, *siktha*, *niśā*, *yaṣṭī*, *naktāhva* (fruits and leaves), *paṭola*, *mālatī* and *nimba* (leaves) is useful for the treatment of ulcers.

---

1. प्रपौण्डरीक इति आदर्शपुस्तकेषु पाठः ।
2. शृतं इति आकरे पाठः ।
3. ०यष्टि० इति आकरे पाठः ।
4. क. ०पत्रैर्व्रण्यघृं: इति द्वितीयपुस्तके पाठः ।
   ख. पत्रैर्हन्ति व्रणं घृतम् इति आकरे पाठः ।
5. स्मृताम् इति चतुर्थपुस्तके पाठः ।

सिन्दूरकष्ठविषहिंगुरसोनचित्रा-
बालांघ्रिलाङ्गलिककल्कविपक्वतैलम्[1] ।
प्रसादमन्त्रयुतहूंकृत[2]तनु[3]न्नफेनः[4]
क्लिन्नव्रणप्रशमनो[5] विपरीतमल्लः ॥१७१॥
खड्गाभिघातगुरुगण्डमहोपदंश-
नाडीव्रणव्रणविचर्चिककुष्ठपामाः[6] ।
एतान्निहन्ति विपरीतकमल्लनाम
तैलं यथेष्टशयनासन[7]भोजनस्य ॥१७२॥
॥ विपरीतमल्लतैलम् ॥"

[भैषज्यरत्नावली : व्रणशोथाधिकार : ६२-६३]

Viparita Malla Taīla

Oil cooked with the paste of *sinddūra*, *kuṣṭha*, *viṣa*, *hiṅgu*, *rasona*, *citrā*, root of *bālā* and *lāṅgalika* and impregnated with auspicious incantations [?] cures ulcers containing sticky matter, ulcers caused by a sword, serious type of *gala gaṇḍa* (goitre). *upadaṃśa* (syphilis), sinus, eczema, *kuṣṭha* (obstinate skin diseases including leprosy) and *pāmā* (scabies). This is called *viparīta malla taila.* The patient using this recipe can have sleep, postures and food as he likes.

---

1. ०बालाङ्० इति ग्राकरे पाठः ।
2. ०फूत्कृत० इति ग्राकरे पाठः ।
3. नु इति द्वितीयपुस्तके पाठः ।
4. फेनं इति ग्राकरे पाठः ।
5. ०प्रशमने इति ग्राकरे पाठः ।
6. कुष्ठहारी इति षष्ठपुस्तके पाठः ।
7. ०नाशन० इति ग्रादर्शपुस्तकेषु पाठः ।

"कुठारकात् पलशतं क्वाथयेन्नल्वणेऽम्भसि[1] ।
तेन पादावशेषेण तैलप्रस्थं विपाचयेत् ॥१७३॥
कल्कैः कुठारापामार्गप्रोष्ठिकामक्षिकासु[2] च ।
एतदङ्गारकं तैलं व्रणशोधनरोपणम् ।
नाडीषु परमाभ्यङ्गो[3] निजास्वागन्तुकीषु[4] च ॥१७४॥"

॥ अङ्गारकतैलम्[5] ॥

[भैषज्यरत्नावली : व्रणशोथाधिकार : ७९-८०]

Aṅgāraka Taila

One hundred *palas* of *kuṭhāraka* should be boiled with one *nalvaṇa* of water till one fourth remains. With this decoction, one *prastha* of oil should be cooked by adding the paste of *kuṭhāraka*, *apāmārga*, *proṣṭhikā* and *makṣikā*. This is called *aṅgāraka taila*. Application of this oil helps in the cleansing and healing of both the exogenous and endogenous types of ulcers and sinus.

"प्रपौण्डरीकं मधुकं काकोल्यौ[6] द्वे सचन्दने[7] ।

---

1. ०क्वाथेल्लल्वणे० इति प्रथमपुस्तके पाठः ।
2. ०मक्षिकायुतैः इति आकरे पाठः ।
3. परमाभ्यङ्गी इति आकरे पाठः ।
4. निजारवागन्तुकीसु इति प्रथमपुस्तके पाठः ।
5. अङ्गाकरकं तैलं इति प्रथमपुस्तके पाठः ।
6. काकोल्ये इति पंचमपुस्तके पाठः ।
7. सचन्दनम् इति चतुर्थषष्ठपुस्तकयोः पाठः ।

सिद्धमेतैः[1] समैस्तैलं[2] तत्परं[3] व्रणरोपणम् ॥१७५॥"

॥ प्रपौंडरीकाद्यं[4] तैलं ॥"

[भारतभैषज्यरत्नाकर : तृतीयोभाग : पृष्ठ ३७२]

Prapauṇḍarīkādya Taila

Oil cooked with *prapauṇḍarīka, madhuka, kākolī, kṣīra kākolī, śveta candana* and *rakta candana* is an excellent healer of ulcers.

"दूर्वास्वरससिद्धं वा तैलं कम्पिल्लकेन च[5] ।
दार्वीत्वचश्च कल्केन प्रधानं व्रणरोपणम् ॥१७६॥
येनैव विधिना तैलं घृतं तेनैव साधयेत् ।
रक्तपित्तोत्तरं ज्ञात्वा सर्पिरेवावचारयेत् ॥१७७॥

॥ दूर्वाद्यं तैलं घृतञ्च ॥"

[भैषज्यरत्नावली : व्रणशोथाधिकार : ७२-७३]

Dūrvādya Taila and Dūrvādya Ghṛta

Oil cooked with the juice of *dūrvā, kampillaka* and the paste of the bark of *dāru haridrā* is an excellent healer of ulcer. In the above mentioned recipe, ghee can be used in the place of oil. This medicated ghee is more useful for ulcers dominated by vitiated blood and aggravated *pitta*.

---

1. सिद्धमेभिः इति आकरे पाठः ।
2. समं तैलं इति आकरे पाठः ।
3. भत्परं इति प्रथमपुस्तके पाठः ।
4. पठोऽयं प्रथमपंचमपुस्तकयोः नोपलभ्यते ।
5. वा इति आदर्शपुस्तकेषु पाठः ।

"मञ्जिष्ठां चंदनं मूर्वां पिष्ट्वा सर्पिर्विपाचयेत् ।

सर्वेषामग्निदग्धानामेतद्रोपणमिष्यते[1] ॥१७८॥

॥ मञ्जिष्ठाद्यं घृतम् ॥

[भारतभैषज्यरत्नाकर : चतुर्थभाग : पृष्ठ ६३]

Mañjiṣṭhādya Ghṛta

Ghee cooked with the paste of *mañjiṣṭhā*, *candana* and *mūrvā* cures all types of ulcers caused by burns.

"सिद्धं कल्ककषायाभ्यां पाटल्या:[2] कटुतैलकम् ।

दग्धव्रण[3]रुजास्रावदाह[4]विस्फोटनाशनम् ॥१७९॥

॥ पाटलातैलम्[5] ॥

[योगरत्नाकर : अग्निदग्धचिकित्सा : पृष्ठ १८७]

Pāṭalā Taila

Mustard oil cooked with the paste and decoction of *pāṭalā* cures pain of burn-ulcers, exudations, burning sensation and pustules.

---

1. मेतेद्रो० इति पंचमपुस्तके पाठ: ।
2. पटोल्या: इति आकरे पाठ: ।
3. दग्धयणुरुजा० इति प्रथमपुस्तके पाठ: ।
4. ०दाहरुविस्फोटकनाशनम् इति षष्ठपुतके पाठ: ।
5. क. कपटोलींतैलम् इति आकरे पाठ: ।
   ख. पाटलीतैलम इति चतुर्थपुस्तके पाठ: ।
   ग. पाटलितैलम् इति षष्ठपुस्तके पाठ: ।

"चन्दनं वटशुङ्गाश्च मञ्जिष्ठां[1] मधुकं तथा ।
प्रपौण्डरीकं दूर्वां च पतङ्गं धातकी[2] तथा ॥१८०॥
एभिस्तैलं[3] विपक्तव्यं सर्पिः[4] क्षीरसमायुतम् ।
अग्निदग्धव्रणे श्रेष्ठं तत्क्षणाद्रोपणं परम् ॥१८१॥
॥ चन्दनाद्यं यमकम् ॥"

[योगरत्नाकर : अग्निदग्धचिकित्सा : पृष्ठ १८७]

Candanādya Yamaka

Oil and ghee together should be cooked along with the paste of *candana*, adventitious roots of *vaṭa*, *mañjiṣṭhā*, *madhuka*, *prapauṇḍarīka*, *pataṅga* and *dhātakī*. This recipe is excellent for ulcers caused by burns which are instantaneously healed.

"मनःशिलाले[5] मञ्जिष्ठा सलाक्षा रजनीद्वयम् ।
प्रलेपः सघृतक्षौद्रस्त्वचः[6] शुद्धिकरः परः ॥१८२॥"

[भैषज्यरत्नावली : सद्योव्रणाधिकार : १६]

Recipes for Correcting Skin Colour

Application of the paste of *manaḥ śilā*, *āla*, *mañjiṣṭhā*, *lākṣā*, *haridrā* and *dāru haridrā* along with ghee and honey corrects the deformities of the skin.

---

1. मञ्जिष्ठा इति आकरे पाठः ।
2. धातकाम् इति प्रथमपुस्तके पाठः ।
3. एतैस्तैलम् इति आकरे पाठः ।
4. गोक्षीरेण समायुतम् इति आकरे पाठः ।
5. मनः शिला समञ्जिष्ठा इति आकरे पाठः ।
6. ०क्षौद्रस्त्वचः सावर्ण्यकृत्परः इति आकरे पाठः ।

अयोरजः सकासीसं[1] त्रिफलाकुसुमानि[2] च ।
प्रलेपः कुरुते काश्न्यं[3] सद्य एव न त्व[4] व चि [?] ॥१८३॥

Application of the paste of *lauha bhasma*, *kāsīsa*, *triphalā* and *jāti puṣpa* makes the discoloured skin black immediately.

कालीयकेन[5] वाम्रास्थिहेमकालारसोत्तमैः ।
लेप सगोमयरसः[6] सवर्णकरणः परः ॥१८४॥

Application of the paste of *kāliyaka*, seed pulp of *āmra*, *hema kālā* [?] and mercury prepared by triturating with the juice of cowdung is excellent for bringing out the appropriate colour of the skin.

चतुष्पदांघ्रित्वग्रोम[7]खुरशृंगास्थिभस्मक ।
तैलाक्ता[8] चूर्णिता भूमिर्भवेद्रोमवती[9] पुनः ॥१८५॥

The ash of the legs, skin, hair, hooves, horn and bone of the cow should be applied along with oil over the baldness caused by a healed ulcer. It causes hair to grow over it.

---

1. सकाशीशम् इति प्रथमपुस्तके पाठः ।
2. ०कुसुमांश्च इति पंचमपुस्तके पाठः ।
3. काश्यें इति षष्ठपुस्तके पाठः ।
4. चल्त्रवचि इति षष्ठपुस्तके पाठः ।
5. कालियकः लताम्रास्थिकालाहेम० इति षष्ठपुस्तके पाठः ।
6. सशोमयरसः इति षष्ठपुस्तके पाठः ।
7. घ्रित्वसोकरणश्रीमयूरश्रृंगा० इति षष्ठपुस्तके पाठः ।
8. तैलाक्तो इति षष्ठपुस्तके पाठः ।
9. ०द्रोमव्रवी इति षष्ठपुस्तके पाठः ।

व्रणग्रंथिं ग्रन्थिवच्च[1] जयेत् क्षारेण[2] वा भिषक् ॥१८६॥

If there are nodules over a healed ulcer, then such nodules are to be treated on the line prescribed for *granthis* (small tumour) Application of *kṣāra* (alkali preparation) is useful in this condition.

"भग्नं[3] समासाद्[4] द्विविधं हुताश-
काण्डे च संधौ[5] वापि[6] तत्र संधौ ।
उत्पिष्टविश्लिष्टविवर्तितं च
तिर्यक्प्रतिक्षिप्तमधश्च[7] षोडा[8] ॥१८७॥

Fractures and Dislocations

Bhagna (fracture and dislocation) is of two types, viz. *kāṇḍa bhagna* (fracture in the shaft of the bone) and *sandhi*

---

1. ग्रंथिवच्च इति चतुर्थषष्ठपुस्तकयोः पाठः ।
2. क्षाण वा इति षष्ठपुस्तके पाठः ।
3. 'कपिलपारार्हिगुलहरितालग्रर्कमूलत्वक् सर्वं सममागं विधाय संचूर्ण्य शरावसम्पुटस्थानामेषां मात्रात्ताक्रमज्ञाते सतिनलिकयां धूमो व्रण-मुखे देयः । अनेन विधिना वातव्याधिग्रन्थिस्फुनिगे फिरंगवाते क्षतेषु हितो भवति पथ्यं तु लवणाम्लंवर्ज्यम् । धूरीशृंगकपिला-पारागंधकमुडदारसींगकपीला द्विगुणघृतेन पुत्त्या सर्वं संमर्द्य नाडी-व्रण दौलापयात् । अवश्यं व्रणशुष्को भवति । मलम । दहेत्यु नोलकतंणुलियौ तुन्दुल्या शकौ तत्र भवेन्मषीयात्त्ल्वुरि तारो हिति-रिष्ट नाडी इष्टो व्रणा वा चीरकालश्च राजमार्तंडात् ।' पाठोऽयं चतुर्थषष्ठपुस्तकयोः अधिकमुपलभ्यते ।
4. क. समासां द्विविधं इति पंचमपुस्तके पाठः ।
   ख. समासाद् द्विविधं इति आकरे पाठः ।
5. संधा इति प्रथमपुस्तके पाठः ।
6. च हि इति आकरे पाठः ।
7. तिर्यग्गतिः क्षिप्त० इति आदर्शपुस्तकेषु पाठः ।
8. षोढात् इति प्रथमपुस्तके पाठः ।

bhagna (fracture and dislocation of bones in a joint). The latter is of six types, viz. *utpiṣṭa* (crushed), *viślīṣṭa* (torn of ligaments), *vivartita* (twisted), *tiryak gata* (sideward dislocation), *prati kṣipta* (upward dislocation) and *adhaḥ kṣipta* (downward dislocation).

प्रसारणाकुञ्चनर्वनोग्रा [?]

रुक्[1] स्पर्शविद्वेषणमेतदुक्तम् ।

[2] सामान्यतः संधिगतस्य लिंग-

मुत्पिष्टसन्धेः श्वयथु[3] समन्तात् ॥१८८॥

विशेषतो रात्रिभवा रुजश्च

विश्लिष्टजे[4] तौ च रुजा च नित्यम् ।

[5] विर्वातिते पार्श्वरुजश्च तीव्रा-

स्तिर्यग्गते तीव्ररुजो भवन्ति ।

---

1. रुक्पार्श्व० इति आदर्शपुस्तकेषु पाठः ।
2. 'आगंतु सामान्याद्भग्नमाहकांडशब्देन । नलककपालवलय तरुण-रुचकानां ग्रहणम् । द्वयोरस्थनः संधानं संधिस्तद्विश्लेषणः संधिभग्नं तत्रेति । तत्र तयोर्मध्ये संधौ मुक्ते लिंगमुच्यते न नु संधिमुक्तं कथं भग्नमुच्यते । अस्न्थां भंगो भग्नं युक्त उच्चते । अस्थिवि-श्लेषोऽत्र न भंगो ऽभिप्रेतः । स च कांडे भग्ने विमुक्ते चालीति न दोषः ।' पाठोऽयं चतुर्थषष्ठपुस्तकयोः अधिकमुपलभ्यते ।
3. स्वथुः य इति प्रथमपुस्तके पाठः
4. विश्लिष्टसंधौ हि रुजा इति प्रथमपुस्तके पाठः ।
5. क. विवर्न्तिते इति प्रथमपुस्तके पाठः ।
   ख. विर्वाजिते इति षष्ठपुस्तके पाठः ।

क्षिप्तेऽतिशूलं विषमा[1] रुजश्च

क्षिप्ते त्वधो[2]रुग्विघटेश्च संधेः ॥१८६॥

Characteristic Features

Extension, contraction, rotation, pain and tenderness—these are the general characteristic features of all types of *sandhi bhagna* (joint fracture). In *utpiṣṭa sandhi* (crushed joint), there will be oedema in all sides and pain specially at night. In *viśliṣṭa sandhi* (torn joint), the above mentioned signs and symptoms along with constant pain are manifested. In *vivartita sandhi* (twisted joint) there will be pain in the sides of the joint. Sideward dislocation (*tiryak gata*) is characterised by excruciating pain. In *kṣipta* (upward dislocation), there will be excessive stabbing and irregular type of pain. In *adhaḥ kṣipta* (downward dislocation) there will be different types of pain.

काण्डे[3] त्वधः कर्कटका[4]श्च कर्ण-

विचूर्णितं पिच्चितम[5]स्थितं च ।

1. विषमं च सक्थनो क्षिप्ते इति आकरे पाठः ।
2. क. रुग्विघटश्च इति आकरे पाठः ।
   ख. त्वधौरुग्विघटैश्च इति षष्ठपुस्तके पाठः ।
3. क. पाठोऽयं आदर्शपुस्तकेषु नोपलभ्यते ।
   ख. उत्पिष्टनामच्चम्यामस्थिभ्यां संधिघर्षण तथा भूतस्य संधे परितः शोथः विश्लिष्टं नाम मनाक संधि विश्लेषः शिथिलमात्रां विवर्त्तितं नाम संधौ द्वयोरस्थ्नोर्विवृत्ते भ्रमणमार्ज्जवं नैति संध्यस्थोः पार्श्वगमनातीव्राः पार्श्व पीडाः । तिर्यगातं नाम पदेकं सांध्यस्थि संधिस्थानं त्पत्कात्तिर्यग्यात्यपरं स्वस्थानं स्थानादिति । क्षिप्तेऽपि शूलमिति । अति शबदः क्षिप्तात्पूर्वं योज्यः तेन अति क्षिप्ते उर्ध्वमिति शेषः । विषमाद्वत्पत्ररुज इत्यध्याहार्य्यं किंचिदधः क्षिप्तेऽधोऽस्थिगमनं व विधर्यविश्लेषः अतः परं काडभग्नमभिधीयते । सर्वस्थिकांडभग्नस्य चिन्हमाहास्रस्तेति कांडेश्त्वतः ।
4. कक्कंटाख इति प्रथमपुस्तके पाठः ।
5. क. पिच्चितमस्थिछल्लिका इति प्रथमपुस्तके पाठः ।
   ख, पिंडितमछल्लिकां इति षष्ठपुस्तके पाठः ।

काण्डेषु भग्नं[1] ह्यतिपातितं च
मज्जागतं च स्फुटितं च वक्रम् ॥१६०॥

[This verse has many errors and the meaning is not clear].

छिन्नं द्विधा द्वादशधा च काण्डे
स्रस्ताङ्गता शोथरुजातिवृद्धिः[2] ।
सम्पीड्यमाने भवतीह शब्दः
स्पर्शासहस्पन्दनतोदशूलाः ॥१६१॥
सर्वास्ववस्थासु न शर्मलाभो[3]
भग्नस्य काण्डे खलु चिह्नमेतत् ।
भग्नं तु काण्डे बहुधा प्रयाति
समासतो नामभिरेव तुल्यम् ॥१६२॥

Chinna (fracture with separation) of the *kāṇḍa* (shaft of the bone) is of two types or twelve types and it is characterised by prostration, oedema, excessive increase in pain, sound production by pressure, tenderness, cramps and pinching pain. In *bhagna* (fracture) the patient does not get peace in any situation. Fracture of the shaft of the bone is of several types and they have similar names.

---

1. क. कांडेषु भिन्नं इति प्रथमपुस्तके पाठः ।
   ख. कांडेषुभग्नंप्यति इति षष्ठपुस्तके पाठः ।
2. शोफरुजा च वृद्धिः इति प्रथमपुस्तके पाठः ।
3. सर्म्मलाभो इति प्रथमपुस्तके पाठः ।

अल्पाशिनोऽनात्मवतो[1] जन्तोर्वातात्मकस्य च ।
उपद्रवैर्वा जुष्टस्य[2] भग्नं कृच्छ्रेण सिध्यति[3] ॥१९३॥

Prognosis

If the patient is unable to take enough of food, if he does not have will-power, if *vāyu* is aggravated and if there are many complications, then such a patient suffering from fracture of bone can be cured with dfficulty.

भिन्नं कपालं कट्यां तु सन्धिमुक्तं तथा च्युतम् ।
जघनं प्रतिपिष्टं च[4] वर्जयेत्[5] च विचक्षणः ॥१९४॥

A wise physician should avoid treatment of fracture of skull or lumber region specially when the joint is separated or displaced. He should also avoid treatment if the bones of the leg are completely crushed.

असंश्लिष्टं कपालं च लालाटे[6] चूर्णितं च यत् ।
भग्नं स्तनान्तरे[7] शङ्खे पृष्ठे मूर्ध्नि विवर्ज्जयेत्[8] ॥१९५॥

If the skull-bone is separated, if the bone of the forehead is reduced to powder form and if fracture has taken place in bet-

---

1. नात्म च तो जतो० इति प्रथमपुस्तके पाठः ।
2. जुष्टं इति आदर्शपुस्तकेषु पाठः ।
3. सिद्धयति इति प्रथमपुस्तके पाठः ।
4. तु इति आकरे पाठः ।
5. वर्जयेच्च विचक्षणः इति आकरे पाठः ।
6. ललाटम् इति आदर्शपुस्तकेषु पाठः ।
7. क. स्तनगुदे इति प्रथमपुस्तके पाठः ।
   ख. नेत्रे गुडेशंखे इति षष्ठपुस्तके पाठः ।
8. च वर्जयेत् इति आकरे पाठः ।

ween the breasts, temporal region, back or chest, then such patients should not be treated.

सम्यक्संधि[1]तमप्यस्थि दुर्निक्षे[2]पनिबन्धनात् ।
संक्षोभाद्वाऽपि यद्गच्छेद्विक्रियां तच्च वर्जयेत् ॥१९६॥

It the bone comes out or gets irregularly aligned because of pressure after the fracture is well set, then the patient should not be treated.

तरुणास्थीनि नम्यन्ते[3] भिद्यन्ते[4] नलकानि तु ।
कपालास्थीनि[5] भज्यन्ते स्फुटन्ति रुचकानि च ॥१९७॥"

[योगरत्नाकर : भग्नव्रणनिदानः पृष्ठ १८८-१९०]

॥ इति भग्ननिदानम्[6] ॥१९८॥

Generally, cartilages get bent, long bones get broken, flat bones get cracked and small bones get scrapped.

Thus, ends the description of the diagnosis of different types of fracture.

"आदौ भग्नं विदित्वा च[7] सेचयेत् शीतवारिणा ।
पङ्केनालेपनं कार्यं बन्धनञ्च कुशान्वितम् ॥१९९॥"

[भैषज्यरत्नावली : भग्नाधिकार : १]

[योगरत्नाकर : भग्नचिकित्सा : पृष्ठ १९०]

---

1. सम्यक्संहितमप्यस्थि इति आकरे पाठः ।
2. दुर्न्निक्षप इति प्रथमपुस्तके पाठः ।
3. नाम्यन्ते इति आकरे पाठः ।
4. भज्यन्ते इति चतुर्थपुस्तके पाठः ।
5. कपोलास्थीनि विभय्यन्ते इति चतुर्थषष्ठपुस्तकयोः पाठः ।
6. पाठोऽयं प्रथमपंचमपुस्तकयोः नोपलभ्यते ।
7. तु सेचयेच्छीतलाम्बुनी इति आकरे पाठः ।

Management of Fracture

After ascertaining the nature of the fracture, the physician should sprinkle the affected area with cold water, apply cold-mud over it and bandage it after applying the splint (*kuśa*).

"[1]भग्नाद्यर्थसाधने पलाशादित्वग्मपि ग्राह्यः ॥२००॥

For correcting the fractured bone, the bark of *palāśa*, etc. may also be used.

उक्तं च सुश्रुते—

पलाशोदुम्बराश्वत्थकदम्बनिचुलत्वचः ।

वंशसर्जवटानां च कुशार्थमुपसंहरेत् ॥२०१॥"

[सुश्रुत : चिकित्सा ३ : ६]

According to Suśruta

For the purpose of splint (*kuśa*), the bark of *palāśa*, *udumbara*, *aśvattha*, *kadamba*, *nicula*, *vaṃśa*, *sarja* or *vaṭa* may be used.

वधमोक्षयोः विधिः सुश्रुते दर्शितम् ।

पदसो(पदस्यो)परिवध्नीयान्नगाढं शिथिलं न च ॥२०२॥

"सप्ताहादथ सप्ताहात् सौम्येष्वृतुषु बन्धनम् ।

साधारणेषु कर्त्तव्यं पंचमे पंचमेऽहनि ।

आग्नेयेषु त्र्यहात् कुर्याद्भग्नदोषवशेन वा[2] ॥२०३॥"

[सुश्रुत : चिकित्सा ३ : ८-९]

1. 'भग्नाद्यर्थ———वा' पाठोऽयं प्रथमपुस्तके नोपलभ्यते ।
2. तथेति इति चतुर्थषष्ठपुस्तकयोः पाठः ।

Suśruta has described the procedure of bandage and its removal as follows :

On the leg, the bandage should be neither too tight nor too loose. In the winter, bandage should be applied for a duration of seven days. After it is removed, it can be applied for seven days more if the healing is incomplete. In moderate seasons (which are neither very cold nor very hot), bandage should be applied for a duration of five days. In summer season, bandage should be applied for a duration of three days only. Duration of the bandage shpuld be determined on the basis of the nature of the fracture.

'[1]कुशशब्देन भग्नबन्धनार्थं वंशवेत्रादिकाण्डाः प्रोच्यन्ते ॥२०४॥'

Splint

The term '*kuśa*' used in the verse no. 201 means a splint prepared of bamboo or cane pieces.

"आलेपनार्थं मञ्जिष्ठां मधुकं रक्तचन्दनम् ।
शतधौतघृतोन्मिश्रं शालिपिष्टं च संहरेत्[2] ॥२०५॥"

[सुश्रुत : चिकित्सा ३ : ७]

Over the fracture, the paste of *mañjiṣṭḥā*, *madhuka* and *rakta candana* or the paste of *śāli* rice should be applied along with *śata dhauta ghṛta*.

किंवामलकमंजिष्ठाकंगु[3]पिष्टं निशायुतम् ।
कुक्कुटाण्डद्रवो[4]पेतं शतधौतघृतान्वितम् ॥२०६॥

---

1. 'कुशशब्देन ——प्रोच्यन्ते' पाठोऽयं आदर्शपुस्तकेषु अधिकमुपलभ्यते ।
2. लेपनम् इति चतुर्थषष्ठपुस्तकयोः पाठः ।
3. ०कुंग० इति चतुर्थपुस्तके पाठः ।
4. ०रसो इति चतुर्थषष्ठपुस्तकयोः पाठः ।

Alternatively, the paste of *āmalaka*, *mañjiṣṭhā*, *kaṅgu*, *niśā* and the liquid portion of hen's egg should be applied along with *śata dhauta ghṛta*.

"लवणं कटुकक्षारमम्लं मैथुनमातपम् ।
व्यायामञ्च न सेवेत भग्नो[1] रूक्षान्नमेव च ॥२०७॥"

[भैषज्यरत्नावली : भग्नाधिकार : ३५]

Diet and Regimens

The patient of bone-fracture should avoid salt, pungent, *kṣāra* (alkali preparation) as well as sour ingredients of food, sexual intercourse, exposure to sun, physical exercise and unctuous food.

अस्थिसंहारकल्कं वा मर्दयेत्[2]ससितासमम् ।
कृत्वा पूपलिकां[3] खादेत्सद्यो संधानमिच्छता ॥२०८॥

If the patient desires to have instantaneous healing, then he should take *pupalikā* (a type of cake) prepared by adding the paste of *asthi samhāra* and equal quantity of sugar.

शालिमांसरसः क्षीरं सर्पिर्यूषः सतीनजः ।
बृंहणं चान्नपानं स्याद्देयं भग्नाय जानता[4] ॥२०९॥
स्मृत्यौजः[5] स्वरहीनानां ज्वरक्षीणक्षतौजसाम् ।

1. क. भग्ने इति प्रथमपुस्तके पाठः ।
   ख. भग्नो चुक्षान्नमेव च इति षष्ठपुस्तके पाठः ।
2. वामर्दयेच्च सतासमम् इति चतुर्थषष्ठपुस्तकयोः पाठः ।
3. वाष्टपिकां इति षष्ठपुस्तके पाठः ।
4. भग्नायजानताम् इति षष्ठपुस्तके पाठः ।
5. स्मृभ्यौजः इति षष्ठपुस्तके पाठः ।

भग्नविश्लिष्टसंधीनां कृशानामल्परेतसाम् ।
आप्पायनः[1] संहननः स्मृतोमांसरसः परम् ॥२१०॥

Wholesome Diet

The patient of bone-fracture should take *śāli* type of rice meat soup, milk, ghee, soup prepared of *satīna* and such other nourishing diet and drinks. Meat-soup provides nourishment and compactness to patients having reduced memory, *ojas* (vitality) and voice, to patients suffering from fever, emaciation and consumption, to patients having fracture or dislocation of joints and to patients suffering from weakness as well as seminal debility.

तत्रातिशिथिले[2] बंधे[3] संधिस्थैर्यं[4] न जायते ।
गाढेनापि त्वगादीनां शोफो रुक् पाक एव च[5] ।
तस्मात् साधारणं[6] बन्धं भग्ने शंसन्ति तद्विदः[7] ॥२११॥

Bandage

If the bandage is applied too loose, then there will be no stability (immobility) of joints and the fractured region. If it is too tight, then there will be oedema in the skin, pain and suppuration. Therefore, bandage should be tied with moderate pressure.

---

1. अप्पायनः इति षष्ठपुस्तके पाठः ।
2. क. शिथिलं इति आकरे पाठः ।
   ख. तत्रापि इति षष्ठपुस्तके पाठः ।
3. बद्धे इति आकरे पाठः ।
4. संधिस्थर्यं इति षष्ठपुस्तके पाठः ।
5. रुक्पाकमाप्नुयात् इति चतुर्थषष्ठपुस्तकयोः पाठः ।
6. साधारणे इति षष्ठपुस्तके पाठः ।
7. क. संशीततद्विद्यः इति प्रथमपुस्तके पाठः ।
   ख. शंसंतत द्विधा इति षष्ठपुस्तके पाठः ।

न्यग्रोधादि[1] कषायं तु सुशीतं परिषेचने[2] ।
पञ्चमूलीविपक्वं तु क्षीरं कुर्यात् सवेदने ॥२१२॥"
लघु[3]पंचमूलीशीतवीर्यत्वात् ॥२१३॥

Excessively cooled decoction of drugs belonging to *nyagrodhādi gaṇa* should be used for sprinkling. If there is pain, then the area should be sprinkled with milk boiled by adding *laghu pañca mūla* because these drugs are cold in potency.

सुखोष्णमवचार्यं वा[4] चक्रतैलं विजानता ।
विभज्यकालं दोषं च दोषघ्नौषधसंयुतम् ।
परिषेकं प्रलेपं[5] च विदध्याच्छीतमेव च ॥२१४॥"

[सुश्रुत : चिकित्सा ३ : ८-१३]

चकाराद्दोषापेक्षया[6] उष्णमपि ॥२१५॥

Over the fractured region, luke-warm *cakra taila* can be applied. Depending upon the season and the nature of *doṣas* involved, sprinkling and paste application should be done with such drugs as would alleviate the aggravated *doṣas*. Such recipes should generally be cooling, but depending upon the nature of the *doṣas uṣṇa* (heating) recipes can also be applied over the fracture.

---

1. न्यग्रोधोदि इति चतुर्थपुस्तके पाठः ।
2. परिषेचनम् इति पंचमपुस्तके पाठः ।
3. पाठोऽयं आकरे नोपलभ्यते ।
4. व चक्रतैलम् इति आदर्शपुस्तकेषु पाठः ।
5. प्रदेह इति आकरे पाठः ।
6. 'चकारा०———उष्णमपि' पाठोऽयं आकरे नोपलभ्यते ।

"गृष्टिक्षीरं सर्पिष्कं मधुरौषधसाधितम् ।
शीतलं लाक्षया युक्तं प्रातर्भग्नः पिबेन्नरः ॥२१६॥"

[सुश्रुतः चिकित्सा ३ : १३-१४]

Gṛṣṭi kṣīra (milk of the cow after first delivery) should be boiled with ghee and drugs belonging to *madhura gaṇa* (sweet drugs), cooled and taken in the morning along with *lākṣā* by the person suffering from fracture.

दाह[1]पीडादियुक्तोऽपि नादौ रक्तं विनिर्हरेत् ।
रक्ताधीनं हि संधानं तस्माद्रक्षे[2]त्प्रयत्नतः ॥२१७॥

The patient having fracture should not be given blood-letting therapy even if he is having burning sensation and pain because the process of healing is dependant upon blood. Therefore, blood should be preserved in the body with utmost care.

कृष्णात्रेयः—

भिषक्[3] सप्तदिनादूर्ध्वं दा[4]हशोफरुजान्वितम् ।
ग्रंथिलं निर्ह[5]रेद्रक्तं यथा दोषं विधानतः ।
स्थितं चैकत्रविज्ञाय नान्यथासृग्विमोक्षयेत् ॥२१८॥

According to Kṛṣṇātreya

If the patient having fracture suffers from burning sensation,

---

1. दारुपीडादि० इति षष्ठपुस्तके पाठः ।
2. तस्मादुक्तेत्प्रयत्नत: इति षष्ठपुस्तके पाठः ।
3. भिषह्युप्त० इति षष्ठपुस्तके पाठः ।
4. दारुहशोफ० इति षष्ठपुस्तके पाठ: ।
5. क. निर्व्जणद्रक्तं इति षष्ठपुस्तके पाठः ।
   ख. निनणं चैव इति चतुर्थपुस्तके पाठः ।

oedema and pain, the physician should administer blood-letting therapy to him to remove the knotted blood only after seven days. For this purpose, the procedure prescribed for blood-letting therapy to eliminate different *doṣas* should be followed. Before administering blood-letting therapy it should be ensured that blood is already accumulated in one place. Otherwise, blood-letting therapy should not be given.

"सव्रणस्य तु भग्नस्य व्रणं सर्पिर्मधूत्तरः[1] ।
प्रतिसार्यं कषायैस्तु शेषं भग्नवदाचरेत्[2] ॥२१९॥
॥ क्षारवर्जम्[3] ॥२२०॥

Open Fracture

If there is an ulcer over the fracture, then it should be anointed with ghee and honey and washed with decoctions. Remaining therapies as indicated for fracture, should then be administered. In the case of open fracture, the patient should avoid *kṣāra* (alkali preparations).

'प्रथमे[4] वयसि त्वेवं भग्नं[5] सुकरमादिशेत् ।
अत्यल्पदोषजन्तोस्तु[6] काले तु[7] शिशिरात्मके ॥२२१॥'

Fracture is easily curable, if the patient is young, if the *doṣas* are less aggravated and if the time is autumn.

1. ०घूकजैः इति चतुर्थषष्ठपुस्तकयोः पाठः ।
2. भग्नवदाचरेत् इति आकरे पाठः ।
3. पाठोऽयं आदर्शपुस्तकेषु अधिकमुपलभ्यते ।
4. 'प्रथमे———शिशिरात्मके' पाठोऽयं षष्ठपुस्तके नोपलभ्यते ।
5. भवम् इति प्रथमपुस्तके पाठः ।
6. अल्पदोषस्य जंतोस्तु इति आकरे पाठः ।
7. च इति आकरे पाठः ।

प्रथमे वयसि त्वेवं मासात् सन्धिः स्थिरो भवेत् ।

मध्यमे द्विगुणात् कालादुत्तरे त्रिगुणात् स्मृतः[1] ॥२२२॥

In young age the fracture heals in one month; in middle age it takes double the time and in old age it takes three months to heal.

[2]अवनामितमुन्नह्येदुन्नतं चावपीडयेत् ॥२२३॥

[सुश्रुत : चिकित्सा ३ : १४-१७]

'[3]अधोगतमुन्न[4]भ्योत्थाप्य वध्नीयादिति वाक्यशेषः' ॥२२४॥

While aligning and setting the fracture, the downwardly bone should be elevated and the elevated bone should be pressed downwards. Thereafter, splint and bandage should be applied.

"[5]आञ्च्छेदतिक्षिप्तमधो गतं चोपरि वर्तयेत् ॥२२५॥"

[सुश्रुत : चिकित्सा ३ : १८]

'[6]अतिक्षिप्तं आञ्च्छेद्विशालं कुर्यात् [7]अञ्चिछ व्यायामे इति धातुः ॥२२६॥'

If the bone has moved upwards, then it should be pulled down and if it has gone downward then it should be pulled up.

---

1. गुणास्मृता इति प्रथमपुस्तके पाठः ।
2. अधस्तान्नतमुन्नमं इति आदर्शपुस्तकेषु पाठः ।
3. 'अधो०———वाक्यशेषः' पाठोऽयं आकरे नोपलभ्यते ।
4. ०न्नभ्योच्छाप्यवध्नी इति पंचमपुस्तके पाठः ।
5. आच्छे० इति प्रथमद्वितीयपुस्तकयोः पाठः ।
6. 'अतिक्षिप्तं———धातुः' पाठोऽयं आकरे नोपलभ्यते ।
7. आंच्छि० इति चतुर्थषष्ठपुस्तकयोः पाठः ।

The term '*āñcched*' used in the text is derived from the root '*āñcchi*' which means physical exhertion (*vyāyāma*). By implication, the bone which has gone up should be pulled down with force.

"आञ्च्छनैः पीडनैश्चैव सङ्क्षोभैर्बन्धनैस्तथा[1] ।
सन्ध्यात्[2] शरीरे सर्वांस्तु चलानप्यचलानपि ॥२२७॥"

[सुश्रुत : चिकित्सा ३ : १८-१९]

By pulling downwards, by pressure, by tilting and by bandage, all the mobile and immobile fractured bones of the body should be correctly set.

"एतैस्तु स्थापनोपायैः[3] स्थापयेन्मतिमान् भिषक् ।
उत्पिष्टमथ विश्लिष्टं सन्धिं वैद्यो न चालयेत्[4] ॥२२८॥
तस्य शीतान् परीषेकान् प्रदेहांश्चावचारयेत् ।
अभिघाते हृते सन्धौ[5] स्वां याति प्रकृतिं पुनः ॥२२९॥

With the above mentioned methods, broken bones should be aligned and correctly set. But if these bones are crushed into small pieces or if the joint is dislocated then the physician should not move them. In such cases, cooling liquids should be sprinkled and cooling pastes should be applied. Once the injury is corrected, the bone and the joint will naturally came to their appropriate positions.

---

1. सङ्क्षेपैर्बन्धनैस्तथा इति आकरे पाठः ।
2. क. सन्धीञ्छरीरे इति आकरे पाठः ।
   ख. संध्याशरीरै इति षष्ठपुस्तके पाठः ।
3. एत्वैः सु स्थापनापायैः इति षष्ठपुस्तके पाठः ।
4. घट्टयेत् इति आकरे पाठः ।
5. सन्धिः इति आकरे पाठः ।

घृतदिग्धेन पट्टेन[1] वेष्टयित्वा यथाविधि[2]ः ।
पट्टोपरि कुशान् दत्वा यथावद्बन्धमाचरेत् ॥२३०॥

The bandage-cloth should be smeared with ghee and wrapped around the fracture. Over this cloth, splints should be placed and tied.

विधि[3] प्रत्यङ्गभग्नस्य अतउर्ध्वं प्रवक्ष्यते ॥२३१॥

Hereafter, management of fracture in minor parts of the body will be described.

नखसंधि समुत्पिष्टं रक्तानुगतमारया[4] ॥२३२॥
'नखे आरया[5] मंथनं दुष्टासृग्गमनार्थम्[6] ॥२३३॥'
अवमथ्य स्रुते रक्तशालिपिष्टेन[7] लेपयेत् ॥२३४॥

If the nail joint is crushed, then with the help of the instrument called *ārā*, the area should be rubbed to take out the vitiated blood. After that, the nail should be smeared with the paste of red variety of *śāli* rice.

भग्नां वा सन्धिमुक्तां वा स्थापयित्वांगुलीं[8] समाम् ।

---

1. पिष्टेन इति आदर्शपुस्तकेषु पाठः ।
2. क. यथाविधि इति षष्ठपुस्तके आकरे च पाठः ।
   ख. 'हांश्चा०———यथावि' पाठोऽयं चतुर्थपुस्तके नोपलभ्यते ।
3. प्रत्यङ्गभग्नस्य विधिरत उर्ध्वं प्रवक्ष्यते इति आकरे पाठः ।
4. रक्तानुगतमारये इति षष्ठपुस्तके पाठः ।
5. आरपामंथनम् इति षष्ठपुस्तके पाठः ।
6. 'नखे———दुष्टासृग्गमनार्थम् ' पाठोऽयं आकरे नोपलभ्यते ।
7. रक्ते शालिपिष्टेन इति आकरे पाठः ।
8. स्थापयित्वाऽङ्गुलीं इति आकरे पाठः ।

अणुनाऽऽवेष्ट्य[1] पट्टेन घृतसेकं[2] प्रदापयेत् ॥२३५॥

If the finger bones are either broken of dislocated, then the hand with the fingers spread should be kept over an even surface and wrapped with the help of a fine cloth. Ghee should then be sprinkled over it.

[3]'अभ्यज्य सर्पिषा पादं तलभग्नं कुशोत्तरम् ।
वस्त्रपट्टेन बध्नीयान्न च व्यायाममाचरेत् ॥२३६॥'

If there is a fracture in the sole of the feet, then the area should be given gentle massage with ghee. After applying splint, it should be tied with the help of a bandage and the patient should refrain from the movement of the leg.

अभ्यज्यायामयेज्जङ्घामूरुं[4] च सुसमाहितः ।
दत्वा वृक्षत्वचः शीता वस्त्रपट्टेन वेष्टयेत् ॥२३७॥

If there is fracture of the bones of the leg or the thigh, then massage should be given and the leg should be stretched for proper alignment of bones. Thereafter, cooling barks of trees should be applied around the area and tied with a bandage.

मतिमांश्चक्रयोगेन ह्याञ्छेद्दूर्वस्थि[5] निर्गतम्[6] ।

---

1. आवध्यचैलखंडेन घृतसैकं इति चतुर्थषष्ठपुस्तकयोः पाठः ।
2. घृतशोकम् इति प्रथमपुस्तके पाठः ।
3. 'अभ्यज्य———व्यायाममाचरेत्' पाठोऽयं षष्ठपुस्तके नोपलभ्यते ।
4. क. अभ्यज्ययमकेयं धामूरुं च इति प्रथमपुस्तके पाठः ।
   ख. अभ्यज्ययमकेजंघामुरुं च इति पंचमपुस्तके पाठः ।
5. आंञ्छेदूर्द्धास्थि भिर्गतम् इति षष्ठपुस्तके पाठः ।
6. निर्गताम् इति प्रथमपुस्तके पाठः ।

स्फुटितं पिच्चितं चापि[1] बध्नीयात् पूर्ववद्भिषक् ॥२३८॥

If the thigh bone has come out of the thigh, then the leg should be tied to a wheel and pulled. If it is cracked or crushed, the same procedure should be employed and tied as described in the above verse.

आञ्छेदूर्ध्वमधो वाऽपि कटिभग्नं तु मानवम् ।
ततः स्थानस्थिते[2] संधौ बस्तिभिः समुपाचरेत् ॥२३९॥

If there is a fracture in the lumber region, then it should be pulled upward or downwards depending upon the nature of the fracture, and after the joint is properly set, the patient should be given medicated enema.

पार्शुकास्वस्थिभग्नासु घृताभ्यक्तस्य तिष्ठतः ।
दक्षिणास्वथवा[4] वामास्वनुमृज्य[5] निबन्धनीः ॥२४०॥
ततः कवलिकां दत्वा वेष्टयेत् सुसमाहितः ।
तैलपूर्णे कटाहे वा द्रोण्यां वा शाययेन्नरम्[6] ॥२४१॥

If there is fracture of the rib bones, gentle massage should be given either on the right or the left side [whereever the fracture has taken place] upto the rib and vertibral joint. A blanket should be wrapped over it and carefully tied. Alter-

1. वापि इति प्रथमपुस्तके पाठः ।
2. स्थानास्थिते इति प्रथमपुस्तके पाठः ।
3. पर्शुकास्वथ इति आकरे पाठः ।
4. दक्षिणाश्चथवा इति प्रथमपुस्तके पाठः ।
5. वामासुन्मज्य इति प्रथमपुस्तके पाठः ।
6. क. स्यपयेन्नरः इति प्रथमपुस्तके पाठः ।
ख. स्थापयन्नरः इति चतुर्थषष्ठपुस्तकोः पाठः ।

natively, the patient should be made to sleep in a pan or bath tub filled with oil.

मुसलेनोत्क्षिपेत्[1] कक्षामांससन्धौ विसंहृते ।
स्थानस्थितं[2] च बध्नीयात्[3] स्वस्तिकेन विचक्षणः ॥२४२॥

If there is injury or dislocation of the shoulder joint, then with the pressure of a pestle placed in the axilla, the defect should be set properly and then tied with *svastika* type bandage.

कौर्परं तु तथा सन्धिमङ्गुष्ठेनानुमार्जयेत्[4] ।
मृदित्वा[5] च ततः सन्धिं पीडयेत् कूर्पराच्च्युतम् ॥२४३॥
प्रसार्याकुञ्चयेच्चैनं स्नेहसेकं च कारयेत्[6] ।
एवं जानुनि[7] गुल्फे च मणिबन्धे च कारयेत् ॥२४४॥

If there is dislocation of the elbow joint, then the joint should be gently rubbed with the help of thumb. Then by applying pressure, the dislocated joint should be set right. Then, after expanding, the hand should be contracted and sprinkled with oil or ghee. Similar procedure should be adopted for fracture or dislocation of knee joint, ankle joint and wrist joint.

---

1. मुशलेनोक्षिपेत् इति प्रथमपुस्तके पाठः ।
2. क. अस्थानस्थितम् इति पंचमपुस्तके पाठः ।
   ख. स्थातस्थिनम् इति षष्ठपुस्तके पाठः ।
3. बध्नीत इति प्रथमपुस्तके पाठः ।
4. ०नतुमार्जयेत् इति षष्ठपुस्तके पाठः ।
5. अनुमृज्य इति आकरे पाठः ।
6. दापयेत् इति आकरे पाठः ।
7. क. जाल्वग्रगुल्मे इति प्रथमपुस्तके पाठः ।
   ख, जान्वग्रगुल्फमुत्थे इति षष्ठपुस्तके पाठः ।

उभे तले समे कृत्वा तलभग्नस्य देह्निः[1] ।
बध्नीयादामतैलेन परिषेकं च कारयेत् ॥२४५॥
प्राग्गोमयमयं पिण्डं धारयेन्मृण्मयं[2] ततः ।
हस्ते जातबले[3] वापि कुर्यात् पाषाणधारणम्[4] ।
'शिरां[5] संकुचितां दृष्ट्वा धारयेत्सैन्धवं क्रमात् ॥२४६॥'

If there is fracture in the palm, then both the palms should be brought to the same level and bandaged. *Āma taila* should then be sprinkled over it. To rehabilitate, first of all the patient should be made to carry and squeeze a bolus of cowdung followed by a bolus of earth. After sufficient strength is regained he should be made to hold a stone. If the vessels are contracted, the patient should hold a piece of rock-salt.

सन्नमुन्नमयेत् स्विन्नमक्षकं मुसलेन तु ।
तथोन्नतं पीडयेच्च बध्नीयाद्गाढमेव च ॥२४७॥

If the clavicle is broken, then fomentation should be given and with a pestle, pressure should be applied to elevate the depressed bone. After its elevation both the pieces of bone should be pressed together and tied tightly.

उरुवद्वापि कर्त्तव्यं बाहुभग्नचिकित्सतम् ॥२४८॥

The fracture in the arm should be treated on the line suggested above for thigh-bone fracture.

---

1. देह्णिः इति षष्ठपुस्तके पाठः ।
2. धारयेन्मृरामये ततः इति षष्ठपुस्तके पाठः ।
3. वातवले इति षष्ठपुस्तके पाठः ।
4. धारणी इति षष्ठपुस्तके पाठः ।
5. शिलासंकुचिताम् इति षष्ठपुस्तके पाठः ।

[1]ग्रीवायां तु विवृतायां प्रविष्टायामधोऽपि[2] वा ।
अवटावथ हन्वोश्च प्रगृह्योन्नमयेन्नरम् ॥२४९॥
ततः[3] कुशाः[4] समं दत्त्वा वस्त्रपट्टेन वेष्टयेत् ।
उत्तानं शाययेच्चैनं[5] सप्तरात्रमतन्द्रितः ॥२५०॥

If the neck has come out of its place or depressed inside [because of damage to the cervical vertibrae], it should be set in its place by pulling the thyroid region and jaw bones. Thereafter, splints should be appropriately applied and tied with a bandage. For seven days, the patient should be made to sleep on his back with his chest elevated. This should be done meticulously.

[6]हन्वस्थिनि समानीय हनुसन्धौ विसंहते ।
स्वेदयित्वा स्थितं सम्यक् पञ्चाङ्गीं विभजेद्भिषक्[7] ।
वातघ्नमधुरैः[8] सर्पिः सिद्धं नस्यं च पूजितम् ॥२५१॥

If there is fracture of the jaw bone, both the jaws should be placed in appropriate position and fomented. Thereafter,

1. 'ग्रीवायां ———वेष्टयेत्' पाठोऽयं षष्ठपुस्तके नोपलभ्यते ।
2. प्रभिन्नयामथोऽपि वा इति चतुर्थपुस्तके पाठः ।
3. तथ्याः कुशाः इति प्रथमपुस्तके पाठः ।
4. कुशादिकं दॉवा इति चतुर्थपुस्तके पाठः ।
5. स्वापयेच्चैनम् इति प्रथमपुस्तके पाठः ।
6. हत्वाशृगालमासीय हनुसन्धौ इति चतुर्थपुस्तके पाठः ।
7. विसृजेद्भिषक् इति चतुर्थषष्ठपुस्तकयोः पाठः ।
8. क. वातघ्नममदैः इति चतुर्थपुस्तके पाठः ।
   ख. वातघ्नमगदै इति षष्ठपुस्तके पाठः ।

pañcāṅga type of bandage should be applied. The patient should be given inhalation therapy with the ghee cooked with drugs that alleviate *vāyu* and are sweet in taste (belonging to *madhura gaṇa*).

[1]अभग्नांश्चलितान् दन्तान् सरक्तानवपीडयेत् ।
तरुणस्य मनुष्यस्य शीतै[2]श्चालेपयेद्बहिः ॥२५२॥
सिक्त्वाऽम्बुभिस्ततः शीतैः सन्धानीयैरुपाचरेत् ।
उत्पलस्य च नालेन क्षीरपानं विधीयते ।
जीर्णस्य तु मनुष्यस्य वर्जयेच्चलितान् द्विजान् ॥२५३॥

If because of injury; teeth are not broken but have become loose and bleeding, then pressure should be applied. In a young patient, the paste of cooling drugs should be applied externally. Cold water should be used for washing the affected teeth, and drugs which help in joining two pieces of bones (*sandhānīya*) should be applied over these teeth. He should take milk by sucking through a stem of lotus (pipe). In an old patient, no effort should be made to settle loose teeth i.e. these teeth should be taken out.

नासां भग्नां[3] विवृत्तां च ऋ[4]ज्वीं कृत्वा शलाकया ।
[5]पृथङ्नासिकयोर्नाड्यौ द्विमुख्यौ संप्रवेशयेत् ।
ततः पट्टेन संवेष्ट्य घृतसेकं प्रदापयेत् ॥२५४॥

---

1. क. भग्नीश्चचलितान् इति प्रथमपुस्तके पाठः ।
   खः भग्नांश्चगलितान् इति चतुर्थषष्ठपुस्तकयोः पाठः ।
2. शीलैश्च० इति षष्ठपुस्तके पाठः ।
3. सन्नाम् इति आकरे पाठः ।
4. आज्वीम् इति प्रथमपुस्तके पाठः ।
5. पृथङ्न्यसिकयोर्नाड्यौ द्विमुख्यौ इति प्रथमपुस्तके पाठः ।

If there is fracture of the nasal bone or if the nose has been blown out, then with the help of rod, it should be set in its appropriate place and two tubes with both ends open should be inserted into the nostrils. Thereafter, it should be wrapped with a bandage and sprinkled with ghee.

भग्नं कर्णं तु[1] बध्नीयात् समं कृत्वा घृतप्लुतम्[2] ।
सद्यः क्षतविधानं च ततः पश्चात् समाचरेत् ॥२५५॥

If the cartilage of the ear is broken, then it should be appropriately set in its original shape, smeared with ghee and tied with a bandage. Thereafter, it should be treated as a fresh injury.

मस्तुलुङ्गाद्विना भिन्ने कपाले मधुसर्पिषी ।
दत्त्वा ततो निबध्नीयात् सप्ताहं च पिबेद्घृतम् ॥२५६॥"

[सुश्रुत : चिकित्सा ३ : १६-४६]

If the skull is broken without the brain-matter coming out of it, then it should be anointed with ghee and honey and bandaged. The patient should take ghee for one week.

विश्लिष्टिते सुकुर्वीत[?]करे वा चरणेऽथवा[3] ।
निखातिते तदुपरि वह्निस्वेदं तु कारयेत् ॥२५७॥

[The meaning of this verse is not clear]

---

1. च इति आदर्शपुस्तकेषु पाठः ।
2. घृताप्लुतम् इति आदर्शपुस्तकेषु पाठः ।
3. पि वा इति चतुर्थषष्ठपुस्तकयोः पाठः ।

लकुटादि प्रहारेषु देहे पंकं प्रलेपयेत् ।
खंटीबोल[1]समायुक्तां सगुडी भक्षयेन्नरः ।
भिन्मिनीं[?]गुडयुक्तां वा भक्षयेद्रक्तमेदिनीम् ॥२५८॥

If the body is injured being beaten by staff, etc. then mud should be applied over the body and the patient should take *khaṇṭī bola* along with jaggery or *rakta medinī* (*gairika*) along with jaggery.

"पतनादभिघाताद्वा सूनमंगं[2] यदक्षतम् ।
शीतान्प्रदेहान्[3]सेकांश्च भिषक् तस्यावचारयेत् ॥२५९॥

If the body is injured by fall or beating without any external wound, then cooling ointments should be applied and cooling liquids should be sprinkled over the affected part.

अथ जंघोरुभग्नानां[4] कपाटशयनं हितम् ।
कीलकाः बन्धनार्थं च पञ्च कार्याः[5] विजानता ॥२६०॥
यथा न चलनं तस्य भग्नस्य क्रियते[6] तथा ।
सन्धेरुभयतो द्वौ द्वौ तले चैकश्च कीलकः ॥२६१॥
श्रोण्यां वा पृष्ठवंशे वा वक्षस्यक्षकयोस्तथा[7] ।
भग्नसन्धिविमोक्षेषु विधिमेनं समाचरेत् ॥२६२॥

---

1. खंटीषोलसमायुक्ती इति षष्ठपुस्तके पाठः ।
2. शूनमङ्गं इति आकरे पाठः ।
3. शितान्प्रदेहात् इति प्रथमपुस्तके पाठः ।
4. ०भग्नानि इति षष्ठपुस्तके पाठः ।
5. पञ्चकार्यं इति आदर्शपुस्तकेषु पाठः ।
6. वृते इति षष्ठपुस्तके पाठः ।
7. वृक्षस्याक्षकयोस्तथा इति आदर्शपुस्तकेषु पाठः ।

In the case of fracture of leg or thigh bones, the patient should be made to sleep over a hard wooden bed having five nails pegged into it—two in each side of the joints and one in between the feet and tied with ropes so that the fractured bones many not be able to move. Similar arrangements should be made for immobility in the case of fracture or dislocation of hip bones, vertibral column, chest and clavicles.

सन्धींश्चिरविमुक्तांस्तु[1] स्निग्धान्[2] स्विन्नान् मृदुकृतान् ।
उक्तैर्विधानैर्बुद्धया च सम्यक् प्रकृतिमानयेत् ॥२६३॥

The physician should utilise his own wisdom and apply the above procedure if there is chronic dislocation of a joint after making the organ soft by the administration of oleation and fomentation therapies so that the defect is corrected.

काण्डभग्ने[3] प्ररूढे तु विषमोल्वणसाधिते[4] ।
आपोथ्योन्मामयेद्भग्नं[5] ततो भग्नवदाचरेत् ॥२६४॥"

[सुश्रुत : चिकित्सा ३ : ४७-५२]

If there is irregular or excessive healing of a fractured long bone, it should be fomented and then broken by bending the bone. Thereafter, the condition should be again treated on the lines suggested for a new bone fracture.

अनुल्वणमनाविद्धं स्वस्थाने पर्यवस्थितम् ।
सुखचेष्टाप्रचारं च सम्यग्रूढस्य लक्षणम् ॥२६५॥

---

1. सन्धीश्चिरविमुक्तांस्तु इति आदर्शपुस्तकेषु पाठः ।
2. स्निग्धाश्चित्रान्मृदूकृतात् इति प्रथमपुस्तके पाठः ।
3. काण्डे भग्ने प्ररुढे वा विमोस्वणसाधिते इति षष्ठपुस्तके पाठः ।
4. विषमोल्वणसंहिते इति आकरे पाठः ।
5. आपोथ्य समयेद्भुग्नम् इति आकरे पाठः ।

Signs of Proper Healing

If there is no elevation or hole, if the bone is in its appropriate place and if the patient is able to work or move with comfort, then this is known as proper healing of the fracture.

"कल्पयेन्निर्गतं[1] शुष्कं व्रणान्तेऽस्थिसमाहितः ।
सन्ध्यन्ते[2] वा क्रियां कुर्यात्सव्रणे व्रणभग्नवत् ॥२६६॥

If there are ulcers above the bones or joints, then such cases should be treated on the lines of open fracture.

ऊर्ध्वकाये तु भग्नानां मस्तिष्क्यं कर्णपूरणम् ।
घृतपानं हितं नस्यं प्रशाखास्वनुवासनम् ॥२६७॥"

[सुश्रुत : चिकित्सा ३ : ५३-५४]

If the fracture takes place in the head and neck, the patient should be given *karṇa pūraṇa* therapy (pouring medicated oil into the ears) along with *ghṛta pāna* (intake of ghee) and inhalation therapy. If, however, there are fractures in the limbs, then *anuvāsana* type of medicated enema therapy should be administered.

"रात्रौ[3] रात्रौ तिलान् कृष्णान् वासयेदस्थिरे जले[4] ।
दिवा दिवा शोषयित्वा गवां क्षीरेण भावयेत् ॥२६८॥
तृतीयं सप्तरात्रं वा भावयेन्मधुकाम्बुना ।

---

1. कल्पयोगतिर्गतम् इति षष्ठपुस्तके पाठः ।
2. संध्यन्ने इति प्रथमपुस्तके पाठः ।
3. राजै राजै तिलाम् इति षष्ठपुस्तके पाठः ।
4. नल इति षष्ठपुस्तके पाठः ।

ततः क्षीरं पुनः पीतान्[1] सुशुष्कांश्चूर्णयेद्भिषक्[2] ॥२६९॥

काकोल्यादिं सयष्ट्याह्वं मञ्जिष्ठां[3] सारिवां तथा ।
कुष्ठं सर्जरसं[4] मांसी सुरदारु सचन्दनम् ।
शतपुष्पां च संचूर्ण्य तिलचूर्णेन योजयेत् ॥२७०॥
पीडनार्थं च कर्त्तव्यं सर्वगन्धश्रृतं पयः ।
चतुर्गुणेन पयसा तत्तैलं विपचेद्भिषक् ॥२७१॥
एलामंशुमती पत्रं जीवकं तगरं तथा ।
रोध्रं प्रपौण्डरीकं च तथा कालानुसारिवा ॥२७२॥
सैरीयकं[5] क्षीरशुक्लामनन्तां समधूलिकाम्[6] ।
पिष्ट्वा[7] श्रृङ्गाटकं[8] चैव पूर्वोक्तान्यौषधानि च ॥२७३॥
'एभिस्तद्विपचेत्तैलं[9] शास्त्रविण्मृदुनाऽग्निना ।
एतत्तैलं सदा पथ्यं भग्नानां सर्वकर्मसु ॥२७४॥

---

1. पीतात् इति प्रथमपुस्तके पाठः ।
2. पीतासुमुष्कम् इति षष्ठपुस्तके पाठः ।
3. मंजिष्ठा सारिवा इति आदर्शपुस्तकेषु पाठः ।
4. क. सर्ज्जरसम् इति प्रथमचतुर्थपंचमपुस्तकेषु पाठः ।
   ख. सर्ज्जनसं इति षष्ठपुस्तके पाठः ।
5. सैरेयकम् इति आकरे पाठः ।
6. समधूयष्टिकाम् इति षष्ठपुस्तके पाठः ।
7. पिस्ता इति प्रथमपुस्तके पाठः ।
8. भृंगारकम् इति षष्ठपुस्तके पाठः ।
9. 'एभिस्तद्विपचेत्तैलम्———पंचशततमो हर्षः । पाठोऽयं षष्ठपुस्तके नोपलभ्यते ।

आक्षेपके पक्षाघाते तालु शोषे तथार्दिते ।
मन्यास्तम्भे शिरोरोगे कर्णशूले हनुग्रहे ॥२७५॥
बाधिर्ये तिमिरे चैव ये च स्त्रीषु क्षयं गताः ।
पथ्यं पाने तथाऽभ्यङ्गे नस्ये बस्तिषु भोजने ॥२७६॥
ग्रीवास्कन्धोरसां वृद्धिरमुनैवोपजायते ।
मुखं च पद्मप्रतिमं स[1] सुगन्धिसमीरणम् ।
गन्धतैलमिदं नाम्ना सर्ववातविकारनुत्[2] ॥२७७॥

[सुश्रुत : चिकित्सा ३ : ५५-६६]

मात्रा[3]वीरादिचूर्णस्य तिलपादे प्रयोजयेत् ।
पीडनार्थं तु पाकार्थं कल्कयोग्या मता पुनः ॥२७८॥
प्रलेपकपरीतानां क्षीणानां मधुमेहिनाम् ।
क्षीणज्वरप्रतप्तानां मन्दाग्नीनां प्रयोजयेत् ॥२७९॥

॥ इति गन्धतैलम् ॥

Gandha Taila

Black variety of *tila* should be kept in flowing water during nights and during days. These seeds should be dried and impregnated with cow's milk. Then for three [?] or seven days these seeds should be impregnated with the decoction of *madhuka*. Again these are to be impregnated with milk, dried in the sun and made to a powder. To this, the powder of

---

1. स सुगंधिसमीरणम् इति आकरे पाठः ।
2. करवीर्यः इति चतुर्थपुस्तके अधिको पाठः ।
3. शतावीरादिक० इति चतुर्थपुस्तके पाठः ।

drugs belonging to *kākolyādi gaṇa*, *madhu yaṣṭi*, *mañjiṣṭhā*, *sārivā*, *kuṣṭha*, *sarja rasa*, *māṃsī*, *sura dāru*, *candana* and *śatapuṣpā* should be added. This powder should be added with milk, boiled with drugs belonging to *sarva gandha gaṇa* and pressed in the oil-press to takeout the oil. This oil should be cooked by adding four times of milk and the paste of *elā*, *aṃśumatī*, *patra*, *jīvaka*, *tagara*, *rodhra*, *prapauṇḍarīka*, *kālānu-sārivā*, *sairīyaka*, *kṣīra śuklā*, *anantā*, *madhulikā*, *śṛṅgāṭaka* and other drugs mentioned before. Cooking should be done over mild fire. This medicated oil is always useful in all therapies for the treatment of fracture. It is also useful for *ākṣepaka*, *pakṣāghāta* (hemiplegia), *tālu śoṣa* (dryness of palate), *ardita* (facial paralysis), *manyā stambha* (torticolis), *śiro roga* (diseases of the head), *karṇa śūla* (earache), *hanu graha* (lock-jaw), deafness, *timira* (cataract) and consumption because of excessive sexual indulgence. It can be used as a drink, for massage, inhalation, medicated enema and in food. Growth of neck shoulder and chest takes place by the use of this recipe. It, gives good complexion to the face and good odour to the body. This is called *gandha taila*. It cures all *vātika* diseases. [The meaning of the verse no. 278 is not clear]. This recipe is also useful for patients suffering from *pralepaka*, consumption, diabetes mellitus, phthisis, fever and suppressed power of digestion.

तैले[1]स्मिन्छागमांसोत्थरसं तैलसमां[2]सकम् ।
हरिद्रे मधुकं तिक्तावराहमधुपर्णिकी ॥२८०॥
बलारास्नाशताह्वा च [3]सहैलाभयचन्दनैः ।
तिक्तातिक्तांगकपटं मञ्जिष्ठोशीरपद्मकैः ॥२८१॥

---

1. तैलेऽस्मिन्छा० इति चतुर्थपुस्तके पाठः ।
2. तैलसमांशकम् इति चतुर्थपुस्तके पाठः ।
3. महैलाभयचन्दनैः इति चतुर्थपुस्तके पाठः ।

क्वाथं तैलसमं दत्वा विपचेत्तैलमुत्तमम् ।
कालेयकोद्भवं तैलं पत्रकल्के प्रयोजयेत् ॥२८२॥

॥ इति महागंधतैलम् ॥

Mahā Gandha Taila

In the above mentioned recipe, the soup of the meat of goat and the decoction of *haridrā, dāru haridrā, madhuka, tiktā, varāha parṇī, madhu parṇī, balā, rāsnā, śatāhvā, elā, abhayā, candana, tiktā* [?], *tiktāṅga, kapaṭa*]?], *mañjiṣṭhā, uśīra* and *padmaka*, (both the meat soup and decoction taken in quantity each equal to that of oil) should be added and cooked. At the end of cooking (*patra kalka*), the oil of *kāleyaka* should be added.

रसराजलक्ष्म्याम्

कान्तं वज्रं हिंगुलाभ्रं रसेन्द्रं
कृत्वा खोटं[1] भूधरे पक्षमेकम् ।
मन्दं मन्दं पाकतः स्याद्गुटीयं
शस्त्रौघं स्याद्वारयेद्यस्य वक्त्रे[2] ॥२८३॥

॥ वज्रगुटिका ॥

Vajra Guṭikā (According to Rasa Rāja Lakṣmī)

Kānta lauha bhasma, vajra bhasma, purified *hiṅgula, abhraka bhasma* and purified *pārada* should be triturated together and cooked in *Bhūdhara yantra* over mild fire for one fortnight. Keeping this pill in the mouth protects the person from any injury by weapons.

1. षोटं इति द्वितीयपुस्तके पाठः ।
2. वक्रे इति चतुर्थपुस्तके पाठः ।

वैक्रान्तं हेमकान्तं च विद्रुमं स्फटिकं तथा ।
[1]मेंमांगंधरसाम्वा[?] च समं खल्वे प्रमर्दयेत् ॥२८४॥
[2]अस्थिसंहारजरसं [3]दत्त्वा दिनत्रयम् ।
मधुना माषमात्रं वा सेवेदग्निबलं प्रति ॥२८५॥
सद्योव्रणोग्निदाहे च भग्ने च विषमज्वरे ।
नाशनार्थं प्रयोक्तव्यो[4] रसोऽयं वज्रशेखरः ॥२८६॥

॥ वज्रशेखरो[5] रसः ॥

Vajra Śekhara Rasa

Vaikrānta bhasma, *svarṇa bhasma*, *kānta lauha bhasma*, *vidruma bhasma*, *sphaṭika bhasma*, *memmāṅgandha rasa* [?] and *amvā* [?]—all taken in equal quantities should be triturated in a pestle and mortar for three days by adding the juice of *asthi saṃhāra*. Depending upon the power of digestion, this recipe should be administered in a dose of one *māṣā* along with honey. It cures fresh wounds, burns, fracture and *viṣama jvara* (irregular fever). This is called *vajra śekhara rasa*.

गोरक्षमतात्—

वातव्याधिविकारोक्तं तैलमत्रापि पूजितम् ।
त्रिकत्रयं[6] निशायुग्मं[7] बला बल्या प्रसारणी ॥२८७॥

---

1. मेंमीगंधरसाम्वा च इति चतुर्थपुस्तके पाठः ।
2. दस्थिसंहारजरसम् इति प्रथमपुस्तके पाठः ।
3. बुधादत्त्वा इति चतुर्थपुस्तके पाठः ।
4. प्रयोक्तव्यां इति पञ्चमपुस्तके पाठः ।
5. पाठोऽयं प्रथमपंचमपुस्तकयोः नोपलभ्यते ।
6. 'य तु' इति प्रथमपुस्तके अधिको पाठः ।
7. निशा वल्या वल्या इति प्रथमपुस्तके पाठः ।

मञ्जिष्ठापार्थयष्ठी च देवदारुपुनर्नवा ।
पृथक् पृथक् शुक्तिसमं[1] पलैकं मृतपारदम् ॥२८८॥
अभ्रं च द्विगुणं देयं त्रिगुणं तु मृतायसम् ।
चतुर्गुणं शुद्धशैलं दत्त्वा[2] संमर्दयेत्ततः[3] ॥२८९॥
अक्षप्रमाणा गुटिका सेव्या नित्यं ततः परम् ।
पिबेन्मांसरसं रोगी सद्योव्रणनिपीडितः[4] ॥२९०॥
[5]मज्जरक्तास्थिवाहीनि व्रणान्याशु प्रयान्ति हि ।
भग्नविश्लिष्टक्षिप्ताद्याः संहतिं[6] यान्ति नान्यथा ॥२९१॥

According to Gorakṣa

Medicated oils prescribed for the treatment of *vāta vyādhi* (diseases caused by *vāyu*) are also useful in the treatment of fracture. One *śukti* of each of *triphalā*, *trikaṭu*, *trimada*, *niśā*, *dāru niśā*, *balā*, *balyā*, *prasāraṇī*, *mañjiṣṭhā*, *pārtha*, *yaṣṭi madhu*, *deva dāru* and *punarnavā*, one *pala* of *pārada bhasma*, two *palas* of *abhra bhasma*, three *palas* of *lauha bhasma* and four *palas* of purified *manaḥ śilā* should be triturated together and pills of one *akṣa* each should be prepared. One such pill should be administered every day followed by meat soup. It quickly

1. श्चक्तिसमम् इति प्रथमपुस्तके पाठः ।
2. सर्वमेकत्र मिश्रयेत् इति चतुर्थपुस्तके पाठः ।
3. 'अस्थि शृङ्खलिकातोये शोधितो यस्तु गुग्गुलुः । सर्वेषां द्विगुणश्चात्र दत्वा संमर्दयेत्ततः ।' पाठोऽयं चतुर्थपुस्तके अधिकमुपलभ्यते ।
4. रोगी चानुदुष्टव्रणनिपीडितः इति चतुर्थपुस्तके पाठः ।
5. पूयरक्तास्थि० इति चतुर्थपुस्तके पाठ : ।
6. संधिग्नाश्चये व्रणः इति चतुर्थपुस्तके पाठः ।

cures freshly occuring ulcers and ulcers secreting bone marrow, blood as well as bone tissue. It also corrects broken, dislocated and displaced bones.

"आभाफलत्रिकव्योषैः सर्वैरेभिः समांशकैः[1] ।
तुल्यो गुग्गुलुरायोज्यो भग्नसन्धिप्रसाधकः ॥२६२॥"

॥ आभागुग्गुलुः ॥

[भैषज्यरत्नावली : भग्नाधिकार : १४]

Ābhā Guggulu

One part of each of *ābhā*, *triphalā* and *trikaṭu* and seven parts of *guggulu* should be pounded together by adding ghee. Intake of this helps in the healing of fracture.

"रसोनमधुकं[2] लाक्षासिताकल्कं समश्नताम् ।
छिन्नभिन्नच्युतास्थीनां सन्धानमचिराद्भवेत् ॥२६३॥"

[भैषज्यरत्नावली : भग्नाधिकार : ६]

Intake of the paste of *rasona*, *madhuka*, *lākṣā* and sugar helps in the setting and healing of cracked, broken and displaced bones.

"लाक्षास्थिसंहृत्ककुभाश्वगन्धा-
श्चूर्णीकृता नागबला पुरश्च ।

1. क. समांशकै इति चतुर्थपुस्तके पाठः ।
   ख. समीकृतैः इति आकरे पाठः ।
2. पाठोऽयं प्रथमपुस्तके नोपलभ्यते ।
3. रसोनमधुलाक्षाज्यसिताकल्कम् इति आकरे पाठः ।

संभग्नामुक्तास्थिरुजं[1] निहन्या-

दंगानिकुर्यात्कुलिशोपमानि ॥२६४॥"

॥ लाक्षागुग्गुलुः ॥

[भैषज्यरत्नावली : भग्नाधिकार : १२]

Lākṣā Guggulu

Intake of *lākṣā*, *asthi saṃhāra*, *kakubha*, *aśvagandhā*, *nāga balā* and *pura* in a powder form corrects pain of broken or dislocated bones. It makes the body strong like a thunderbolt.

'श्वेतखैरटं[2] ३ एकत्रकं तिलतैल दी ग्राकरिते हिमांस जँहा फाटं तहाँ खपरव पाच्छे द्वं चूर्ण मेलव पूरै व्यथा न करै: ॥२६५॥'

Three *ṭaṅkas* of *śveta khadira* should be mixed with sesame oil and applied over the area where the bone is broken. This relieves pain and helps in the healing of fracture.
[This prose paragraph is in old Hindi).

विश्लेषितायास्त्वथ[3] नासिकायाः वक्षामि[4] संधानविधिं यथावत् ।

नासाप्रमाणं पृथिवीरुहाणां पत्रं गृहीत्वा त्वविलंवितस्य ॥२९६॥

1. संभिन्नमुक्तास्थिरुजम् इति चतुर्थपुस्तके पाठः ।
2. 'श्वेतखैरट——०करै' पाठोऽयं चतुर्थपुस्तके नोपलभ्यते ।
3. क. श्वेतखदिर टंकतीन चूर्ण कृत्वा तिल तैलेन शस्त्रहतक्षते लेपनं कृत्वा व्रणपूर्तिर्भवति । रालचूर्णटंक ५ उत्तम खदिरटंक २ तुरटी भर्जित टंक १, अतसी तैल टंक १२ सर्व कांस्य पत्रेण मर्द्य (*continued on next page*)
4. वक्ष्यामि इति चतुर्थपुस्तके पाठः ।

तेन प्रमाणेन हि गंडपार्श्वादुत्कृत्य वद्धं त्वथ नासिकाग्रम्[1] ।
विलिख्य चाशु प्रतिसंदधीत तं साधुवैद्यैर्भिषगप्रमत्तम् ॥२९७॥
सुसंहितं सम्यगथो यथा वा नाडीद्वयेनापि समात्तबध्वा ।
प्रोन्नम्य चैनामवचूर्णयेच्च पतंगयष्ठिमधुकांजनैश्च ॥२९८॥
संछाद्य सम्यक् पिचुनासितेन
तैलेन सिंचेदसकृत्तिलानाम् ।
(स)घृतं च पाथ्यः सनरः प्रजीर्णे
स्निग्धं विरेच्यः सयथोपदेशम् ॥२९९॥
रूढं च संधानमुपागतं च तदर्द्धशेषं च पुनर्न्निकृते ।
हीनां पुनर्वर्द्धयितुं यतेत समां च कुर्यादतिवृद्धमांसम् ॥३००॥

Rhinoplasty

Now the appropriate method of correcting the detached nose will be described. If the nose is cut and separated, then

---

(*Continued from last page*)

किंचिज्जलं दत्वा पुनर्मंद्य प्रहरपर्यन्तं ज्जलतपक्वा तद् द्रव्यं व्रणे लेपः ।। मलम ।। पाठोऽयं चतुर्थपुस्तके अधिकमुपलभ्यते ।

ख. पारागन्धकसेंदरमरिचतुत्थमुरदाशंख सुहागाकबीला नीकें कैंपलैधीतो लावं व्रणकण्डू जाई सर्वथा । राल चूर्ण रं ५ पपरीरवयरटं २११ फटकरी रं १ तीसी र १ कातैलरं १२ थारी महमेग्लिमथ पानि देयी करि प्रहर एक पर्यंतं मथना भल्लेभव्रणसाबजपूरई । पुरानापनहीजलावै धावैकैं फूलजलावै ऐहं चूर्ण कितीसी के तेल से फाहा देरते हि पर चूर्ण देहव्रणनीक हाई मनुष्य वा घोरेका पाठोऽयं पंचमपुस्तके अधिकमुपलभ्यते ।

1. हिंगडपार्श्वं० इति पञ्चमपुस्तके पाठः ।

without any delay, leaf of a tree should be made to the shape of the nose. A piece of the muscle should be taken from the cheek with its contact with the face intact. This should be made to the shape of the nose. Then the stump of the original nose should be scraped and immediately, over it, the artificially prepared nose with the cheek muscle should be placed. This artificially prepared nose should have two pipes for nostrils. Having placed over the area of the original nose, it should be slightly elevated by pressure of fingers to shape the tip of the nose and to make it compact. Over the wound, the powder of *pataṅga*, *yaṣṭi madhu* and *añjana* should be sprinkled. It should then be covered with cotton wool, and over it, oil of the black variety of sesame seed should be frequently sprinkled. The patient should be given food with ghee, and after its digestion, he should be given unctuous type of purgation therapy. After the ulcer is healed and the nose is united, the portion of the flesh connected with the cheek should be severed. If the reconstructed nose has become smaller than the original, then effort should be made to enlarge it and the bigger one should be brought to normal size and shape.

नाडीयोगं[1] विनौष्ठस्य नासासंधानवद्विधिम् ॥३०१॥

Repairing Lip

If the lip is severed, then the procedure prescribed for rhinoplasty should be adopted except that the fixation of tube is not necessary.

इति श्रीमहाराजाधिराजटोडरमल्लविरचिते[2] टोडरानन्दे आयुर्वेदसौख्ये शोफव्रणशारीरव्रणसद्योव्रणनासिकासंधानवह्नि-[3]

---

1. नाडीयुतं इति चतुर्थपुस्तके पाठः ।
2. 'महाराजा०——विरचिते' पाठोऽयं चतुर्थपुस्तके नोपलभ्यते ।
3. शोथ० इति चतुर्थपुस्तके पाठः ।

दग्धनिदानचिकित्साकथनं नाम त्रिपंचाशत्तमो हर्षः ॥३०२॥'

Thus, ends the 53rd Chapter dealing with the diagnosis and treatment of *śopha vraṇa* (ulcer with oedema), *śārīra vraṇa* (endogenous ulcer), *sadyo vraṇa* (fresh wound caused by exogenous factors), *nāsikā sandhāna* (repairing of mutilated nose) and burns in *Āyurveda saukhya* of *Ṭodarānanda* composed by the great king Ṭoḍara Malla.

Index I

Appendix I

(Authors and Books Quoted)

Index II

Appendix II

(Recipes Described)

Index III

Appendix III

(**Drugs described :** *For Bot. names refer to Appendices of previous volumes)*

Index IV
Appendix IV

(Diseases Described)

Index V

(Glossary of Technical Terms)

Abhighāta, 515
Injury.

Abhighātaja, 390, 94
Caused by external injury.

Abhiṣyandi, 172, 422
Which obstruct channels of circulation. *Ref.* Glossary in Basic Principles of Āyurveda, p. 581.

Ācārya, 233
The author.

Adhaḥ kṣipta, 563, 64
Downward dislocation of joint.

Āḍhaka, 137, 140, 187, 206, 307, 355, 377, 385, 409, 412, 433
Unit of measurement. Four *prasthas* make one *āḍhaka* which is equivalent to 3,072 Kg. or Ltr. *Ref.* Index IV in p. 495 of Diagnosis and Treatment of Diseases in Āyurveda, Part Two.

Ādhmānā, 8, 108, 172, 321
An ailment characterised by excessive accumulation of wind or gas in the gastro-intestinal tract. It is one of the eighty *vāta rogas*, and generally caused by the suppression of the manifested urges for passing flatus; stool and urine. *Ref.* Index IV in p. 495 of Diagnosis and Treatment of Diseases in Āyurveda, Part Two.

Āgantu, 505
Exogenous.

Āgantuja, 483
Caused by exogenous factors.

Agni, 301, 320, 464

Enzymes responsible for digestion and metabolism in the body. *Ref.* Glossary in p. 585 of Basic Principles of Āyurveda.

Agni māndya, 87

Suppression of the activities of enzymes responsible for digestion and metabolism. It is generally used to mean the suppression of digestive power.

Agnyāśaya, 512

Small intestine including duodenum; often denotes pancreas

Agra vakra, 247

A metallic rod with a curved top; surgical equipment for the removal of stone.

Agropaharṇīya, 246

Preparatory measures; drugs equipments etc., required to be kept in the operation theatre before operation; name of a chapter of *Sus. Saṃhitā* dealing with this topic.

Akṣa, 62 71, 198, 205, 206, 237, 239, 277, 282, 307, 356, 385, 395, 409, 435, 475, 492, 550

Unit of weight approx. 12 Gm. This term is used as as syn. of *bibhītaka* (*Terminalia belerica* Roxb.). Weight of the fruit of this plant is also implied by this term.

Āma, 2, 9, 26, 27, 102, 371, 401, 487, 499, 504

Product of improper digestion and metabolism. *Ref.* Glossary in p. 587 of Basic Principles of Āyurveda.

Āmaja, 1, 7

The ailment caused by *āma.*

Āmāśaya, 30, 86, 226, 395, 512

Anatomically, it implies stomach, and physiologically, it covers both the stomach and the upper part of the small-intestine where the food remains in undigested form. For details ref. Glossary in Basic Principles of Āyurveda, p. 588.

Āma taila, 581

Freshly extracted oil. Generally oil after extraction from the oil seed is cooked over fire to promote its shelf-life, taste and smell. The uncooked oil is called *āma taila* which is more useful for application over injuries and ulcers.

Ambu, 256, 320

Water. For details, ref. pp. 210-240 in Materia Medica of Ayurveda.

Ānāha, 13, 47, 88, 93-95, 102-105, 124, 126, 134, 282

Constipation. *Ref.* p. 586 of Glossary in Diagnosis and Treatment of Diseases in Ayurveda, Part-I.

Aṅgulas, 456, 471

Unit of measurement equivalent to 1/2″ approx. *Ref.* Glossary in p. 587 of Diagnosis and Treatment of Diseases in Ayurveda, Part-I.

Antraja (*vṛddhi*), 418

Inguinal hernia into which the intestines protrude.

Anulomana, 114

Downward movement of *vāyu*; mostly refers to wind in the abdomen. Generally a laxative or purgative is administered with *vāyu*-alleviating drugs for this purpose.

Anupāna, 44, 85, 87, 151, 153, 154, 189, 291-93, 307, 374, 383

Vehicle or post-prandial drink. *Ref.* Glossary in p. 591 of Basic Principles of Ayurveda.

Anuvāsana, 251, 327, 334, 335, 432, 587

A type of medicated enema. *Ref.* Glossary in p. 591 of Basic Principles of Ayurveda.

Apacī, 437, 441, 453, 455, 478, 550

Adenitis, specially inflammation and suppuration of lymph glands in the neck.

Apāna vāyu, 193, 320

One of the five varieties of *vāyu* located in the lower abdomen. It regulates the movement of urine, stool, foetus and menstrual fluid, and any derangement of this *vāyu* causes local ailments including pain in lumber region.

Apatānaka, 519

Emprosthotonos. One of the serious diseases caused by the aggravation of *vāyu*.

Apatarpaṇa, 524

Cooling applications; also fasting therapy.

Ārā, 577

A surgical instrument; a saw.

Āranāla, 405, 471, 472

A type of sour-vinegar.

Arbuda, 297, 437, 444, 461-465, 472, 478

Tumour.

Armaṇa, 139, 281

Unit of measurement. Approx. 12.288 Kg. or Ltr.

Ariṣṭa, 25, 335

A type of alcoholic preparation.

Āsava, 161, 375, 496

The medicines or drinks prepared by fermentation are called *āsava*. *Ref.* Glossary in p. 592 of Basic Principles of Ayurveda.

Aśmarī, 99, 176, 203, 209, 211, 215, 227-29, 231, 235-37, 239, 241-43, 249, 253, 282, 284, 387, 407, 432

Stone in urinary or biliary tract. *Ref.* Glossary in p. 593 in Basic Principles of Ayurveda.

Asra, 256

Blood.

Aṣṭamikā, 133

Unit of weight equivalent to 24 G. approximately.

Āsthāpana, 95, 251

This is one of the two types of medicated enema. *Ref.* Glossary in p. 593 of Basic Principles of Ayurveda.

Asthi, 481, 535

Bone tissue. *Ref.* Glossary in p. 589 of Diagnosis and Treatment of Diseases in Ayurveda, Part-I.

Aṣṭhilā, 130

Enlargement of prostate gland. Sometimes it refers to any hard growth in the abdomen and pelvis.

Asvapna, 302

Remaining awake at night; sleeplessness.

Ati-sthūla, 302

Excessively fatty or suffering from obesity.

Avasecana, 520
Sprinkling of medicated liquids.

Āvṛtta, 264
Obstructed.

Ayaskṛti, 335
Specially processed iron.

Baḍiśa, 251, 450
A type of forceps.

Bali, 246
Sacred offerings

Balla, 44
Unit of weight approx. 375 mg. Also written as *valla*.

Basti, 210, 225, 252
Generally refers to urinary bladder, but also includes kidneys and ureters; also refers to medicated enema therapy.

Basti śiras, 216, 225
Kidneys.

Bhasma, 31, 35, 36, 39, 40, 43, 53, 61, 63, 64, 66, 185, 188, 189, 200, 288, 289, 292, 294, 295, 358, 373, 461
Calcined powder of metals, menerals, etc. *Ref.* Glossary in p. 597 of Basic Principles of Ayurveda.

Bhasmaka, 476
Voracious appetite.

Bhinna, 511
Perforated (Ulcer).

Bhūdhara puṭa, 151
N. of a pharmaceutical process specially used for preparing *bhasmas* (calcined powder) of metals etc.

Bhūdhara yantra, 591
An implement used for the preparation of medicines. *Ref.* Glassary in p. 592 of Diagnosis and Treatment of Diseases in Ayurveda, Part-I.

Bīja doṣa, 263
Defective genes.

Blood-letting therapy, 523, 524, 574

San : *rakta mokṣaṇa*; one of the five specialised ayurvedic therapies together called *pañca karma*. Caraka has included *nasya* or inhalation therapy in its place.

Bradhna, 422, 430-432, 434

Tumour in the inguinal region.

Brīhi mukha yantra, 425

Trochar and canula.

Cauterization therapy, 121

One of the surgical measures; San : *agni karma.*

Chinna, 511, 565

Cut (Wound).

Cleansing therapy, 459

Emetic, purgation therapy, etc., for removing waste products from the body.

Coṣa, 4

Sensation as if parched by strong héat.

Darvī pāka, 80

A stage of cooking linctus or syrup; when the preparation sticks to the stirrer.

Dhātu, 264

Tissue elements of the body which according to Āyurveda are of seven categories. *Ref.* Glossary in p. 600 of Basic Principles of Ayurveda.

Doṣa, 2, 6, 11, 12, 25, 34, 35, 37, 42, 58, 66, 76, 77, 80, 100, 110, 111, 123, 157, 163, 173, 198, 207, 210, 213, 216, 255, 257, 262, 264, 267, 284, 316, 17, 20, 21, 324-26, 329-31, 369, 390, 393 395, 400, 410, 422, 438, 444, 445, 447, 462, 470, 485, 489, 490, 503, 505, 508, 572, 574

Factors responsible for the regulation of all the functions of the body. *Ref.* Glossary in p. 601 of Basic Principles of Ayurveda.

Droṇa, 143, 145, 187, 206, 238, 385, 387, 433

Unit of weight. Approx. 12.288 Kg.

Dūṣya, 257, 462

see *dhātu.*

Dvandvaja, 506

Caused by the simultaneous vitiation of two *doṣas.*

Emetic therapy, 13, 22, 25, 60, 86, 180-81, 327, 363

One of the five specialised therapies taken together called *Pañca Karma.*

Fomentation therapy, 14, 180, 234, 250, 424, 425, 433, 448, 459, 471, 490, 491, 523, 524, 586

San : *Svedana*; One of the preparatory therapies administer ed before *Pañca Karma*; also used separately.

Gaja puṭa, 41, 43, 350

Ref. Glossary in p. 596 of Diagnosis and Treatment of Diseases in Ayurveda, Part-I

Gaṇḍū pada, 542

Earth-worm.

Gara viṣa, 307, 324, 341

Artificially prepared poisons.

Gharṣaṇa, 515

rubbing.

Ghṛṣṭa, 511, 515

Abraison (Wound)

Ghṛta pāna, 587

Intake of medicated ghee.

Glāni, 516

Fatigues. *Ref.* Glossary in p. 596 of Diagnosis and Treatment of Diseases in Ayurveda, Part-I.

Gonī, 238

Unit of measurement; equivalent to four ***droṇas.***

Guḍa pāka, 76, 81, 200, 225, 252

Cooking drugs into a thick syrup or linctus from with the help of jaggery (also sugar); the final stage of such cooking.

Gulma, 73, 85, 92, 95, 97, 102, 104, 106-08, 118, 120, 123, 124, 127, 128, 130-32, 138-40, 143, 145, 148-50, 155, 165, 166, 188, 236, 281, 310, 333, 341, 343, 344, 345, 350, 352, 354, 355, 363, 364, 370, 373, 374, 376, 377, 381, 382, 387, 407, 409, 414, 415, 432, 475, 484, 489, 550,

Phantom tumour.

Guñjā, 37, 38, 39, 40, 41, 149, 150, 151, 189, 370, 373, 374

Unit of weight. Approx. 125 mg.

Hanu graha, 518, 590

Lock-jaw.

Hṛd roga, 158, 159, 160, 163, 166, 167, 168

Heart disease.

Indra basti, 456

N. of a *marma* (vital place in the body) located in the calf-region, (13 *aṅgulas* above the ankle joint) and in the fore-arm.

Indra gopa, 517

Red insect found during rainy season; the insect cochineal of variaus kinds.

Inhalation therapy, 25, 309, 452, 453, 454, 583

Caraka includes this under *Pañca Karma*; used for elimination of waste products from head and neck.

Jaraṇa, 59

Digestion; cooking.

Kajjalī, 84

Physical mixture of mercury and sulpher which is in the form of a black powder and which looks like *kajjala* or collyrium.

Kākolyādi gaṇa, 117, 459, 590

Group of drugs-vide *Suśtruta*: *Sūtra* : 38:17

Kaṁsa, 240, 413, 415

Unit of measurement. Approx. 3.072 Kg. or Ltr.

Kāṇḍa, 565

Shaft of the bone.

Kāñjī, 21, 29, 79, 304, 308, 430, 431, 455, 473, 475, 476, 479, 521
Sour vinegar or sour gruel.

Kapha, 8, 11, 12, 29, 31, 42, 47, 50, 51, 56, 64, 65, 66, 68, 75, 78, 86, 93, 97, 107, 116, 138, 141, 152, 156, 172, 181, 195, 197, 198, 207, 209, 210, 213, 215, 216, 217 218, 219, 227, 230, 232, 242, 255, 256, 261, 276, 279, 287, 300, 304, 307, 309, 325, 332, 343, 347, 350, 381, 389, 390, 403, 426, 427, 431, 438, 440, 441, 446, 469, 470, 474, 475, 478, 523
One of the three *doṣas*—the other two being *vāyu* and *pitta.* It is the cohesive force in the body. *Ref.* Glossary in p. 606 of Basic Principles of Ayurveda.

Kapha alleviating drugs, 233
Generally those having pungent and bitter taste.

Kaphaja, 1, 25, 26, 27, 28, 110, 120, 121, 122, 126, 130, 133, 148, 158, 160, 163, 181, 183, 215, 217, 232, 255, 256, 262, 271, 279, 321, 390, 393, 399, 400, 419, 420, 424, 427, 439, 443, 463, 468, 473, 481, 482, 492, 493, 499, 502, 506, 522, 528
Diseases caused by aggravated *kapha.*

Karṇa puraṇa therapy, 587
Ear drop used in the treatment of ear diseases.

Karṣa, 20, 38, 41, 44, 74, 80, 82, 97, 120, 132, 134, 136, 140, 144, 151, 286, 287, 291, 293, 339, 350, 356, 366, 374, 375, 377, 403, 407, 411, 476, 477, 478
Unit of weight. Approx. 12Gm.

Khaḍa, 115
A sour preparation.

Kleda, 255
Sticky metabolic by products.

Kola, 73, 83, 366, 407
Unit of weight Approx. 6 Gm.

Koṣṭha, 301, 545
Alimentary tract. It is generally used to indicate viscera of alimentary and respiratory systems.

Kṛmi, 547, 551
Parasitic infection.

Kṛmija, 159, 160
Disease caused by parasitic infection.

Kṛśarā, 5, 14, 417
A preparation of rice added with pulses.

Kṛśa roga, 312
Excessive Emaciation.

Kṣāra, 26, 27, 35, 40, 43, 46, 48, 65, 68, 85, 98, 99, 124, 147, 165, 188, 204, 229, 232, 233, 236, 237, 243, 259, 335, 343, 344, 350, 351, 364, 365, 366, 377, 380, 381, 387, 391, 454, 462, 463, 464, 465, 500, 527, 562, 570, 574
Alkali preparation.

Kṣata, 511, 514
Lacerated wound.

Kṣataja, 481, 483, 493
Caused by injury.

Kṣirī vṛkṣa, 249, 250
Collective name of a group of plants having milky latex like *nyagrodha*, *udumbara*, *aśvattha*, *pāriṣa* and *plakṣa*.

Kuḍava, 53, 75, 81, 144, 187, 199, 241, 356, 412
Unit of measurement. Approx. 192 Gm. or ml.

Kukkuṭa pūṭa, 373
Fire-place for the calcination of metals; cow dung cakes are used as fuel.

Kulaja, 263
Familial.

Kumadya, 169
Alcoholic drink not fermented properly.

Kuṇḍala, 144
Movement of wind in the abdomen.

Kuśa, 568, 569
Splint.

Kuśa patra, 450
A thin scalpel.

Kuṣṭha, 91, 96, 102, 123, 132, 136, 141, 143, 145, 167, 281, 287, 307, 310, 341, 352, 354, 407, 475, 509, 556
Obstinate skin diseases including leprosy.

Laghu pañca mūla, 572
Collective name for five drugs, namely, *śāla parṇi*, *pṛśni parṇī*, *bṛhatī*, *kaṇṭakārī* and *gokṣura*.

Laghu puṭa, 37, 38
Half in size *gaja puṭa Ref. gaja puṭa* in this glossary.

Lājā, 22
Fried paddy.

Lālā yukta, 259
Extremely slimy.

Lasikā, 257, 260
Lymph.

Leha, 143
Linctus,

Lepana, 470
External application of drugs in a paste form.

Madhura gaṇa, 573
Group of drugs having sweet taste—vide *Aṣṭāṅga hṛdaya*: *Sūtra* 10 : 22-25.

Mādhvīka, 121
A type of wine.

Madya, 126, 147, 161
A type of alcoholic drink.

Maha srotas, 247
Alimentary tract.

Mahātyaya, 256
Serious ailment.

Majjā, 257, 260, 509
Bone-marrow.

Māṁsa, 255, 441, 444, 478, 481
Muscle tissue.

Māṁsa marma, 519
A group of vital parts in the body involving muscles.

Maṇḍa, 82, 86, 339
Water which is strained out after boiling rice.

Mandāgni, 319, 321
Suppression of the power of digestion and metabolism.

Maṅgala, 246
Auspicious invocation.

Maṇi, 193
Glans penis or external urethral sphincter.

Mantha, 101
Thin gruel.

Marma, 462
Vital part of the body.

Māṣa, 43, 82, 85, 86, 153, 154, 293, 592
Unit of weight. Approx. 1 Gm.

Mastuluṅga, 509
Brain matter.

Matsyāṇḍa nibha jāla, 456
Net-work like fish eggs; a structure below the calf region.

Meda, 255, 256, 267, 424, 440, 441, 443, 446, 478, 481, 509
Fat tissue.

Meḍhra, 33, 178, 222
Male genital organ.

Medoja, 419, 420, 443, 444
Caused by fat tissue.

Modaka, 60, 61, 67, 365, 476
Large size pills mostly sweet in taste.

Muṣka srotas, 252
Vas deferns.

Muṣṭi, 489
Unit of weight. Approx. 48 gms.

Mūtrāghāta, 190, 191, 198, 202, 203, 205, 239, 241, 282, 284, 287
Anuria.

Mūtraja, 419
Caused by urine.

Mūtra Kṛcchra, 99, 171, 173-175, 180-182, 192, 202
Dysuria.

Mūtrāśaya, 512
Urinary bladder.

Mūtra vaha srotas, 252, 253
Urinary channel.

Nāḍi sveda method, 462
A fomentation therapy in which a tubular structure is attached to the kettle in which drugs are boiled and by the steam which comes out of the tube, fomentation is performed.

Nirūha, 180, 234, 327, 332, 335
This is a variety of medicated enema prepared of decoction of drugs etc.

Niṣka, 39, 48, 85, 152, 294, 297, 371, 383
Unit of weight ; Approx. 4 Gm.

Niṣpāva, 4
Different types of beans.

Nyagrodhādī gaṇa, 275, 528, 572
Group of drugs—vide *Suśruta* : *Sūtra* 38 : 48-49

Ojas, 257, 571
Essence of all tissue elements.

Oleation therapy, 117, 121, 143, 234, 245, 327, 341 471
One of the *pre-Pañca Karma* therapies involving external and internal use of oil, ghee etc.

Pācana, 229
Cooking of uncooked food; promotion of metabolic activities; carminative action.

Pacymāna, 504
Beginning stage of suppuration.

Paittika, 1, 21, 24, 28, 37, 57, 72, 109, 110, 120, 130, 133, 151, 158, 161, 162, 177, 178, 179, 184, 186, 209, 218, 231, 232, 255, 262, 272, 279, 321, 390, 392, 394, 398, 399, 419, 424, 442, 459, 468, 469, 472, 481, 482, 483, 492, 499, 505, 522, 528, 534, 538, 539
Caused by *pitta*, Ref. *pitta*.

Pakvāṣaya, 30, 86, 395, 485, 487, 488, 501, 504, 512
Colon.

Pala, 43, 46, 63, 69, 70, 71, 72, 75, 77, 105, 115, 116, 120, 132, 134, 136, 137, 138, 139, 140, 141, 142, 143, 144, 167, 187, 188, 189, 200, 241, 281, 288, 307, 350, 351, 352, 354, 355, 358, 369, 373, 374, 382, 385, 403, 407, 411, 414, 415, 433, 453, 476, 557

Unit of weight and measurement ; Approx. 48 Gm. or ml.

Palala, 147, 169

Immature curd or cheese.

Pāna, 337

Drink.

Pañca kola, 351, 380, 400, 408

Collective name of five drugs, namely, *pippalī*, *pippali mūla*, *cavya*, *citraka* and *nāgara*.

Pañca kṣāra, 350

Five types of alkali preparations.

Pañca lavaṇa, 341, 350, 430, 478

Five types of salt.

Pañca mūla, 99, 105, 121, 140, 142, 162, 397

Five plants whose roots are used in medicine; of two types, namely *bṛhat pañca mūla* and *kṣudra pañca mūla*.

Pañcāṅga type of bandage, 583

Specially used for fracture of jaw-bone.

Pañca valkala, 492, 532, 553

Group of five barks of trees, namely *nyagrodha*, *udumbara*, *aśvattha*, *pāriṣa* and *plakṣa*.

Pañcoṣaṇa, 408

Same as *Pañca kola*.

Paribhāṣā, 136, 281

The text explaining technical terms.

Pārṣṇi, 456

Calcaneum bone.

Pāṭana, 520

Opening the wound by incission.

Pātra, 239, 351

Unit of measurement; Approx. 3.072 Kg. or Ltr.

Pātāla yantra, 433
Equipment used under ground for extraction of oil.

Pāyasa, 14, 348, 399
A type of milk preparation.

Peyā, 22, 114, 304, 339, 356
Thin gruel.

Phuphusa, 512
Lungs.

Piccita, 511, 514
Contusion.

Picu, 354
Cotton; usually in a swab-form.

Piḍakā, 265
Pimples

Pīnasa, 262, 381, 441
Chronic rhinitis.

Piṇḍikā, 525
Bolus form.

Pippali vardhamāna kalpa, 338
A special rejuvenating therapy in which long pepper is used in a gradually increased and decreased quantity.

Piśita, 257
Muscle tissue.

Piṣṭānna, 208
Pastry; food ingredients prepared of paste of corn flour, rice etc.

Piṣṭi, 43
Amalgam.

Pitta, 9, 11, 12, 22, 23, 24, 28, 29, 42, 56, 66, 75, 77, 86, 97, 107, 116, 117, 136, 151, 157, 162, 169, 170, 181, 194, 195, 198, 207, 210, 212, 218, 227, 232, 242, 255, 256, 261, 276, 279, 287, 325, 343, 369, 389, 390, 441, 472, 483, 503, 506, 536, 542, 558
One of the three *doṣas*—the other two being *vāyu* and *kapha*. For details *Ref.* Glossary in p-616 of Basic Principles of Āyurveda.

Pittaja, 1, 215, 420
Caused by *pitta*.

Pradeha, 523
Application of ointment.

Prahara, 551
Unit of measurement of time, equivalent to three hours.

Prāṇa vāyu, 320
One of the five varieties of *vāyu*, It is located in the heart and it regulates breathing, among others.

Prāṇāyāma, 41
A serious type of *vātika* disease in which *vāyu* causes contraction of the body with great force. In *yoga*, this term pertains to breath control ; one of the steps of *Aṣṭāṅga yoga*.

Prastha, 69, 70, 75, 80, 81, 105, 137, 138, 140, 143, 145, 168, 188, 206, 241, 281, 282, 288, 307, 351, 352, 354, 355, 356, 380, 382, 385, 387, 411, 412, 414, 415, 433, 435, 436, 477, 478, 553, 557
Unit of measurement; Approx. 748 Gm.

Prati kṣipta, 563
Upward dislocation.

Pūpa, 338
Cake.

Pūpalikā, 455, 570
A type of cake.

Purgation therapy 21, 60, 103, 117, 147, 166, 177, 181, 327, 330-31, 334-36, 339, 363, 371
One of the *Pañca Karmas* for elimination of waste products through downward tract.

Puruṣakādī gaṇa, 232
Group of drugs—vide *Suśruta* : *Sūtra* 38 : 43-44.

Puṣpa netra, 249
Catheter.

Puṣya, 456
N. of a constellation.

Puṭa pāka, 82 103, 166, 189, 262, 343, 359, 360, 361, 362, 374
Preparation of *bhasma* etc., of metals by keeping inside a pit dug in the earth. The pit is filled with cowdung cakes and ignited. It is of several types and the dimension of pits varies.

Raktaja, 419, 424, 444, 445, 481, 493, 499, 506, 522
Caused by the vitiation of blood.

Rasa, 157, 159, 257
(a) Plasma, chyle and lymph.
(b) Digestive-end-product.

Rasa dhātu, 157
Plasma, chyle and lymph.

Ratha, 251
Cart; chariot

Ratti, 296
Syn. of *guñjā* – unit of weight; Approx. 125 mg.

Ropaṇa, 118, 520
Healing therapy.

Rudhirāśaya, 512
Liver and spleen.

Rūkṣa, 534
Ununctuous; not greasy.

Sakṣāra, 243
Having action of the alkalis.

Śakti, kunta, 512
Spear.

Śālasārādi gaṇa, 275, 284, 290
Group of drugs – vide *Suśruta* : *Sūtra* 38 : 8-9

Sālvaṇa, 114
A type of bath.

Samtarpaṇa, 22, 304
Nourishing therapy.

Samvāhana, 234
Gentle massage.

Śāṇa 129, 287, 355
Unit of weight; Approx. 3 Gm.

Sandhāniya, 583
Drugs which help in joining two pieces of bones.

Sandhi, 535
Joints.

Śaṅkara sveda, 326
A type of fomentation by medicated steam.

Sānnipātika, 1, 133, 152, 158, 181, 182, 279, 321, 324, 332, 343, 390, 393, 398, 400, 401, 468, 469, 481, 482, 484, 488, 489, 506
A disease caused by the simultaneous vitiation of all the three *doṣas*.

Śarāva (sampuṭa), 38, 41, 103, 238, 288
Recipe closed inside two earthen plates and sealed.

Śārira, 505
Endogenous.

Śarkarā, 176, 183, 214, 223, 224, 234, 235, 236, 284
Gravelluria.

Sarva gandha gaṇa, 590
Group of drugs having good aroma—vide *Aṣṭāṅga saṅgraha* 8 : 72.

Śaśa, 22
Rabbit.

Śastra, 464
Surgical instrument

Seka, 177, 337
Sprinkling of water.

Śephas, 225
Pudendum.

Sevanī, 217, 246, 252, 253, 425
Suture between umbilicus and pelvic region.

Simbī dhānya, 42
Legumes; pulses.

Śirā, 535
Vessels.

Sirāja, 443
Caused in a vessel.

Siro vireka, 424
Elimination of *doṣas* from head.

Śiśira, 5
First half of winter.

Skandana, 537
Coagulation

Snāyu, 517, 535
Ligaments including nerves.

Sneha (dravya), 327, 493, 534, 539, 546
Oleation therapy; oil, ghee, etc.

Śodhana, 520
Cleansing the wound by medicated decoctions.

Spandana, 112
Palpitation.

Sramsana, 117
Mild laxative.

Staimitya, 7
A feeling as if covered with wet-cloth.

Śukra, 256
Semen in general and sperm in paticular. One of the seven groups of tissue elements.

Śukraja, 183, 209, 215
Seminal.

Śukra vaha srotas, 252, 253
Semen carrying channel

Śukti, 239, 415, 593
Unit of weight; Approx. 24 Gm.

Surasādi gaṇa, 309, 547
Group of drugs—vide *Suśruta* : *Sūtra* 38 : 18-19.

Svastika type of bandage, 580
Used for fracture or dislocation of shoulder joint.

Svasti vācana, 246
Recitation of incantations for the welfare of the patient.

Svedana, 358
Fomentation (therapy).

Svinna, 537
Liquefied; also fomented.

Tama, 120
A feeling as if entering into darkness.

Tīkṣṇa, 4, 31, 173, 180, 307, 336, 391, 473
Ingredients having sharp attributes.

Tiryak gata, 563, 564
Sideward dislocation.

Tridoṣaja, 130
Caused by the simultaneous vitiation of all the three *dosas*.

Trijātaka, 81
Collective name of three aromatic drugs, namely, ***tvak***, ***elā*** and *patra*.

Trika, 220
Lumbo-sacral joint.

Trikaṭu, 33, 34, 35, 38, 40, 43, 44, 60, 104, 125, 201, 283, 294, 305, 333, 370, 475, 475, 550, 593, 594
Collective name for three pungent drugs, namely *śuṇṭhī*, *pippali* and *marica*.

Trimada, 305, 593
Collective name for three drugs, namely ***mustā***, *viḍaṅga* and *citraka*.

Triphalā, 24, 29, 31, 35, 48, 66, 73, 76, 79, 120, 131, 133, 135, 137, 141, 144, 161, 166, 199, 200, 206, 207, 238, 275-78, 281-83, 286, 294, 304, 305, 307 308, 333, 337, 341, 342, 346, 356, 362, 385, 398, 407, 427, 435, 475-77, 492, 493, 548, 549, 550. 561, 593, 594
Collective name for three fruits, namely ***harītakī***, ***bibhitakī*** and *āmalakī*.

Trisugandhi, 288, 415
Collective name of three aromatic drugs, namely, ***tvak***, ***elā*** and ***patra***.

Tṛṇa pañca mūla, 178, 187
Group of five roots, namely, ***kuśa***, ***kāsa***, ***sara***, ***darbha*** and ***ikṣu***.

Tryūṣaṇa, 48, 63, 73, 135, 147, 166, 332, 387, 409, 411
See ***trikaṭu***.

Vāluka yantra, 253
An implement used for the preparation of medicine by sublimation. *Ref. Sikatā yantra* in p. 616 of the Glossary in Diagnosis and Treatment of Diseases in Ayurveda, Part-I.

Varatī, 315
Wasp.

Varti, 531, 532
Elongated pill generally used for collyrium and suppository.

Varuṇādi gaṇa, 232, 290, 494
Group of drugs—vide *Suśruta* : *Sūtra* 38 : 10-11.

Vāruṇī maṇḍa, 19, 115
A type of alcoholic preparation.

Vasā, 257, 260, 491
Muscle fat.

Vātaja, 215, 421, 427, 468
Caused by *vāyu*.

Vātānulomana, 113
Which helps in the downward movement of wind.

Vātika, 1, 20, 40, 57, 72, 89, 91, 109, 115, 126, 130, 133, 134, 135, 150, 158, 163, 183, 202, 209, 212, 219, 229, 230, 263 321, 341, 390, 392, 397, 398, 410, 411, 419, 438, 442, 458, 462, 469, 481, 82, 491, 499, 505, 521, 528, 590
Diseases by aggravated *vāyu*.

Vāyu, 2, 3, 6, 8, 9, 10, 11, 12, 16, 21, 28, 29, 31, 42, 44, 56, 64, 65, 66, 68, 77, 88, 90, 92, 93, 97, 100, 107, 111, 114, 138, 141, 156, 161, 165, 167, 172, 177, 182, 190, 191-197, 207, 212, 214, 219, 221-224, 227, 229, 230, 255, 256, 261, 264, 284, 287, 301, 307, 322, 325, 330, 332, 333, 341, 343, 346, 350 369, 381, 389, 390, 403, 418, 419, 421, 426, 427, 431, 438, 441, 443, 474, 475, 476, 478, 483, 503, 516, 517, 523, 532, 533 560, 566, 583, 593
One of the three *doṣas*. *Ref. vāta* in p. 625 of Glossary in Basic Principles of Āyurveda.

Vidagdha, 4
Putrefied.

Vidagdhatva, 488
Over matured or over suppurated.

Vidāhi, 4, 109, 325, 417
Ingredients causing burning sensation.

Vidāri gandhādi gaṇa, 140
Group of drugs—vide *Suśruta* : *Sūtra* 38 : 4-5.

Viddha, 511, 514
Punctured wound.

Vidradhi, 480, 481-483, 488, 489, 490-493, 534, 538
Abscess.

Viparita rati, 221
Having sexual intercourse with the man sleeping below and woman above him.

Viratarvādi gaṇa, 202, 243
Group of drugs –vide *Suśruta* : *Sūtra* 38 : 12-13.

Vimlāpana, 520, 523
Dissolution of Oedema or the accumulated material.

Vīrya, 536
Potency.

Viṣaja, 390, 594
Caused by poisoning.

Visarpa, 534
Erysipelas.

Viśliṣṭa, 563, 564
Torn ligaments.

Vivartita, 563, 564
Twisted.

Vṛddhi, 47, 67, 287, 373, 419-427, 436, 478
Hydrocele and hernia.

Vṛṣaṇa, 225
Testicle.

Vyoṣa, 27, 45, 104, 127, 134, 142, 146, 286, 303, 304, 341, 370, 385, 406, 407, 412, 414, 415, 451, 457
See *trikaṭu*.

Vyāyāma, 576
Physical exhertion or exercise.

Yama, 209, 228
The god of death.

Yava, 246
Unit of measurement; thickness of a barley grain; also refers to barley.

Yavāgū, 101, 144, 200, 232, 233, 250. 545
Thick gruel.

Yojana, 289
Unit of measuring distance equivalent to four *Krośas* or eight miles.

Yoni, 252
Female genital organ.

Yoni viśodhana, 147
Cleansing of female genital organ.